Chet Wyman

1995
YEAR BOOK OF
ANESTHESIOLOGY AND
PAIN MANAGEMENT®

Statement of Purpose

The YEAR BOOK Service

The YEAR BOOK series was devised in 1901 by practicing health professionals who observed that the literature of medicine and related disciplines had become so voluminous that no one individual could read and place in perspective every potential advance in a major specialty. In the final decade of the 20th century, this recognition is more acutely true than it was in 1901.

More than merely a series of books, YEAR BOOK volumes are the tangible results of a unique service designed to accomplish the following:

- to *survey* a wide range of journals of proven value
- to *select* from those journals papers representing significant advances and statements of important clinical principles
- to provide *abstracts* of those articles that are readable, convenient summaries of their key points
- to provide *commentary* about those articles to place them in perspective

These publications grow out of a unique process that calls on the talents of outstanding authorities in clinical and fundamental disciplines, trained literature specialists, and professional writers, all supported by the resources of Mosby, the world's preeminent publisher for the health professions.

The Literature Base

Mosby subscribes to nearly 1,000 journals published worldwide, covering the full range of the health professions. On an annual basis, the publisher examines usage patterns and polls its expert authorities to add new journals to the literature base and to delete journals that are no longer useful as potential YEAR BOOK sources.

The Literature Survey

The publisher's team of literature specialists, all of whom are trained and experienced health professionals, examines every original, peer-reviewed article in each journal issue. More than 250,000 articles per year are scanned systematically, including title, text, illustrations, tables, and references. Each scan is compared, article by article, to the search strategies that the publisher has developed in consultation with the 270 outside experts who form the pool of YEAR BOOK editors. A given article may be reviewed by any number of editors, from one to a dozen or more, regardless of the discipline for which the paper was originally published. In turn, each editor who receives the article reviews it to determine whether or not the article should be included in the YEAR BOOK. This decision is based on the article's inherent quality, its probable usefulness to readers of that YEAR BOOK, and the editor's goal to represent a balanced picture of a given field in each volume of the YEAR BOOK. In addition, the editor indicates when to include figures and tables from the article to help the YEAR BOOK reader better understand the information.

Of the quarter million articles scanned each year, only 5% are selected for detailed analysis within the YEAR BOOK series, thereby assuring readers of the high value of every selection.

The Abstract

The publisher's abstracting staff is headed by a physician-writer and includes individuals with training in the life sciences, medicine, and other areas, plus extensive experience in writing for the health professions and related industries. Each selected article is assigned to a specific writer on this abstracting staff. The abstracter, guided in many cases by notations supplied by the expert editor, writes a structured, condensed summary designed so that the reader can rapidly acquire the essential information contained in the article.

The Commentary

The YEAR BOOK editorial boards, sometimes assisted by guest commentators, write comments that place each article in perspective for the reader. This provides the reader with the equivalent of a personal consultation with a leading international authority—an opportunity to better understand the value of the article and to benefit from the authority's thought processes in assessing the article.

Additional Editorial Features

The editorial boards of each YEAR BOOK organize the abstracts and comments to provide a logical and satisfying sequence of information. To enhance the organization, editors also provide introductions to sections or individual chapters, comments linking a number of abstracts, citations to additional literature, and other features.

The published YEAR BOOK contains enhanced bibliographic citations for each selected article, including extended listings of multiple authors and identification of author affiliations. Each YEAR BOOK contains a Table of Contents specific to that year's volume. From year to year, the Table of Contents for a given YEAR BOOK will vary depending on developments within the field.

Every YEAR BOOK contains a list of the journals from which papers have been selected. This list represents a subset of the nearly 1,000 journals surveyed by the publisher and occasionally reflects a particularly pertinent article from a journal that is not surveyed on a routine basis.

Finally, each volume contains a comprehensive subject index and an index to authors of each selected paper.

The 1995 Year Book Series

Year Book of Allergy and Clinical Immunology: Drs. Rosenwasser, Borish, Gelfand, Leung, Nelson, and Szefler

Year Book of Anesthesiology and Pain Management: Drs. Tinker, Abram, Chestnut, Roizen, Rothenberg, and Wood

Year Book of Cardiology®: Drs. Schlant, Collins, Engle, Gersh, Kaplan, and Waldo

Year Book of Chiropractic: Dr. Lawrence

Year Book of Critical Care Medicine®: Drs. Parrillo, Balk, Calvin, Franklin, and Shapiro

Year Book of Dentistry®: Drs. Meskin, Berry, Currier, Kennedy, Leinfelder, Roser, and Zakariasen

Year Book of Dermatologic Surgery®: Drs. Swanson, Glogau, and Salasche

Year Book of Dermatology®: Drs. Sober and Fitzpatrick

Year Book of Diagnostic Radiology®: Drs. Federle, Clark, Gross, Madewell, Maynard, Latchaw, and Young

Year Book of Digestive Diseases®: Drs. Greenberger and Moody

Year Book of Drug Therapy®: Drs. Lasagna and Weintraub

Year Book of Emergency Medicine®: Drs. Davidson, Dronen, King, Niemann, Roberts, and Wagner

Year Book of Endocrinology®: Drs. Bagdade, Braverman, Horton, Kannan, Landsberg, Molitch, Morley, Nathan, Odell, Poehlman, Rogol, and Ryan

Year Book of Family Practice®: Drs. Berg, Bowman, Davidson, Dexter, Dietrich, and Scherger

Year Book of Geriatrics and Gerontology®: Drs. Beck, Burton, Goldstein, Reuben, Small, and Whitehouse

Year Book of Hand Surgery®: Drs. Amadio and Hentz

Year Book of Hematology®: Drs. Spivak, Bell, Ness, Quesenberry, Wiernik, and Blume

Year Book of Infectious Diseases®: Drs. Keusch, Barza, Bennish, Gelfand, Klempner, Skolnik, and Snydman

Year Book of Infertility and Reproductive Endocrinology®: Drs. Mishell, Lobo, and Sokol

Year Book of Medicine®: Drs. Bone, Cline, Epstein, Greenberger, Malawista, Mandell, O'Rourke, and Utiger

Year Book of Neonatal and Perinatal Medicine®: Drs. Fanaroff and Klaus

Year Book of Nephrology®: Drs. Coe, Curtis, Favus, Henderson, Kashgarian, and Luke

Year Book of Neurology and Neurosurgery®: Drs. Bradley and Wilkins

Year Book of Neuroradiology: Drs. Osborn, Eskridge, Grossman, Hudgens, and Ross

Year Book of Nuclear Medicine®: Drs. Gottschalk, Blaufox, McAfee, Wacker, and Zubal

Year Book of Obstetrics and Gynecology®: Drs. Mishell, Kirschbaum, and Morrow

Year Book of Occupational and Environmental Medicine®: Drs. Emmett, Frank, Gochfeld, and Hessl

Year Book of Oncology®: Drs. Simone, Bosl, Glatstein, Ozols, and Steele

Year Book of Ophthalmology®: Drs. Cohen, Adams, Augsburger, Benson, Eagle, Flanagan, Grossman, Laibson, Nelson, Rapuano, Reinecke, Sergott, Tasman, Tipperman, and Wilson

Year Book of Orthopedics®: Drs. Sledge, Cofield, Dobyns, Griffin, Poss, Springfield, Swiontkowski, Wiesel, and Wilson

Year Book of Otolaryngology–Head and Neck Surgery®: Drs. Paparella and Holt

Year Book of Pain: Drs. Gebhart, Haddox, Jacox, Marcus, Rudy, Shapiro, and Janjan

Year Book of Pathology and Laboratory Medicine®: Drs. Mills, Bruns, Gaffey, and Stoler

Year Book of Pediatrics®: Dr. Stockman

Year Book of Plastic, Reconstructive, and Aesthetic Surgery: Drs. Miller, Cohen, McKinney, Robson, Ruberg, and Whitaker

Year Book of Podiatric Medicine and Surgery®: Dr. Kominsky

Year Book of Psychiatry and Applied Mental Health®: Drs. Talbott, Breier, Frances, Meltzer, Schowalter, Tasman, and Yudofsky

Year Book of Pulmonary Disease®: Drs. Bone and Petty

Year Book of Rheumatology®: Drs. Sergent, LeRoy, Meenan, Panush, and Reichlin

Year Book of Sports Medicine®: Drs. Shephard, Drinkwater, Eichner, Torg, Col. Anderson, and Mr. George

Year Book of Surgery®: Drs. Copeland, Bland, Deitch, Eberlein, Howard, Luce, Seeger, Souba, and Sugarbaker

Year Book of Thoracic and Cardiovascular Surgery®: Drs. Ginsberg, Lofland, and Wechsler

Year Book of Transplantation®: Drs. Sollinger, Eckhoff, Hullett, Knechtle, Longo, Mentzer, and Pirsch

Year Book of Ultrasound®: Drs. Merritt, Babcock, Carroll, Fagin, Finberg, and Fleischer

Year Book of Urology®: Drs. deKernion and Howards

Year Book of Vascular Surgery®: Dr. Porter

1995

The Year Book of
ANESTHESIOLOGY AND PAIN MANAGEMENT®

Editor-in-Chief

John H. Tinker, M.D.
Professor and Head, Department of Anesthesia, University of Iowa College of Medicine, Iowa City, Iowa

Editors

Stephen E. Abram, M.D.
Professor and Vice Chairman, Department of Anesthesiology, Pain Management Center, Medical College of Wisconsin, Milwaukee, Wisconsin

David H. Chestnut, M.D.
Alfred Habeeb Professor and Chairman, Department of Anesthesiology; Professor of Obstetrics and Gynecology, University of Alabama, Birmingham, Alabama

Michael F. Roizen, M.D.
Professor and Chair, Department of Anesthesia and Critical Care; Professor of Medicine, University of Chicago, Chicago, Illinois

David M. Rothenberg, M.D.
Associate Professor of Anaesthesia; Director, Division of Anesthesia–Critical Care, Rush-Presbyterian/St. Luke's Medical Center, Chicago, Illinois

Margaret Wood, M.D.
Professor of Anesthesia, Department of Anesthesia, Vanderbilt University School of Medicine, Nashville, Tennessee

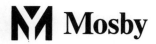 Mosby

St. Louis Baltimore Boston Carlsbad Chicago Naples New York Philadelphia Portland
London Madrid Mexico City Singapore Sydney Tokyo Toronto Wiesbaden

Vice President and Publisher, Continuity Publishing: Kenneth H. Killion
Director, Editorial Development: Gretchen C. Murphy
Manager, Continuity–EDP: Maria Nevinger
Developmental Editor: Bernadette Bucholz
Acquisitions Editor: Jennifer Roche
Illustrations and Permissions Coordinator: Lois M. Ruebensam
Senior Production Editor: Wendi Schnaufer
Senior Project Manager, Production: Max F. Perez
Freelance Staff Supervisor: Barbara M. Kelly
Director, Editorial Services: Edith M. Podrazik, R.N.
Senior Information Specialist: Terri Santo, R.N.
Information Specialist: Nancy R. Dunne, R.N.
Senior Medical Writer: David A. Cramer, M.D.
Vice President, Professional Sales and Marketing: George M. Parker
Marketing Coordinator: Lynn Stevenson

1995 EDITION
Copyright © August 1995 by Mosby-Year Book, Inc.

Printed in the United States of America
Composition by Reed Technology and Information Services, Inc.
Printing/binding by Maple-Vail

Mosby-Year Book, Inc.
11830 Westline Industrial Drive
St. Louis, MO 63146

Editorial Office:
Mosby-Year Book, Inc.
200 North LaSalle Street
Chicago, IL 60601

International Standard Serial Number: 1073-5437
International Standard Book Number: 0-8151-5987-0

Table of Contents

Mosby Document Express

Copies of the full text of the original source documents of articles abstracted or referenced in this publication are available by calling Mosby Document Express, toll-free, at 1 (800) 55-MOSBY.

With Mosby Document Express, you have convenient, 24-hour-a-day access to literally every article on which this publication is based. In fact, through Mosby Document Express, virtually any medical or scientific article can be located and delivered by FAX, overnight delivery service, international airmail, electronic transmission of bitmapped images (via Internet), or regular mail. The average cost of a complete, delivered copy of an article, including up to $4 in copyright clearance charges and first-class mail delivery, is $12.

For inquiries and pricing information, please call the toll-free number shown above. To expedite your order for material appearing in this publication, please be prepared with the code shown next to the bibliographic citation for each abstract.

Journals Represented

Mosby subscribes to and surveys nearly 1,000 U.S. and foreign medical and allied health journals. From these journals, the Editors select the articles to be abstracted. Journals represented in this YEAR BOOK are listed below.

ASAIO Journal
Acta Anaesthesiologica Scandinavica
Acta Ophthalmologica
American Journal of Cardiology
American Journal of Emergency Medicine
American Journal of Infection Control
American Journal of Obstetrics and Gynecology
American Journal of Respiratory and Critical Care Medicine
Anaesthesia
Anaesthesia and Intensive Care
Anesthesia and Analgesia
Anesthesiology
Annals of Internal Medicine
Annals of Surgery
Annals of Thoracic Surgery
Annals of Vascular Surgery
Annals of the Royal College of Surgeons of England
Archives of Otolaryngology–Head and Neck Surgery
Archives of Physical Medicine and Rehabilitation
Archives of Surgery
British Journal of Anaesthesia
Canadian Journal of Anaesthesia
Chest
Circulation
Circulatory Shock
Clinical Journal of Pain
Clinical Orthopaedics and Related Research
Clinical Pharmacology and Therapeutics
Clinical Science
Critical Care Medicine
Environmental Research
Epilepsia
European Journal of Obstetrics, Gynecology and Reproductive Biology
European Journal of Surgery
European Journal of Vascular Surgery
Experimental Hematology
Hepatology
Intensive Care Medicine
International Journal of Gynaecology and Obstetrics
International Journal of Obstetric Anesthesia
Journal de Chirurgie
Journal of Arthroplasty
Journal of Bone and Joint Surgery (American Volume)
Journal of Bone and Joint Surgery (British Volume)
Journal of Clinical Anesthesia
Journal of Clinical Epidemiology
Journal of Clinical Pharmacology
Journal of Emergency Medicine
Journal of Hand Surgery (American)
Journal of Hand Surgery (British)

Journal of Neurology, Neurosurgery and Psychiatry
Journal of Pain and Symptom Management
Journal of Pediatric Orthopedics
Journal of Reproductive Medicine
Journal of Thoracic and Cardiovascular Surgery
Journal of Trauma
Journal of Vascular Surgery
Journal of the American College of Surgeons
Journal of the American Medical Association
Lancet
Life Sciences
Mayo Clinic Proceedings
Medical Care
Medical Journal of Australia
Metabolism
New England Journal of Medicine
Obstetrics and Gynecology
Ophthalmology
Pain
Paraplegia
Pediatric Emergency Care
Pediatrics
Postgraduate Medical Journal
Proceedings of the National Academy of Sciences
Psychopharmacology
Regional Anesthesia
Southern Medical Journal
Spine
Stroke
Surgery
Thrombosis and Haemostasis
Transfusion
Urology

Standard Abbreviations

The following terms are abbreviated in this edition: acquired immunodeficiency syndrome (AIDS), cardiopulmonary resuscitation (CPR), central nervous system (CNS), cerebrospinal fluid (CSF), computed tomography (CT), deoxyribonucleic acid (DNA), electrocardiography (ECG), health maintenance organization (HMO), human immunodeficiency virus (HIV), intensive care unit (ICU), intramuscular (IM), intravenous (IV), magnetic resonance (MR) imaging (MRI), and ribonucleic acid (RNA).

Introduction

This past year has been a "stabilizing" one for anesthesiology. As the reader may painfully recall, 1993–1994 was filled with turmoil, with President and Mrs. Clinton telling us that the health care profession is "sick," coupled with our own tendencies toward self-flagellation, resulting in what can best be described as an "unholy mess." In addition, the Clinton's health care bill collapsed, due to, if nothing else, its own weight. It's not exactly business as usual, but we are back in business again, and it's nice to be there. This past year, steady and solid clinical, scientific, and technical advances have been achieved in anesthesiology.

In pain management, preemptive analgesia is probably the hottest topic. I don't see solid agreement on whether it works, however. Considerable progress has been made in the pathophysiology and treatment of reflex sympathetic dystrophy. Animal models now exist, and this is a big step forward. Clonidine, given intrathecally and epidurally, still holds a spotlight (as it did last year). There is continuing interest in refining our techniques of epidural opioids and local anesthetics both for postoperative and chronic pain. There are still not any really exciting new drugs in this area, and I think that may be what we need next. Perhaps remifentanyl will be of interest from the standpoint of postoperative pain, but it is too early to tell.

With respect to the clinical pharmacology of anesthesiology, propofol is of interest as usual, but this year it has been shown to have potential for being abused. Remifentanyl is also of great interest as an inhaled nitric oxide. Probably the most talked about development in this field is sevoflurane. It is widely used in Japan, as our readers know. Anesthesiologists are clearly impatient to get their hands on it in the United States. It is reported by many to have excellent clinical characteristics, i.e., fast on the uptake and recovery, with little or no potential for airway irritation, with perhaps less hypotension than desflurane. The problems are, of course, its breakdown in soda lime to "compound A," which is toxic, and its breakdown by the liver into flouride ion, also toxic. These 2 potential toxicities are widely discussed now because we will likely get sevoflurane in the United States soon. Compound A comes off soda lime in very low concentrations if flows are high enough, and, from the standpoint of flouride-related nephrotoxicity, no such definitive link has been shown as yet with respect to sevoflurane. Still, some may remember that it took 7 years, from 1959 to 1966, before methoxyflurane was linked to nephrotoxicity, and another decade before we agreed that flouride was the culprit. Therefore, we are understandably wary of introducing a new anesthetic that undergoes high levels of biotransformation. This edition of the YEAR BOOK contains many articles on these subjects.

Awareness under anesthesia, coupled with learning and memory, are still hot topics, as they were last year. Another area of considerable interest has to do with latex allergies and their prevalence in and around the operating room. How one keeps patients from being exposed to latex is not all that easy in today's operating room.

With respect to obstetrical anesthesia, the hottest topic has to do with whether relatively early epidural analgesia application affects the progress and outcome of labor, especially in nulliparous women. This year's edition of the YEAR BOOK contains some solid definitive studies that clearly indicate that early performance of epidural analgesia in these women *does not* impede the progress of labor, indeed possibly just the opposite. This is very encouraging news for those who have seen primigravida women truly agonizing in labor, waiting for their epidurals while their cervices dilated to some magic number, usually 5 cm. The anesthesiologist who does obstetrical anesthesia will want to read carefully about this, but I think you will come to the conclusion that you can perform epidural analgesia earlier than at 5 cm of cervical dilation.

This year's edition of the YEAR BOOK also has a good number of mechanistic scientific studies that do take legitimate scientific looks at mechanisms of various phenomena of interest to anesthesiologists (e.g., various pain mechanisms, the nature of nociception, pharmacokinetics of various anesthetic agents). I am very happy to see this level of science and interest in science in our specialty.

I think this has been a solid year in critical care medicine as well. Nitric oxide is now becoming possible to use, and a number of papers in this edition discuss its efficacy and safety. There is considerable interest in the augment of systemic oxygen in delivery during sepsis and trauma. Ethical issues of withdrawal of life support and physician-assisted suicide are also addressed. There may be a new drug, namely tirilazad, that can reduce cerebral infarct size, although we've heard about these kinds of drugs before.

One disturbing development that I will risk comment about, despite the fact that it is not a publication from which we can abstract here, has to do with the television show "Day One" with Diane Sawyer and Forrest Sawyer, which aired in February 1995. On that particular show, which was obviously heavily edited, the organized medicine side of our specialty attempted to use this program to scare the public about nurse-administered anesthesia. I think they succeeded in doing that. To their surprise, however, the Sawyers used the show to present a point of view that anesthesiologists' supervision of nurse anesthetists is far from ideal. Indeed, several instances more were described in which nurse anesthetists were "supervised" by physicians from another hospital, i.e., supervision was nonexistent. They even managed to film guilty-looking anesthesiologists who refused to answer questions while escaping to their cars in parking lots.

The results of this television show were 3, in my opinion. First, doubt about the safety of nurse-administered anesthesia was broadcast to the public. Second, physician anesthesiologists were portrayed as greedy, lazy, crooked, or all 3, despite disclaimers that only a small minority were involved in the fraudulent practices described. Third, and by far the most important long-term potential effect of this television show and others like it is to alarm the viewers and public enough to consider even whether they should have surgery (and anesthesia) *at all.* I think there is a disturbing trend toward convincing the public that surgery in general should somehow be avoided. This is dangerous for many reasons, not the least because it will result in our having to care for patients who are older, sicker, or both. I decry this kind of turf battling through the media.

In our science, there were no shocking or terrifying events, i.e., none of our drugs or techniques were found to cause cancer or some other horrible outcome. After a year of economic turmoil that had a distressingly negative effect on the job market for new graduates in anesthesiology, I think it is fair to say that the situation with respect to our specialty is leveling out again and things are more stable. As I said last year, there still are sick patients and they still need our care.

John H. Tinker, M.D.

1 Preoperative Evaluation

Patients' Desire for Information About Anaesthesia: Australian Attitudes

Farnill D, Inglis S (Univ of Sydney, Australia; Manly Hosp, Sydney, Australia)
Anaesthesia 48:162–164, 1993   101-95-1–1

Purpose.—The balance between the principles of informed consent and nonmaleficence can lead to dilemmas about providing preoperative information. A previous study of Canadian and Scottish patients suggested that patients vary by country, sex, and age in the amount of information they desire about anesthesia. Australian patients' desires for information about anesthesia were assessed using a preoperative questionnaire.

Methods.—Forty consecutive patients who were scheduled for surgery that required general anesthesia completed the questionnaire. The results were compared with those of the previous study of Canadian and Scottish patients.

Results.—The Australian and Canadian patients wanted more information than the Scottish patients. Eighty-two percent of the Australian patients wanted information about dangerous complications compared with 66% of the Canadian and 40% of the Scottish patients. Ninety-two percent of the Australian patients wanted information about all complications compared with 72% of the Canadian and 43% of the Scottish patients. Many elderly patients did not want to hear about unpleasant aspects of perioperative procedures or potential complications. In all countries, patients younger than 50 years of age wanted more information than older patients. All 3 national groups gave the highest priority to meeting with the anesthetist before surgery.

Conclusion.—In most cases, preoperative patients should receive sufficient information to enable them to understand the serious and common risks associated with general anesthesia. Most patients prefer to receive this information, and many believe they have a right to receive it. However, some patients—especially the elderly—prefer not to know. Ultimately, the clinician must take a judgment on behalf of the individual patient, including the extent to which possibly distressing details should be disclosed.

▶ Patients in Australia and Canada wanted more information than those in Scotland about anesthesia risks, and they also wanted to meet their anesthesiologist. It is clear that patient education and information will be 2 of the new areas for much future research through the information superhighway.

Although this article has some deficits—such as not indicating what types of patients were questioned, specifically the type of operations they were about to undergo and whether the results would have been different if they were undergoing oncologic surgery vs. cosmetic surgery—it highlights and emphasizes again the importance of the individual interaction between the anesthesiologist and the patient. Such interaction is vital, and I believe that a medically validated informational procedure that summarizes the patient's history should be provided to anesthesiologists in advance so that each of the minutes they spend with the patient can be used most effectively to inquire about things they need to know more about, to allay the patient's anxiety, to answer the patient's questions, and to provide information about perioperative procedures and postoperative pain relief.

Currently, patients are dissatisfied with the information they receive from doctors, and they think they are interrupted by physicians 19 seconds into an answer. A medically validated informational procedure that provides anesthesiologists with a summary of the patient's medical history could facilitate this communication and help instill more confidence in the patients regarding their anesthesiologist and enable them to undergo their surgical procedures in more comfort. It could even lead to earlier and faster recovery.

This article also says a great deal about the future of health care reform not only in this country, but worldwide. The information revolution can potentially be used by patients to seek more information regarding who does what best, who possesses what qualities, and who provides what type of pain relief, thereby rendering the managed care competition and the current health care reform movement in the United States but a passing fad on the way to informed decision making and the empowerment of patients and physicians through greater information access.—M.F. Roizen, M.D.

Patient's Knowledge of Anaesthetic Practice and the Rôle of Anaesthetists
Swinhoe CF, Groves ER (Royal Hallamshire Hosp, Sheffield, England)
Anaesthesia 49:165–166, 1994   101-95-1–2

Background.—Despite increasing public interest in medicine, public knowledge of anesthetic practice remains limited. The latest studies of this issue appeared in 1978; changes in public knowledge about anesthetic practice and the role of anesthetists since that time were assessed by questionnaire.

Methods and Results.—One hundred consecutive patients completed the 7-question instrument as part of their routine preoperative assessment. All were adults; 62 were women. Thirty-five percent of the respondents did not believe that the anesthetist was a "qualified doctor." Seventy-nine percent were aware that the anesthetist had primary responsibility for the patient's well-being during the operation, and 60% knew of the anesthetist's role in monitoring during surgery. However, only 25% could name an area of hospital care other than the operating room where anesthetists play a major role.

Conclusion.—Public knowledge of anesthesia practice continues to be limited, especially the anesthetist's involvement in numerous areas of hospital care. An information sheet concerning the anesthetist's role and training and the conduct of anesthesia is being developed for distribution to all patients before surgery.

▶ This is an important study, because if we have done as bad a job as the British have done (and I guess we have) of informing patients about our role, we will not have the respect of the patient in the information age. As a result, we will not have political clout needed to insist on quality care or to make changes that are appropriate for patient well-being.—M.F. Roizen, M.D.

Parental Knowledge and Attitudes Toward Discussing the Risk of Death From Anesthesia
Litman RS, Perkins FM, Dawson SC (Univ of Rochester, New York)
Anesth Analg 77:256–260, 1993   101-95-1–3

Introduction.—There is disagreement about the amount of detail required for informed consent for anesthesia, particularly concerning disclosure of the rare risk of death in healthy children undergoing minor surgery. Parental knowledge of the risks associated with anesthesia and parental opinions about hearing about the risk of death were assessed.

Methods.—Parents of healthy infants and children undergoing outpatient surgery completed a questionnaire before their preoperative discussion with the anesthesiologist that assessed their knowledge and attitudes toward full disclosure of the risk of death from anesthesia. Another group of parents of healthy infants and children undergoing outpatient surgery was accompanied to the preoperative interview with the anesthesiologist to determine how often anesthesiologists mention the risk of death in this situation. After the interview, the parents were asked whether they wanted to know about this risk or whether they would have preferred not to know.

Results.—Of the 115 parents who completed the questionnaire, 87% wanted to know about the risk of death and 13% did not. Regarding the preferred extent of disclosure, 74% wanted to know all possible risks, 24% wanted to know only probable risks, and 2% wanted to know only about risks that could result in significant complications. Mothers were more likely than fathers to want to know all possible risks. Regarding parental knowledge, 13% believed there was no possible risk of death attributable to anesthesia, 68% believed death was extremely rare, and 19% believed that death occurred occasionally. The patient's age or previous surgery in the patient or siblings did not influence any of the answers. The risk of death was mentioned to 44 parents, implied to 30 parents, and not implied or mentioned to 47 parents during the preoperative interview with the anesthesiologist. Among those to whom the risk was mentioned or implied, 88% of the parents preferred hearing about the risk and 11% would have preferred not hearing about it. Among those who did not hear about the risk of death, 38% of the parents were satisfied, 47% would have preferred discussion of the risk, and 15% said it did not matter.

Conclusion. —Most parents are aware that a very small risk of death is associated with anesthesia and would like to discuss it in the preoperative interview with the anesthesiologist.

▶ In Iowa, a State Supreme Court decision in an anesthesia case mandates that all patients (or their guardians, if they are children) receive information regarding the risk or at least the possibility of death caused by or during anesthesia. This law must be taken very seriously. Once it became a state law, we learned how easy it is to include an honest discussion of the possibility of death (however inaccurate our risk estimates might be) in our preoperative conference with patients. It is honest and appropriate, and this study clearly shows that it is desired by most parents of children undergoing anesthesia. The truth is, it is something that is on people's minds. The notion that you will scare patients unnecessarily or drive them away from needed surgery is simply not valid. I think we should be discussing this important topic with our patients. I would not let you anesthetize me if we did not discuss it first.—J.H. Tinker, M.D.

Users' Guides to the Medical Literature: III. How to Use an Article About a Diagnostic Test: B. What Are the Results and Will They Help Me in Caring for My Patients?
Guyatt GH, for the Evidence-Based Medicine Working Group (McMaster Univ, Hamilton, Ont, Canada)
JAMA 271:703–707, 1994   101-95-1-4

Introduction. —After deciding whether an article in the medical literature regarding a diagnostic test is valid, the physician must then try to understand and use the results of the study. Two clinical scenarios were presented that required the interpretation of ventilation-perfusion (V/Q) scanning. Results of studies and their relevance to individual cases were assessed according to specific principles.

Probability.—Patients included a woman 78 years of age 10 days after surgery and an anxious man 28 years of age with shortness of breath and nonspecific chest pain after a 10-hour auto trip. The pretest probabilities of pulmonary embolus (PE) were very different in the 2 cases. Results of a V/Q scan modified the pretest probability and yielded a new post-test probability. The test's properties determined the direction and magnitude of this change. The property focused on was the likelihood ratio (LR).

Likelihood Ratios.—A study of the value of the V/Q scan in acute PE included 251 patients with proven PE and 630 in whom PE had been excluded. Calculation of the LR yields a number by which high probability or low probability can be assumed. The LR is the ratio of 2 likelihoods: that of a high-probability scan among patients who have PE and that of a high-probability scan among patients who are suspected to have PE but who do not. A nomogram is provided that enables the clinician to obtain the post-test probability by anchoring a ruler at the pretest probability and rotating it until it lines up with the LR for the observed test result. For the elderly woman, both high-probability and intermediate V/Q scans would yield a high probability of PE. For the young man, only a high-probability scan result would yield a high probability of PE. This approach is recommended as being simpler and more efficient than the concepts of sensitivity and specificity.

Application.—The test may not have the same accuracy among other patients as it did in these patients. For example, it would be most useful if all the patients with the target disorder have severe disease. The test would not be very useful if most patients had test results with LRs near 1, thereby altering probability to a minor degree. Results should be applicable if they are used in a setting similar to that of the investigation and the patient meets all the study inclusion criteria and does not violate any exclusion criteria. An increasing number of tests are now publishing LRs, thereby allowing this approach to be applied directly to daily practice.

▶ This article is perhaps the most important of the 300 or so I was privileged to read as my editorial assignment for the 1995 YEAR BOOK, and it is clearly the most important of the 70 or so about which I wrote comments. Nonetheless, it is also one of the hardest to review and about which to write. I urge everyone to read the article more than once, but I will comment on some of its highlights.

The authors observe that "the ultimate criterion for the usefulness of a diagnostic test is whether it adds information beyond that otherwise available, and whether this information leads to a change in management that is ultimately beneficial to the patient." They cite the pretest probability and its modification by the LR, based on the test result, to derive the post-test probability. Therefore, the LRs indicate how much a given diagnostic test, whether it is a clotting test we obtained intraoperatively or the results of an ECG we see pre- or postoperatively, will raise or lower the pretest probability of the diagnostic probability. Then, a decision must be made about whether we should change the care on the basis of that finding.

The authors of this article demonstrate how knowledge of the LR of a test result is better than knowing the sensitivity and the specificity. Thus, whereas this article is of particular importance to anyone who is studying the qualities of tests, such as dipyridamole thallium, it is also incredibly important to each of us who practices clinical medicine. I have decided to keep it by my bedside, read it several more times, and then start trying to apply it in daily practice. Although I assume that this attempt to apply it in daily practice will be difficult, I think it also will make me a better clinician.—M.F. Roizen, M.D.

Preoperative Laboratory Screening Based on Age, Gender, and Concomitant Medical Diseases
Velanovich V (Madigan Army Med Ctr, Tacoma, Wash)
Surgery 115:56–61, 1994   101-95-1–5

Introduction.—A wide variety of laboratory screening tests that are performed routinely before surgery have come under scrutiny. Some studies have found the tests to be underused once they are obtained and to be neither cost-effective nor predictive of postoperative complications. Patients undergoing elective surgery were followed up to determine the most effective laboratory screening.

Methods.—The study group consisted of 520 patients who were undergoing elective operations in the general, vascular, thoracic, and head and neck surgical services. The data evaluated included patient age, gender, race, American Society of Anesthesiologists (ASA) physical status classification, ponderal index, and presence of concomitant respiratory disease, coronary artery disease, and other significant conditions. Preoperative screening included tests for electrolytes and levels of blood urea nitrogen, creatinine, and glucose; a hemogram; nutrition; coagulation; urinalysis; an ECG; and a chest radiograph. The results were examined by univariate analysis and by multivariate analysis with stepwise logistic regression.

Results.—In univariate analysis, age, gender, and the specific concomitant illness were associated with specific abnormal preoperative laboratory results. Correlations were generally high between the univariate and multivariate analyses. According to the findings here, only certain preoperative screening tests would be required for certain patients. For example, for those with an associated malignancy, the hemogram and nutritional studies would be useful. A hemogram, testing of levels of glucose and blood urea nitrogen/creatinine, nutritional studies, coagulation studies, an ECG, and a chest radiograph are suggested for patients in ASA physical status III or IV. Unless otherwise indicated by a specific condition, a chest radiograph is recommended only for patients older than age 60 years.

Conclusion.—Many items included in routine preoperative laboratory testing are neither useful nor cost-effective. Data on patient age, gender, concomitant medical disease, and type of operation to be performed can be used as the basis for appropriate preoperative laboratory screening.

▶ I think this article is valuable, because it confims our studies and hypotheses that laboratory tests should be done for specific indications that are based on a medical history of concomitant disease.

We have used this approach in our HealthQuiz system and also used statistical analyses that are somewhat more sophisticated than the one used by Velanovich to select testing. Thus, the data we published in the 1994 edition of Miller's *Anesthesia* (1), together with these and other data, indicate that selective testing can reduce the incidence of laboratory tests by about 50% and improve usefulness as long as a detailed, comprehensive, and validated history is obtained.

Even more important than these reduced laboratory test data are data on outcome that show which of these preoperative test abnormalities lead to beneficial changes either in perioperative care or in general health care for the patient. Although we and others have begun to do use this approach, I think this study by Velanovich is an appropriate first step toward others doing so.—M.F. Roizen, M.D.

Reference

1. Miller RD (ed): *Anesthesia*, ed 4. New York, Churchill-Livingstone, 1994.

Value of Routine Preoperative Chest X-Rays: A Meta-Analysis
Archer C, Levy AR, McGregor M (Conseil d'évaluation des Technologies de la santé du Québec, Montréal)
Can J Anaesth 40:1022–1027, 1993   101-95-1–6

Objective.—The need for routine chest radiography before all surgery that requires anesthesia has been questioned in recent years. Although most studies have looked at the frequency of abnormal radiographs, none has evaluated the clinical relevance of information obtained from this expensive procedure. In a meta-analysis, 21 reports were examined for the frequency with which new information was obtained from routine chest radiography.

Methods.—All English, French, and Spanish reports published from 1966 through 1993 were identified. The 21 reports with appropriate information, involving 14, 390 patients, were analyzed.

Results.—The average rate of detection of a preoperative abnormality was 10%, with unsuspected intrathoracic abnormalities averaging 1.3%.

The findings were sufficient to cause the medical team to take action in only .1% of the cases.

Conclusion.—Because is costs approximately $23,000 to detect the 1 abnormality in 1,000 chest radiographs that influences management in any way, discontinuance of routine chest radiographs appears to be justified, except in special circumstances.

▶ In a meta-analysis of preoperative chest x-rays (CXRs), the maximum benefit of a CXR would be to the 1 out of every 1,000 patients in whom a CXR resulted in a change in patient management. The authors believe that the likelihood that those changes in management are beneficial would range from 5% to 20% and that the cost of that benefit would range from $115,000 to $460,000 per CXR taken, assuming a cost of $23 per CXR.

They clearly establish that there are dangers to getting CXRs, such as the pursuit of false positives, that may outweigh the benefits. The authors further note that the harm would result in a 1–2 in 100,000 risk of cancer from a preoperative CXR. As a result, they came to the reasonable conclusion that unless there is an increase in asymptomatic disease that can be discovered by CXR or an increase in the inability to gather a history from preoperative patients, asymptomatic patients probably should not have preoperative screening CXRs.

I think some comments are essential. The authors acknowledge the lack of age variation in their findings and note that the elderly may be more at risk for disease and therefore receive greater benefit from screening CXRs. Whereas it is acknowledged in a small part of the study, I think more emphasis is needed to show that data are not presented to indicate that the elderly would benefit from CXRs and that they would not incur greater harm from the pursuit of these abnormalities. The authors also observe that the long-term health benefits and risks of screening CXRs have been largely unstudied. Thus, perhaps the most important point we can get from this article is that a large series of studies has shown very small benefits, if any, from screening CXRs and that these small benefits may be outweighed by the small harms, irrespective of the cost of the screening program. Although there have been many studies on the issue, this is one area where we can cut back on costs and at the same time improve the health of the nation. Further study of the exact benefits and harms of CXR is needed if we are to definitely establish the risk-benefit ratio of a screening program.—M.F. Roizen, M.D.

Pulmonary Function Tests Before and After Laparoscopic Cholecystectomy

Freeman JA, Armstrong IR (Western Gen Hosp, Edinburgh, Scotland)
Anaesthesia 49:579–582, 1994   101-95-1-7

Introduction.—Patients who undergo laparoscopic cholecystectomy require less postoperative analgesia, have shorter hospital stays, and return to full activity earlier than patients who undergo conventional cholecystectomy. Although conventional cholecystectomy is known to alter pulmonary function, the pulmonary effects of laparoscopic cholecystectomy are unknown. Postoperative changes in pulmonary function were studied prospectively in patients who underwent laparoscopic cholecystectomy.

Methods.—Spirometric readings of forced expiratory volume in 1 second (FEV_1), forced vital capacity, vital capacity, residual volume, total lung capacity, and functional residual capacity were obtained the day before and 24 hours after surgery in 22 adult patients who were scheduled for laparoscopic cholecystectomy and at 6 weeks postoperatively in 12 of the patients. Inspiratory and expiratory mouth pressures were premeasured and postoperatively. Arterial blood measurements of oxygen pressure (PO_2) and carbon dioxide pressure (PCO_2) were obtained the day before and 1 and 24 hours after surgery.

Results.—The patients experienced significant postoperative reductions in FEV_1 (to 75%), forced vital capacity, inspiratory and expiratory mouth pressures (to 66% and 63%, respectively), functional residual capacity (to 92%), vital capacity (to 73%), and total lung capacity (to 83%), whereas residual volume did not change. Although arterial concentrations of PO_2 decreased significantly 24 hours after surgery, arterial PCO_2 did not change significantly postoperatively. The 6-week follow-up lung function tests and measurement of inspiratory and expiratory mouth pressures revealed that all values had returned to preoperative levels.

Discussion.—The reductions in the various lung function indices were small but statistically significant, suggesting only minor restriction. The reductions in inspiratory and expiratory mouth pressures combined with reduced vital capacity and FEV_1 and the unchanged FEV_1 forced vital capacity ratio suggest that reduced respiratory muscle activity played a more important role in respiratory change than airway restriction.

▶ This article addresses the main reasons for laparoscopic cholecystectomy: less morbidity and faster return to function. In these patients, functional residual capacity and total lung capacity were decreased the first day after surgery but not to the levels seen with open cholecystectomy. Whereas the major changes with open cholecystectomy occur on days 2 and 3 and only slowly improve, we don't know what happens with laparoscopic cholecystectomy.

Like all good studies, this one provides more questions than answers. I wish that there was an open cholecystectomy control group and that further day-by-day study could have been done to see whether the proposed benefits of laparoscopic cholecystectomy and pulmonary function are realized. My gut feeling, based on looking at patients and in following my patients' courses, is that these benefits are realized, but many a feeling is debunked when studied in a rigorous fashion.—M.F. Roizen, M.D.

Preoperative HIV Testing: Is It Less Expensive Than Universal Precautions?

Lawrence VA, Gafni A, Kroenke K (Univ of Texas Health Science Ctr at San Antonio; McMaster Univ, Hamilton, Ont, Canada; Uniformed Services Univ of the Health Sciences, Bethesda, Md)
J Clin Epidemiol 46:1219–1227, 1993   101-95-1–8

Background.—Universal precautions, a set of barrier practices, are officially recommended to prevent the transmission of HIV in the health care setting. A previous economic evaluation has indicated these precautions are very expensive and not cost-effective for hospitals. An economic evaluation of universal precautions vs. routine preoperative HIV testing was undertaken.

Methods.—Conservatively, equal effectiveness in prevention of HIV transmission was assumed for both routine testing and universal precautions. Using the literature to establish costs and standard procedures, a minimized estimated cost for routine HIV testing was compared with a maximized average cost of universal precautions per elective operation.

Results.—Per elective surgical precedure, the minimized estimate for routine testing was $57 (United States) compared with $36 for universal precautions. Even with variations in the assumptions underlying the analysis (e.g., testing sensitivity and specificity), these results remained stable or were strengthened.

Conclusion.—Routine preoperative testing for HIV infection does not appear to have an economic advantage over routine universal precautions for preventing HIV transmission in health care settings. Although universal precautions are not cost-effective, they are less expensive and no less effective than routine testing. This comparative methodology can be used as a preliminary strategy for reviewing future suggestions for preventing HIV transmission in health care settings.

▶ This very interesting study looks only at the cost of universal precautions vs. the cost of preoperative HIV testing. Failure to counsel in screening programs for HIV infection is considered unethical; therefore, the patient who has either a negative or positive test must be counseled as to the meaning of that test result. This entails approximately 1 ½ hours of counseling (at the unbelievably low rate of $10 per hour for psychological counseling). However, the principal expense is the actual cost of the first test, $40, and not the cost of follow-up tests or of other aspects such as azidothymidine treatment or psychological counseling for the false positives.

Although I think, and the authors imply, that these elements may be more expensive, they do not even have to be calculated because the initial test and the minimal counseling that are offered cost more than the mandatory use of universal precautions, which the authors found to be approximately $36 per patient for the extra eye shields, water-impermeable gowns, booties, and gloves. On the other hand, the cost of the universal testing is $57 per patient.

Through this analysis, the authors do not even have to go into the ethical dilemmas about false positive and false negative tests and whether diseases other than HIV infection are also prevented by using universal precautions. The authors agree with the Centers for Disease Control recommendation that everyone should use universal precautions and the universal preoperative HIV testing should not be done because it is less cost-effective than universal precautions.

I recommend that all anesthesiologists read this article to understand the logic in the mind of the public health physician and public health economist. I found that it presented an enlightening view of the way medicine might be practiced in the future, where economic decisions may come before clinical ones. It is almost as though the authors give a technical answer to an ethical dilemma rather than exploring the clinical implications of the question and the problem at hand.—M.F. Roizen, M.D.

Outpatient Internal Medicine Preoperative Evaluation: A Randomized Clinical Trial
Macpherson DS, Lofgren RP (Univ of Pittsburgh, Pa; Pittsburgh Veterans Affairs Med Ctr, Pa)
Med Care 32:498–507, 1994   101-95-1–9

Background.—Although considerable effort has been devoted to shift care from the inpatient to outpatient setting, the effects of such a shift on health care use, patient outcome, and patient satisfaction have not been rigorously investigated. The effect of an outpatient internal medicine preoperative evaluation program on resource use was analyzed.

Methods.—One hundred seventy-nine inpatients and an equal number of outpatients were enrolled in the 2-arm, parallel-design, randomized, clinical trial. The outpatient internist preoperative assessment was done 2–3 weeks before admission for surgery in the experimental arm, with preoperative laboratory and radiology testing being performed during the visit; the control group was admitted for surgery with no outpatient assessment. The length of stay was the main outcome measure.

Findings.—The preoperative length of stay was decreased from 2.9 days in the inpatient group to 1.6 days in the outpatient group, a significant difference. The postoperative length of stay in the outpatient group was slightly but nonsignificantly longer than that of the inpatient group. The groups did not differ significantly in the total length of stay. Unnecessary admissions, that is, patients who were admitted but did not have surgery, were significantly reduced in the inpatient arm compared with the outpatient arm.

Conclusion.—A program of outpatient internal medicine preoperative assessment reduced the preoperative length of stay significantly. Its effect on the total length of stay was not so marked. The program also reduced the unnecessary admission of patients for elective surgery.

▶ It is hard for me to conceive of this article being published at this time. To claim that it is successful to decrease the preoperative length of stay from 2.9 to 1.6 days seems unusual to me. Perhaps it relates to this study having been done in a VA hospital.

Although I think that an outpatient internal medicine preoperative evaluation might shorten things in a VA hospital, I firmly believe that outpatient perioperative medicine consultations by anesthesiologists are less expensive both in terms of resource utilization and total care than the internal medicine care pattern used here. Macpherson and Lofgren are to be congratulated for trying to eliminate some of the waste in a VA hospital.—M.F. Roizen, M.D.

Efficacy of Radiographic Evaluation of the Cervical Spine in Emergency Situations

Lindsey RW, Diliberti TC, Doherty BJ, Watson AB (Baylor College of Medicine, Houston)
South Med J 86:1253–1255, 1993   101-95-1–10

Background.—In the emergency assessment of the cervical spine, it is usually standard procedure to use radiographs; however, this results in many unnecessary or inadequate imaging studies and may delay appropriate treatment while it ties up personnel and equipment time. In previous research, the physician's clinical judgment was correct in determining that a fracture was not present 94% of the time, but it could only appropriately predict the presence of fracture 50% of the time. An algorithm has been developed that may accurately determine which patients do not need radiographs. The number of undiagnosed fractures identified with the current indiscriminate use of radiographic studies was determined, as well as whether the use of clinical criteria (Fisher's clinical criteria: neck pain, neurologic deficit, and altered consciousness) included in the algorithm is appropriate in the clinical setting.

Materials and Methods.—The records of one group of patients were retrospectively reviewed to determine the efficacy of indiscriminate radiographs. A second group was observed prospectively to determine the specificity of radiographs. These patients were also assessed using the algorithm.

Results.—In the first group, 32 (1.9%) patients with cervical injuries were identified by indiscriminate radiographs. In group 2, 597 patients were evaluated for cervical spine injury. Whereas 2.8% of these patients were assessed as having cervical injury by indiscriminate radiographs, further evaluation revealed that the actual injury rate was only .8%. All true positive and false positive findings were accompanied by the clinical signs included in the algorithm.

Discussion.—These results, although they may be considered preliminary, support the use of Fisher's clinical criteria in these trauma patients. The finding that a high percentage of the initial radiographic assessments were false positives further decreased the cost-effectiveness of indiscriminate radiography. Larger studies would be appropriate.

▶ Although the authors' cause is noble, given the cost of potentially unnecessary emergency cervical spine x-rays, their ability to apply specific clinical criteria to the ordering of these films is tainted by their lack of any statistical analysis. Should a future prospective study validate that an altered consciousness, neck pain and/or tenderness, or neurologic symptoms are indeed independent variables, and if in such a large series these variables offer a high degree of predictability, then perhaps time and money can be saved. Until then, medicolegally speaking, most of us will continue to prefer to have the cervical spine "cleared" in the trauma setting before any airway manipulation.—D.M. Rothenberg, M.D.

A Methodology to Evaluate Motion of the Unstable Spine During Intubation Techniques
Donaldson WF III, Towers JD, Doctor A, Brand A, Donaldson VP (Univ of Pittsburgh, Pa)
Spine 18:2020–2023, 1993   101-95-1–11

Background.—Airway management of patients with an unstable cervical spine is a well-known problem that has not been well studied. Although many methods have been recommended for intubating the unstable cervical spine, measurements have not been reliably recorded. A technique that accurately records and measures motions of the unstable cervical spine during various airway maneuvers was investigated.

Methods.—Video fluoroscopy was performed in 5 cadavers with the cervical spine in the neutral position, flexion, and extension and during various airway maneuvers. Neck flexion and extension, chin life/jaw thrust, and cricoid pressure were performed. Intubation methods studied included forced direct oral intubation, direct oral, lighted nasal stylet, and tracheostomy. Unstable cervical spines were created in the cadavers through the posterior surgical release of the interspinous ligaments, facet capsule, ligamentum flavum, and posterior half of C5–6. Translation was recorded as the difference in the measures between the stable and unstable cervical spine for each maneuver in each cadaver.

Findings.—The largest motion for the direct crash oral maneuver was 4.77 mm. The least motion, during the indirect, blind nasal technique, was .39 mm. Spinous process distraction was greatest with the in-line head stabilization direct oral method (2.3 mm) and least with the blind nasal method (.7 mm). Because of technical problems, all recordings of measurement could not be used, and statistical analysis could not be applied. However, the direct oral intubations generally caused the most distraction and translation of the unstable spine. Indirect nasal methods showed the least translation and distraction. Some of these airway maneuvers, such as chin lift/jaw thrust and cricoid pressure, may cause as much motion as some intubation maneuvers do.

Conclusion.—The assessment of airway methods in unstable cervical spines can be facilitated by direct observation, recording, and measurement of the spine's motion. Direct fluoroscopy enables accurate measurement, standardization, and comparison. Indirect nasal intubation apparently causes less motion than direct unsupported oral techniques. Airway maneuvers such as cricoid pressure and jaw thrust/chin lift frequently result in as much motion as intubation techniques.

▶ The optimal technique for establishing tracheal intubation in the patient with an unstable cervical spine remains controversial. All techniques (e.g., blind nasal, orotracheal with in-line axial traction, fiberoptic, cricothyroidotomy) can be associated with certain degrees of cervical spine mobility and the potential for neurologic sequelae after intubation.

This study is significant not because of the results (indeed, this was a very poor study in which application of statistical analyses was impossible because of very small numbers and technical difficulties), but because of the new technology of video fluoroscopy. Once refined, this technique offers a unique, dynamic way to experimentally ascertain the optimal way to secure the airway in a patient with a traumatic cervical spine injury. The potential risks of such maneuvers as cricoid pressure can also be addressed.

Despite the authors' contention that blind nasal intubation causes the least cervical mobility, it is most likely that skill and experience are more important in managing the airways of these patients. I have no doubt that were the authors to assess their future data (assuming they repeat this study), they would conclude that an anesthesiologist's expertise makes the difference, irrespective of the technique chosen. In a combative trauma patient, I think we would strongly discourage an attempt at blind nasal intubation by an orthopedic surgeon! —D.M. Rothenberg, M.D.

Dobutamine Stress Echocardiography for Assessment of Perioperative Cardiac Risk in Patients Undergoing Major Vascular Surgery
Poldermans D, Fioretti PM, Forster T, Thomson IR, Boersma E, El-Said E-SM, du Bois NAJJ, Roelandt JRTC, van Urk H (Univ Hosp Rotterdam-Dijkzigt, The Netherlands; Erasmus Univ, Rotterdam, The Netherlands)
Circulation 87:1506–1512, 1993   101-95-1–12

Background.—Many perioperative cardiovascular complications can be avoided in patients who are having major noncardiac surgery if those at high risk can be identified. This is especially true for patients having major elective vascular operations, who are at particular risk of cardiovascular complications.

Methods.—The predictive value of dobutamine stress echocardiograpohy was studied in 136 patients (mean age, 68 years) who were scheduled for major vascular surgery and were unable to exercise. Dobutamine, from 10–40 μg/kg/min, was infused at increasing rates. Atropine was given intravenously in a dose of .25–1 mg if needed to achieve 85% of the age-predicted maximum heart rate without the development of ischemia. The clinical risk was estimated using Detsky's modification of Goldman's risk factor analysis. Two observers who had no knowledge of the clinical data examined the echocardiographic images.

Results.—Technically adequate images were acquired in all but 2 patients. The 1 major complication was ventricular fibrillation. Three tests were discontinued because of side effects. The test was positive, as evidenced by new or worsening wall motion abnormality, in 35 of the 131 evaluable patients. Five patients died of myocardial infarction postoperatively, 9 had unstable angina, and 1 had pulmonary edema. All 15 patients had a positive dobutamine stress test, and no patient with a negative test had a cardiac event. On multivariate analysis, the only significant predictors of perioperative cardiac events were age older than 70 years and a new wall-motion abnormality during the test.

Conclusion.—Echocardiography using dobutamine-induced stress is a safe and effective means of predicting the risk of perioperative cardiac complications in patients who are scheduled to undergo major vascular surgery.

▶ The excellent article by Mantha in the September 1994 issue of *Anesthesia and Analgesia* shows that the odds ratio for predicting an adverse effect perioperatively after vascular surgery is greatly increased by dobutamine stress echocardiography and that it appears to have a higher likelihood of being an accurate measure than dipyrodamole thallium, Holter monitoring, or radionuclide scanning. Nevertheless, I wonder what a simple clinical test, such as the ability to exercise to a heart rate of 100 with a hand bicycle ergometer, or other similar measures might yield in this setting.—M.F. Roizen, M.D.

Preoperative Clinical Assessment and Dipyridamole Thallium-201 Scintigraphy for Prediction and Prevention of Cardiac Events in Patients Having Major Noncardiovascular Surgery and Known or Suspected Coronary Artery Disease
Younis L, Stratmann H, Takase B, Byers S, Chaitman BR, Miller DD (St Louis Univ, Mo; VA Med Ctr, St Louis, Mo)
Am J Cardiol 74:311–317, 1994   101-95-1-13

Introduction.—Patients who are undergoing major noncardiovascular surgery are often evaluated for cardiac risk because of the possibility of reinfarction during surgery. The prognostic value of preoperative clinical risk evaluation and of IV dipyridamole thallium-201 scintigraphy was assessed in patients with an intermediate-to-high likelihood of having coronary artery disease (CAD) develop. In addition, the impact of preoperative medical interventions or coronary revascularization on the development of cardiac complications was assessed.

Methods.—Within a 3-year period, 161 patients scheduled for major noncardiovascular surgery were prospectively studied. They were screened preoperatively with clinical cardiac evaluation and IV dipyridamole thallium-201 scintigraphy. Perioperative events were derived from retrospective review, patient follow-up, and physician interview. Data were collected on cardiac events, including cardiac death, nonfatal myocardial infarction, unstable angina, and acute pulmonary edema.

Results.—Sixty patients had documented CAD, more than half of the patients had at least 2 risk factors for CAD, and 45% had an abnormal dipyridamole thallium-201 myocardial perfusion scan. Twenty-five of the 161 patients experienced cardiac events, including 9 cardiac deaths, 6 nonfatal myocardial infarctions, 4 with unstable angina, and 6 with acute pulmonary edema. These patients were significantly more likely to have a history of myocardial infarction or congestive heart failure, abnormal ECGs, abnormal thallium-201 myocardial scans, reversible thallium-201 perfusion defects, and more frequent segmental thallium-201 perfusion abnormalities. Thirty-six of the 72 patients who had abnormal thallium-201 studies were treated with preoperative interventions—coronary angioplasty in 6 patients and adjusted antianginal medication in 30. Perioperative cardiac events were significantly reduced in this group of patients.

Discussion.—Dipyridamole thallium-201 myocardial scintigraphy significantly increases the predictive value of clinical risk evaluation. In addition, the risk of perioperative cardiac events in patients with abnormal thallium-201 studies may be significantly mitigated by preoperative medical therapy or coronary revascularization.

▶ The basis for this article was the low rate of adverse effects from coronary angiography. It might be that we will reach the day when the cost of coronary angiography and its complications is so low that all patients who undergo major vascular surgery and have age or any other risk factor for CAD will have it as a first step, thereby skipping the dipyridamole thallium forerunner. I don't think that the dipyridamole studies have added much to simply going straight to coronary angiography for every patient.—M.F. Roizen, M.D.

Preoperative Prediction for the Use of Cardiopulmonary Bypass in Lung Transplantation

de Hoyos A, Demajo W, Snell G, Miller J, Winton T, Maurer JR, Patterson GA (Univ of Toronto)
J Thorac Cardiovasc Surg 106:787–796, 1993   101-95-1-14

Background.—The use of cardiopulmonary bypass during single- and double-lung transplantation is based on either preoperative indications, such as pulmonary hypertension or concurrent cardiac repair, or intraoperative parameters. The advent of sequential lung transplantation has reduced reliance on the bypass. The increased technical demands, operative time, and ischemia time argue against routine use of the bypass procedure. Preoperative variables that could accurately predict the need for the bypass procedure would be useful.

Methods.—Of 109 lung transplantations, 69 patients with obstructive or restrictive lung disease had cardiopulmonary bypass initiated because of intraoperative hemodynamics; only patients with restrictive lung disease needed bypass. The preoperative data of these 69 patients were analyzed to determine whether any data could predict the eventual use of the bypass. Preoperative tests included pulmonary function, exercise tolerance, and radionuclear cardiac tests. Exercise tolerance included the distance walked in 6 minutes and arterial oxygen desaturation during a 3- to 5-minute walk on a treadmill at 1 mile per hour at a 4% grade. Cardiac tests included resting and exercise technetium-99m–gated angiographic studies. Right ventricular ejection fraction was determined from gated first-pass and equilibrium tests. Intraoperatively, cardiac output, index, pulmonary vascular resistance, and systemic vascular resistance were obtained through a pulmonary artery catheter using standard methods.

Results.—In patients receiving single-lung transplantation, those with obstructive lung disease had a significantly lower forced expiratory volume in 1 second than the restrictive patients, but this test did not predict who would eventually need bypass. Patients with restrictive disease and with no bypass procedure walked more than 400 m in 6 minutes, whereas patients with restrictive disease who underwent bypass walked 256 m. There was no difference between the patients with obstructive disease and those with restrictive disease. The oxygen desaturation and oxygen requirement were greatest in the restrictive patients who underwent bypass. The right ventricular ejection fraction was lower in restrictive than obstructive patients, regardless of bypass status determined by either first-pass or resting equilibrium methods. The differences were magnified during exercise. The left ventricular ejection fraction did not discriminate between the groups. Intraoperatively, restrictive patients who had bypass had a significantly lower cardiac index and a higher pulmonary artery pressure and vascular resistance as well as an alveolar-arterial oxygen gradient. There were no systematic variations in patients who underwent double-lung transplantation.

Conclusion.—Many patients can have lung transplantation without the need for cardiopulmonary bypass. No preoperative measures predicted the need for bypass in patients with obstructive lung disease. For patients with restrictive disease, a combination of less than 300 m in the 6-minute walk, exercise oxygen saturation of less than 85% when supplemented with oxygen, right ventricular ejection fraction of less than 27%, and oxygen requirements during the treadmill test of greater than .5 L per minute predicts the need for cardiopulmonary bypass. Six of 9 bypass patients satisfied these criteria; 1 of 17 patients who did not have bypass and none of the obstructive patients met all 4 criteria. Intraoperative factors dictate the need for bypass in double-lung transplantation.

▶ At our institution, we usually decide whether to use cardiopulmonary bypass intraoperatively and always have a perfusionist in the operating room. Although this study defines "patients at risk" for cardiopulmonary bypass, I do not think it will change our current practice.—M. Wood, M.D.

Pulmonary Risk Factors of Elective Abdominal Aortic Surgery

Calligaro KD, Azurin DJ, Dougherty MJ, Dandora R, Bajgier SM, Simper S, Savarese RP, Raviola CA, DeLaurentis DA (Univ of Pennsylvania, Philadelphia; Drexel Univ, Philadelphia)
J Vasc Surg 18:914–921, 1993   101-95-1-15

Background.—Few reports have addressed the prevalence of and the risk factors for postoperative pulmonary complications in elective abdominal aortic surgery. The preoperative and intraoperative pulmonary risk factors were identified in patients undergoing elective abdominal aortic surgery in which a midline incision was used.

Methods.—A retrospective record review was conducted for 181 consecutive patients who underwent this procedure at a large university hospital between July 1986 and December 1992.

Results.—Mortality was 1.7% (3 of 181), and 2 of the 3 deaths were the result of pneumonia. Pulmonary complications affected 97 (54%) of the patients, with major complications occurring in 29 (16%) and minor complications (atelectasis) occurring in 68 (38%). Pneumonia was the most common major complication (16 patients). Nine patients required prolonged intubation because of respiratory complications, and 4 required reintubation as a result of pulmonary insufficiency. The strongest correlation of a preoperative risk factor with a major complication was being classified as American Society of Anesthesiologists physical status IV. A forced vital capacity of 80% of normal or less, a forced expiratory flow rate (25–75) of 60% of normal or less, and an age greater than 70 years were also significant risk factors for postoperative pulmonary complications. Intraoperative risk factors that correlated significantly with major pulmonary complications included an operative time of more than 5 hours and administration of more than 6 L of crystalloid during surgery. Minor complications were significantly correlated only with administration of greater than 5 L of crystalloid during surgery. Patients with major complications experienced significantly longer stays in both the ICU and the hospital compared with those who did not experience pulmonary complications. Those with minor complications did not experience significantly longer stays in either the ICU or the hospital.

Conclusion.—Pulmonary risk factors may play as important a role as cardiac factors in the outcome of elective abdominal aortic surgery. The most notable risk factors are age older than 70 years, decreased forced vital capacity and forced expiratory flow rate, American Society of Anesthesiologists physical status IV, operative time of greater than 5 hours, and crystalloid replacement of greater than 6 L.

▶ Clearly, American Society of Anesthesiologists physical status IV had the highest specificity for predicting pulmonary complications, but the authors did not evaluate patient symptoms such as the ability to walk 2 blocks, walk up 1 flight of stairs without shortness of breath, or pedal a bicycle ergometer to a heart rate of 100 without shortness of breath. I think these simpler tests that use patient symptoms may be both more specific and sensitive than those the authors evaluated. I wonder when physicians will return to talking to patients and incorporating risk factors of patient symptoms into their "computerized databases."—M.F. Roizen, M.D.

Sugarless Gum Chewing Before Surgery Does Not Increase Gastric Fluid Volume or Acidity
Dubin SA, Jense HG, McCranie JM, Zubar V (Med College of Georgia, Augusta)
Can J Anaesth 41:603–606, 1994   101-95-1–16

Introduction.—Anesthetists have sometimes canceled or delayed surgery when a patient arrives chewing gum, assuming that gum chewing could increase gastric volume and acid production. This assumption was tested in a prospective, controlled study.

Methods.—Seventy-seven patients with an American Society of Anesthesiologists physical status I or II who were scheduled for elective outpatient surgery arrived after fasting. The first 31 patients were randomly assigned to either the control group (group 1) or to chew sugarless gum until 20 mintues before the induction of anesthesia (group 2). The remaining 46 patients (group 3) were given sugarless gum and allowed to chew it until immediately before the induction of anesthesia. After the induction of anesthesia, gastric contents were aspirated, and the volume and pH were measured.

Results.—The mean gastric volumes were 26 mL for group 1, 40 mL for group 2, and 28 mL for group 3. The mean gastric pH values were 1.8 for group 1, 1.6 for group 2, and 1.7 for group 3. There was no correlation between gastric volume or gastric pH and the time interval between discarding the gum and the induction of anesthesia or the length of time the patient chewed gum.

Discussion.—Gastric contents and pH did not differ significantly among the 3 groups of patients, indicating that there was no correlation between gum chewing and gastric volume and acid production, regardless of the duration of chewing or the time interval between gum chewing and the induction of anesthesia. Surgery does not have to be delayed if a patient arrives chewing gum.

▶ Although this study indicates that sugarless gum does not increase gastric volume or acidity, it should be noted that the mean value of gastric volume and of gastric pH was less than 2.5 for pH and greater than .4 mL/kg for volume, which are known as trigger values for serious aspiration pneumonitis. The authors also point out 3 other problems and 1 benefit of chewing sugarless gum. The risks included increased salivation, laryngospasm, and aspiration; the benefit was a reduction in anxiety. Therefore, although this article tends to be edifying, it does not answer the basic risk vs. benefit question of permitting gum chewing until the time of surgery. Perhaps if aspiration prophylaxis with an H_2-antagonist, or by some other means such as metoclopramide or a combination thereof, were instituted, the risk of aspiration from gum would all but disappear.—M.F. Roizen, M.D.

Gastric Volume and pH in Infants Fed Clear Liquids and Breast Milk Prior to Surgery

Litman RS, Wu CL, Quinlivan JK (Univ of Rochester, NY)
Anesth Analg 79:482–485, 1994   101-95-1–17

Background.—Preoperative fasting intervals in pediatric patients undergoing elective surgery have recently been shortened. Because there is little information on the safety of this practice in infants younger than 1 year of age, residual gastric volumes and pH were measured in infants who were fed either clear liquids or breast milk approximately 2 hours before anesthesia induction.

Methods.—Seventy infants were studied prospectively; 46 were fed 2–8 oz of clear liquids, and 24 were breast-fed 2 hours before anesthesia induction. After induction and tracheal intubation, a "blinded" investigator aspirated gastric fluid with a syringe and measured its volume and pH.

Results.—Sufficient gastric fluid for analysis was aspirated from 10 (22%) of the infants who were fed clear liquids and 8 (33%) of the breast-fed infants. In the group given clear liquid, the mean residual gastric volume was .3 mL/kg and the mean pH was 2.1. In the breast-fed group, the mean residual gastric volume was .71 mL/kg and the pH was 2.6. Eight (33%) breast-fed infants had from .9 to 3 mL of residual gastric contents per kg.

Conclusion.—Infants younger than 1 year of age can safely ingest clear liquids until 2 hours before anesthesia induction. Breast-feeding fewer than 3 hours before surgery is not recommended, because some infants may have relatively large residual gastric volumes.

▶ Guidelines for fasting intervals in pediatric patients are rapidly changing, and I think that we all agree that the old way of fasting children for prolonged periods is not necessary and may not be beneficial. I believe that allowing even small children to ingest fluids up to 2 hours before surgery is sensible. I also am cautious regarding breast-feeding.—M. Wood, M.D.

Preoperative Autonomic Function Abnormalities in Patients With Diabetes Mellitus and Patients With Hypertension
Charlson ME, MacKenzie CR, Gold JP (Cornell Univ, New York)
J Am Coll Surg 179:1–10, 1994   101-95-1–18

Introduction.—Autonomic neuropathy has been implicated in patients with diabetes mellitus who die of cardiorespiratory arrest after the induction of anesthesia or who experience intraoperative cardiovascular hypotension. The relative risk of autonomic function abnormalities for postoperative cardiac arrest was assessed prospectively in patients with diabetes mellitus.

Methods.—Autonomic function was evaluated preoperatively with a series of tests in 74 patients with diabetes mellitus and 118 patients with hypertension and no diabetes. Blood pressure was monitored intraoperatively, and vasopressor requirements were recorded by an independent observer. For 7 days postoperatively, the patients were evaluated clinically and with ECGs and serum analysis by another independent observer. The observers in each phase were unaware of the findings in the other phases.

Results.—Preoperative autonomic function abnormalities were not significantly associated with intraoperative hypotension or vasopressor requirements in either the patients with diabetes or hypertension. Five patients had postoperative cardiac arrest or death; all 5 had diabetes mellitus and at least 2 abnormal autonomic function tests. In addition, 15 patients had myocardial infarction and 8 had postoperative heart failure. The risk of cardiovascular complications was increased in patients with diabetes mellitus who had at least 2 abnormal autonomic function tests or a history of infarction or cardiomegaly; autonomic neuropathy was not a risk factor for postoperative complications in patients with hypertension.

Discussion.—In assessing the risk of patients with diabetes mellitus having postoperative cardiovascular complications, the positive predictive value of autonomic function tests or previous infarction and cardiomegaly was 17% to 22%; for both, it was 38%. These data justify close postoperative surveillance of patients with diabetes mellitus who have at least 2 autonomic function test abnormalities preoperatively and a history of myocardial infarction or cardiomegaly.

▶ This study confirms my long-held belief that patients with diabetes who have autonomic insufficiency should be kept in an ICU or recovery room setting for 24 hours after surgery. Seven percent of the patients with diabetes experienced cardiorespiratory arrest or death, and all had abnormal autonomic nervous system function tests preoperatively. Five of the 8 patients with a history of myocardial infarction or cardiomegaly who had 2 or more abnormal tests died suddenly in the postoperative period, and 3 of 21 patients who did not have a myocardial infarction or cardiomegaly but had 2 or more abnormal tests had a myocardial infarction postoperatively. As a result, autonomic insufficiency should be one of the outcomes that is routinely sought in diabetics, and it should evoke a heightened level of care, responsiveness, and discussion of risk with the patient.—M.F. Roizen, M.D.

Autonomic Reflex Dysfunction in Patients Presenting for Elective Surgery Is Associated With Hypotension After Anesthesia Induction
Latson TW, Ashmore TH, Reinhart DJ, Klein KW, Giesecke AH (Univ of Texas, Dallas; Dallas; Ogden, Utah)
Anesthesiology 80:326–337, 1994   101-95-1–19

Introduction.—Alterations in autonomic nervous system (ANS) reflex function are found in patients with advanced age and in association with a variety of drug therapies and medical conditions. In patients with diabetes, ANS dysfunction is associated with an increased incidence of hypotension after induction of anesthesia. Patients in for general day surgery were evaluated for hypotension after anesthesia induction.

Methods.—Study participants included 26 consecutive day-surgery patients older than 39 years of age (mean, 52 years); 19 were women. Ten had concomitant hypertension and 4 were diabetic. Tests of autonomic function were performed before any sedative agents were administered. Preoperative tests included the Valsalva maneuver, change in heart rate with forced breathing, change in heart rate and blood pressure with standing, and spectral analysis of heart rate variability. Thiopental, fentanyl, vercuronium, and isoflurane were the anesthetic agents used. The mean blood pressure was measured every minute for 10 minutes after induction, then every 3 minutes until skin incision.

Results.—Hypotension, which was defined as a mean blood pressure of less than 70 mm Hg, developed in 12 patients who had autonomic reflex function measurements that were significantly more abnormal than those of patients without hypotension. Based on critical test values, the incidence of hypotension ranged from 67% to 83% in patients with ANS dysfunction vs. 9% to 17% in those with negative autonomic tests. Normotensive and hypotensive patients did not differ significantly in the baseline mean blood pressure or in the incidence of specific medical conditions. These 2 groups showed highly significant differences for most autonomic tests.

Conclusion.—Preexisting ANS dysfunction, as measured by several autonomic tests, was associated with an increased incidence of postinduction hypotension in these day-surgery patients. The association between hypotension and ANS dysfunction was greater than that between hypotension and any specific medical condition. Preoperative ANS reflex dysfunction can be identified by simple noninvasive tests and may be a significant factor in the hemodynamic response to anesthetic induction.

▶ Simple preoperative tests that have the power to predict adverse events would be extremely valuable, but we must know how good the test is at predicting abnormality. This very nice study demonstrates that autonomic reflex dysfunction occurs in relatively young patients and is associated with an increased incidence of postinduction hypotension.

The various tests the authors used did not show a very high sensitivity and specificity. The incidence of hypotension was 67% to 83% in patients with positive tests, and whole hypotension occurred in 9% to 17% of patients with negative tests.

It is difficult to achieve 100% sensitivity and specificity, because if sensitivity is increased, specificity decreases. I think that we need to debate what sensitivity and specificity are required to modify out treatment plan. Although we would accept lower specificity for maximum sensitivity in malignant hyperthermia testing, I am not certain what is reasonable for anesthesia induction techniques.—M. Wood, M.D.

Call Mosby Document Express at **1 (800) 55-MOSBY** to obtain copies of the original source documents of articles featured or referenced in the YEAR BOOK series.

2 Anesthetic Technique, Procedures, and Equipment

A Prospective, Randomized, Double-Blind Comparison of Epidural and Intravenous Sufentanil Infusions
Miguel R, Barlow I, Morrell M, Scharf J, Sanusi D, Fu E (Univ of South Florida, Tampa)
Anesthesiology 81:346–352, 1994   101-95-2-1

Background.—Opioids are frequently administered epidurally to control postoperative pain. Those that are water-soluble, such as morphine,

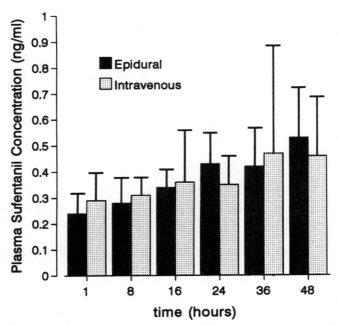

Fig 2–1.—Plasma sufentanil concentrations found in the patients in the 2 groups. Values are expressed as the mean ± the standard deviation. The differences between the patients in the groups were not statistically significant. (Courtesy of Miguel R, Barlow I, Morrell M, et al: *Anesthesiology* 81:346–352, 1994.)

act mainly at the dorsal horn ganglia of the dorsal spinothalamic tract. The site of action of lipid-soluble opioids such as fentanyl and sufentanil is less certain.

Objective.—In 50 patients who were to have intra-abdominal surgery under combined epidural and general anesthesia, a double-blind, prospective study was performed to compare the effects of sufentanil that was given epidurally and intravenously in equivalent doses and volumes.

Methods.—Twenty-four patients received an epidural infusion of sufentanil, .2 μg/kg/hr, and an IV infusion of saline at the same rate. The remaining 26 patients received IV sufentanil and an epidural saline infusion at the same rate. All patients were eligible to receive IV morphine in increments of 2 mg postoperatively. Subsequently, a patient-controlled IV pump was used to provide morphine on demand in doses of 1 mg with a 10-minute lockout.

Results.—Patients in the 2 groups had similar levels of pain and required comparable amounts of supplemental morphine. Sedation scores were similar at most intervals, but 6 of the patients who received IV sufentanil and only 1 in the epidural sufentanil group had to have their dose reduced. None of the patients in either group had respiratory depression develop. There were no significant group differences in nausea scores or in the frequency or severity of pruritus. Plasma sufentanil levels were similar at all intervals (Fig 2–1).

Conclusion.—No substantial differences were found between the IV and epidural routes for delivering sufentanil, except for more frequent excessive sedation with the IV route.

▶ Are there really only minor differences between epidural and IV sufentanil administration? Many anesthesiologists believe that for the lipid-soluble opioids, there is really very little difference between epidural and IV administration. This study seems to support this concept. Acute postoperative pain relief using epidural infusions has become very popular, but large epidemiologic trials are required with sufficient patients studied to enable statistical analysis.—M. Wood, M.D.

Early and Late Recovery After Major Abdominal Surgery: Comparison Between Propofol Anaesthesia With and Without Nitrous Oxide and Isoflurane Anaesthesia
Kalman SH, Jensen AG, Ekberg K, Eintrei C (Univ Hosp, Linköping, Sweden)
Acta Anaesthesiol Scand 37:730–736, 1993   101-95-2-2

Introduction.—A search for new anesthetic techniques has been underway because halogenated agents and nitrous oxide are a threat to the ozone layer, and because recovery after anesthesia and surgery has been a focus of interest in recent years. The early and late recovery of patients after major surgery was compared under 3 forms of anesthesia: IV anesthesia with propofol; propofol/nitrous oxide; and isoflurane/nitrous oxide.

Methods.—Sixty patients who were scheduled for major lower abdominal surgery were randomly assigned to 1 of the 3 groups. All 60 also received fentanyl and vecuronium. For comparison, the preoperative values of all tests were gathered 1–4 days before surgery. Recovery was monitored during the first 2 hours after extubation and on days 1, 2, 3, 7, and 30 after surgery. The Steward recovery scale, orientation in time and place, collaboration and comprehension, and degree of sedation were assessed by a blinded observer every 30 minutes during the first 2 postoperative hours (early recovery scores). In 32 patients, the psychomotor function was evaluated by computerized simple reaction time and finger tapping speed.

Results.—In all 60 patients, an improvement was noted in the early recovery scores with regard to the Steward recovery scale, sedation, orientation, and collaboration and comprehension. No statistically significant differences emerged among the 3 groups. Late recovery of psychomotor function showed a statistically significant prolongation of simple reaction time on all postoperative days when compared with the values in 32 preoperative patients. By comparison, early and late recovery of psychomotor function showed no statistically significant differences among the 3 groups. After surgery, all 60 patients demonstrated an increase in adverse symptoms. The isoflurane/nitrous oxide group showed the most pronounced increase, and the propofol/nitrous oxide group showed the smallest. When vegetative symptoms were analyzed, the difference between the propofol and isoflurane groups appeared to be greatest on day 7, when the 2 groups that received propofol had almost resumed preoperative values, but those in the isoflurane group remained affected. In all 3 groups, the average mood score decreased after surgery. When compared with patients who were anesthetized with isoflurane, patients who received propofol indicated better subjective control and social orientation. On day 7, patients who received propofol and isoflurane/nitrous oxide showed significant differences in the mood scales hedonic tone, social orientation, calmness, and average mood.

Conclusion.—The results of early recovery in all 3 groups were similar. Late recovery was better after propofol-based anesthesia than after isoflurane anesthesia. The use of nitrous oxide did not affect the results of the study. Continuing the use of nitrous oxide could be questioned because it adds to ozone depletion and the greenhouse effect.

▶ These authors clearly want to believe that the subjective positive findings in favor of propofol might somehow translate into decreased costs. They note that "it is interesting to speculate whether the improved mood and reduction in postoperative symptoms could reduce the need for hospital care. We have not been able to show this." Despite this, they are still "true believers." In the very next sentence, they observe that "propofol anesthesia is costly, but if one takes into account the costs of maintaining the tubing for central gases and the supply of gases, the difference is small and perhaps in favour of propofol." If you believe that last statement, I've got some land under a bridge somewhere to sell you!

The "tubing" through which the gases in hospitals are piped and its maintenance are part of the hospital's overall general budget, which includes the far-reaching areas to which oxygen and other gases are piped, certainly not just the operating room. Much of that maintenance budget would be there whether or not there were any other operations in progress. Propofol is costly compared with volatile anesthetics. The question is whether its subjective benefit, as reported in this study, is worth the cost. It's as simple as that.—J.H. Tinker, M.D.

Propofol Infusion and the Suppression of Consciousness: Dose Requirements to Induce Loss of Consciousness and to Suppress Response to Noxious and Non-Noxious Stimuli

Dunnett JM, Prys-Roberts C, Holland DE, Browne BL (Princess Margaret, Hosp, Swindon, England; Univ of Bristol, England; Southmead Hosp, Bristol, England)
Br J Anaesth 72:29–34, 1994   101-95-2–3

Background.—Propofol is widely accepted as an appropriate drug for induction and maintenance of anesthesia. Dose-response requirements based on somatic or visceral motor responses to surgical stimuli have been described, and it has been noted that smaller infusion doses are needed for older patients. Correlations between infusion rate and blood concentration, consciousness, and electroencephalographic data have

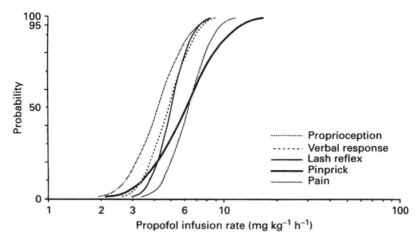

Fig 2–2.—Log dose-response curves, derived from probit analysis, relating the probability of a positive response to sensory stimuli to the final infusion rate for propofol infusion. (Courtesy of Dunnett JM, Prys-Roberts C, Holland DE, et al: *Br J Anaesth* 72:29–34, 1994.)

also been published. The dose-response relationship in the suppression of consciousness during stable blood concentrations of propofol was determined.

Methods.—Patients undergoing minor surgical procedures were divided into 2 groups. The younger group, 18–40 years of age, included 52 patients, whereas the older group, 41–65 years of age, included 32 patients. The younger sample was divided into 5 groups, whereas the older sample was divided into 4 groups. Each group received a different infusion scheme, which had previously been shown to result in stable blood levels of propofol after 20 minutes. At 10 and 20 minutes, each patient was asked a series of more complex questions. When no response was given, the eyelash reflex was tested followed by increasingly more noxious stimuli. Data were subjected to probit analysis, and a 95% confidence interval for each dose-response was determined.

Results.—In the younger group the infusion rate to abolish responses to proprioception and verbal response in 50% of the patients was less at 20 minutes than at 10 minutes. No differences were seen in the infusion rates to abolish responses in 95% of the younger patients. For the older patients, the infusion rates to abolish responses to pinprick or verbal response in 50% were less at 20 minutes than at 10 minutes. No differences were seen in the infusion rates to abolish responses in 95% of the older patients. Calculated dosages to suppress proprioception, verbal response, and painful stimuli in 50% and 95% of patients indicated that the dose-response curve shifted to the right (Fig 2–2). Proprioception and finger counting were suppressed at a lower dose than were verbal responses. Larger doses were required to suppress painful stimuli such as pinprick and supraorbital pain, whereas the corneal reflex was not suppressed in any patient.

Conclusion.—The infusion values for loss of consciousness in 50% and 95% of patients over a wide range of ages were defined. The dose-response curve for noxious stimuli was shifted to the right of the curves representing consciousness. The dose-response curves for suppression of proprioception, light touch, and finger counting were shifted to the left of the curves for the eyelash reflex and consciousness.

▶ I have always thought that movement in response to a noxious stimulus was a rather crude, although extremely reproducible, end point. This study describes infusion regimens for the suppression of consciousness. Although we must always titrate a drug to an individual clinical effect, infusion schemes such as this constitute a good starting point.—M. Wood, M.D

Control of Plasma Glucose With Somatostatin Analogue (SMS 201-995) During Surgical Removal of Insulinomas

Utas C, Kelestimur F, Boyaci A, Saglam A (Erciyes Univ, Kayseri, Turkey)
Postgrad Med J 69:920–921, 1993   101-95-2–4

Introduction.—Because hypoglycemia must be avoided during surgical treatment of insulinoma, large volumes of parenteral glucose-containing solutions are usually administered during surgery. However, volume overload is contraindicated in patients with severe cardiac failure. Octreotide has been used successfully to inhibit insulin secretion in patients undergoing medical therapy for insulinoma. The efficacy of octreotide in preventing hypoglycemia during surgery for insulinoma was studied.

Methods.—Two female patients with hypoglycemic episodes had pancreatic masses diagnosed with CT. They both underwent surgery to excise the tumors. Histopathologic examination of the tumors confirmed the diagnosis of insulinoma. The patients were managed preoperatively with octreotide, and no further hypoglycemic episodes occurred. One hour before surgery, the patients were given 100 μg of octreotide subcutaneously; their glucose profiles were monitored every 15 minutes.

Results.—Neither patient registered hypoglycemic values at any time during or after surgery. Neither patient required IV glucose infusion.

Discussion.—Hypoglycemia must be prevented before and during surgery for insulinomas. The risk of hypoglycemia is especially high during manipulation of the tumor, which secretes insulin. A single dose of octreotide administered subcutaneously 1 hour before surgery controlled glucose values throughout and after surgical excision of the insulinomas, without administration of large volumes of glucose solutions. Therefore, octreotide therapy is a safe and effective option for patients who cannot tolerate fluid administration.

▶ Somatostatin is a peptide that has been shown to inhibit the release of regulatory peptides such as growth hormone, insulin, glucagon, and gastrin (1). Long-acting analogues of somatostatin (octreotide) have now been developed (2). These long-acting analogues are very useful, because the half-life of octreotide is about 45 minutes after IV and 80 minutes after subcutaneous injection, whereas the half-life of somatostatin is very short, necessitating administration by continuous infusion.

Octreotide has been used successfully in the medical management of patients with insulinomas, and its use is now advocated for the control of blood glucose during surgical removal of insulin-secreting tumors. Continuous monitoring and control of plasma glucose during surgery for removal of insulinomas are still, of course, mandatory, and glucose-containing solutions may be required.—M. Wood, M.D.

References

1. Bloom SR, Polak JM: *BMJ* 295:288, 1987.
2. Kvols LK, et al: *N Engl J Med* 315:663, 1986.

Perioperative Glucocorticoid Coverage: A Reassessment 42 Years After Emergence of a Problem
Salem M, Tainsh RE Jr, Bromberg J, Loriaux DL, Chernow B (Johns Hopkins Univ, Baltimore, Md; Florida Hosp Med Ctr, Orlando; Med Univ of South Carolina, Charleston; et al)
Ann Surg 219:416–425, 1994   101-95-2-5

Background.—Forty years ago, 2 case reports were published that prompted recommendations for perioperative glucocorticoid coverage. These recommendations became the standard of care. Although the understanding of the role of the hypothalamic-pituitary-adrenal-cortical (HPA) axis in the stress response has subsequently been refined, recommendations for perioperative glucocorticoid coverage have not changed. The historical basis for providing perioperative glucocorticoid coverage was reviewed, as well as the evolution in the understanding of the role of the HPA axis in response to physical stressors. New recommendations were proposed for glucocorticoid-dependent patients who needed anesthesia and surgery.

Methods and Results.—Reports of the physiologic actions of the adrenal glands that first appeared in 1855 and descriptions and clinical uses of cortisone that appeared between 1930 and 1993 were identified. Studies were selected for review if they involved or assessed the provision of stress-related glucocorticoid administration. All clinical research was assessed to determine the basis for the provision of perioperative glucocorticoid coverage and the validity of the data used to justify the conclusions. Evidence suggested that the current amount of perioperative glucocorticoid coverage was excessive and was based on anecdotal reports.

Conclusion.—The amount and duration of glucocorticoid coverage should be determined by the preoperative dose of glucocorticoid taken by the patient, the preoperative duration of glucocorticoid administration, and the nature and anticipated duration of surgery.

▶ I selected this article because it is always useful to have current recommendations for perioperative glucocorticoid coverage at hand. These new recommendations are lower than some anesthesiologists may be using at this time. However, it is still important to be aware of complications resulting from inadequate glucocorticoid coverage, such as postoperative hypotension. Of course, in an ideal world, individualization of therapy would be the norm, and each patient would have HPA cortical axis function assessed before surgery.—M. Wood, M.D.

Anesthesiologists' Management of Isolated Limb Perfusion With "High-Dose" Tumor Necrosis Factor α

Sigurdsson GH, Nachbur B, Lejeune FJ (Univ of Berne, Switzerland; Univ Hosp, Lausanne, Switzerland)
Anesthesiology 79:1433–1437, 1993   101-95-2–6

Introduction.—Human recombinant tumor necrosis factor-α (TNFα) has exhibited activity against advanced malignancies in humans, but its severe systemic side effects have limited the clinical benefit that can be achieved. The efficacy of perfusing the isolated extremity with a high dose of cytotoxic drug suggested the use of this approach to deliver recombinant TNFα in a high dosage. Encouraging results have been reported in patients with advanced malignant melanoma or sarcoma of the extremities.

Case Report.—Man, 62, with a history of hypertension, received high-dose recombinant TNFα as well as interferon and melphalan by perfusion for a rhabdomyosarcoma of the left leg. After induction of general isoflurane anesthesia, indomethacin, heparin, and dopamine were administered; a tourniquet was applied; and the patient was given 4 mg of recombinant TNFα, .2 mg of recombinant interferon-γ, and 85 mg of melphalan by femoral cannula. Subsequently, the leg was perfused with dextran 40 and Ringer's lactate, and 5% IV human albumin was given to elevate the pulmonary capillary wedge pressure from 9 to 12 mm Hg before releasing the tourniquet. The patient remained clinically stable throughout the perfusion. Leakage of perfusate into the systemic circulation peaked at 3% after 1 hour. Intravenous gelatin was given after perfusion when oxygen saturation decreased. When signs, including a hyperdynamic circulation, marked hypotension, and tachycardia, suggested severe septic shock had developed, the patient was given pentoxifylline, and he did well subsequently. The patient was discharged 8 days postoperatively and was doing well when he was readmitted 7 weeks later for surgical removal of the tumor, which was 90% necrotic.

Discussion.—This patient had severe toxicity from perfusion therapy, most of which probably was caused by TNFα. Inhibitors of arachidonic acid metabolism and pentoxifylline, which inhibits phosphodiesterase, may counter the side effects of TNFα. Only patients in good general health should be accepted for TNFα treatment.

▶ This case report demonstrates the usual practice for isolated limb perfusion with TNF and what happens when a reaction occurs with the use of an unusual agent—pentoxifylline—rather than the usual agent—epinephrine—to treat such reactions. Pentoxifylline is a phosphodiesterase inhibitor that may have special benefits in treating TNF overdoses. Although therapy with TNF for lung disease and isolated limb perfusions promises to increase, its exact role has yet to be established. Furthermore, whether patients will need anesthesia for this procedure and the role of the anesthesiologist or intensivist in these isolated limb perfusions remain to be established.

It would be nice if the editors of *Anesthesiology* would insist, as do those of many other anesthesia journals, on indicating who sponsored the study. That way, we would know whether the work is prejudiced and the extent of its bias. For instance, if Hoechst had sponsored the study, it might be obvious why pentoxifylline was chosen rather than epinephrine. I have no idea whether that was done or who was the sponsor because it was not indicated in *Anesthesiology.*—M.F. Roizen, M.D.

An Assessment of a Blood Warmer for High and Low Flows

Johnson ALM, Morgan M (Hammersmith Hosp, London)
Anaesthesia 49:707–709, 1994   101-95-2–7

Background.—Heat loss commonly occurs during anesthesia and surgery. Hypothermia can result in increased mortality and morbidity from metabolic derangements, abnormal hemostasis, or ventricular arrhythmias. The efficacy of a new disposable set for use with the level 1 H-250 blood warmer, which was designed to warm fluids over a wide variety of flows, was investigated in the laboratory.

Methods and Findings.—The effectiveness of the D-60 HL disposable set in the level 1 H-250 blood warmer was compared with that of the D-100 standard disposable giving set for warming at high flows and with the Fenwal blood warmer. The temperature of the infusing saline ranged from 21.7° to 22.4°C for room temperature fluids and 3.8° and 4.3°C for refrigerated fluids, except at a flow of 750 mL/min^{-1}. The Fenwal warmer automatically shut off at flows of 500 and 750 mL/min^{-1} with the cold saline, because the heating elements could not maintain operational temperatures. At 22°C, the D60 HL achieved warming to more than 35°C at flows of 1 to 500 mL/min^{-1} and warming to 33° to 35°C at other flows. Warming to 33.4°C was achieved at a maximum flow of 750 mL/min^{-1}. The D100 giving set warmed to more than 35°C with flows between 50 and 500 mL/min^{-1}. With the Fenwal, the maximum warming temperature was only 34°C at 50 mL/min^{-1}, and it warmed to above 30°C only at flows of 15 to 250 mL/min^{-1}.

Conclusion.—The H-250 level 1 warmer with its new disposable D-60HL set effectively warms fluids at flows of 1 to 500 mL/min^{-1} for room temperature fluids and of 5 to 100 mL/min^{-1} for fluids at 4–5°C. This system is easy to set up and use.

▶ This well-done study of technology points out the limitations of flow rates for this level 1 warmer with its new disposable set. For fluids at room temperature, it could handle up to 500 mL/min^{-1}, which is just about the maximum needed; even with cold fluids, it handled them at 100 mL/min^{-1}. At both these flows, citrate intoxication would seem to be more of a problem than lack of volume status.—M.F. Roizen, M.D.

The New Tec 6 Desflurane Vaporizer

Andrews JJ, Johnston RV Jr (Univ of Texas, Galveston)
Anesth Analg 76:1338–1341, 1993   101-95-2–8

Introduction.—Desflurane is a new inhaled anesthetic with a low blood gas solubility coefficient, which allows rapid recovery. However, its vapor pressure is 3–4 times higher than that for other inhaled anesthetic agents, and it boils at 23.5°C. Therefore, it cannot be used with currently available vaporizers. A new vaporizer, the Tec 6, has been introduced that can be used for desflurane administration.

Operating Principles.—Heat and pressure are electrically controlled in the Tec 6 vaporizer so that the vaporization of desflurane can be adequately controlled. The fresh gas and vapor circuits are independent, and pressure in the vapor circuit is regulated so that it equals that in the fresh gas circuit, whereas the flow rate in the vapor circuit is regulated proportionally with that in the fresh gas circuit. The 2 circuits are then interfaced through differential-pressure transducers, control electronics, and a pressure-regulating valve. The fresh gas flow rate, which is regulated by the operator, is directly related to the working pressure.

Effects.—To maintain the necessary anesthetic partial pressure at altitudes other than sea level, the operator must manually adjust the concentration control dial. The Tec 6 vaporizer is designed to be used with 100% oxygen as the carrier gas. Use of air or nitrous oxide as the carrier gas will result in output decreases.

Safety Features.—The anesthetic-specific filling system prevents overdoses and hypoxemia, and, by interlocking the vaporizer and the dispensing bottle, it prevents anesthetic spillage. If conditions occur that alter the normal operation of the vaporizer, the shut-off valve closes to prevent output and an alarm sounds.

▶ As the reader can see, this is a complex "high-tech" vaporizer. Subsequent to the publication of this article, this vaporizer was voluntarily recalled because of a small number of instances in which the vaporizer issued concentrations of desflurane that were considerably in excess of what was indicated on the dial. Nonetheless, despite these probably inevitable difficulties with a new high-tech device, this vaporizer does quite a remarkable job with an agent that is certainly different from earlier volatile anesthetics.—J.H. Tinker, M.D.

Laryngeal Mask Airway Cuff Pressure and Position During Anaesthesia Lasting One to Two Hours

Brimacombe J, Berry A (Cairns Base Hosp, Australia; Royal Berkshire Hosp, England)
Can J Anaesth 41:589–593, 1994   101-95-2–9

Introduction.—The cuff of the laryngeal mask airway (LMA) is highly permeable to nitrous oxide. When this airway is used during nitrous oxide/oxygen anesthesia, the cuff pressure increases significantly. Previous studies have examined the extent of these changes and their effect on LMA position in short procedures only. The effects of 1 or 2 hours of nitrous oxide/oxygen anesthesia on cuff pressure, LMA position, and pharyngeal morbidity were assessed.

Methods and Findings.—Twenty-four men received spontaneous ventilation anesthesia with 66% nitrous oxide in oxygen and isoflurane. After a no. 4 LMA was inserted and inflated with 30 mL of air, the mean cuff pressures increased immediately, from 107 to 145 mm Hg. This was followed by a slower increase for 90 minutes to a peak of 215 mm Hg. The nitrous oxide concentration correlated significantly with the final cuff volume. In no case did the LMA cuff become displaced. A mild sore throat was reported by 3 of 19 patients at follow-up.

Conclusion.—The increase in the LMA cuff pressure during nitrous oxide/oxygen anesthesia appears to be self-limiting for a 1- to 2-hour period. No LMA displacement occurs during procedures of this length. Thus, monitoring and limitation of cuff pressure appear to be unnecessary during LMA anesthesia.

▶ I included this article to remind readers of the increasing use of the LMA, a device that will, as the years go by, come under increasing scrutiny as complications occur. One of these complications may be that nitrous oxide can increase its cuff volume in a fashion similar to what occurs in endotracheal tube cuffs. Although the authors believe this is not a problem, I would argue that as the use of this device increases, we will understand more and more about its limitations.—J.H. Tinker, M.D.

3 Complications Related to Anesthesia

Seizures Associated With Propofol Anesthesia
Mäkelä JP, Iivanainen M, Pieninkeroinen IP, Waltimo O, Lahdensuu M (Univ of Helsinki; Jorvi Hosp, Espoo, Finland)
Epilepsia 34:832–835, 1993

101-95-3-1

Background.—The short-acting anesthetic agent propofol is rapidly metabolized, so psychomotor performance is quickly restored for a rapid recovery of the surgical patient. Propofol is used to induce and maintain anesthesia as well as sedation of patients in the ICU. Few side effects, beyond hypotension and dose-dependent breathing depression, have been reported. Convulsions were neither caused nor prevented in animals, but human data are lacking. Five cases of seizures associated with propofol were reported.

Case 1.—Woman, 23, an active athlete with a history of seizures controlled by valproate, had previously undergone orthopedic surgery twice with no seizures. Anesthesia for knee arthroscopy was introduced with 150 mg of propofol. Twenty minutes after surgery, she had systemic clonic seizures followed by 2 more seizures within the next 2 hours. Myoclonic jerks occurred 3 hours after anesthesia. Despite diazepam infusion, 1-minute seizures occurred every 5–10 minutes. An ictal electroencephalogram showed epileptic activity. Phenytoin, valproate, and hydrocortisone were administered. The patient was clumsy and weak on the left side. Her signs and symptoms subsided during the 21-day hospital stay.

Case 2.—Woman, 29, was examined because of infertility. A previous laparoscopy had been uneventful. During a subsequent laparoscopy, with anesthesia induced using 130 mg of propofol, a 20-second tonic-clonic seizure of the left side of the trunk occurred. Neurologic examination showed transient, slight left-sided tendon jerks. The patient had an unremarkable recovery.

Case 3.—Woman, 35, had an abortion. Anesthesia was induced with 100-mg and 50-mg IV injections of propofol. Both injections were followed by brief clonic seizures. Her recovery was normal.

Case 4.—Woman, 49, underwent uterine dilation and curettage for metrorrhagia. After premedication, anesthesia was induced with 140 mg of propofol followed by a 20-mg dose. Low-frequency clonic seizures followed the first injection; the second caused no reactions.

Case 5.—Woman, 20, underwent uterine dilation and curettage for an unwanted pregnancy. Anesthesia was started with 150 mg of propofol. Her recovery was normal. A repeat procedure was performed 2 days later because of residual bleeding; this time 120 mg of propofol was used. After injection, slight limb movement and tension of the trunk and jaw were noted. Muscular tension and twitches occurred over the 1.5-hour recovery period. On awakening, the patient's strength was reduced, her speech was disturbed, and she learned she had bitten her tongue. Right gluteal pain and right finger paresthesias were noted the next day. Five days later, physical and neurologic examinations were normal.

Conclusion.—Propofol was administered in combination with other drugs, so no direct relationship to seizures can be demonstrated. Case 1 had an epileptic seizure, cases 2 and 3 also probably had epileptic seizures, whereas cases 4 and 5 might have been dystonic. However, case 1 had undergone previous surgery without seizures, and in 3 other patients, the responses occurred on infusion, suggesting a role for propofol in the convulsions. Because all cases were women, gender differences cannot be ruled out. Thus, propofol should be avoided in patients with epilepsy.

▶ A fairly common side effect of IV anesthesia is the occurrence of excitatory phenomena (e.g., tremor, hypertonus, spontaneous involuntary movement) that can easily be confused with tonic-clonic seizures. However, in last year's YEAR BOOK (p 82), Dr. Stoelting commented on an article that described delayed seizures after sedation with propofol and suggested that a preexisting seizure disorder probably might be a reason to consider the risk-benefits of this drug (1). It is difficult to conduct prospective studies to evaluate whether propofol causes seizures in patients with preexisting seizure disorders, and I think we must be content with making up our own minds on this issue.—M. Wood, M.D.

Reference

1. Finley GA, et al: *Can J Anaesth* 40:863, 1993.

A Clinical Prediction Rule for Delirium After Elective Noncardiac Surgery
Marcantonio ER, Goldman L, Mangione CM, Ludwig LE, Muraca B, Haslauer CM, Donaldson MC, Whittemore AD, Sugarbaker DJ, Poss R, Haas S, Cook EF, Orav EJ, Lee TH (Brigham and Women's Hosp, Boston; Harvard Med School, Boston)
JAMA 271:134–139, 1994   101-95-3–2

Introduction.—Postoperative delirium carries increased mortality and complication rates, poor functional recovery, and an increased length of stay. There is no valid rule for the clinical prediction of delirium in a surgical population. An attempt was made to develop such a rule that used clinical data that were available preoperatively.

Methods.—The prospective cohort study included 1,341 patients who were admitted for major elective general, orthopedic, or gynecologic surgery within a 17-month period. Preoperative assessment included a medical history, physical examination, laboratory testing, and physical and cognitive function tests, including the Specific Activity Scale and the Telephone Interview for Cognitive Status. The Confusion Assessment Method or data from the medical record or nursing intensity index was used to make the diagnosis of postoperative delirium.

Results.—Nine percent of patients had postoperative delirium. Factors that were independently associated with this complication included age 70 years or older; self-reported alcohol abuse; poor cognitive status; poor functional status; marked preoperative abnormalities in serum sodium, potassium, or glucose level; noncardiac thoracic surgery; and aortic aneurysm surgery. These factors were used to develop a simple predictive rule, which was tested in an independent population. Using this rule, rates of postoperative delirium were classified as low, 2%; medium, 8% to 13%; or high, 50%. The development of postoperative delirium was associated with increased rates of major complications, longer lengths of stay, and higher rates of discharge to long-term care or rehabilitation facilities.

Conclusion.—This predictive rule can assess a patient's risk of postoperative delirium using data that are available preoperatively. For patients at high risk, interventions may be able to reduce the risk of postoperative delirium and thereby improve the overall surgical outcome.

▶ According to the "Letters to the Editor," this classic article has anesthesia input, even though none of the authors are anesthesiologists. The article reports that if you are age 70 or older, have self-reported alcohol abuse, poor cognitive status, poor functional status, or markedly abnormal preoperative sodium potassium or glucose level and are undergoing major thoracic or aortic surgery, you have a high degree of likelihood of postoperative delirium. If any 3 of these conditions are present, or if you are having aortic aneurysm surgery and have 1 of these conditions, you have a 50% chance of delirium developing. I find this rate astonishing, because virtually all our current aortic aneurysm patients are older than age 70. Therefore, there would be a 50% chance of delirium, and that is not what happens in our practice. Maybe the article isn't as interesting as the subsequent "Letters to the Editor."—M.F. Roizen, M.D.

Stroke Complicating Percutaneous Coronary Revascularization

Brown DL, Topol EJ (Cleveland Clinic Found, Ohio)
Am J Cardiol 72:1207–1209, 1993   101-95-3–3

Background.—The indications and devices for percutaneous coronary revascularization have increased. Most earlier reports of complications have focused on untoward events that occurred after standard balloon angioplasty of the instrumented vessel, especially abrupt closure. Few have looked at stroke as a complication of angioplasty. The incidence, clinical characteristics, and outcome of stroke among patients who are undergoing various percutaneous revascularization procedures were reported.

Patients.—Within an 18-month period at a single institution, 2,679 percutaneous revascularization procedures were performed. Of these, 9 patients had a new neurologic deficit that persisted for more than 24 hours after the intervention. Those who had an intervening procedure that appeared to be responsible for the stroke were excluded. Therefore, the overall incidence of stroke was .3%. Age, sex, left ventricular function, and the presence of hypertension, diabetes, or hypercholesterolemia did not appear to affect the development of stroke. Two thirds of the patients with stroke had previous bypass surgery compared with about one fourth of the controls. The incidence of stroke was .2% in patients who received thrombolytic therapy vs. .3% in those who did not receive such therapy. Two of the 4 patients with stroke who received thrombolytic therapy and all 5 patients with stroke who did not receive thrombolytic therapy had ischemic strokes. In 6 of 9 patients, the symptoms began within 24 hours of leaving the laboratory.

Outcomes.—Four of the 9 patients with stroke died in the hospital; 7% of procedure-related deaths in the overall sample were caused by stroke. Of the 5 surviving patients, 4 were left with severe neurologic impairments that required transfer to a rehabilitation facility. Only 1 patient, who had a mild residual hemiparesis, was discharged home.

Conclusion.—The incidence of stroke among patients who are undergoing percutaneous coronary interventions appears to be increased, possibly because of the shift toward older patients with more extensive disease. Previous bypass surgery and treatment with thrombolytic agents appear to predispose patients to stroke. However, percutaneous revascularization appears to be associated with lower overall cerebrovascular mortality than surgical revascularization.

▶ It seems that stroke complicating percutaneous angioplasty of coronary arteries occurred in at least .3% of the patients at the Cleveland Clinic. However, this was detected only if the patient had a severe outcome such as death, as 4 of the 9 with strokes did; the need for referral to a rehabilitation facility, as another 4 of the 9 did; or significant hemiparesis. How many of these patients had more subtle neurologic deficits is not clear from this article, and it is not evident how routinely neurologic problems were sought postoperatively.

As an old clinician once said, if you don't look for something, you won't find it, and it isn't clear how well they looked for neurologic complications. Nevertheless, if those patients who had neurologic complications after being referred for coronary artery bypass are included, the rate doubles to approximately .6%. Furthermore, in most of these cases, the stroke was embolic as might be thought in relation to things that were dislodged from the aorta. Although this incidence is more than fivefold greater than that reported in the initial 1,500 angioplasties that were documented at the National Heart, Lung, and Blood Institute, it would be expected, because angioplasties are now being done in sicker patients with disease in more than 1 vessel, in older patients, and in those with worse left ventricular function and more unstable symptoms and hemodynamics. I would guess that if one looked carefully for neurologic symptoms and sequelae with routine neurologic evaluation by trained individuals immediately before and after angioplasty, the complication rate would not only be significantly higher, but it might be higher in those patients for the next 6 months if they did not undergo the angioplasty. The greater risk of angioplasty is not to be minimized, but it must be compared with the alternatives of no therapy or coronary artery bypass grafting.

Although the data provided are informative, they do not help us answer the question of whether patients are better off with this therapy than with alternative therapies.—M.F. Roizen, M.D.

Traumatic Aneurysm of the Internal Jugular Vein Causing Vagal Nerve Palsy: A Rare Complication of Percutaneous Catheterization
Nakayama M, Fujita S, Kawamata M, Namiki A, Mayumi T (Sapporo Med Univ, Japan; Hokkaido Univ, Sapporo, Japan)
Anesth Analg 78:598–600, 1994   101-95-3–4

Purpose.—Percutaneous catheterization of the internal jugular vein (IJV) is commonly used for central venous catheter placement. Reported complications of this technique include hematoma, pneumothorax, aortic dissection, hemothorax, and air embolization. A case of traumatic aneurysm of the IJV that caused vagal nerve palsy after percutaneous catheterization was reported.

Case Report.—Man, 73, with grade 3 aortic insufficiency was admitted for elective aortic valve replacement. He underwent placement of a 16-gauge double-lumen central venous catheter through the right IJV under general anesthesia. This catheter was removed on the fifth postoperative day; the patient was discharged without complications 1 month after surgery. A few days later, he complained of hoarseness with a swelling on the right side of his neck. The cystic mass measured 5 × 4 cm, with no pulsation or audible bruit. The right vocal cord was completely palsied. Ultrasound showed an aneurysm with turbulent flow located between the right IJV and the common carotid artery. Venography of the IJV could not demonstrate the feeding vessels. At surgical exploration 3 days later, the aneurysm was filled with thrombus and tightly adhered to the IJV, with no feeding vessels. A definite diagnosis of venous aneurysm of the IJV was made surgically; the hoarseness resulted from aneurysmal compression of the vagal nerve. The clot of the aneurysm was removed, and the entry from the IJV was closed. The hoarseness resolved within 1 week after the operation.

Discussion.—Venous catheterization can lead to traumatic aneurysm, and aneurysm of the IJV may result in vagal nerve palsy. Several weeks may pass between catheterization and symptoms. Ultrasound is the initial diagnostic approach to suspected venous aneurysm; early surgical excision should be performed to prevent pulmonary embolism and rupture.

▶ In our quality assurance studies of postoperative complications, hoarseness occurs 2–4 times per 10,000 cases postoperatively. Most of these cases that persist for 10 days go away over a period of months, but about 1 per 10,000 persists and is associated with decreased vocal cord function.

I can't remember ever looking for the incidence of jugular venous catheterization in these cases or whether an IJV aneurysm had recently occurred, as happened with these patients. Thus, this article is important because it indicates a potentially curable entity. In this case, the aneurysm could at least be seen as a mass on the side of the neck, but I imagine that such a mass would not be present in many cases.—M.F. Roizen, M.D.

Valve Injury: A New Complication of Internal Jugular Vein Cannulation
Imai M, Hanaoka Y, Kemmotsu O (Hokkaido Univ, Sapporo, Japan)
Anesth Analg 78:1041–1046, 1994   101-95-3–5

Introduction.—The valve of the internal jugular vein (IJV), which is located somewhere near the point of the junction of the IJV with the subclavian vein, is the only valve between the brain and the heart. As such, it plays a key role in the control of transmission of increases in intrapleural pressure to the brain during coughing or positive-pressure ventilation. Any damage to the IJV valve would allow increases in intrapleural pressure to be conveyed directly to the brain. The anatomical appearance and competency of IJV valves were evaluated in a cadaver and surgical study.

Methods.—The appearance of the IJV valves was observed after dissection of the vessel in 20 cadavers. The movements of the IJV valves were assessed in 2 adult patients using an intravascular fiberoptic endoscope, pulsed Doppler ultrasound, and venography. In addition, the competence of the IJV valve was examined using transvalvular pressure gradients in 10 adult surgical patients.

Findings.—Of 19 valves that were available for assessment in the cadaver specimens, all were located directly above the termination of the IJV in the inferior valve. The valves were usually situated bilaterally. Sixteen of the cadaver valves were bicuspid and semiluminar. The other 3 specimens showed valves with 3 leaflets or 2 valves placed vertically or side by side. Both fiberscopy and real-time ultrasound demonstrated the opening and closing of the valves. Of the 10 surgical patients, 8 had normal central venous pressure and competent IJV valves; the mean cough-induced transvalvular pressure gradient in this group was 45 mm Hg. In a fresh cadaver experiment, 4 valves from 2 cadavers remained competent at a mean pressure of 75 mm Hg. After a hole was made with a 14-gauge needle, these valves became incompetent at a mean pressure of 6 mm Hg.

Conclusion.—The IJV valve, which is situated .5 to 2 cm above the union of the subclavian vein and the IJV and is usually bicuspid, plays an important role in preventing retrograde blood flow to the brain. Very little attention is paid to the presence of this valve during internal jugular venipuncture, but puncture injury to the valve can result in incomplete valve closure, depending on the location of the puncture. Such injuries may be preventable by performing venipuncture at the level of the cricoid ring or higher.

▶ This interesting article gave me information on a new subject. However, how important these IJVs are to preserving brain function is unclear to me at this time. Obviously, if we are going to do retrograde perfusion of the brain during aortic artery reconstructive surgery, these valves must be bypassed, but whether retrograde brain perfusion is a benefit or a detriment in daily life is not clear.—M.F. Roizen, M.D.

Complications of Labor Analgesia: Epidural Versus Combined Spinal Epidural Techniques

Norris MC, Grieco WM, Borkowski M, Leighton BL, Arkoosh VA, Huffnagle HJ, Huffnagle S (Thomas Jefferson Univ, Philadelphia)
Anesth Analg 79:529–537, 1994   101-95-3–6

Background.—Both epidural and combined spinal epidural (CSE) analgesia can alleviate pain during labor. Few studies have compared the risks and complications of these 2 methods.

Methods and Findings.—The incidence and severity of complications associated with anesthetic were recorded in 1,022 laboring parturients. Ninety-eight women chose parenteral or no analgesia, 388 opted for epidural, and 536 chose CSE. Women who received CSE analgesia were usually given an intrathecal injection of sufentanil, 10 μg, when the epidural catheter was inserted. As the intrathecal analgesia waned, the epidural catheters were dosed as needed. Compared with women who received epidural analgesia only, women who received CSE analgesia were more likely to experience itching, nausea, or vomiting. Women who requested only epidural analgesia were more likely to have an unintentional dural puncture. Hypotension occurred in less than 10% with either technique. The risk of headache was comparable with both anesthetics and did not differ in women who were not given neuraxial analgesia. An epidural blood patch was needed for moderate-to-severe postural headache in 6 patients; 4 of these women sustained a dural puncture with an 18-gauge Hustead epidural needle, and the other 2 had uncomplicated epidural and CSE analgesia.

Conclusion.—The incidence of minor complications associated with epidural and CSE analgesia is low. Hypotension occurs in about 10% of women who receive intrathecal opioid or epidural local anesthetic labor analgesia. Therefore, careful monitoring is needed during induction of either analgesic technique. Intentionally puncturing the dura with a small-gauge pencil-point needle during CSE analgesia induction does not increase the risk of postpartum headache.

▶ I am sold on the utility of the combined spinal-epidural analgesia technique for selected laboring women. (I used this technique to provide analgesia for my wife when she recently gave birth to our fifth child.) I find this technique especially useful in 3 patient populations: nulliparous women who request analgesia during early labor; parous women who request analgesia during advanced labor; and women in whom I want to provide a rapid onset of analgesia *without* a rapid onset of sympathectomy (e.g., severe pre-eclampsia, selected forms of cardiovascular disease).—D.H. Chestnut, M.D.

Nausea: The Most Important Factor Determining Length of Stay After Ambulatory Anaesthesia. A Comparative Study of Isoflurane and/or Propofol Techniques
Green G, Jonsson L (Östersund Hosp, Sweden)
Acta Anaesthesiol Scand 37:742–746, 1993   101-95-3-7

Background.—Both isoflurane and propofol are promising agents for use in outpatient anesthesia where there is a need for rapid recovery without side effects. Propofol has been proven to be superior in shorter-term anesthesia, but for longer procedures, the situation is unclear.

Objective.—Propofol and isoflurane were used as the chief anesthetic agents in 95 ambulatory patients who underwent laparoscopic or arthroscopic procedures lasting 30–60 minutes.

Methods.—Thirty-two patients received isoflurane in an end-tidal concentration of .7%. Thirty-one others received IV propofol, 10 mg/kg/hr, for the first 25 minutes, followed 10 minutes later by a dose of 8 mg/kg/hr for 10 minutes and then 6 mg/kg/hr for 5 minutes. Isoflurane was then administered for the rest of the anesthesia. Thirty-two patients received an infusion of propofol throughout the procedure. All patients also received a nitrous oxide and oxygen mixture, and IV meperidine was given if the pulse or blood pressure increased by more than 30%.

Results.—All patients had similar awakening times, but the time to extubation was shortest in patients who were given isoflurane only. Patients in this group tended to do less well in tests of psychomotor recovery than those who were given propofol or combined anesthesia. Postoperative pain was comparable in all groups. Patients who were given isoflurane only required more treatment for protracted nausea and/or vomiting than those in the other groups; 3 patients were hospitalized overnight for this reason. No patient reported having been aware, and nearly all the patients would be willing to have the same anesthesia again.

Conclusion.—Propofol appears to minimize the risk of prolonged nausea and vomiting in patients who have same-day surgery. Patients without nausea recover as rapidly as those who are given isoflurane.

▶ This is one of several articles that have been recently published that call into question the notion that the short-acting drugs will prove seminal in allowing the patients to go home sooner after ambulatory surgery. This article debunks that notion and indicates that nausea is the single most important impediment to early exit from an ambulatory surgery center. This article also adds to the growing collection of data that indicate propofol may indeed be a genuine antinauseant and not simply associated with less nausea.—J.H. Tinker, M.D.

Autoantibodies to Hepatic Microsomal Carboxylesterase in Halothane Hepatitis

Smith GCM, Kenna JG, Harrison DJ, Tew D, Wolf CR (Ninewells Hosp and Med School, Dundee, Scotland; St Mary's Hosp Med School, London; Univ of Edinburgh, Scotland; et al)
Lancet 342:963–964, 1993   101-95-3–8

Introduction.—Halothane hepatitis can be life-threatening, severe adverse reaction that may be caused by an immune process. The severe form can lead to massive hepatic necrosis and death, a rare complication that occurs in 1 in 10,000 cases. In previous rat studies, several of the trifluoroacetylated proteins implicated were purified from halothane-treated rats and characterized biochemically. One of the proteins corresponded to a carboxylesterase isozyme.

Patients and Methods.—Serum was obtained from 20 patients with halothane hepatitis (defined clinically as otherwise unexplained hepatitis within 28 days of halothane anesthesia) from 9 halothane-exposed controls and from 33 patients with liver disease caused by fulminant hepatic failure, autoimmune chronic active hepatitis, alcoholic liver disease, primary biliary cirrhosis, or jaundice resulting from the use of flucloxacillin. All the patients with halothane hepatitis had received halothane anesthesia between 1 and 8 times previously, and they ranged in age from 32 to 60 years. Antibodies to carboxylesterase were determined by enzyme-linked immunosorbent assay (ELISA).

Results.—Thirteen of the 20 patients in the halothane hepatitis group had liver failure and 12 died. In 17 of these patients (85%), autoantibodies to purified human liver microsomal carboxylesterase were detected. Autoantibodies were not detected in the 9 halothane-exposed controls and were found at low levels in only 2 patients with primary biliary cirrhosis. The test results in the other 31 patients with nonhalothane liver disease were negative. In immunohistochemical studies, the carboxylesterase was localized in the centrilobular region of the liver sections, which is consistent with the area affected by halothane hepatitis.

Conclusion.—In halothane hepatitis, the human hepatic microsomal carboxylesterase is a target antigen, and in liver damage, an immune response to this protein may be involved. A diagnosis of halothane hepatitis can be confirmed by testing for antibodies to trifluoroacetylated liver proteins; however these assays are technically demanding, whereas a carboxylesterase ELISA is a quick, simple, and sensitive test.

▶ Just about the time we are (perhaps) going to get sevoflurane and as a result (again perhaps) allow halothane to pass into history (at least in the United States), we are beginning to understand the mechanisms of halothane hepatotoxicity. This work will enable us to test future anesthetics quickly and to screen them for possible hepatotoxicity. I think this article reports extraordinary findings, because we are beginning to nail down this long-sought mechanism.—J.H. Tinker, M.D.

Absence of Agonist Effects of High-Dose Flumazenil on Ventilation and Psychometric Performance in Human Volunteers

Forster A, Crettenand G, Klopfenstein CE, Morel DR (Univ Hosp of Geneva)
Anesth Analg 77:980–984, 1993   101-95-3–9

Background.—Flumazenil, the first clinically available specific benzodiazepine antagonist, reverses both the sedative and respiratory depressant effects of benzodiazepines. Previous studies have suggested that flumazenil may be associated with inverse agonist effects, such as anxiety, or agonist activity, such as drowsiness or anticonvulsant properties. Whether a large dose of flumazenil causes respiratory depression or altered psychomotor performance was determined.

Methods.—Eight young male volunteers took part in 3 different study sessions. In the first, the men received a 1-mg dose of flumazenil per kg—which is 7–15 times the clinically recommended dose—by IV injection over 5 minutes followed by placebo. In the second session, the volunteers received the same dose of flumazenil followed by midazolam, .1 mg/kg, injected over 5 minutes. Finally, in the third session, the volunteers received placebo then midazolam in the same dose as in session 2.

Results.—Tidal volume decreased by 40% and minute ventilation and inspiratory flow by 25% during the placebo-midazolam session compared with baseline and with the other 2 study sessions. Psychometric performance was significantly altered as well. During the flumazenil-placebo and flumazenil-midazolam sessions, there were no significant changes in either respiratory or psychometric variables.

Conclusion.—Even at 10 times the recommended clinical dose, flumazenil appears to have no agonist effects on resting ventilation or psychomotor performance in healthy volunteers. As a result, flumazenil should not depress respiration when it is given for diagnostic and therapeutic purposes in patients with unknown intoxication or patients who are in comatose states that are unrelated to benzodiazepine ingestion. However, flumazenil could potentiate the ventilatory depressant effects of opiates or other centrally acting drugs.

The Effects of Large-Dose Flumazenil on Midazolam-Induced Ventilatory Depression
Flögel CM, Ward DS, Wada DR, Ritter JW (Univ of Calif, Los Angeles; Univ of Rochester, NY)
Anesth Analg 77:1207–1214, 1993   101-95-3-10

Introduction.—The ability of the benzodiazepine antagonist flumazenil to reverse midazolam-induced hypnosis and sedation has clearly been demonstrated. However, its ability to completely reverse the ventilatory depressant effects of midazolam is less clear. The dose-response characteristics and duration of flumazenil's effects on midazolam-induced ventilatory depression and hypnosis were assessed in a randomized, double-blind, placebo-controlled study.

Methods.—Thirty-two healthy, nonsmoking men received a computer controlled continuous infusion of midazolam to titrate and then maintain the predicted midazolam plasma concentration at which the men failed to respond to verbal commands. Ventilation and hypnosis were assessed at intervals before midazolam administration; before administration of flumazenil, 1, 3, or 10 mg; and at 5 to 180 minutes afterward. An isocapnic hyperoxia clamp at an end-tidal pressure of carbon dioxide ($PETCO_2$) of 46 mm Hg was used to measure ventilation ($\dot{V}_E46$) and tidal volume (V_T46). The hypercapnic ventilatory response (HCVR) slope and ventilation intercept at a $PETCO_2$ of 58 mm Hg ($\dot{V}_E58$) were measured by a pseudorebreathing technique.

Results.—The $\dot{V}_E46$, V_T46, $\dot{V}_E58$, and hypnosis scores were reduced by midazolam in all groups; only in the overall group was the HCVR slope significantly reduced. Within 5 minutes, all 3 doses of flumazenil reversed hypnosis and the reduction in $\dot{V}_E46$ and V_T46; reversal of the reduction in $\dot{V}_E58$ was less consistent. The effects of the 2 lower doses of flumazenil on $\dot{V}_E46$ and V_T46 paralleled their effects on hypnosis. At the higher dose, flumazenil $\dot{V}_E46$ and V_T46 decreased to placebo and midazolam and control values by 120 minutes, whereas reversal of sedation lasted for 154 minutes. The groups were similar in their midazolam plasma concentrations, which remained constant throughout the study. At the highest dose of flumazenil, plasma concentrations remained elevated even after hypnosis and ventilatory depression had returned, possibly indicating the development of acute tolerance to flumazenil.

Conclusion.—At an IV dose of 1 mg, flumazenil fully reversed midazolam-induced hypnosis and ventilatory depression. The full acute effects were achieved at larger doses with longer durations, although the results of high doses were consistent with the development of acute tolerance. At a flumazenil dose of 10 mg, the results indicated discordance between the duration of hypnosis and the reversal of ventilatory depression.

▶ In very high doses, flumazenil has weak benzodiazepine-like agonist activity in animals, and there has always been concern that if flumazenil was given to overdose patients (e.g., in coma, intoxicated), it might potentiate the effects of hypnotic drugs and produce respiratory depression as well as fail to produce prolonged reversal. These 2 articles (Abstracts 101-95-3–9 and 101-95-3–10) address the use of high-dose flumazenil. I do not recommend the use of flumazenil to hasten discharge from the recovery room.—M. Wood, M.D.

A Potentially Hazardous Interaction Between Erythromycin and Midazolam
Olkkola KT, Aranko K, Luurila H, Hiller A, Saarnivaara L, Himberg J-J, Neuvonen PJ (Univ of Helsinki; Univ of Turku, Finland)
Clin Pharmacol Ther 53:298–305, 1993   101-95-3–11

Background.—Midazolam, a short-acting hypnotic, is often used to induce anesthesia. It has extensive first-pass metabolism, and its oral bioavailability is less than 50%. Erythromycin inhibits the metabolism of midazolam in vitro. Recently, a child who received both oral midazolam and IV erythromycin became deeply unconscious and was found to have a very high plasma midazolam level.

Study Design.—Twelve persons, 18–29 years of age, received either 500 mg of erythromycin base or a placebo 3 times a day by mouth for 1 week in a randomized, double-blind, crossover design. On day 6, they ingested 15 mg of midazolam 2 hours after receiving erythromycin. After 4 months, 6 of the same individuals again received erythromycin or placebo for a week, and on day 6 they were given IV midazolam, .05 mg/kg.

Results.—Plasma midazolam levels after oral dosing were much higher in patients given erythromycin than in placebo recipients (Fig 3–1). Erythromycin prolonged the elimination half-life of midazolam from 2.4 to 5.7 hours. Individuals who were given erythromycin were profoundly sedated, as evidenced by psychomotor test findings and measurements

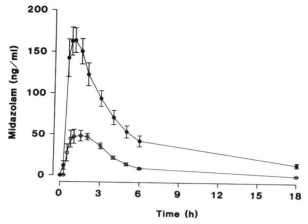

Fig 3–1.—Concentrations (mean ± standard error of the mean) of midazolam in plasma after an oral dose of 15 mg after pretreatment with oral erythromycin (500 mg 3 times a day) or placebo for 1 week to 12 healthy volunteers. *Open circles* are concentrations of midazolam after placebo; *filled circles* are concentrations of midazolam after erythromycin. (Courtesy of Olkkola KT, Aranko K, Luurila H, et al: *Clin Pharmacol Ther* 53:298–305, 1993.)

of peak saccadic velocity. At the time midazolam was given, the plasma erythromycin level was 3 mg/L. Erythromycin reduced the plasma clearance of intravenously injected midazolam by 54%. Psychomotor test performance was not markedly affected, but saccadic eye movements were unrecordable for 2 hours after midazolam injection. The mean plasma erythromycin level at the time of midazolam injection was 1.2 mg/L.

Implications.—Midazolam is more than a short-term hypnotic agent in patients who are receiving erythromycin; their ability to drive the next morning may be compromised. Either erythromycin should be avoided in patients who are to receive midazolam or the dose of midazolam should be reduced by 50% to 75%.

▶ Many drugs are metabolized by cytochrome P450 enzymes in the liver. The P450 superfamily comprises families and subfamilies; each P450 enzyme is encoded by a separate gene. The cytochrome P450 3A subfamily metabolizes many drugs, including alfentanil, nifedipine, erythromycin, and midazolam. If 2 drugs that are metabolized by CYP3A are given together, they will both compete for the enzyme. This can lead to serious drug interactions such as were described in this report. Unconsciousness after midazolam and erythromycin has been reported (1). Chronic administration of erythromycin decreases alfentanil clearance (2), so that recovery from alfentanil might be prolonged (3, 4).—M. Wood, M.D.

References

1. Hiller A, et al: *Br J Anaesth* 65:826, 1990.
2. Bartkowski RR, et al: *Clin Pharmacol Ther* 46:99, 1989.

3. Bartkowski RR, McDonnell TE: *Anesthesiology* 73:566, 1990.
4. Yate PM, et al: *Br J Anaesth* 58:1091, 1986.

Latex Allergy: An Unfamiliar Cause of Intra-Operative Cardiovascular Collapse

Hodgson CA, Andersen BD (Oregon Health Sciences Univ, Portland)
Anaesthesia 49:507–508, 1994   101-95-3–12

Introduction.—Latex allergy is increasingly reported as a cause of severe intraoperative anaphylaxis. It has been more commonly reported in the United States than in the United Kingdom. A case of severe latex allergy leading to intraoperative circulatory collapse was described.

Case Report.—Girl, 8 years, with cerebral palsy was undergoing adductor tendon release and femoral osteotomy. The patient was quadriplegic and blind and received fluids through a gastrostomy tube. She had no history of allergy to rubber products or of repeated catheterization. Forty minutes after induction of anesthesia and paralysis, the patient demonstrated sudden and profound cardiorespiratory collapse. The surgery was halted; total obstruction of the tracheal tube was initially suspected, but it proved to be patent. Severe anaphylaxis was considered, even though it had been a long time since induction and no recent drug boluses had been given. The child received resuscitative procedures for 1 hour, including administration of 14.5 mL of adrenaline 1:10,000. The patient's condition stabilized within 12 hours in the ICU. She had a very strongly positive IgE radioallergosorbent test for latex allergy. The femoral osteotomy was performed uneventfully 2 weeks later. At this surgery, neoprene surgical gloves were used, all latex materials were removed from the anesthetic equipment, and latex contact was strictly avoided during drug preparation and administration.

Discussion.—Patients who are at high risk should be asked specifically about allergies to rubber products. Latex anaphylaxis can be distinguished from that caused by anesthetic agents, because it usually appears at least 20 minutes after induction. Patients with demonstrated latex allergy must be subsequently managed by strict avoidance of latex exposure.

▶ Worrisome allergies to latex are cropping up all over the place these days. When you need to eliminate latex, it is amazing how much there is to which patients can theoretically be exposed. When our nursing colleagues first began to call our attention to this problem, I tended to dismiss its importance. However, cases like this should make anesthesiologists listen. For example, IV injection ports are usually stoppered with latex. Does the use of IVs with them constitute exposure to latex in a patient with a known latex allergy? I wonder whether it is even possible to perform a 100% latex-free anesthetic and surgical procedure.—J.H. Tinker, M.D.

Latex Allergy in Spina Bifida Patients: Prevalence and Surgical Implications

Tosi LL, Slater JE, Shaer C, Mostello LA (Children's Natl Med Ctr, Washington, DC)

J Pediatr Orthop 13:709–712, 1993   101-95-3–13

Background.—A high prevalence of latex sensitivity has been reported in patients with spina bifida. The prevalence of this sensitivity in a pediatric population was documented.

Methods and Findings.—Ninety-three consecutive children with spina bifida were interviewed between 1989 and mid-1992. All were undergoing surgery. In addition to the prevalence of latex sensitivity, predictors of anaphylactic reaction and the risk of type I hypersensitivity reaction perioperatively were determined. Ten percent of the children were clinically allergic. Radioallergosorbent testing (RAST) had a sensitivity of 89%. In cases of known latex allergy, children were premedicated and latex exposure was rigorously avoided. There were no intraoperative anaphylatic reactions. One patient, who had a history of latex sensitivity but negative RAST results, had a postoperative reaction.

Conclusion.—Surgery can be performed safely in children with latex allergy. Children with spina bifida should be screened carefully by history and, when available, RAST. During surgery, latex exposure should be rigorously avoided. Premedication, which ideally should begin at home the night before surgery and continue for 12 hours after surgery, may ameliorate the reponses of patients who have positive histories or RAST results.

▶ Latex (rubber) allergy or anaphylaxis has become an important problem for operating room staff in the 1990s (1). Antigen, in this case latex, that is capable of stimulating IgE antibody production causes IgE-mediated anaphylaxis after initial sensitization and subsequent reexposure. Contact dermatitis to rubber products such as gloves has been recognized for many years. Certain groups are more at risk for anaphylaxis; for example, health care workers and patients who have frequent exposure to latex (e.g., pediatric patients with meningomyelocele and spina bifida who require frequent urinary catheterization).

If previous sensitization to latex has occurred, it would then appear prudent to avoid latex products. Many operating rooms now have a cart of latex-free products available. However, I believe that a number of questions now require answers. To whom should stringent latex avoidance precautions be directed? Should all patients be routinely questioned about a history of latex allergy? Who should undergo skin testing or RAST and when?

These authors suggest that all spina bifida children should be protected from sensitization by avoiding the use of latex whenever possible. In addition, all their patients are monitored for clinical evidence of latex allergy and a conversion in their RAST status. They follow rigorous latex avoidance precautions for all clinically latex-allergic individuals. However, they do not believe that children with latex allergy should be denied surgery. Other workers may not agree with all these recommendations.

Are health care workers who work in the operating room and wear gloves on a daily basis at increased risk of anaphylaxis when they undergo surgery? Although it is well recognized that contact dermatitis secondary to latex allergy can occur, the clinical significance of serious latex anaphylaxis requires careful scientific evaluation.—M. Wood, M.D.

Reference

1. Holzman RS: *Anesth Analg* 76:635, 1993.

Call Mosby Document Express at **1 (800) 55-MOSBY** to obtain copies of the original source documents of articles featured or referenced in the YEAR BOOK series.

---

4 Physiology and Pathophysiology Related to Anesthesia

Blood Volume Redistribution During Cross-Clamping of the Descending Aorta
Gelman S, Khazaeli MB, Orr R, Henderson T (Harvard Med School, Boston; The Univ of Alabama at Birmingham)
Anesth Analg 78:219–224, 1994   101-95-4-1

Introduction.—Occlusion of the descending aorta has been hypothesized to be associated with changes in the blood flow, which cause relative hypervolemia in organs and tissues proximal to the site of occlusion. This hypothesis was tested by studying blood flow in various target organs and tissues with aortic occlusion at 2 different levels in dogs.

Methods.—The aorta was randomly cross-clamped just above the renal arteries and at the level of the diaphragm for 30 minutes in 6 anesthetized, splenectomized dogs; the aorta was not occluded in 3 control dogs. Whole body scintigraphic recordings were made after IV injection of albumin labeled with technetium-99m. Activity was counted in the brain, left and right ventricles, left and right lungs, left and right deltoid muscles, liver, and intestines at baseline, in the first and last 10 minutes of the occlusion periods, and between and after the occlusion periods.

Results.—In the control dogs, activity in all measured regions decreased in a linear fashion to 75% of the baseline values at the final observation period. No significant changes in blood volume occurred in any of the measured regions when the aorta was occluded suprarenally. Blood volume increased by 15% to 25% in deltoid muscles, 8% to 15% in the lungs, 18% to 30% in the brain, and 17% to 38% in the heart when the aorta was occluded at the level of the diaphragm. All blood volumes returned to normal when the aorta was unclamped.

Discussion.—The hypothesized association between aortic occlusion and relative hypervolemia in the organs and tissues proximal to the occlusion was supported. These changes may cause increased preload and blood flow above the occlusion, increasing the cardiac burden and interfering with all microcirculatory gas exchange.

▶ I included this article because I wanted to jerk the authors' chains a bit. They hypothesized that if the aorta is clamped above the renals, blood flow will be redistributed above the diaphragm. Does that really surprise anyone? I can't imagine why anyone would have thought otherwise! I was hoping this article would address (but it did not) why we get so much renal failure after *infra*renal cross-clamping. One would think that when the aorta is clamped below the renals, renal blood flow would be massively enhanced. If this does not happen, renal failure can occur instead. One theory suggests there is so much renal blood flow that perivascular edema and subsequent diminished glomerular filtration and/or renal blood flow occur. Anyway I don't think this article tells us much we didn't already know or strongly suspect. It sure has plenty of data though.—J.H. Tinker, M.D.

Sodium-Calcium Exchange in Neonatal Myocardium: Reversible Inhibition by Halothane

Baum VC, Wetzel GT (Univ of California, Los Angeles)
Anesth Analg 78:1105–1109, 1994   101-95-4–2

Background.—The myocardium of neonates is more sensitive to depression by volatile anesthetics than that of adults. It appears that the neonatal myocardium relies on calcium entry across the sarcolemma through a reversible sodium-calcium exchange channel to support contraction rather than entry from sarcoplasmic reticular stores. The effect of halothane on sodium-calcium exchange was determined to explore a possible mechanism for enhanced neonatal myocardial sensitivity to the anesthetic.

Methods.—The sodium-calcium exchange current was determined on isolated neonatal rabbit myocardial cells using the whole cell voltage clamp before and after exposure to culture medium that was equilibrated with air containing 1.5% or 3% halothane.

Results.—The sodium-calcium current was reduced by 49% and 66% after exposure of cells to 1.5% and 3% halothane, respectively; however, the difference between the 1.5% and 3% treatment did not reach statistical significance. The effect was reversed when the cells were washed with halothane-free medium.

Conclusion.—Halothane, at clinically realistic concentrations, can reversibly inhibit sodium-calcium exchange in neonatal myocardial cells. Because of neonatal myocardial reliance on transsarcolemmal calcium exchange, this halothane exposure may result in a more marked inhibition of contractility in the neonatal than the adult myocardium.

▶ Now that halothane is nearly "extinct" at least in the United States, we are finally beginning in a "molecular" way to understand the mechanisms of its long-known myocardial depression. Whether these mechanisms apply to other anesthetics is less clear.—J.H. Tinker, M.D.

The Influence of Anesthesia on Myocardial Oxygen Utilization Efficiency in Patients Undergoing Coronary Bypass Surgery
Hoeft A, Sonntag H, Stephan H, Kettler D (Univ of Göttingen, Germany)
Anesth Analg 78:857–866, 1994   101-95-4-3

Introduction.—Because patients with coronary artery disease have limited oxygen delivery to the heart, it is important to maintain minimum myocardial oxygen consumption and efficient myocardial oxygen use. It would be expected that anesthesia and surgical stimulation would have opposing effects on myocardial efficiency. The influence of various anesthetic protocols on myocardial oxygen use during coronary bypass surgery was investigated in a retrospective study.

Methods.—Measurements of myocardial blood flow, myocardial oxygen uptake, and standard hemodynamics were reviewed for 65 patients with an ejection fraction of greater than 50% and no valvular disease who underwent coronary bypass surgery. The data sets were obtained before and after the induction of anesthesia and during sternotomy and sternal spread. Eight patient groups were defined by anesthetic protocol: halothane nitrous oxide, enflurane nitrous oxide, morphine, high-dose fentanyl, fentanyl midazolam, high-dose sufentanil, sufentanil nitrous oxide, and propofol.

Results.—All groups experienced a decrease in blood pressure during the induction of anesthesia, which was most pronounced in the enflurane group and least pronounced in the high-dose narcotics groups. The stroke volume index and the cardiac index were also decreased with the induction of anesthesia in all groups, but the systemic vascular resistance was unchanged. The decreases in stroke volume index and blood pressure resulted in a decrease in both external cardiac work and myocardial oxygen consumption. However, the external cardiac work decreased proportionally more than myocardial oxygen uptake, so the efficiency of myocardial oxygen use was decreased by the induction of anesthesia in all groups. During sternotomy and sternal spread, blood presssure and myocardial oxygen consumption increased with high-dose morphine, fentanyl, and sufentanil anesthesia, whereas blood pressure and myocardial oxygen consumption decreased with halothane and enflurane anesthesia. Nevertheless, the efficiency of myocardial oxygen use was similarly decreased in all groups compared with awake values.

Discussion.—The efficiency of myocardial oxygen use decreased uniformly after induction of anesthesia and decreased again during sternotomy or sternal spread using all anesthetic protocols. Therefore, particular anesthetic techniques do not influence the efficiency of myocardial

MYOCARDIAL ENERGY TRANSFORMATION

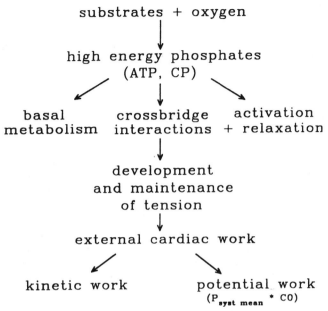

Fig 4–1.—Myocardial energy transformation. Several steps of energy transformation are involved in myocardial metabolism. First, the energy contained in substrates is converted to high-energy phosphates by oxidative metabolism. In the active heart, this energy is used for basal metabolism, cross-bridge interactions, and electrophysiologic processes, i.e., ion fluxes for activation and relaxation of the contractile system. Only the energy that is converted to crossbridge interactions will contribute to mechanical energy in the form of myocardial wall tension. In terms of myocardial efficiency, the other forms of energy are lost because they do not contribute to external cardiac work. External cardiac work results from conversion of wall tension into muscle shortening and ejection of the stroke volume. Total external work can be divided into kinetic work, which results from the acceleration of the stroke volume, and into potential work, which is equivalent to pressure-volume work. The kinetic work is usually very small and can be neglected. Assuming a constant relation between oxidative fat and carbohydrate metabolism, energy intake can be determined from oxygen uptake. Thus, a reasonable physiologic definition of myocardial efficiency is the ratio of myocardial oxygen consumption to external pressure volume work. *Abbreviations:* ATP, adenosine triphosphate; CP, creatine phosphate; CO, cardiac output. (Courtesy of Hoeft A, Sonntag H, Stephan H, et al: *Anesth Analg* 78:857–866,1994.)

oxygen use, which is defined by a multistep energy transformation mechanism (Fig 4–1).

▶ Hydraulic work, as used in cardiac physiology, is really power, namely, pressure × flow; this is the business end of the pump. It has always seemed logical to try to understand the oxygen costs, i.e., the efficiency of the delivery of that power (work).

I have done animal experiments in this regard and agree with Sonntag and colleagues that when defined this way, the "efficiency" of the "human engine" is low. In animals, I have come up with numbers ranging from 12% to 20%, and Sonntag and colleagues report similarly low numbers in this study. They assume that values are "depressed" in these patients who are undergoing major cardiac surgery. I wonder whether they are really depressed. It is entirely possible that this is relatively normal "efficiency," at least when it is measured this way. That would make the human cardiac "engine" even more amazing, lasting 70 or 80 years and operating at only 20% efficiency!

I applaud the authors' approach and hope that more studies using this measure will emerge, because I think it may help us develop drugs that can more objectively improve cardiac condition.—J.H. Tinker, M.D.

The Electrophysiologic Effects of Volatile Anesthetics and Sufentanil on the Normal Atrioventricular Conduction System and Accessory Pathways in Wolff-Parkinson-White Syndrome

Sharpe MD, Dobkowski WB, Murkin JM, Klein G, Guiraudon G, Yee R (Univ of Western Ontario, London, Canada)
Anesthesiology 80:63–70, 1994   101-95-4-4

Background.—Although nonsurgical catheter techniques are now available for the ablation of accessory pathways in patients with Wolff-Parkinson-White (WPW) syndrome, some of these patients, particularly children, continue to require a general anesthetic. There is little information on the effects of volatile agents and sufentanil anesthesia on the incidence of intraoperative tachyarrhythmias in patients with WPW syndrome. The electrophysiologic effects of these agents were studied in patients with WPW syndrome undergoing surgical ablative procedures.

Methods.—Twenty-one adult patients with WPW syndrome were undergoing surgical ablation. Anesthesia was with sufentanil, 20 μg/kg; lorazepam, .06 mg/kg; and vecuronium, 20 mg. Electrophysiologic studies were performed preoperatively; during antegrade and retrograde stimulation; and after the patients had received 1 minimum alveolar concentration of halothane, isoflurane, or enflurane in a randomized fashion.

Results.—Initial anesthesia with sufentanil-lorazepam resulted in only mild prolongation of the effective refractory period of the accessory pathway and the shortest cycle length of the atrioventricular node. With isoflurane and, particularly enflurane, significant prolongation occurred in all electrophysiologic parameters related to refractoriness during antegrade conduction. Isoflurane prolonged the effective refractory period of the right ventricle and accessory pathway and the shortest cycle length of the accessory pathway during retrograde conduction. By contrast, enflurane prolonged only the accessory pathway effective refractory period and shortest cycle length. Refractoriness was least affected by halothane, which prolonged the atrioventricular node effective refractory period and the shortest cycle length of the accessory pathway during antegrade conduction only. Halothane and isoflurane, but not enflurane, prolonged the coupling interval, which reflects the period of vulnerability to supraventricular tachycardia. However, supraventricular tachycardia could still be obtained in all patients.

Conclusion.—In patients with WPW syndrome, sufentanil-lorazepam anesthesia had no significant effects on the electrophysiology of the accessory pathway. The volatile anesthetic enflurane caused the greatest increases in refractoriness of the accessory and atrioventricular pathways, followed by isoflurane and halothane. As a result, giving volatile anesthetics during ablative procedures may confound the interpretation of postablative studies. On the other hand, for patients who require general anesthesia for nonablative procedures, volatile agents may reduce the incidence of perioperative refractoriness. In this situation, enflurane, which yields the greatest prolongation in refractoriness but does not prolong the coupling interval, would be the best choice.

▶ This article contains a fascinating dichotomy. If you are doing cardiac surgery for ablative procedures for WPW syndrome and trying to detect locations of aberrant conduction systems, according to this study, you don't want the volatile agents. These authors would contend that the exact opposite should be done in patients who have WPW syndrome and require general anesthesia for noncardiac surgery. In those patients, use of the volatile agents may specifically suppress the aberrant conduction pathway, thereby protecting the patient against runaway tachycardia. I have seldom read an article that contained a more clinically relevant yet seemingly opposing set of findings.—J.H. Tinker, M.D.

Effect of Diabetes Mellitus on the Cardiovascular Responses to Induction of Anaesthesia and Tracheal Intubation
Vohra A, Kumar S, Charlton AJ, Olukoga AO, Boulton AJM, McLeod D (Manchester Central Hosps and Community Care NHS Trust, England)
Br J Anaesth 71:258–261, 1993   101-95-4–5

Background.—Increased operative morbidity and mortality have been observed in diabetics and ascribed to the systemic dysfunction associated with diabetes. Autonomic neuropathy could alter cardiovascular responses during anesthesia, thereby increasing the risk of cardiovascular morbidity.

Objective.—Cardiovascular responses during anesthesia were compared in 10 patients with diabetes, 8 of whom were insulin-dependent, and 10 American Society of Anesthesiologists physical status I patients who were matched with the diabetics for age, gender, and body size. The patients, all of whom underwent vitreous surgery, had no cardiovascular disease.

Methods.—The patients were premedicated with 20 mg of tempazepam 2 hours before surgery. Anesthesia was induced with propofol,

2.5 mg/kg, and pancuronium and maintained with .8% enflurane and 50% nitrous oxide in oxygen. The trachea was intubated 3 minutes after induction, and ventilatory assistance was provided.

Results.—Heart rate tests of autonomic function were abnormal in all the patients with diabetes. The heart rate increased after induction of anesthesia in the controls only. In diabetics, it increased significantly only at the time of tracheal intubation. The cardiac index decreased in both groups after induction, but it did so significantly in controls only. The mean cardiac index was greater in controls than in diabetics. Patients in both groups had a significant decline in the mean arterial pressure after induction of anesthesia. After intubation, the pressure increased more in diabetics. Systemic vascular resistance decreased in both groups after induction, but after intubation, it increased more in the diabetic patients.

Discussion.—An exaggerated pressor response to tracheal intubation was observed in patients with diabetes, and it may indicate autonomic dysfunction. A study of cardiovascular responses to sympathomimetic drugs in this setting would be of interest.

▶ Many patients with diabetes mellitus have an autonomic neuropathy develop, so the finding that they show an exaggerated response to tracheal intubation is not surprising. Diabetic patients often have cardiovascular disease (e.g., hypertension), even though the authors attempted to study patients with no cardiac disease; of course, hypertensive patients also have an abnormal response to tracheal intubation. It would be interesting to look at vascular responses to sympathetic drugs in this group of patients.—M. Wood, M.D.

Response to Repeated Phlebotomies in Patients With Non-Insulin-Dependent Diabetes Mellitus

Bofill C, Joven J, Bages J, Vilella E, Sans T, Cavallé P, Miralles R, Llobet J, Camps J (Hosp de Sant Joan de Reus, Spain; Boehringer-Mannheim Labs, Barcelona)
Metabolism 43:614–620, 1994   101-95-4–6

Introduction.—Because diabetes mellitus, regardless of the type, causes disruption of metabolic homeostasis, physicians treating patients with diabetes may be reluctant to perform the repeated phlebotomies necessary for participation in a predeposited autologous blood transfusion program (PABTP). However, alternative sources for blood transfusion are less than ideal as well. As a result, biochemical and hematologic variables, particularly serum erythropoietin (EPO) concentration, were monitored during repeated phlebotomies.

Methods.—Standard laboratory tests were performed on 42 patients with type II diabetes mellitus who were enrolled in a preoperative predeposited PABTP. Six phlebotomies were performed at 2- to 4-day intervals. Venous blood was obtained immediately before each donation for analysis of albumin, prealbumin, cholesterol, triglycerides, phospholipids, apoproteins A-I and B, hemoglobin A_{1c}, and EPO. The values in the patients with diabetes were compared with those found in controls without diabetes who were enrolled in the PABTP.

Results.—There were no significant differences between the diabetic and control groups in serum transferrin and iron concentrations; both groups experienced a significant reduction in serum iron after acute blood loss. The patients with diabetes had higher serum ferritin concentrations than the controls. Serum lipids were higher at baseline in patients with diabetes, but they decreased with repeated phlebotomies, a response that did not occur in controls. Neither group exhibited changes in high-density lipoprotein cholesterol, albumin, or prealbumin. The 2 groups had similar hemoglobin concentrations and hematologic profiles. In both groups, reticulocyte increases correlated with hemoglobin A_{1c} proportions. Increases in the serum EPO levels of controls were between 1.5 and 3.2 times the initial values; serum EPO increases in patients with diabetes ranged widely between no increase and a 12-fold increase, which did not correlate with hemoglobin levels. Strict glycemic control produced a better EPO response.

Discussion.—The PABTP seems to be a safe practice for patients with diabetes. However, strict glycemic control should be maintained whenever possible in these patients. The lack of correlation between the serum EPO and hemoglobin levels suggests that additional factors may mediate EPO changes. The EPO response requires further study.

▶ It is surprising that there are any restrictions on predeposition of blood in diabetes. The risks/benefits would seem to favor the latter for predeposits in avoiding homologous transfusion, which carries with it immunodepression and higher susceptibility to infections. Thus, this article reinforces the notion that diabetics have a favorable benefit-risk ratio for predeposition of blood they need for major surgery.—M.F. Roizen, M.D.

Components of the Inspiratory-Arterial Isoflurane Partial Pressure Difference
Landon MJ, Matson AM, Royston BD, Hewlett AM, White DC, Nunn JF (Clinical Research Centre, Harrow, England; Northwick Park Hosp, Harrow, England)
Br J Anaesth 70:605–611, 1993   101-95-4–7

Background.—The concept of minimum alveolar concentration presupposes that alveolar partial pressure is transmitted to the arterial blood without change. Recent studies cite arterial-to–end-expiratory partial pressure ratios ranging (after equilibration) from .79 to .86. The effects of venous admixture and alveolar dead space provide partial but not sufficient explanations for the gradient.

Objective.—Eger's hypothesis that high-molecular-weight anesthetics may not become uniformly mixed in the alveoli was tested. The alveolar-pulmonary end-capillary partial pressure difference of isoflurane was measured simultaneously with the shunt and physiologic dead space in 6 patients, 57–79 years of age, who underwent major vascular operations.

Methods.—The partial pressure of isoflurane was measured simultaneously in inspired and end-expired gas, mixed-expired gas, and arterial and mixed venous blood. The patients also received nitrous oxide in oxygen. Measurements were repeated after the partial pressure in end-expired gas had been stable for 15 minutes or longer. The alveolar dead space dilution of end-expired gas was calculated for carbon dioxide, and this dilution factor was used to estimate the "ideal" alveolar partial pressure of isoflurane from the observed inspired and end-expired concentrations. Shunt fraction, which was measured for oxygen, was used to calculate the partial pressure of isoflurane in pulmonary end-capillary blood from the partial pressures in arterial and mixed venous blood.

Results.—The mean ideal alveolar-to-pulmonary end-capillary partial pressure difference was .12 kPa, a highly significant value. The arterial partial pressure was substantially less than the value in end-expired gas, but the difference was fairly constant. The effects of shunting and dead space accounted in part for the difference, but a failure of isoflurane to equilibrate between the alvoelar gas and pulmonary end-capillary blood was also a factor.

Conclusion.—A failure of isoflurance to be uniformly distributed within the alveolus may be the chief reason for the observed end-expired–to–arterial partial pressure gradient. The existence of a gradient can be expected to hinder the achievement and reversal of anesthesia.

Diaphragmatic Function Before and After Laparoscopic Cholecystectomy

Erice F, Fox GS, Salib YM, Romano E, Meakins J, Magder SA (Univ of Trieste, Italy; McGill Univ, Montreal)
Anesthesiology 79:966–975, 1993   101-95-4–8

Introduction.—Laparoscopic surgery has recently increased in popularity because it is less invasive and less costly and may reduce postoperative pulmonary complications by avoiding the restrictive pattern of breathing that usually follows upper abdominal surgery. A primary cause of ventilatory impairment after upper abdominal surgery is diaphragm dysfunction. Less dysfunction may be caused by laparoscopic procedures. The theory that ventilatory performance remains impaired after laparoscopic cholecystectomy because the site of surgery is adjacent to reflexogenic splanchnic areas was evaluated.

Methods.—Diaphragmatic function was tested in 10 healthy adult patients who had elective laparoscopic cholecystectomy and in 5 who had laparoscopic hernia repair. Three hours before and after surgery, respiratory gas exchange ventilation and breathing patterns were measured. The relationship of end-tidal carbon dioxide during tidal breathing was measured to determine respiratory drive. Diaphragmatic contractile function was measured from maximal transdiaphragmatic pressure and during a maximal sniff maneuver.

Results.—After surgery, oxygen consumption and carbon dioxide production did not change. In the laparoscopic cholecystectomy group, maximal diaphragmatic pressure decreased by more than 50%, but the maximal sniff maneuver did not change. The tidal volume decreased by 30%, and the ratio of inspiratory time over the total cycle time decreased by 13%; the end-tidal carbon dioxide increased by 9%, and minute ventilation did not change. In the group that had laparoscopic hernia repair, there was no variation in ventilatory function. Depressed respiratory drive and contractile failure of the diaphragm were discounted, because the maximial sniff maneuver did not change.

Conclusion.—Laparoscopic cholecystectomy impairs diaphragmatic function, but it does not increase metabolic demands in the early postoperative period. The critical variable determining diaphragmatic inhibition after laparoscopic abdominal surgery is the internal site of surgical intervention. A very likely mechanism for the depressed diaphragmatic activity after laparoscopic cholecystectomy is reflex inhibition of phrenic nerve output. Postoperative pulmonary complications may result in patients who have preexisting limited cardiorespiratory performance.

▶ Laparoscopic cholecystectomy is very popular in 1995, partly because it is said to result in less postoperative pulmonary disturbance. This study shows that ventilatory performance can still be impaired after laparoscopic cholecystectomy. We have known for years that upper abdominal surgery carries a higher respiratory complication rate than lower abdominal surgery and that nonthoracic, nonabdominal surgery has an even lower complication rate. Among other things, postoperative respiratory complications are related to the specific operation, and a cholecystectomy is still a cholecystectomy.—M. Wood, M.D.

Effect of Sevoflurane on Hypoxic Pulmonary Vasoconstriction in the Perfused Rabbit Lung

Ishibe Y, Gui X, Uno H, Shiokawa Y, Umeda T, Suekane K (Tottori Univ, Japan; Kinki Univ, Osaka, Japan)
Anesthesiology 79:1348–1353, 1993   101-95-4–9

Background.—A number of inhalational anesthetics, including halothane, enflurane, and isoflurane, inhibit hypoxic pulmonary vasoconstriction (HPV) with similar potency. This effect is often not evident clinically, because secondary effects of anesthetics may modulate the HPV response. Sevoflurane has been reported not to inhibit HPV in intact dogs.

Objective and Methods.—The effect of sevoflurane on HPV in vitro was studied in lungs from adult rabbits that were perfused at constant flow. Baseline HPV responses were measured as the pulmonary artery pressure increased after decreasing the inspired oxygen concentration from 95% to 3% for 5 minutes. The preparations were then exposed to isoflurane in concentrations of .5, 1, and 2 minimum alveolar concentration (MAC) and to sevoflurane in concentrations of .4, .8, and 1.2 MAC. Some animals received ibuprofen, a cyclooxygenase inhibitor, in a dose of 12.5 mg/kg before the lungs were exposed to sevoflurane.

Results.—Isoflurane and sevoflurane depressed the HPV response in a dose-related manner and to similar degrees. Sevoflurane in a concentration of 1 MAC inhibited the HPV response by 50%. Pretreatment with ibuprofen did not alter the effect of sevoflurane, although the absolute pressor response was greater than without pretreatment.

Conclusion.—Sevoflurane directly inhibits the pulmonary vascular response to alveolar hypoxia.

▶ Many studies over the years have shown that inhalational anesthetics inhibit hypoxic pulmonary vasoconstriction. Although this is true in the laboratory, especially for in vitro or in vivo nonintact models, the inhibitory effect is not often clinically evident in human studies. Therefore, it is important to recognize that this study evaluates the effect of a new investigational inhalational anesthetic, sevoflurane, on hypoxic pulmonary vasoconstriction in the perfused rabbit lung where it appears to have an effect similar to that of isoflurane. The effects of sevoflurane in patients undergoing thoracotomy during one-lung ventilation have not been studied. If they are still similar to those produced by isoflurane, a marked effect on arterial oxygenation might not be expected.—M. Wood, M.D.

Comparison of Low Concentrations of Halothane and Isoflurane as Bronchodilators

Brown RH, Zerhouni EA, Hirshman CA (Johns Hopkins Med Institutions, Baltimore, Md)
Anesthesiology 78:1097–1101, 1993   101-95-4–10

Background.—All current inhalational anesthetics are considered to be effective bronchodilators when administered in high concentrations. Conventional measures of airway tone have failed to demonstrate differences in airway responsiveness with the inhalation of halothane, enflurane, and isoflurane.

Objective and Methods.—A sensitive method of determining airway responsiveness, which is based on high-resolution CT, was used to com-

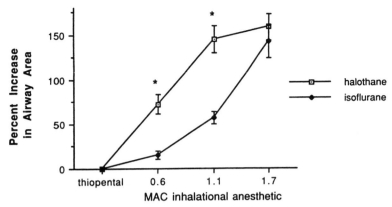

Fig 4–2.—Dose-response dilation of histamine-preconstricted airways to increasing concentrations of halothane (*upper line, open boxes*) and isoflurane (*lower line, filled diamonds*). The airways were significantly more dilated at the lower concentrations of anesthetic by halothane than by isoflurane (*P < .001). At the higher concentration, there was no difference between halothane and isoflurane in the amount of dilation in the airways. (Courtesy of Brown RH, Zerhouni EA, Hirshman CA: *Anesthesiology* 78:1097–1101, 1993.)

pare the ability of halothane and insoflurane to dilate histamine-con-stricted airways at minimum alveolar concentration (MAC)–equivalent levels. Dogs were anesthetized with thiopental, intubated, and mechanically ventilated before administering IV histamine at a rate of 200 µg/min. The dogs received halothane and insoflurane on alternate days in concentrations of .6, 1.1, and 1.7 MAC. The study was repeated in dogs that were given .2 mg of atropine per kg after histamine infusion.

Results.—Histamine infusion reduced the airway area by 34% on average. All preconstricted airways dilated significantly in a dose-related manner at all concentrations of both anesthetics (Fig 4–2). At .6 and 1.1 MAC, halothane was significantly more effective, but no major difference was noted at 1.7 MAC. The difference that was in effect at the lower concentration was noted only for airways 7 mm and less in diameter. Atropine reversed the histamine-induced airway constriction.

Implications.—In low concentrations, halothane is a more potent bronchodilator than isoflurane. Therefore, it may be a better choice for inducing anesthesia in patients who have reactive airway disease.

▶ The relatively lower concentrations of volatile agents that are often used today, for example, .5–1 MAC (or less), are worthy of study vis-à-vis airway constriction. Halothane comes off better, but I strongly doubt we will see a resurgence of it, even in asthmatic patients. Is it really valid to anesthetize an asthmatic adult with halothane? For that matter, is it valid to anesthetize any adult with halothane? How much risk of hepatotoxicity are you willing to take? Can the administration of halothane be justified on the basis of its somewhat better performance in asthma (at least in dogs)?

The problem with all of this is Murphy's law. It circles over all our heads, and as surely as Murphy was born, the patient you choose to anesthetize with halothane because of his or her asthma will be the one who turns yellow several days or weeks later! I don't think this article will bring halothane back.—J.H. Tinker, M.D.

Nitrous Oxide-Isoflurane Anesthesia Causes More Cerebral Vasodilation Than an Equipotent Dose of Isoflurane in Humans

Lam AM, Mayberg TS, Eng CC, Cooper JO, Bachenberg KL, Mathisen TL (Univ of Washington, Seattle)

Anesth Analg 78:462–468, 1994   101-95-4–11

Objective.—When it is used in neuroanesthesia, nitrous oxide has the potential for dilating cerebral vessels and increasing intracranial pressure when intracranial elastance is increased. Accordingly, the cerebrovascular effects of nitrous oxide in a minimum alveolar concentration (MAC) of .6 in isoflurane were compared with those of an equipotent dose of isoflurane.

Methods.—Six healthy American Society of Anesthesiologists physical status I men, 25–39 years of age, who were to undergo minor orthopedic procedures participated in the study. Anesthesia was induced with thiopental, and after intubation it was maintained with isoflurane alone or combined with nitrous oxide. The flow velocity in the right middle cerebral artery was monitored using a Doppler probe under 4 steady-state conditions: .5 MAC of isoflurane; .5 MAC isoflurane plus .6 MAC of nitrous oxide; 1.1 MAC of isoflurane plus .6 MAC of nitrous oxide; and 1.1 MAC of isoflurane. The cerebral arteriovenous oxygen content difference ($AVDO_2$) and cerebral metabolic equivalent (CME) were also determined.

Results.—Compared with 1.1 MAC of isoflurane alone, combined anesthesia correlated with a higher flow velocity and increased values of $AVDO_2$ and CME. Changes in electroencephalographic (EEG) activity were consistent with increased cerebral metabolism. Adding .6 MAC of nitrous oxide to low-dose isoflurane had variable effects on the flow velocity, but there was no overall change. The $AVDO_2$ decreased 14% and EEG activity changed only slightly. There was no significant change in CME. By contrast, when nitrous oxide was added to 1.1 MAC of isoflurane, the flow velocity increased 25% overall. The $AVDO_2$ decreased in 5 of 6 patients, but the overall change was not significant. The CME and EEG activity remained unchanged.

Conclusion.—Nitrous oxide is a stronger cerebral vasodilator than an equipotent dose of isoflurane when it is used along with isoflurane in moderate-to-high doses. The final state of cerebral blood flow may reflect both direct vasodilation and metabolically conditioned vasoconstriction.

▶ I included this article because, although we have been studying cerebral vasodilation caused by anesthetics for more than 40 years, we still aren't sure what to do with nitrous oxide. I also included it to point out that a major problem with these kinds of studies is the use of MAC as the measure of "potency." Where is it written in stone that simply because MAC, as a measure of potency, predicts that 50% of the patients will and 50% will not move in response to skin incision at that concentration, "equipotent" doses of isoflurane vs. nitrous oxide will have similar effects on cerebrovasculature?—J.H. Tinker, M.D.

Exaggerated Anesthetic Requirements in the Preferentially Anesthetized Brain
Antognini JF, Schwartz K (Univ of California, Davis)
Anesthesiology 79:1244–1249, 1993   101-95-4–12

Background.—How and where inhalational anesthetics exert their effects remain unknown. The brain is assumed to be the site of anesthetic action, but these agents also exert effects in other areas, including the spinal cord. The arrangement of the cerebral circulation of the goat makes it convenient for studies that require isolating the cerebral vessels.

Objective and Methods.—A goat brain was preferentially anesthetized by ligating the occipital arteries to prevent vertebral blood from entering the carotid system. The minimum alveolar concentration (MAC) of isoflurane was determined using a dew-claw clamp as a painful stimulus. Cranial venous blood was then drained into a bubble oxygenator, where an isoflurane vaporizer was in line with the gas flow. Inhalation of the anesthetic was discontinued. The partial pressure of isoflurane in blood delivered by the carotid artery was increased as needed to encompass the partial pressures that permitted and prevented movement in response to stimulation. The MAC was again estimated after the native circulation was restored.

Results.—The isoflurane requirement increased from 1.2% to 2.9% when anesthesia was isolated to the head and brain, and it decreased to 1.3% after the native circulation was restored. A mild, nonprogressive metabolic acidosis developed. Marked electroencephalographic suppression accompanied bypass. The systemic mean arterial pressure decreased from 88 to 83 mm Hg during bypass, and the cranial mean arterial pressure decreased from 76 to 48 mm Hg.

Implications.—Subcortical cerebral structures modulated movement in response to painful stimulation during general anesthesia. Different end points of anesthesia, such as movement and unconsciousness, may be related to different sites of anesthetic action.

▶ Anesthetic potency is traditionally defined as the MAC, the minimal anesthetic concentration required to prevent movement in 50% of patients or research subjects in response to a noxious or surgical stimulus. This definition implies that there is a motor response at the spinal level.

In this study, MAC was 1.2% when isoflurane was delivered to the goat's whole body and 2.9% when only the goat's brain was exposed to isoflurane, so that the cortex was not the important site of anesthetic action. It makes us think about exactly what we mean by anesthetic potency as defined by MAC.

As Kendig pointed out in the accompanying editorial, the converse experiment, in which only the spinal cord was exposed to isoflurane, was not done (1). However, Rampil and associates (2) have also shown that in acutely decerebrated rats, MAC for isoflurane is independent of forebrain structures and is probably determined by anesthetic action at the midbrain or lower, in the spinal cord and/or brain stem, because MAC for the decerebrated rats was the same as MAC for the same rats intact. Although the brain is assumed to be the site of anesthetic action, anesthetics act at other sites, such as the spinal cord.

All these studies make intuitive sense, and it is satisfying to see the idea that different end points (e.g., hypnosis and movement during anesthesia) may be associated with different sites of action that are actually being tested.—M. Wood, M.D.

References

1. Kendig JJ: *Anesthesiology* 79:1161, 1993.
2. Rampil IJ, et al: *Anesthesiology* 78:707, 1993.

Anesthetic Potency is Not Altered After Hypothermic Spinal Cord Transection in Rats
Rampil IJ (Univ of California, San Francisco)
Anesthesiology 80:606–610, 1994   101-95-4–13

Background.—Blockade of the somatic motor response to painful stimulation is commonly accepted as an indicator that adequate anesthesia has been achieved. The level of anesthetic needed to achieve this, or the minimum alveolar concentration (MAC), is the standard measure of anesthetic potency. Evidence suggests that precollicular decerebration in the rat does not alter the MAC of isoflurane, indicating that the forebrain is not a major site of action.

Objective and Methods.—The relative importance of the brain stem and spinal cord as sites of anesthetic effect in blocking somatic responsiveness was examined in 7 rats that were anesthetized with isoflurane in oxygen. The MAC was estimated by monitoring responses to tail clamping and toe pinch in the fore and hind limbs after intubation, cervical laminectomy, and staged transection of the spinal cord using liquid nitrogen.

Results.—Tail-clamp estimates of MAC did not change during the various stages of the study. Most of the variance in the postlesioning values was explained by a decrease in the MAC from 1.2% to .25% in a single animal, in which the paw-pinch MAC value was unchanged. Toe-pinch estimates of MAC remained unchanged after spinal transection in all animals.

Conclusion.—In animals such as the rat that generate complex, autonomous spinal motor patterns, anesthetics may inhibit motor responses in the spinal cord. It is possible that these responses exist independent of perceived pain.

▶ This study provides further evidence that the site of anesthetic inhibition of the motor response, such as seen in the determination of MAC, is at the spinal cord level. The author also postulates that the somatic motor response exists independent of the "perception of pain."

The concept of the "perception of pain" is worth further thought. Does this mean that the use of a physiologic response to noxious stimuli as a surrogate for anesthetic depth is flawed? Studies such as this raise intriguing questions and are certainly changing how we view the concept of MAC.—M. Wood, M.D.

The Association Between Foot Temperature and Asymmetrical Epidural Blockade

Griffin RP, Reynolds F (St Thomas' Hosp, London)
Int J Obstet Anesth 3:132–136, 1994   101-95-4-14

Background.—Asymmetric and unilateral analgesia are complications of epidural blockade that lead to inadequate pain relief in labor. The hypothesis that an asymmetric sensor block is associated with an asymmetric sympathetic block was investigated. Clinical experience has shown that differences in foot temperature can be a convenient and effective means of detecting the development of sympathetic block.

Methods.—Sixty parturients who requested epidural analgesia had epidural catheters placed at L3–4 while in the lateral position. A test dose was followed 5 minutes later by a main dose of 25–30 mg of plain bupivacaine. A thermistor thermometer was applied to the dorsum of both feet, and the temperature was recorded before and 5, 10, 15, 20, and 30 minutes after the end of the main dose. The upper and lower limits of sensory blockade on both the left and right sides were recorded at the same time intervals. The relationship between foot temperature difference and sensory block asymmetry was calculated using Spearman's coefficient of rank correlation. The medical staff, which was blinded to foot temperature, was asked whether it could detect foot asymmetry during the 30 minutes after administration of the main dose.

Results.—Spearman's coefficient of rank correlation between sensory block asymmetry and foot temperature difference was .4 at 5 minutes, .39 at 10 minutes, .54 at 15 minutes, .59 at 20 minutes, and .6 at 30 minutes. This correlation was significant at 5 and 10 minutes and highly significant at 15, 20, and 30 minutes. Most of the staff physicians could detect a difference between the temperature of the feet when it was greater than 1°C.

Conclusion.—A clear relationship was demonstrated between sensory block asymmetry and the difference between the temperature of the feet. Touching the feet was a simple means of detecting sensory block asymmetry, and it may be useful in determining the appropriate patient positioning to reduce sensory block asymmetry and provide more effective analgesia during labor.

▶ The authors concluded that early detection of a difference in the temperature of the feet may be useful "to determine appropriate patient positioning in order to reduce sensory block asymmetry. . . ." The rationale for this statement is their belief that "if patients remain on one side without turning a more extensive and longer lasting block will develop on the dependent side." I disagree. Posture has little effect on the spread and development of symmetric epidural analgesia. Malposition of the catheter is a more likely cause of unilateral sensory blockade.—D.H. Chestnut, M.D.

Effects of Inhalant Anesthesia on the Middle Ear as Measured by Tympanometry
Chinn K, Brown OE, Manning SC (Univ of Texas at Dallas; Southwestern Med Ctr, Dallas)
Arch Otolaryngol Head Neck Surg 119:283–287, 1993   101-95-4-15

Introduction.—Nitrous oxide and halothane are typically used to produce anesthesia during myringotomy procedures. There have been inconsistent reports of the effects of halothane and nitrous oxide on the status of the middle ear. Middle ear pressure was measured using tympanometry to assess the effects of either nitrous oxide alone or nitrous oxide and halothane on middle ear pressure and to test the validity of tympanometric assessment.

Methods.—A total of 138 children who underwent myringotomy with grommet placement were divided into 2 groups. Group 1 received nitrous oxide and halothane anesthesia; group 2 received halothane only. Patients were examined preoperatively with a handheld otoscope. Tympanometry was performed on both ears before and immediately after the induction of anesthesia and when the patient reached the depth of anesthesia required for surgery. Middle ear status was recorded during myringotomy and compared with that on tympanograms. Twenty-seven patients in each group were matched for age, sex, and type of preanesthesia tympanogram to assess any differences between the 2 anesthesia protocols.

Results.—Of the 163 ears studied in group 1, 115 had effusion at myringotomy, whereas 56 of 92 ears in group 2 had effusion. Tympanography recorded changes in 62 of 163 ears (38%) in group 1 and in 42 of 92 ears (46%) in group 2; however, the changes were minimal. Type A or A′ preanesthesia tympanograms correlated with the absence of effusion in 19 of 26 cases in group 1 and in 16 of 21 cases in group 2, and type B tympanograms correlated with effusion in 65 of 68 cases in group 1 and in 24 of 26 cases in group 2. Within the subset of matched patients from each group, there were no significant anesthesia-related differences in tympanogram changes.

Discussion.—There were nonsignificantly more tympanogram changes in the group that received halothane only than in the group that received both halothane and nitrous oxide, which challenges the belief that nitrous oxide causes middle ear changes. Although there appear to be anesthesia-related middle ear changes, they are not significant and do not appear to affect effusion states. The preanesthesia tympanometry sensitivity was 57% for group 1 and 44% for group 2; specificity was 93% for group 1 and 95% for group 2. The postanesthesia tympanometry sensitivity was 61% for group 1 and 55% for group 2; specificity was 85% for group 1 and 97% for group 2.

▶ As the authors indicate, myringotomy with tube placement is the most common surgical procedure performed in children in the United States. I don't know the percentages, but I'm sure that halothane/nitrous oxide has been used for more of these procedures than any other combination of anesthetics. Numerous other studies have shown no real problem with this anesthetic in terms of middle ear pressure. I cannot figure out why the authors chose to study it again. I included this article because readers might wish to be brought up to date with respect to studies of anesthetics and middle ear pressure, a subject about which we haven't read much lately. It may be reassuring to know that there isn't much new on this subject.—J.H. Tinker, M.D.

5 Pharmacology and Toxicology of Anesthetics, Sedatives, and Other Drugs Except Relaxants

Rapid Increase in Desflurane Concentration Is Associated With Greater Transient Cardiovascular Stimulation Than With Rapid Increase in Isoflurane Concentration in Humans
Weiskopf RB, Moore MA, Eger El II, Noorani M, McKay L, Chortkoff B, Hart PS, Damask M (Univ of California, San Francisco)
Anesthesiology 80:1035–1045, 1994   101-95-5–1

Purpose.—During induction of anesthesia, transient increases in arterial blood pressure and/or heart rate can result from increases in desflurane and isoflurane concentrations. A recent nonrandomized study suggested that increasing the concentration of desflurane, but not isoflurane, increased mean arterial blood pressure and muscle sympathetic nerve activity. The effects on sympathetic activity, hormonal variables, heart rate, and arterial blood pressure were assessed for a rapid increase of desflurane vs. isoflurane concentration in humans.

Methods.—Twelve healthy young men were randomized to receive desflurane and isoflurane on separate occasions. At each session, anesthesia was induced with propofol, 2 mg/kg, and maintained at a .55 minimum alveolar concentration (MAC) for 32 minutes. Normocapnia was maintained with mechanical ventilation. Anesthetic concentrations were then rapidly increased to 1.66 MAC, maintained at that level for 32 minutes, then rapidly decreased again and maintained at .55 MAC for another 32 minutes. Throughout the study, the mean arterial blood pressure and heart rate were continuously recorded, and arterial blood samples were taken for measurement of plasma catecholamine and vasopressin (AVP) concentrations and plasma renin activity.

Results.—During the first period at .55 MAC, neither anesthetic resulted in sympathetic or cardiovascular stimulation. With both agents, increasing the concentration to 1.66 MAC resulted in increases in the

71

mean arterial blood pressure, heart rate, and plasma epinephrine and norepinephrine concentrations; these responses were usually greater with desflurane than with isoflurane. Only desflurane resulted in an increase in the plasma AVP concentration.

The mean arterial blood pressure returned to control levels within 4 minutes. The heart rate decreased 50% of the difference between its peak and the value at 32 minutes at 1.66 MAC within 2 to 4 minutes; however, with neither anesthetic did it return to the value at .55 MAC. Plasma epinephrine and AVP concentrations decreased quickly with desflurane and remained elevated for 8 minutes. Decreasing concentrations of both agents resulted in a rapid decrease in heart rate and increased mean arterial pressure. After 32 minutes, the only measurement that remained increased compared with the values during the initial period of anesthesia was the heart rate.

Conclusion.—Increasing desflurane or isoflurane concentrations from .55 to 1.66 MAC appears to increase sympathetic and renin-angiotensin activity in normal volunteers. Transient increases in arterial blood pressure and heart rate occur at the same time. Greater increases occur with desflurane, which also causes a transient increase in plasma AVP concentration. The increased sympathetic activity may increase the mean arterial pressure and heart rate. The increased plasma AVP concentration may also play a role in increasing the mean arterial pressure. The delayed increase in plasma renin activity probably represents a response to the ensuing hypotension and/or earlier inhibition by AVP.

▶ With the introduction of desflurane, the first truly rapid-acting volatile anesthetic, came a disturbing complication, namely, worrisome tachycardia during the relatively large increases in concentrations necessary to change levels of anesthesia. Desflurane is considerably less potent than isoflurane and requires larger absolute changes in inspired concentrations.

The authors demonstrated that the transient cardiovascular stimulation is secondary to sympathetic discharge. It may be that this is the result of airway irritation, although currently there isn't really proof. The authors speculate that the transient nature of these responses may be caused by airway receptor "adaptation," whatever that means.—J.H. Tinker, M.D.

Minimum Alveolar Concentration of Desflurane in Patients Older Than 65 Yr

Gold MI, Abello D, Herrington C (Univ of Miami, Fla)
Anesthesiology 79:710–714, 1993   101-95-5–2

Objective.—Previous studies have indicated that the minimum alveolar concentration (MAC) of desflurane, alone or combined with nitrous oxide, is less in middle-aged patients than in young adults; older persons also have lower MACs of other volatile anesthetics. Whether patients older than 65 years of age require less desflurane was studied in a series of 39 such patients who were in American Society of Anesthesiologists physical status II or III and were scheduled for elective surgery that necessitated a skin incision.

Methods.—Anesthesia was induced by inhaled desflurane in nitrous oxide/oxygen or in oxygen only. Starting concentrations of desflurane were 3% in nitrous oxide/oxygen and 6% in oxygen. The inspired concentration was increased at a rate of about 2% per minute until intubation was possible without a neuromuscular blocking agent. Gas flow then was adjusted to maintain a stable end-tidal level for at least 10 minutes, using lack of patient movement as a criterion of adequate anesthesia.

Results.—The MAC was 5.17% for desflurane in oxygen and 1.67% for desflurane in nitrous oxide/oxygen. Patients in the 2 groups did not differ significantly with respect to age or body size.

Conclusion.—The MAC of desflurane was less in patients who were older than 65 years of age than in younger individuals.

▶ I included this paper to once again point out something that we all know intellectually but tend to forget or ignore: Elderly patients do not need very much anesthesia. We get deceived by their apparent health, especially if they are characterized by loved ones as being "spry."—J.H. Tinker, M.D.

Relative Potency of Eltanolone, Propofol, and Thiopental for Induction of Anesthesia

Van Hemelrijck J, Muller P, Van Aken H, White PF (Katholieke Universiteit Leuven, Belgium; Univ of Texas, Dallas)
Anesthesiology 80:36–41, 1994   101-95-5-3

Background.—A number of structurally related pregnanes, such as pregnenolone (eltanolone), have been found to have sedative and hypnotic activity but no endocrinologic effects.

Study Plan.—The potency and safety of eltanolone compared with those for propofol and thiopental when it was used to induce anesthesia in generally healthy individuals were determined. The study group included 175 American Society of Anesthesiologists physical status I or II individuals, 18–50 years of age, who were in good general health and nonobese. Patients who were premedicated with lorazepam initially received 5 different doses of either eltanolone or propofol. The highest dose of each drug that consistently led to a loss of consciousness was administered. Each dose was injected into a forearm vein in 30 seconds.

Results.—Eltanolone had a relative potency of 3.2 compared with propofol, and it was sixfold more potent than thiopental (Fig 5–1). Eltanolone increased the heart rate significantly, but the decline in blood pressure was significantly greater after propofol injection. Apnea was

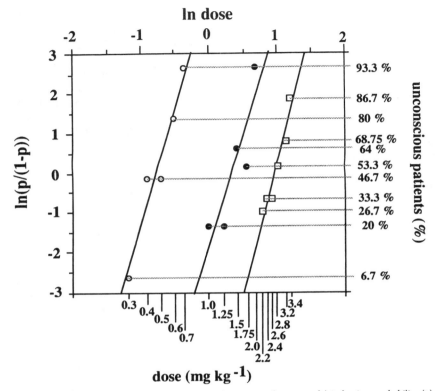

Fig 5-1.—Relationship between the logit transformation of a successful induction probability (p) (the percentage of patients not responding to verbal commands) and the logarithm of the dose of eltanolone (*open circles*), propofol (*filled circles*), and thiopental (*squares*). (Courtesy of Van Hemelrijck J, Muller P, Van Aken H, et al: *Anesthesiology* 80:36–41, 1994.)

more frequent in patients who were given propofol. Two patients who received eltanolone transiently had involuntary muscle movements. Pain in the arm was much more prevalent after the injection of propofol.

Conclusion.—Eltanolone is an effective means of inducing anesthesia in healthy adults. It is more potent than either propofol or thiopental.

▶ The hypnotic properties of steroids have been recognized for many years. When I was a junior resident in the United Kingdom, I remember using the steroid anesthetic induction agent, Althesin, which was a mixture of steroids, alphaxalone, and alphadolone. Unfortunately, it was solubilized in cremophor EL, a vehicle that is known to cause hypersensitivity reactions. Rapid induction of anesthesia and high potency are associated with the free 3α-hydroxy group on the steroid molecule, but these compounds are very insoluble. Althesin was an effective IV anesthetic agent, but it produced serious hypersensitivity reactions, which were manifested as severe cardiovascular collapse, bronchospasm, and a generalized erythematous reaction. It was suggested that these reactions might be the result of the solubilizing agent, cremophor EL. Thus, when the new anesthetic propofol was formulated in an emulsion, interest was renewed in the possibility of other agents of low water solubility being prepared in this way.

Eltanolone or pregnenolone is a new steroid IV anesthetic agent that is 3.2 times more potent than propofol and 6 times more potent than thiopental in relative hypnotic potency. Its future role will be determined by its pharmacokinetic and pharmacodynamic properties when it is given as a continuous IV infusion for maintenance of anesthesia. I think that we might see other "old" insoluble IV anesthetic agents such as propanidid formulated in this manner.—M. Wood, M.D.

Propofol and Autonomic Reflex Function in Humans
Ebert TJ, Muzi M (Medical College of Wisconsin, Milwaukee; VA Med Ctr, Milwaukee, Wis)
Anesth Analg 78:369–375, 1994   101-95-5–4

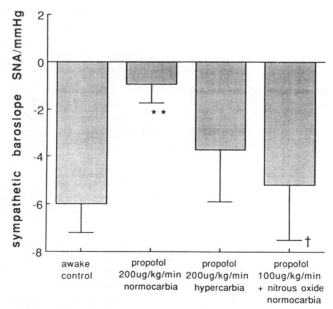

Fig 5–2.—Sympathetic baroreflex sensitivity (baroslope) derived from the linear relationship between diastolic pressure (DP) and sympathetic nerve activity (SNA). Propofol infusion at 200 μg/kg^{-1}/min^{-1} during normocarbia nearly abolished the reflex response of SNA. However, during hypercarbia and during lower infusion rates of propofol combined with nitrous oxide administration, reflex sensitivity was restored to awake levels. $**P < .01$ vs. awake; $\dagger P < .05$ vs. propofol at 200 μg/kg^{-1}/min^{-1}, normocarbia. (Courtesy of Ebert TJ, Muzi M: *Anesth Analg* 78:369–375, 1994.)

Background.—A number of animal studies indicate that relatively large doses of propofol limit both the range and gain of baroreceptor reflex control of heart rate. Two persuasive studies of infused propofol in humans, however, found little, if any, effect of propofol on baroreflex control of the heart rate.

Objective and Methods.—The hemodynamic and sympathetic neural effects of infused propofol were studied in 7 men, 19 to 26 years of age, who were normotensive and in excellent health. The heart rate and radial artery pressure were monitored along with efferent sympathetic vasoconstrictor outflow in the peroneal nerve. The men received a bolus IV injection of 100 μg of nitroprusside and 150 μg of phenylephrine while conscious and after anesthesia was induced with propofol, 200 μg/kg/min. In addition, data were collected under hypercarbic conditions and when a reduced rate of propofol, 100 μg/kg/min, was given in combination with 70% nitrous oxide.

Results.—Propofol initially almost abolished muscle sympathetic nerve activity (SNA) and significantly reduced the mean arterial pressure. The heart rate did not change significantly. The blood pressure declined further during hypercarbia. Muscle SNA returned to waking levels when the rate of propofol infusion was reduced, and blood pressure increased toward the baseline level. Sympathetic baroslopes were nearly abolished during propofol anesthesia under normocarbic conditions (Fig 5–2). Both hypercarbia and the addition of nitrous oxide to a lesser rate of infused propranolol restored sympathetic reflex responsiveness to waking levels.

Conclusion.—Propofol infusion markedly lessened reflex responses to hypotension in healthy men, but reflex sympathetic responsiveness was well maintained under hypercarbic conditions or when a lower dose of propofol was given in conjunction with nitrous oxide. Vagal responses were well preserved during propofol infusion.

▶ These are very elegant studies of sympathetic function in humans using recordings of efferent sympathetic nerve traffic from the peroneal nerve. It is always satisfying to see clinical research such as this being carried out in humans, and it proves that it still can be done.

Propofol markedly attenuates the reflex sympathetic response to hypotension so that during anesthesia using propofol, 200 μg/kg/min, we may not see tachycardia in response to a fall in blood pressure. However, it is important to recognize that if lower doses, such as propofol, 100 μg/kg/min, are given, autonomic reflex function is much better preserved.—M. Wood, M.D.

Inhibition of Volatile Sevoflurane Degradation Product Formation in an Anesthesia Circuit by a Reduction in Soda Lime Temperature

Ruzicka JA, Hidalgo JC, Tinker JH, Baker MT (Univ of Iowa, Iowa City)
Anesthesiology 81:238–244, 1994   101-95-5–5

Objective.—The volatile products known as compounds A and B are formed by reaction of sevoflurane with soda lime or other carbon dioxide absorbents. Other products, known as compounds C, D, and E, have been detected only in heated-sealed systems. The effects of soda lime temperature on formation of compounds A to D were assessed, including the possibility that a lower soda lime temperature could eliminate the formation of these products.

Methods.—Sevoflurane at 1.5% was circulated in oxygen at 6 L/min in a partially closed, low-flow anesthesia circuit. The circuit included a canister containing 1.2 kg of fresh soda lime. After carbon dioxide was released into the circuit at a rate of 200 mL/min, gas samples were taken at the opening of an attached artificial lung for analysis of sevoflurane, compounds A to D, and carbon dioxide. For 8 hours, the circuit was operated to allow the soda lime temperature to increase freely or with the soda lime chilled by ice.

Results.—When the soda lime temperature was allowed to increase, it reached a maximum of about 46°C. With time, concentrations of compounds A and B peaked at 23 and 9 ppm, respectively. Compounds C and D formed after 4½ hours of circuit operation. When the soda lime was chilled, its peak temperature was 26°C, preventing the formation of compounds C or D. The circuit concentration of compound A remained at about 10 ppm at all times. Regardless of soda lime chilling, carbon dioxide levels remained constant at 5%.

Conclusion.—The release of volatile sevoflurane degradation products depends in great part on the temperature of soda lime in the circuit. Chilling the soda lime may be a simple and effective way to prevent the release of significant levels of compounds A to D without affecting carbon dioxide absorption or altering sevoflurane concentration.

▶ It is probably not valid to comment about an article of which I am an author, but I will do it anyway! The possibilities that excessive fluoride might be released by hepatic metabolism and that sevoflurane might break down in soda lime into a toxic compound that is also volatile, namely "compound A," prompted us to launch an assault on these 2 problems with sevoflurane, because we and others believed that sevoflurane itself has interesting and potentially useful clinical characteristics.

To solve the problem of fluoride release, we synthesized deuterated sevoflurane, wherein the fluoromethoxy carbon was substituted using 2 deuterium atoms instead of 2 hydrogens. This dramatically slowed the metabolism both in vitro, i.e., with rat liver microsomes, and in vivo (again in rats). We believe the other worrisome part of the molecule, namely its reaction with soda lime, can be ameliorated by removal of the heat generated by the exothermic carbon dioxide/soda lime reaction. Soda lime heats up to about 50°C during typical, modern relatively low-flow situations. Cooling the soda lime to somewhere between 25°C–30°C effectively stops the formation of compound A. Other approaches have attempted to remove compound A after its formation, and still others have tried to use a passive heat exchanger. We believe the latter will prove problematic in operating rooms where the temperature is necessarily kept warm, for example, in the treatment of burns and pediatric patients. Nothing like taking a shot at criticizing one's own paper. Mike Royko would be proud of me.—J.H. Tinker, M.D.

Clinical Enflurane Metabolism by Cytochrome P450 2E1

Kharasch ED, Thummel KE, Mautz D, Bosse S (Univ of Washington, Seattle; Seattle Veteran Affairs Med Ctr)
Clin Pharmacol Ther 55:434–440, 1994   101-95-5-6

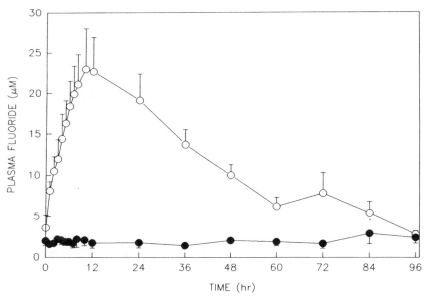

Fig 5–3.—Plasma fluoride concentration (mean ± standard error of the mean) in controls (*open circles*) and disulfiram-treated (*filled circles*) patients. Enflurane was given from 0 to 3 hours, unless the surgical procedure ended before 3 hours. The mean fluoride concentrations in controls were significantly different from preanesthetic values at all time points between 1 and 72 hours. The mean fluoride concentrations in disulfiram-treated patients were not significantly different from preanesthetic values at any time point. The mean fluoride concentrations in disulfiram-treated patients were significantly different from those for controls (P < .05) at all time points between 1 and 36 hours. Each group initially consisted of 10 patients, but the number of patients remaining after day 2 decreased because some patients were discharged from the hospital. (Courtesy of Kharasch ED, Thummel KE, Mautz D, et al: *Clin Pharmacol Ther* 55:434–440, 1994.)

Introduction.—The CYP2E1 isoform of cytochrome P450 is responsible for catalyzing the volatile anesthetic enflurane to the inorganic fluoride ion in human liver microsomes in vitro. Previously, chlorzoxazone and acetaminophen were the only known therapeutic substrates for this enzyme. Whether P450 2E1 is implicated in vivo is unknown. To study this further, enflurane was administered to patients whose P450 2E1 was inhibited with disulfiram.

Methods.—Twenty patients who were undergoing elective surgery lasting fewer than 3–5 hours were divided into 2 groups: 10 who would receive 500 mg of disulfiram the night before surgery and 10 who would receive nothing. All patients were free of hepatic or renal insufficiency, ethanol abuse, or drugs that would alter hepatic drug metabolism. Anesthesia was induced using propofol, fentanyl, and succinylcholine. Once intubated, the anesthesia was maintained with enflurane at a 2.2% end-tidal concentration. Muscle relaxants were avoided when possible. If the surgery lasted more than 3 hours, enflurane was discontinued and anesthesia was maintained with nitrous oxide and fentanyl. Inspired and end-tidal enflurane concentrations were noted every 15 minutes while the patient was intubated. Blood samples for the determination of plasma fluoride and enflurane levels were obtained before induction and hourly for 10 hours after induction of enflurane. More blood samples were collected at 12-hour intervals until 96 hours or hospital discharge, after the start of enflurane administration. Urine was obtained before and for consecutive 24-hour intervals for 96 hours or until hospital discharge. Fluoride concentrations in plasma and urine were determined using an ion-selective electrode.

Results.—Blood levels of enflurane were similar in control and disulfiram-treated patients. Predictably, the plasma fluoride concentrations increased in controls (Fig 5–3), peaking at 10.5 hours after the start of enflurane anesthesia. Disulfiram treatment eliminated the plasma fluoride concentration increase, resulting in no significant time factor changes. Urine fluoride excretion was also abolished with disulfiram treatment.

Conclusion.—A single dose of disulfiram resulted in a nearly complete inhibition of enflurane metabolism, supporting the results of previous in vitro studies. Substantial reductions in plasma fluoride and urinary excretion were demonstrated. These data implicate the P450 2E1 isoform of cytochrome P450 as being the enzyme responsible for enflurane metabolism. Patients with elevated P450 2E1, either from obesity or from long-term isoniazid therapy, could have rapid enflurane metabolism and be at risk for enflurane-associated toxicity. The inhibition by disulfiram may suggest a clinical intervention for minimizing the risk of anesthetic toxicity in sensitive patients.

Identification of Cytochrome P450 2E1 as the Predominant Enzyme Catalyzing Human Liver Microsomal Defluorination of Sevoflurane, Isoflurane, and Methoxyflurane

Kharasch ED, Thummel KE (Univ of Wash, Seattle)
Anesthesiology 79:795–807, 1993   101-95-5-7

Introduction.—Inorganic fluoride ions from the metabolism of volatile fluorinated ether anesthetics may cause subclinical nephrotoxicity or, at excessive concentrations, renal insufficiency. In addition, idiosyncratic hepatic necrosis can be triggered when fluoride metabolites bind to liver proteins. This limits the clinical development of fluorinated anesthetics. The metabolism of such compounds in humans is estimated either by recovery of urinary metabolites or mass balance studies or determined directly in vitro. Of the 14 isoforms of liver cytochrome P450, the 2E1 isoform is implicated in the in vitro metabolism of enflurane, methoxyflurane, and sevoflurane by human liver microsomes. In vivo metabolism of these 3 anesthetics was tested.

Methods.—Hepatic microsomes were prepared from livers of 12 kidney donors, and evidence of anesthetic metabolism was obtained by measuring fluoride metabolism. To evaluate the role of P450 2E1, correlations between P450 2E1 content and defluorination rate, as well as between P450 2E1 catalytic activity and defluorination rate, were determined; chemical inhibitors of P450 isoforms were also determined.

Results.—Anesthetic metabolism was determined by fluoride production, and the rank order of anesthetic defluorination rates was methoxyflurane, sevoflurane, enflurane, isoflurane, and desflurane. There was a significant correlation between P450 2E1 content and defluorination of sevoflurane and methoxyflurane, no matter what method of analysis was used. Defluorination of enflurane, which is known to be metabolized by P450 2E1, was highly correlated with the defluorination rate of sevoflurane. Selective inhibition of P450 2E1 by diethyldithiocarbamate inhibited defluorination of sevoflurane, methoxyflurane, and isoflurane.

Conclusion.—In liver microsomes, the predominant, if not the sole, enzyme that catalyzes the defluorination of sevoflurane is P450 2E1. This enzyme is the primary but not the sole enzyme responsible for the metabolism of methoxyflurane, which is also catalyzed by other isoforms. The enyzme is also accountable for a significant amount of isoflurane metabolism. The high content and activity of P450 2E1 in obese patients are probable mechanisms for their elevated fluoride concentrations.

Serum Inorganic Fluoride Levels in Mildly Obese Patients During and After Sevoflurane Anesthesia

Higuchi H, Satoh T, Arimura S, Kanno M, Endoh R (Natl Defense Med College, Saitama, Japan; Central Hosp of Self Defense Force, Tokyo; Mishuku

Hosp, Tokyo)
Anesth Analg 77:1018–1021, 1993

101-95-5–8

Background.—Sevoflurane is a fluorinated derivative of ethyl isopropyl ether that releases fluoride ion when it is metabolically biodegraded, potentially creating a risk of nephrotoxicity.

Objective.—The extent to which sevoflurane is metabolized to inorganic fluoride was compared in 15 obese men whose body weights were more than 20% greater than ideal and in 16 nonobese patients. All were in good general health and were not taking drugs that induced liver enzymes or altered renal function.

Methods.—Anesthesia was induced with thiopental and was maintained with sevoflurane and 66% nitrous oxide in oxygen for 3½ hours. Blood samples were taken at hourly intervals during anesthesia and for as long as 48 hours afterward.

Results.—The 2 groups of patients received statistically similar doses of sevoflurane, but serum inorganic fluoride levels increased more rapidly and were significantly higher in the obese patients than in nonobese persons at all sampling intervals (Fig 5–4). Eleven obese and 4 nonobese patients had peak fluoride levels greater than 50 μmol/L. No patient had a prolonged change in renal function. Urine osmolality was reduced in the obese patients on the first day after anesthesia, but not significantly. The urinary β_2-microglobulin level increased significantly but remained within normal limits.

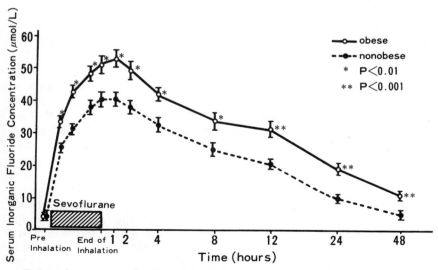

Fig 5–4.—Serum inorganic fluoride levels in 15 obese patients and 16 nonobese patients during and after sevoflurane anesthesia. Data points shown are mean ± standard error. The mean peak value for obese patients is 51.7 ± 2.5 μmol/L. *P < .01; **P < .001 for obese patients compared with nonobese patients. (Courtesy of Higuchi H, Satoh T, Arimura S, et al: *Anesth Analg* 77:1018–1021, 1993.)

Conclusion.—Patients who are mildly obese who receive sevoflurane anesthesia have relatively high serum levels of fluoride ion.

▶ We have known for many years that the cytochrome P450 enzyme system in the liver is important for drug metabolism. Recently, we have become aware that the P450 group of enzymes is made up of more than 30 individual isozymes that have been classified into families and subfamilies. I selected the preceding 3 articles (Abstracts 101-95-5-6 to 101-95-5-8) because of what they tell us about cytochrome P450 2E1 (CYP 2E1), an isoenzyme that is readily induced by ethanol and isoniazid and is responsible for the metabolism of a variety of carcinogens and hepatotoxins. The content of CYP 2E1 is also increased in obesity. It now appears that CYP 2E1 is important in the metabolism of the volatile anesthetics: enflurane, sevoflurane, isoflurane, and methoxyflurane (Abstract 101-95-5-6).

Now we have an explanation for many earlier findings. Chronic isoniazid therapy has been shown to induce enflurane metabolism (increasing fluoride levels) (Abstract 101-95-5-7), and for years, ethanol has been known to stimulate anesthetic metabolism. Finally, fluoride levels are higher after sevoflurane anesthesia in obese patients (Abstract 101-95-5-8), indicating that there is an increased biotransformation of sevoflurane to fluoride. We do not know the effect of ethanol and isoniazid on sevoflurane metabolism, but it might have important implications for toxicity.—M. Wood, M.D.

Closed-Circuit Anesthesia With Sevoflurane in Humans: Effects on Renal and Hepatic Function and Concentrations of Breakdown Products With Soda Lime in the Circuit
Bito H, Ikeda K (Hamamatsu Univ, Japan; Univ Hosp, Hamamatsu, Japan)
Anesthesiology 80:71–76, 1994   101-95-5-9

Background.—Sevoflurane has been widely used in Japan without hepatotoxic or nephrotoxic effects being described. A potential disadvantage of this anesthetic is the generation of possibly toxic breakdown products as a result of its reaction with carbon dioxide (CO_2) absorbent materials. Two such materials, compounds A and B, have been described after heating liquid sevoflurane with soda lime at 70°C for 3 hours.

Objective and Methods.—Breakdown products of sevoflurane were determined in 10 patients with an American Society of Anesthesiologists physical status I or II who received closed-circuit sevoflurane anesthesia for 5 hours or more. The mean duration of anesthesia was 6.9 hours. Anesthesia was induced with thiopental and vecuronium and maintained with sevoflurane in oxygen, adjusted for an end-tidal CO_2 of 30–40 mm Hg. Breakdown products in gas samples taken from the inspiratory limb of the circuit were estimated by gas chromatography.

Results.—Compound A [$CF_2 = C(CF_3)\text{-O-}CH_2F$] was consistently detected. Its concentration peaked at 19.5 ppm 1 hour after anesthesia and

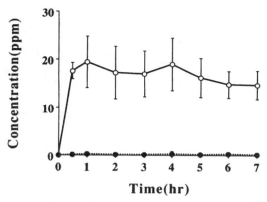

Fig 5–5.—Concentration of breakdown products in the anesthesia circuit. *Open circles* denote concentration of compound A; *filled circles* denote concentration of compound B. All values are means ± 1 SD; *n* = 10. (Courtesy of Bito H, Ikeda K: *Anesthesiology* 80:71–76, 1994.)

declined after 5 hours (Fig 5–5). The highest level recorded was 30 ppm. Compound B [$CH_3OCF_2CH(CF_3)OCH_2F$] was detected in 7 of 10 cases. A level of .17 ppm was present after 30 minutes of anesthesia. The peak mean temperature of the soda lime was 46°C (Fig 5–6). None of the patients had hepatic or renal functional abnormalities that could be attributed to anesthesia.

Conclusion.—Breakdown products of sevoflurane were detected after prolonged closed-circuit anesthesia, but no organ damage resulted.

▶ This is one of many papers that are now emerging from the Japanese experience with sevoflurane. Several ways of ameliorating or eliminating the possibility that sevoflurane might react with soda lime are under investiga-

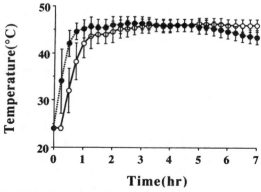

Fig 5–6.—Temperature of soda lime. *Open circles* indicate the temperature of soda lime at the upper point in the lower compartment of the canister; *filled circles* denote the temperature at the lower point in the lower compartment of the canister. All values are means ± 1 SD; *n* = 10. (Courtesy of Bito H, Ikeda K: *Anesthesiology* 80:71–76, 1994.)

tion. Obviously, one way to do it is to eliminate the soda lime! This has been the case for several years now in Japan, simply by using high-flow circuitry and (further) polluting the air in that country.

This article represents an attempt to again resurrect closed-circuit anesthesia. I think it is important to understand why closed-circuit anesthesia has not become popular. It is perceived as dangerous, and it is certainly more difficult to control in less experienced hands.

I don't think this is the way to control the reaction between soda lime and sevoflurane. However, I am biased, because our group has developed another way—heat removal from the CO_2/soda lime reaction.—J.H. Tinker, M.D.

Toxicity of Compound A in Rats: Effect of Increasing Duration of Administration
Gonsowski CT, Laster MJ, Eger EI II, Ferrell LD, Kerschmann RL (Univ of California, San Francisco)
Anesthesiology 80:566–573, 1994   101-95-5–10

Introduction.—Compound A is an olefin, $CF_2 = C(CF_3)OCH_2F$, that results from the degradation of sevoflurane by alkali such as soda lime and Baralyme. Previously, rats exposed to compound A for 3 hours were found to have sustained renal injury and died at an olefin concentration of 331 ppm, which is lower than the concentrations previously reported as producing these effects. The impact of the duration of olefin exposure was assessed in another study.

Methods.—Twenty-three groups of 10 Wistar rats were exposed to compound A concentrations ranging from 0 to 250 ppm in oxygen for periods of 6 or 12 hours. Surviving animals were killed on the first or fourth day after olefin exposure. At those times, specimens of brain, kidney, lung, liver, and small intestine were taken for light microscopic examination, using hematoxylin and eosin stain and a proliferating cell nuclear antigen stain to assess regeneration.

Results.—The mean olefin concentrations that were lethal in 50% of animals were 203 ppm in those exposed for 6 hours and 127 ppm in those exposed for 12 hours. Signs of injury in olefin-exposed rats were detected only in kidney and lung tissue, with pulmonary injury occurring only at near-lethal concentrations. Exposures required to produce renal injury—defined as necrosis of the outer medullary layer or corticomedullary junction—were at or greater than 25 ppm with a 6-hour exposure and 50 ppm with a 12-hour exposure. At these concentrations, cell regeneration was stimulated in a dose-dependent manner.

Conclusion.—The lethal and renal injury–producing concentrations of compound A in rats were inversely related to olefin exposure. These concentrations were 2–4 times greater than those achieved in clinical practice. Minimal nephrotoxicity can occur at concentrations equal to those that can be produced in clinical practice; however, these threshold effects would probably not affect renal function in humans. The lethal and toxic effects are dose related, but they are not simply a function of cumulative dose, that is, concentration over time. Further studies are recommended to assess the issue of safety in humans.

▶ This is one of the more controversial articles presented this year. It is controversial because one of the authors, E.I. ("Ted") Eger, one of the most respected and best-known scholars in our specialty, has been a paid consultant for the Ohmeda Pharmaceutical Company for many years. Dr. Eger has made no secret of this and has forthrightly declared his potential biases because he is such an outstanding scholar.

Ohmeda's patented anesthetic, desflurane, may soon come into direct competition with sevoflurane. Therefore, studies of the potential toxicity of sevoflurane by Dr. Eger could be construed as reflecting conflicts of interest, especially if they indicate, as they do in this article, that compound A, which results from sevoflurane, is more toxic than we thought. The more toxic compound A proves to be, the less desirable sevoflurane might be if it were used with soda lime. Nonetheless, I believe, based on my own bias, that Dr. Eger and his colleagues are correct; sevoflurane's breakdown by soda lime into compound A will be problematic and the threshold levels for toxicity of compound A are probably lower, that is, worse, than previously thought.

One final note. Having offered my opinion about a conflict of interest, I must indicate my own. I have invented an alternative anesthetic to sevoflurane, namely, deuterated sevoflurane. We are also working on a process by which we believe compound A production can be completely inhibited. Therefore, I have my own biases, but they favor sevoflurane, at least in its deuterated form. Ah, such complex webs we weave!—J.H. Tinker, M.D.

Sevoflurane Does Not Increase Intracranial Pressure in Hyperventilated Dogs
Takahashi H, Murata K, Ikeda K (Hamamatsu Univ, Japan)
Br J Anaesth 71:551–555, 1993   101-95-5-11

Introduction.—Because of its low blood-gas partition coefficient and its ability to permit rapid induction and recovery, sevoflurane may be suitable for neurosurgery. However, because it is an ether anesthetic, it may affect intracranial pressure (ICP) and cerebral perfusion pressure, especially in patients with hypocapnia. The effects of sevoflurane, enflurane, and halothane on ICP, cerebral perfusion pressure, and the cardiovascular system were compared in hypocapnic dogs.

Methods.—The mean arterial pressure (MAP), heart rate, central venous pressure, ICP, end-tidal concentrations of volatile anesthetic, carbon dioxide, and oxygen, and arterial blood-gas tensions were measured in 24 anesthetized dogs. The cerebral perfusion pressure was calculated by taking the difference between the MAP and ICP. The measurements were taken 30 minutes after anesthesia was induced with sodium pentobarbitol and pancuronium, with normocapnia being maintained. The dogs were then hyperventilated for at least 15 minutes and randomly assigned to receive halothane, enflurane, or sevoflurane at .5 minimum aveolar concentration (MAC), followed by 1 MAC and 1.5 MAC. Measurements were obtained 15 minutes after induction of each anesthetic concentration. Twenty minutes after the volatile anesthetic was withdrawn, measurements were repeated using only nitrous oxide.

Results.—Baseline measurements revealed no differences in ICP between the groups. Hyperventilation did not change the cerebral perfusion pressure or MAP. The ICP increased significantly with all concentrations of enflurane and halothane, but it remained steady with all concentrations of sevoflurane. The ICP remained high after discontinuation of enflurane and halothane. The CPP and MAP decreased similarly with all 3 agents and remained low after discontinuation of halothane. Decreases in the heart rate were seen after 1 and 1.5 MAC of sevoflurane and halothane and at all concentrations of enflurane.

Discussion.—Sevoflurane did not affect ICP at any concentration, but all concentrations of enflurane and halothane induced increased ICP. The ICP increased before arterial pressure decreased, suggesting that enflurane and halothane directly dilate cerebral vessels. Thus, sevoflurane seems to be suitable during neurosurgery as long as arterial pressure is carefully monitored.

▶ This is one of many articles from Japan that catalogue the massive experience with sevoflurane, a drug that probably will soon be introduced in the United States.—J.H. Tinker, M.D.

Effects of Sevoflurane on Cerebral Circulation and Metabolism in Patients With Ischemic Cerebrovascular Disease
Kitaguchi K, Ohsumi H, Kuro M, Nakajima T, Hayashi Y (Natl Cardiovascular Ctr, Osaka, Japan)
Anesthesiology 79:704–709, 1993   101-95-5–12

Introduction.—The features of rapid induction and recovery that are characteristic of sevoflurane anesthesia make it an attractive agent for neurosurgical anesthesia. However, the effects of sevoflurane on cerebral circulation and metabolism have not been studied in humans. The effects of sevoflurane on cerebral blood flow (CBF) and cerebral metabolic rate for oxygen ($CMRO_2$) were studied in patients with ischemic cerebrovascular disease.

Methods.—Anesthesia was maintained with .99 minimum alveolar concentration sevoflurane in 10 patients who were undergoing extracranial-intracranial arterial anastomosis for correction of unilateral carotid artery stenosis. Cerebral blood flow was measured using the Kety-

Schmidt technique, with 33% argon inhalation during 5 conditions: normocapnea-normotension, hypocapnea-normotension, hypercapnea-normotension, normocapnea-normotension, and normocapnea-hypertension. The measurements were taken with the partial pressure of carbon dioxide in arterial blood ($PaCO_2$) at levels of 40, 35, and 45 mm Hg and with the mean arterial pressure (MAP) increased by 20–25 mm Hg with a methoxamine infusion.

Results.—During normocapnic-normotensive conditions, CBF was 28/100 g^{-1}/min^{-1} and $CMRO_2$ was 1.34 mL/100 g^{-1}/min^{-1}. Cerebral blood flow decreased when $PaCO_2$ decreased and increased when $PaCO_2$ increased. No significant change occurred in CBF in response to MAP increases.

Discussion.—The CBF was directly reactive to $PaCO_2$ concentrations during sevoflurane anesthesia. However, CBF was unaffected by MAP changes, indicating that cerebral autoregulation was adequately maintained during anesthesia with .88 MAP sevoflurane.

▶ A major drug company expects to market sevoflurane in the United States in 1995. Criticism of the drug involves its release of relatively large amounts of flouride, because the anesthetic is highly metabolized by hepatic cytochrome P450. The agent also reacts with soda lime to produce "compound A," which may be toxic if it is inhaled in sufficient quantities. As far as I know, there have been no questions raised regarding sevoflurane's effects on cerebral circulation or metabolism, which this article confirms.—J.H. Tinker, M.D.

Plasma Inorganic Fluoride Levels With Sevoflurane Anesthesia in Morbidly Obese and Nonobese Patients
Frink EJ Jr, Malan TP Jr, Brown EA, Morgan S, Brown BR Jr (Univ of Arizona, Tucson)
Anesth Analg 76:1333–1337, 1993   101-95-5–13

Introduction.—Metabolism of sevoflurane produces an elevated plasma inorganic fluoride ion concentration. With inhaled anesthetics, inorganic fluoride levels are typically higher in obese than nonobese patients, which makes the obese patients more vulnerable to renal toxicity. Plasma inorganic fluoride ion concentrations were measured during and after sevoflurane anesthesia, and the levels in obese and nonobese patients were compared.

Methods.—Thirteen patients who were morbidly obese and 10 patients who were not obese underwent sevoflurane anesthesia for approximately 1.4 minimum alveolar concentration (MAC) hours. Venous blood was sampled to measure plasma fluoride concentrations and monitor renal and hepatic function preoperatively, hourly during anesthesia, at anesthetic discontinuation, and at 1, 2, 4, 6, 12, and 24 hours after anesthetic discontinuation. Arterial blood was sampled to measure sevoflurane concentrations.

Results.—There were no signs of decreased renal function in either patient group at any time. The 2 groups had similar hepatic function studies pre- and postoperatively. Plasma inorganic fluoride concentrations and the rate of increase in those concentrations were similar in the 2 groups during and after anesthesia. Arterial blood sevoflurane concentrations were nonsignificantly lower in nonobese patients until 30 minutes after induction and were similar thereafter.

Discussion.—There were no significant differences in plasma fluoride concentrations between morbidly obese and nonobese patients with sevoflurane anesthesia, suggesting that obese patients are not at increased risk of anesthesia-related renal dysfunction. The low blood gas solubility coefficient exhibited by sevoflurane and its rapid elimination may protect against prolonged elevations of inorganic fluoride levels in patients, regardless of their body mass index.

▶ A potential for nephrotoxicity from inorganic fluoride released by the metabolism of sevoflurane has been a concern because the fluoromethoxy carbon it contains is relatively easily metabolizable. This study does not indicate that particular difficulties will occur with obese or morbidly obese individuals.—J.H. Tinker, M.D.

Antiemetic Efficacy of Prophylactic Ondansetron in Laparoscopic Surgery: Randomized, Double-Blind Comparison With Metoclopramide
Raphael JH, Norton AC (Pilgrim Hosp, Boston, England)
Br J Anaesth 71:845–848, 1993   101-95-5–14

Background.—Women who undergo gynecologic laparoscopic surgery have a high rate of postoperative nausea and vomiting (PONV) of about 50%. Most of the antiemetics commonly used in these patients are of limited efficacy. Placebo-controlled studies have suggested that ondansetron may be a promising antiemetic in such a setting. Ondansetron and metoclopramide were assessed for their prophylactic antiemetic efficacy in patients undergoing gynecologic laparoscopy as day-case surgery.

Methods.—The randomized, double-blind study included 123 patients undergoing general anesthesia for elective day-case gynecologic laparoscopic surgery. Patients were assigned to receive either ondansetron, 4 mg IV, or metoclopramide, 10 mg IV, immediately before a standard anesthetic regimen. The 2 groups were stratified to ensure that an equal number of patients with previous PONV, the occurrence of which was assessed by observation and questionnaire, were included in each group.

Results.—In the first 6 hours postoperatively, 87% of the ondansetron group and 60% of the metoclopramide group had no PONV. Proportions for the first 24 hours were 82% and 47%, respectively. Among patients with postoperative nausea, the degree of nausea tended to be less in the ondansetron group, including those patients who had experienced PNOV. Those in the 2 groups were no different in their time to awakening or postoperative sedation.

Conclusion.—In patients undergoing day-case gynecologic laparoscopy, ondansetron appeared to be superior to metoclopramide for the prevention of PONV. Clinically and economically, patients with a history of PONV may be an important group to target for ondansetron treatment.

Ondansetron Decreases Emesis After Tonsillectomy in Children
Litman RS, Wu CL, Catanzaro FA (Univ of Rochester, NY)
Anesth Analg 78:478–481, 1994   101-95-5–15

Objective.—A double-blind, randomized, placebo-controlled trial was designed to investigate the efficacy of ondansetron in preventing vomiting after tonsillectomy in children. This recently introduced serotonin antagonist has already been shown to prevent postoperative emesis in adults and chemotherapy-induced emesis in children.

Methods.—Eligible patients were older than 3 years of age, American Society of Anesthesiologists physical status I or II, and scheduled for outpatient tonsillectomy with or without adenoidectomy. Children with a history of motion sickness or preoperative vomiting were not excluded. All 60 study participants were premedicated with oral midazolam, .5 mg/kg, and underwent inhaled induction and maintenance of anesthesia with halothane and nitrous oxide. After IV catheter placement, IV morphine, .075 mg/kg; vecuronium, .1 mg/kg; and either ondansetron, .15 mg/kg, or saline placebo were administered. The 2 patient groups were similar in mean age, weight, male-female ratio, proportion with adenoid removal, time to intubation, duration of anesthesia, and duration of surgery.

Results.—Thirty children in each group completed the protocol. Postoperative emesis occurred in 23% of the ondansetron group vs. 73% of the placebo group. More than half (57%) of the children who received placebo compared with 7% of those who received ondansetron had 2 or more episodes of vomiting. More children in the ondansetron group (8 vs. 1) had received dexamethasone, but analysis limited to those who did not receive dexamethasone yielded similar results.

Conclusion.—Vomiting is common after tonsillectomy, and many regimens have been used to prevent its occurrence. When given shortly after induction of anesthesia, IV ondansetron, .15 mg/kg, safely and effectively reduced the incidence of vomiting in these children after tonsillectomy, with or without adenoidectomy. A lower dose of the drug might also be beneficial and would reduce the cost of treatment.

Prophylactic Antiemetic Therapy With Patient-Controlled Analgesia: A Double-Blind, Placebo-Controlled Comparison of Droperidol, Metoclopramide, and Tropisetron

Kaufmann MA, Rosow C, Schnieper P, Schneider M (Univ of Basel, Switzerland; Harvard Med School, Boston)

Anesth Analg 78:988–994, 1994
           101-95-5-16

Introduction.—Opioid-induced nausea remains a major problem for patients who use a patient-controlled analgesia (PCA) system for severe postoperative pain. In a placebo-controlled trial, 3 prophylactic antiemetic regimens were compared for their effects on postoperative nausea and vomiting (PONV) during PCA with morphine.

Patients and Methods.—Eligible patients were adults who were scheduled for major orthopedic surgery. All were American Society of Anesthesiologists physical status I or II and candidates for postoperative PCA. The anesthetic regimen used varied according to the type of surgery. Group 1 (67 patients) controls received only morphine from the PCA device; group 2 (71 patients) received metoclopramide mixed with morphine in the PCA syringe; group 3 (70 patients) had droperidol mixed with morphine; and group 4 (78 patients) received tropisetron, not in the PCA device, but as a single IV dose. Patients were assessed postoperatively for frequency and severity of PONV, need for rescue, side effects of the antiemetics, and overall patient satisfaction. A symptom-severity score (STS) based on intensity and duration measured the severity of PONV.

Results.—The average total doses of the antiemetics were 53.8 mg of metoclopramide, 5.99 mg of droperidol, and 6.1 mg of tropisetron. The incidence of PONV over the initial 36-hour postoperative period was 54% in group 1, 40% in group 2, 17% in group 3, and 33% in group 4. Dropiderol (group 3) significantly reduced both the incidence and severity of PONV for the entire 36-hour study. Although tropisetron (group 4) also had a significant antiemetic result, a single bolus was effective for only 18 hours. The benefits of metoclopramide were only marginally significant. Only droperidol reduced the need for rescue medication, but patients who received this agent tended to be sleepier and recalled somewhat more anxiety. The 3 antiemetic prophylaxis groups reported similar side effects and satisfaction scores.

Conclusion.—Administration of opioids with a PCA system for postoperative pain can aggravate PONV. The addition of droperidol to PCA morphine was very effective in reducing the incidence and severity of PONV. Tropisetron was also a useful antiemetic, but more than 1 dose was required during the 36-hour postoperative study.

▶ Nausea and vomiting are common and important problems after anesthesia and surgery, especially in these days of increased outpatient anesthesia costs, accountability, and the need for operating room efficiency. Postoperative nausea and vomiting may be as high as 70% after some operations. Thus, antiemetic drugs are often used to both prevent and treat PONV, but they may have adverse side effects.

Droperidol has been shown to be effective, but it may be associated with sedative and extrapyramidal symptoms. A new class of drugs, the 5-hydroxy-tryptamine$_3$ (5-HT$_3$) receptor antagonists, such as ondansetron, granisetron, and tropisetron, has recently been developed in an attempt to produce antiemetic drugs with fewer side effects. Ondansetron has been shown to be effective in decreasing PONV (Abstracts 101-95-5–14 and 101-95-5–15) when compared with placebo (1, 2), and we are now observing the publication of comparative trials, for example, with metoclopramide.

The study that compared droperidol, metoclopramide, and tropisetron in the prevention of PONV during patient controlled analgesia with morphine (Abstract 101-95-5–16) once again confirmed the high incidence (about 50%) of PONV when opioids are administered.

I think that the careful use of opioids can be very helpful in preventing PONV. Should antiemetics only be given to treat PONV, or should they be given prophylactically to prevent nausea and vomiting in specific clinical settings (3)? For example, the administration of antiemetics such as droperidol to a patient who might not have had nausea and vomiting develop may cause sedation and delay discharge from an outpatient facility. New drugs with fewer side effects may mean that it is beneficial to give them routinely, but we need further information. Therefore, although this new class of drugs, which is exemplified by ondansetron, may indeed have fewer sedative and extrapyramidal side effects, its exact role in clinical practice remains to be defined.—M. Wood, M.D.

References

1. McKenzie R, et al: *Anesthesiology* 78:21, 1993.
2. Dershwitz M, et al: *Clin Pharmacol Ther* 52:96, 1992.
3. White PF, Watcha MF: *Anesthesiology* 78:2, 1993.

Use of *Drosophila* Mutants to Distinguish Among Volatile General Anesthetics
Campbell DB, Nash HA (Natl Inst of Mental Health, Bethesda, Md)
Proc Natl Acad Sci U S A 91:2135–2139, 1994   101-95-5–17

Background.—The potency of anesthetic gases is largely differentiated by their solubility in olive oil. Should these gases be thought of as equivalent entities that can be discriminated only by their solubility, or do these gases produce their clinical effects in a distinctive manner? Gases could be discriminated among if their potency differed with genetic variations. The fruit fly *Drosophila melanogaster* is affected by a variety of volatile agents. Halothane-resistant (har) genetic mutations of *Drosophila* especially show altered postural responses to halothane. Eight volatile gases were tested on 4 mutant strains of har fruit flies to seek differences among anesthetic agents.

Methods.—Mutant har fruit flies of the OreR strain were used. The tail-flick assay was performed in a rectangular glass chamber. Ten flies were placed inside, and a beam of light was projected into the chamber. Untreated flies walked out of the beam. When anesthesia was introduced, some flies walked out, others jumped out and exhibited paroxysmal movements, and still others showed no movement in response to the light. This last response was the behavior of interest. An inebriometer assay was performed on large groups (20–100) of male flies. The inebriometer is a tall glass column containing mesh baffles on which flies can rest. When an anesthesia is pumped into the chamber, flies lose control of their posture and fall out of the column. Data were recorded as percentages of flies eluted after 30 minutes. The gases studied were methoxyflurane, trichloroethylene, chloroform, halothane, enflurane, isoflurane, diethyl ether, and desflurane.

Results.—Within the 4 strains of flies, the agents enflurane, isoflurane, and desflurane had similar potencies; thus, they probably have similar mechanisms of action. The similarity in chemical structure suggests that the targets of anesthesia are sensitive to that structure. The postural assay results argued against a pharmacokinetic mechanism in any of the mutations.

Conclusion.—Significant information was provided regarding the theoretical debate about the diversity of action of anesthetic agents at their target. That 3 methyl ethyl ethers tested were similar in their interactions with each other but differed from the other gases tested lends credence to this hypothesis.

▶ The reader is referred to *Anesthesia and Analgesia* for an article by Allada and Nash on this subject (1). These authors are first-class molecular geneticists, who believe that the vast knowledge base that geneticists have established for *Drosophila* can be used to separate various *Drosophila* mutants that are more rather than less resistant to anesthetics. Because so much is known about the genetics of each mutant, their theory is that they might be able to figure out the genetics of "anesthetic resistance." If they could do that, they might be able to nail down the genuine molecular site of action of the volatile anesthetic. In my editorial, entitled "Ice crystals to fruit flies," which accompanied their article, I worried that these authors might simply prove to be the latest in a long line of brilliant investigators from other fields who have attempted to solve the "mystery" of the mechanism of general anesthesia. Although I wish them the best, truly great biological minds going all the way back to that of Claude Bernard have tackled this problem. Nonetheless, theirs is a fascinating approach. I will stay tuned.—J.H. Tinker, M.D.

Reference

1. Allada R, Nash HA: *Anesth Analg* 77:19, 1993.

Effects of Halothane on EDRF/cGMP-Mediated Vascular Smooth Muscle Relaxations

Hart JL, Jing M, Bina S, Freas W, Van Dyke RA, Muldoon SM (George Mason Univ, Fairfax, Va; Uniformed Services Univ of the Health Sciences, Bethesda, Md; Henry Ford Hosp, Detroit)
Anesthesiology 79:323–331, 1993   101-95-5–18

Introduction.—Halothane appears to have a number of direct and indirect effects on vascular smooth muscle. In a variety of vessels, this volatile anesthetic is reported to inhibit endothelium-dependent relaxation. Whether this inhibition is caused by interference with synthesis, release, or action of endothelium-derived relaxing factor on cyclic guanosine monophosphate (cGMP) levels within the vascular smooth muscle was determined.

Methods.—Thoracic aortas were removed from halothane-anesthetized male Sprague-Dawley rats. Aortic rings were suspended in aerated Krebs solution and contracted to a stable plateau with EC_{60-70} norepinephrine (NE). Relaxations caused by acetylcholine (ACh), nitric oxide (NO), or nitroglycerine (NG) in the aortic rings contracted with NE were compared in the absence and presence of halothane (.5, 1, and 2 minimum alveolar concentration [MAC]). A radioimmunoassay kit was used to analyze the frozen tissues for cGMP content.

Results.—The ACh-induced relaxations were significantly attenuated in the presence of halothane, an effect that was reversible and occurred

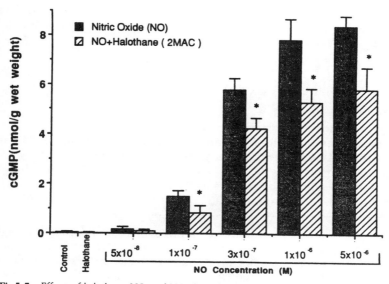

Fig 5–7.—Effects of halothane, NO, and NO plus halothane on cGMP content (nm/g wet weight) of rat aortic rings without endothelium. *Significant difference from NO-treated vessels. $P < .05$ and $n = 4-5$. (Courtesy of Hart JL, Jing M, Bina S, et al: *Anesthesiology* 79:323–331, 1993.)

in a concentration-dependent manner. Halothane (2 MAC) significantly attenuated NO-induced relaxations at all concentrations and NG-induced relaxations at low concentrations in denuded vessels. Halothane alone did not significantly change cGMP content, but it significantly decreased NO stimulation of cGMP concentrations of 10^{-7} M and greater (Fig 5-7).

Conclusion.—Halothane significantly inhibited vascular relaxation induced by ACh, NO, and the nitrovasodilator NG in rat aortic ring preparations. Thus, the site of action of halothane in this experimental setting is within the vascular smooth muscle, and its action may involve interference with guanylate cyclase activation. The inhibitory effect of halothane on the guanylate cyclase–mediated relaxation pathway in vascular smooth muscle is dose-related.

▶ Vascular tone is regulated by opposing factors that mediate vasodilation and vasoconstriction. Over the past 10 years, we have seen tremendous advances in our understanding of the factors that modulate vascular tone. Nitric oxide causes smooth muscle relaxation through the NO-signaling pathway: L-arginine/NO synthase/NO/cGMP (1). We know that halothane inhibits endothelium-dependent relaxation, but we do not know the mechanism. At what site(s) on the NO cascade does halothane exert its effect? Does halothane inhibit the synthesis and release of NO, or does halothane interfere with guanylate cyclase?

This report by Hart and colleagues shows that halothane decreases NO stimulation of cGMP in vitro. They suggest that halothane might bind to guanylate cyclase at the NO-binding site and make it unresponsive to NO. These experiments do not rule out inhibition of NO production by inhalational anesthetics.—M. Wood, M.D.

Reference

    1. Moncada S, Higgs A: N *Engl J Med* 329:2002, 1993.

Pharmacokinetics of Remifentanil (GI87084B) and Its Major Metabolite (GI90291) in Patients Undergoing Elective Inpatient Surgery
Westmoreland CL, Hoke JF, Sebel PS, Hug CC Jr, Muir KT (Emory Univ, Atlanta, Ga; Glaxo Inc, Research Triangle Park, NC)
Anesthesiology 79:893–903, 1993   101-95-5–19

Purpose.—The new synthetic μ-opioid agonist, remifentanil, is highly potent, with a rapid onset and short duration of action because of its rapid hydrolysis by esterases in blood and tissue. Its major metabolite, GI90291, is much less potent than remifentanil itself. The pharmacokinetics of remifentanil and GI90291 were assessed in 24 patients undergoing elective inpatient surgery.

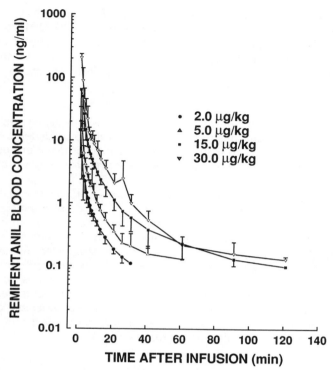

Fig 5–8.—Mean (± standard deviation) blood concentration time curves after a 1-minute infusion of remifentanil at doses of 2 (*circle*), 5 (*open triangle*), 15 (*square*), and 30 μg/kg (*open upside-down triangle*); *n* = 6 for each dose. (Courtesy of Westmoreland CL, Hoke JF, Sebel PS, et al: *Anesthesiology* 79:893–903, 1993.)

Methods.—After the induction of anesthesia and tracheal intubation, the patients received a 1-minute infusion of remifentanil, 2, 5, 15, or 30 μg/kg (Fig 5–8). Within the subsequent 6 hours, arterial blood samples were collected and assayed for remifentanil and GI90291.

Results.—The total remifentanil clearance was 250 to 300 L/hr, independent of dose, and was about 3 or 4 times greater than normal hepatic blood flow. The volume of distribution at a steady state, also independent of dose, was 25 to 40 L. Remifentanil's terminal half-life ranged from 10 to 21 minutes. The total remifentanil clearance was unaffected by patient weight, age, and gender, suggesting that it did not have to be dosed according to weight for adult patients. A simulation study showed that the time required for a 50% reduction in the effect-site concentration was fewer than 4 minutes compared with 34 minutes for sufentanil, 59 minutes for alfentanil, and 262 minutes for fentanyl. The pharmacokinetics of GI90291, which had a mean terminal half-life of 88–137 minutes, were independent of the dose of remifentanil.

Conclusion.—The pharmacokinetics of remifentanil reflect its rapid elimination by blood and tissue esterases. Although GI90291, its major metabolite, is eliminated more slowly, its low potency makes it unlikely to have any significant effect. With its rapid onset and short-lasting action, remifentanil is well suited for titration of an infusion rate to achieve the desired degree of effect.

▶ Remifentanil is a unique new opioid that is selective for the μ-receptor. An ester linkage in its chemical structure means that the drug undergoes rapid hydrolysis by circulating and tissue esterases in a manner that is analogous to the metabolism of the ultra-short-acting selective β-adrenergic blocking agent, esmolol.

I selected this article because remifentanil has the potential to be an important new drug in the anesthesiologist's armamentarium. Its pharmacokinetic profile results in a rapid onset and a short duration of effect so that it can be given by continuous IV infusion and titrated according to each patient's requirements. However, much more remains to be determined, for example, the side effects in a large number of patients. The advantages of remifentanil in certain clinical settings such as outpatient surgery are obvious. As Rosow points out in an accompanying editorial (1), it is also of interest to determine how remifentanil is metabolized in patients with renal and hepatic disease. More clinical trials of remifentanil are under way, so we will probably be hearing more of this interesting drug.—M. Wood, M.D.

Reference

1. Rosow L: *Anesthesiology* 79:875, 1993.

Ethnic Differences in Response to Morphine

Zhou HH, Sheller JR, Nu H, Wood M, Wood AJJ (Vanderbilt Univ, Nashville, Tenn; Hunan Med Univ, Changsha, People's Republic of China)
Clin Pharmacol Ther 54:507–513, 1993   101-95-5–20

Background.—Increased attention has recently been devoted to ethnic differences as an important determinant of interindividual variability in drug response. The interethnic difference in the disposition or response to morphine between Chinese and white healthy males was studied.

Patients and Methods.—Eight Chinese and 8 white males, with a mean age of 29 and 27.5, respectively, were evaluated. All individuals were nonsmokers, did not regularly drink alcohol, and were not taking medications. Intravenous morphine, .15 mg/kg, was given to each participant over a 10-minute period. Blood samples were obtained over a 12-hour period, and urine was collected over a 48-hour period. Partial metabolic and renal clearances were analyzed, as was the respiratory response to morphine, which was determined by measuring minute ventilation and end-tidal carbon dioxide at rest and in response to rebreathing carbon dioxide.

Results.—Chinese individuals showed a significantly higher clearance of morphine than white participants, because of an increase in the partial metabolic clearance by glucuronidation. No interethnic difference in the metabolism to normorphine was noted. Morphine depressed the respiratory response to rebreathing carbon dioxide to a greater degree in white participants, leading to a greater decrease in resting ventilation and resting end-tidal partial pressure of carbon dioxide (PCO_2) compared with Chinese participants. The slope of the ventilation/PCO_2 response curve (a measure of carbon dioxide sensitivity) was also more greatly reduced in white participants, resulting in a greater depression in ventilation at a PCO_2 of 55 mm Hg compared with Chinese participants. Morphine-induced reductions in blood pressure were also higher in white than in Chinese participants.

Conclusion.—Chinese and white individuals differ in their ability to metabolize morphine. Therefore, ethnicity is an important determinant of the disposition and effects of morphine.

▶ Given the authorship, I almost did not select this article, but in the end I decided to go for it! For many years, anecdotal reports have suggested that Chinese patients are more sensitive to opioids, including morphine; however, this study shows the exact opposite. White subjects had a greater depression in ventilation, whereas a morphine-induced reduction in blood pressure was also greater in white subjects than in Chinese subjects. However, the gastrointestinal effects were greater in the Chinese subjects.

I selected this article because pharmacogenetics, ethnicity, and pharmacoanthropology are important new areas in pharmacology. With a new understanding of the genetic determinants of drug metabolism, scientists can now predict some interethnic differences in drug metabolism and response. A recent Food and Drug Administration advisory committee also emphasized the importance of looking for interethnic differences in drug metabolism and sensitivity.—M. Wood, M.D.

Augmented Thermic Effect of Amino Acids Under General Anaesthesia: A Mechanism Useful for Prevention of Anaesthesia-Induced Hypothermia

Selldén E, Brundin T, Wahren J (Karolinska Hosp, Stockholm)
Clin Sci 86:611–618, 1994   101-95-5–21

Background.—Hypothermia commonly develops in patients receiving anesthesia. By some unknown mechanism, IV infusion of amino acids stimulates energy expenditure and heat accumulation in normal humans. If this process works during general anesthesia, giving amino acids might prevent anesthesia-induced hypothermia. Thermogenesis was measured

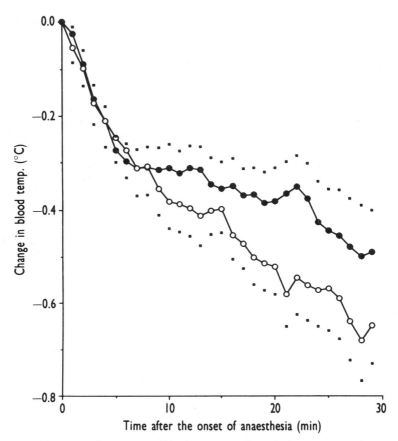

Fig 5–9.—Changes in pulmonary arterial blood temperature during the first 30 minutes of anesthesia in 11 controls (*open circles*) and 10 patients (*filled circles*) receiving IV infusion of amino acids (4 kJ/min) started at the onset of anesthesia. *Squares* indicate ± of stand error of the mean of mean changes. (Courtesy of Selldén E, Brundin T, Wahren J: *Clin Sci* 86:611–618, 1994.)

before, during, and after anesthesia and surgery in patients receiving IV infusion of an amino acid solution or a nutrient-free standard saline infusion.

Methods.—Twenty-one men were scheduled for abdominal surgery. During anesthesia, 10 patients received a mixture of 19 amino acids, 240 kJ/hr, by IV infusion; the other 11 received saline. Cardiac output, arteriovenous oxygen difference, pulmonary oxygen uptake, and mixed blood temperature were measured using pulmonary and systemic artery catheters.

Results.—Blood temperature during anesthesia and surgery decreased at a rate of .67°C/hr in the controls vs. .38°C/hr in the amino acid group (Fig 5-9). The temperature difference between the 2 groups became sig-

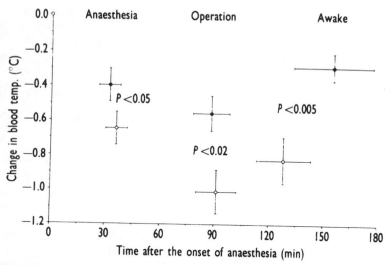

Fig 5–10.—Changes in pulmonary arterial blood temperature during anesthesia, operation, and awakening in 11 controls (*open circles*) and 10 patients (*filled circles*) receiving IV infusion of amino acids (4 kJ/min) started at the onset of anesthesia. *Vertical bars* indicate ± standard error of the mean (SEM) of mean changes. *Horizontal bars* indicate ± SEM of time after the onset of anesthesia. (Courtesy of Selldén E, Brundin T, Wahren J: *Clin Sci* 86:611–618, 1994.)

nificant 20 minutes after the onset of anesthesia and remained so throughout the study (Fig 5–10). Anesthesia, which was given at a mean of 34 minutes before surgery, resulted in reductions in pulmonary oxygen uptake: 145 mL/min in controls and 81 mL/min in the amino acid–treated patients. These reductions corresponded to reductions in the total energy expenditure of 47 W and 26 W, respectively. The 21-W difference between the 2 groups represented the thermogenic action of the amino acids and compared with a 4-W value observed in unanesthetized individuals who were given the same amino acid infusion for 30 minutes. When the patients awoke, oxygen consumption increased to 71% more than the preanesthetic level in the amino acid group. These patients quickly returned to normothermia without shivering. By contrast, oxygen uptake remained slightly below the preanesthetic level in the controls, even with sustained hypothermia and vigorous shivering.

Conclusion.—General anesthesia with muscle relaxation augments fivefold the thermic effect of amino acids. Giving a balanced mixture of amino acids by IV infusion effectively prevents anesthesia-induced hypometabolism and hypothermia. More research is needed to define the optimal duration of the preanesthetic infusion period.

▶ This article comes under the "too good to be true" category. Could we really "jazz up" our patients' temperatures when we see them falling off during anesthesia simply by infusing amino acids? There must be a down side to this. This article is an example of a truly innovative combination of facts about awake patients in the nutrition literature and our knowledge about hypothermia during anesthesia. I hope it generates further controversy and/or confirmation, because if there aren't any particularly problematic side effects, it would be an important addition to our armamentarium.—J.H. Tinker, M.D.

Methionine Prevents Nitrous Oxide-Induced Teratogenicity in Rat Embryos Grown in Culture

Fujinaga M, Baden JM (Stanford Univ, Calif)
Anesthesiology 81:184–189, 1994   101-95-5-22

Introduction.—Nitrous oxide–induced teratogenicity is well documented in rats. Its mechanisms are unknown, but they may involve decreased tetrahydrofolate, resulting in decreased DNA synthesis. Decreased methionine and the sympathomimetic effects of nitrous oxide were studied using a rat whole-embryo culture model.

Methods.—Whether supplemental methionine or folic acid could prevent nitrous oxide–induced teratogenicity, and whether α_1-adrenergic stimulation mediates nitrous oxide–induced situs inversus were determined. Rat embryos were explanted on the ninth day of ingestion. Those at the late primitive streak stage, or stage 10b, were cultured with or wihout nitrous oxide and various chemicals: methionine, 25 μg/mL^{-1}; folinic acid, 5 μg/mL^{-1}; phenylephrine, .5 to 50 μM; and prazosin, 10 μM. For those exposed to nitrous oxide, the concentration was 75% for the first 24 hours of culture. Situs inversus and other abnormalities were evaluated after 50 hours of culture.

Results.—Malformations and growth retardation were more common in embryos treated with nitrous oxide alone. These abnormalities were almost entirely prevented by methionine but not by folinic acid or prazosin. Situs inversus did not result from nitrous oxide per se, but nitrous oxide exposure increased the incidence of this abnormality in embryos that were exposed to phenylephrine. Prazosin blocked this additive effect.

Conclusion.—Decreased methionine rather than decreased tetrahydrofolate plays the most important role in nitrogen oxide–induced teratogenicity in rats. Nitrous oxide stimulation of the α_1-adrenergic pathway in rat embryos results in an increased incidence of phenylephrine-induced situs inversus. Nitrous oxide–induced teratogenicity is obviously a multifactorial process. Further studies are needed to examine its molecular mechanisms in detail.

▶ Most anesthesiologists agree that patients in early pregnancy should not be anesthetized at all if possible. However, if it is necessary to anesthetize a patient during early pregnancy, there may be an increased incidence of spontaneous abortion or worse. Whether methionine, when it is given prophylactically to patients who are in early pregnancy and must undergo anesthesia and surgery, will be beneficial is certainly open to question, but one wonders whether it might not prove efficacious. There seems to be considerable interest in methionine this year.—J.H. Tinker, M.D.

Preoperative Methionine Loading Enhances Restoration of the Cobalamin-Dependent Enzyme Methionine Synthase After Nitrous Oxide Anesthesia

Christensen B, Guttormsen AB, Schneede J, Riedel B, Refsum H, Svardal A, Ueland PM (Armauer Hansens hus, Bergen, Norway)
Anesthesiology 80:1046–1056, 1994   101-95-5–23

Introduction.—Individuals who have prolonged exposure to nitrous oxide show adverse effects similar to those of cobalamin deficiency, which is the result of irreversible oxidation of cobalamin bound to methionine synthase. Nitrous oxide's inactivation of methionine synthase in cultured human fibroblasts is decreased at high methionine concentrations in the culture medium. The potential of preoperative methionine loading to protect against cobalamin inactivation in patients undergoing nitrous oxide anesthesia was assessed.

Methods and Results.—The study sample included 14 patients who received nitrous oxide anesthesia for 75 to 230 minutes. Two hours before the start of anesthesia, half the patients received an oral loading dose of methionine. All patients showed considerable inactivation of methionine synthase in mononuclear white blood cells after nitrous oxide exposure, which reached a nadir at 5–48 hours. Enzyme activity did not recover completely within 1 week in the patients who were not pretreated with methionine. For those who did, the kinetics of methionine synthase activation were similar; however, the rate and extent of enzyme recovery were higher. For 4 patients in the methionine-loading group, the enzyme activity exceeded even the preoperative level.

Methionine synthase inactivation was associated with a transient increase in plasma homocysteine, which was still elevated 1 week after anesthesia in the patients who did not receive methionine. The homocysteine concentration peaked markedly immediately after anesthesia in the methionine group, and it was still elevated at 1 week. Neither nitrous oxide exposure nor methionine loading affected the activity of methylmalonyl coenzyme A mutase in the mononuclear white blood cells or the serum concentration of methylmalonic acid.

Conclusion.—Patients with brief exposure to nitrous oxide show selective impairment of the cobalamin-dependent enzyme methionine synthase. Preoperative methionine loading can counteract the adverse effects of nitrous oxide. Long-term follow-up studies of methionine prophylaxis in patients who are receiving prolonged nitrous oxide anesthesia are needed.

▶ The authors have shown that nitrous oxide's well-known inhibition of methionine synthase can be counteracted by loading the patient with methionine. However, when they get to the clinical implications, things get really weak. They talk about the "debilitated or cobalamin-deficient patient undergoing prolonged anesthesia." Do they mean "general debility"? Would you seriously consider giving methionine for "general debility"? I wouldn't. The next sentence under "Clinical Implications" is even more amazing. The authors note that "methionine administration protects monkeys or fruits bats against neurologic impairment caused by nitrous oxide. . . ." I wasn't aware that either monkeys or fruit bats are usually included under the rubric "clinical." The truth is that nitrous oxide anesthesia probably doesn't really hurt very much. However, I doubt that methionine prophylaxis will catch on.—J.H. Tinker, M.D.

Efficacy and Kinetics of Extradural Ropivacaine: Comparison With Bupivacaine

Morrison LMM, Emanuelsson BM, McClure JH, Pollok AJ, McKeown DW, Brockway M, Jozwiak H, Wildsmith JAW (Royal Infirmary of Edinburgh, Scotland; Astra Pain Control AB, Sodertalje, Sweden)
Br J Anaesth 72:164–169, 1994   101-95-5-24

Introduction.—The new local anesthetic drug, ropivacaine, is considered to be an alternative to bupivacaine. Early studies suggest that extradural injection of each produced similar sensory blocks, with ropivacaine producing a less intense and shorter motor block. The hypothesis that a small volume of a high concentration might produce a less variable block compared with a larger volume of a lower concentration was tested. Drug kinetics were also studied.

Methods.—Ninety-one patients, aged 19–70, undergoing elective surgery for varicose veins or inguinal hernia repair were randomly divided into 3 groups: 20 mL of ropivacaine at 5 mg/mL, 10 mL of ropivacaine at 10 mg/mL, and 20 mL of bupivacaine at 5 mg/mL. Extradural injections at the second or third lumbar space were performed in a double-blinded manner. Drugs were injected in 25% increments in slightly more than 3 minutes; surgery followed at least 30 minutes later. During this time, sensory block was tested at 2 and 5 minutes post injection as well as every 5 minutes for the full 30 minutes. The block was judged every 30 minutes until it was deemed to have completely regressed. Motor block was assessed at similar intervals using a modified Bromage scale, where 0 stood for able to raise extended leg and 3 stood for unable to move leg. Assessments were performed by an investigator who was blinded to the grouping. Blood pressure and heart rate were recorded for the first 3 hours. Hypotension and bradycardia were treated according to standard practices. A decision about the quality of the block was made before surgery. If it was judged to be inadequate, general anesthesia was administered. In 10 patients from each group, drug kinetics, including peak concentration, time to peak concentration, and area under the curve, were determined over a 28-hour period.

Results.—All solutions produced an effective block within 30 minutes, with a median onset time of 5–20 minutes for all groups across various dermatomal levels. The cephalad level of block was at the seventh thoracic vertebra in 25 minutes for all groups. There was no significant difference in onset times of motor block; however, the duration of grade I motor block with the .5% bupivacaine group exceeded that of the .5% ropivacaine group. The quality of the block was judged to be unsatisfactory in nearly one third of the 1% ropivacaine group vs. half of the other 2 groups. The most common adverse effects were hypotension and postoperative headache and backache. None of the events were severe, and all patients recovered normally. The peak concentration of ropivacaine was significantly higher than that of bupivacaine, whereas the time to peak was similar across groups. The half-life of ropivacaine was 5.3 and 5.5 hours for the 1% and .5% groups, respectively, whereas that of bupivacaine was 10.6 hours (significantly longer than that of the ropivacaine groups).

Conclusion.—Equal doses and concentrations of ropivacaine and bupivacaine produced virtually identical sensory blocks. There were no differences in duration at any dermatomal level. The motor block from ropivacaine was of less intensity and duration than that of bupivacaine. A smaller volume of ropivacaine at a higher concentration produced poorer-quality anesthesia. Ropivacaine kinetics did not differ by concentration, but they were different from those for bupivacaine.

▶ The systemic cardiotoxicity of bupivacaine has stimulated a search for new local anesthetics. Ropivacaine is a new amide local anesthetic that has a chemical structure similar to that of bupivacaine, but it is less potent and less lipid-soluble. Clinical trials appear promising, and although no patients showed any symptoms of systemic toxicity in this study, ropivacaine's role in clinical practice remains to be determined.—M. Wood, M.D.

A Multicentre Randomized Study of Single-Unit Dose Package of EMLA Patch vs EMLA 5% Cream for Venepuncture in Children
Chang PC, Goresky GV, O'Connor G, Pyesmany DA, Rogers PCJ, Steward DJ, Stewart JA (Alberta Children's Hosp, Calgary, Canada; British Columbia's Children's Hosp, Vancouver, Canada; Izaak Walton Killam Hosp for Children, Halifax, NS, Canada)
Can J Anaesth 41:59–63, 1994
101-95-5–25

Background.—Eutectic mixture of local anesthetics (EMLA) cream, which contains lidocaine and prilocaine as well as an emulgent and thickener, reportedly relieves pain associated with skin procedures in both children and adults. The total concentration of local anesthetics in the emulsion is only 5%, but each droplet of cream contains a high concentration. A patch has been developed to make it easier to apply the active product. It is a prepackaged dressing that contains 1 g of 5% EMLA emulsion surrounded by an adhesive ring.

Study Plan.—An open, randomized trial was carried out at 5 pediatric centers to compare the EMLA patch with EMLA cream in 178 children aged 3–10 years, who required venipuncture. Either an EMLA patch or half the contents of a 5-g tube of EMLA cream plus the standard occlusive dressing, Tegaderm, was applied to the dorsum of 1 hand or antecubital fossa for 1 hour or longer before venipuncture. Both the patient and an observer quantified pain on a 3-point verbal rating scale.

Results.—No more than slight pain occurred in 95% of children who were given an EMLA patch and 94% of those treated with EMLA cream. Observers agreed in 95% and 97% of the cases, respectively. Patients found no difference in the discomfort that occurred when the patch or Tegaderm was removed, but observers found that removing the patch was more painful. There was no overall group difference in local reactions.

Conclusion.—Use of the EMLA patch is a convenient form of limiting pain in children who require venipuncture.

ACE Inhibitor Premedication Attenuates Sympathetic Responses During Surgery

Böttcher M, Behrens JK, Møller EA, Christensen JH, Andreasen F (Univ of Aarhus, Denmark; Aarhus Municipal Hosp, Denmark)
Br J Anaesth 72:633–637, 1994   101-95-5–26

Objective.—The hemodynamic and catecholamine responses to surgery after premedication with a normal antihypertensive dose of an angiotensin-converting enzyme (ACE) inhibitor or a β_1-adrenoreceptor blocker were studied for 3 days in patients undergoing abdominal hysterectomy.

Study Design.—In a double-blind, randomized, double-dummy design, 27 patients received either the ACE inhibitor ramipril, 5 mg; the β_1-blocker metoprolol, 10 mg; or placebo on the night before and again 2 hours before surgery. Anesthesia was induced with meperidine followed by thiopental and maintained with halothane, nitrous oxide in oxygen, and meperidine.

Results.—In both the actively treated groups, the mean diastolic arterial pressure was lower by approximately 10 mm Hg during surgery, and increases in heart rate and arterial pressure caused by the skin incision were attenuated. During surgery, stroke volume and cardiac output increased significantly in the ramipril group but not in the metoprolol group. The ramipril group did not show the anticipated increase in plasma norepinephrine concentrations in response to skin incision, and it had persistently lower urinary norepinephrine concentrations during surgery. In the metoprolol group, plasma norepinephrine concentrations were similar to those of the placebo group, and urinary excretion of norepinephrine was decreased only on day 1.

Discussion.—Premedication with an ACE inhibitor attenuates the release of norepinephrine during surgery. This can be mediated by a combination of a reduction in the concentration of angiotensin II in circulating blood and a decrease in sympathomimetic activity, as reflected by low concentrations of norepinephrine in plasma and urine.

▶ Perioperative myocardial ischemia is a major cause of morbidity and death after anesthesia and surgery. The response to surgical stress-induced changes in catecholamines and increased cardiac sympathetic activity has been implicated in the etiology of myocardial ischemia by many investigators. Therapeutic regimens such as the use of α_2-adrenoceptor agonists and β-adrenergic blocking agents have been advocated.

Excessive activation of the sympathetic nervous system is well recognized in congestive cardiac failure, and ACE inhibitor therapy has been shown to have beneficial effects on outcome in this clinical setting. Prejunctional angiotensin II receptors have recently been shown to facilitate norepinephrine release (1). Therefore, it is interesting that ACE inhibitor therapy attenuates sympathetic responses during surgery. However, the authors studied only a small group of patients, and large epidemiologic studies are required to evaluate whether ACE inhibitor therapy represents a new strategy to attenuate the stress response and reduce perioperative cardiac morbidity. It should be emphasized that surrogate end points, such as hemodynamic parameters, transient ECG changes, and a decrease in catecholamines, are not the same as showing a change in outcome.—M. Wood, M.D.

Reference

1. Clemson B, et al: *J Clin Invest* 93:684–691, 1994.

Inhaled Nitric Oxide: Selective Pulmonary Vasodilation in Cardiac Surgical Patients

Rich GF, Murphy GD Jr, Roos CM, Johns RA (Univ of Virginia, Charlottesville)
Anesthesiology 78:1028–1035, 1993   101-95-5–27

Background.—No selective pulmonary vasodilating agent has been available for patients with pulmonary hypertension, but there is increasing evidence that low levels of inhaled nitric oxide (NO), which seems to be an endothelium-derived relaxing factor, have the effect of dilating pulmonary vessels without altering systemic hemodynamics. The effect is

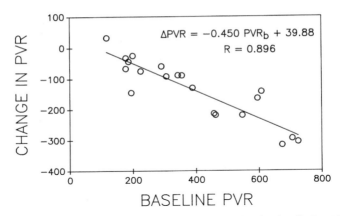

Fig 5–11.—Changes in pulmonary vascular resistance (PVR) (dyne/cm/sec^{-5}) after inhalation of nitric oxide vs. the baseline PVR before cardiopulmonary bypass. (Courtesy of Rich GF, Murphy GD Jr, Roos CM, et al: *Anesthesiology* 78:1028–1035, 1993.)

dose-dependent, but it is not clear whether it correlates with the baseline level of pulmonary vascular resistance (PVR).

Objective and Methods.—Hemodynamic function was monitored in 20 patients who underwent mitral valve replacement and/or coronary bypass graft surgery and who had varying levels of PVR. Five patients who were supported by a ventricular assist device (VAD) were also studied. The participants inhaled 20 ppm of NO for 6 minutes before sternal incision and again after sternal closure.

Results.—Inhalation of NO reduced the pulmonary artery pressure by 7 mm Hg before and by 5 mm Hg after cardiopulmonary bypass and from 68 to 55 mm Hg in patients with a VAD. The PVR decreased substantially in all settings. The reduction in PVR after NO inhalation was proportional to the baseline value (Fig 5–11).

Conclusion.—Inhalation of a low level of NO selectively dilates pulmonary blood vessels in patients undergoing cardiac surgery and also in those whose circulation is supported by a VAD.

▶ We continue to hear more about NO. It is amazing how quickly the discovery that vascular endothelial cells produce NO has progressed to therapeutic use in the operating room. Nitric oxide appears to be a selective pulmonary vasodilator in cardiac patients before and, more important, after cardiopulmonary bypass. Although I think that everyone is looking forward to being able to use NO, it is not an easy gas to administer, and it will have to be introduced into clinical practice very carefully through effective teaching and training.—M. Wood, M.D.

Amrinone Enhances Myocardial Contractility and Improves Left Ventricular Diastolic Function in Conscious and Anesthetized Chronically

Instrumented Dogs
Pagel PS, Hettrick DA, Warltier DC (Med College of Wisconsin, Milwaukee; Zablocki VA Med Ctr, Milwaukee, Wis)
Anesthesiology 79:753–765, 1993   101-95-5–28

Introduction.—Left ventricular mechanical performance is decreased by volatile anesthetics through alterations in intracellular calcium regulation. The negative inotropic effects of volatile anesthetics can be reversed by amrinone; however, the effects of this phosphodiesterase fraction III inhibitor on anesthetic-induced diastolic dysfunction are unknown. Conscious and anesthetized dogs were studied to assess the direct effects of amrinone on left ventricular systolic and diastolic function.

Methods.—Experiments were conducted in 9 dogs that were chronically instrumented for measurement of aortic and left ventricular pressure, maximum rate of increase in left ventricular pressure (dP/dt_{max}), subendocardial segment length, diastolic coronary blood flow velocity, and cardiac output. Measures of myocardial contractility and diastolic function were assessed as well. On 3 different occasions, the dogs received a bolus of amrinone, 1 mg/kg, followed by an infusion of amrinone, 10–80 μg/kg/min^{-1}, while conscious or receiving isoflurane or halothane anesthesia, 1.25 minimum alveolar concentration. At each amrinone dose, hemodynamics and ventricular pressure segment–length loops and waveforms were recorded after a 15-minute equilibration period. All animals were studied during autonomic nervous system blockade, because autonomic activity can influence the hemodynamic actions of both volatile anesthetics and amrinone.

Results.—In the conscious state, amrinone significantly increased the dogs' myocardial contractility in a dose-dependent fashion. The slope of the preload recruitable stroke work relationship was 65 vs. 108 mm Hg at the high amrinone dose. A dose-related shortening of isovolumic relaxation and enhancement of rapid ventricular filling were noted as well. In conscious animals, amrinone reduced regional-chamber stiffness, from a constant of .49 to .31 mm/sec at the high dose. In the same dose, amrinone also enhanced left ventricular systolic function and diastolic function when administered to anesthetized dogs.

Conclusion.—In dogs with autonomic nervous system blockade, both conscious and anesthetized, amrinone has both positive inotropic and lusitropic effects. Amrinone-induced improvements in left ventricular performance appear to result from actions in diastole as well as systole, suggesting that amrinone yields increases in cyclic adenosine monophosphate, which led to enhanced Ca^{2+} availability during systole and simultaneous improvements in Ca^{2+} sequestration during diastole.

▶ There is increasing interest in the use of amrinone these days. Its ability to lower diastolic arterial pressure (and sometimes systolic arterial pressure), despite an increased dynatropic state, has heightened interest in the possibility that amrinone might improve diastolic ventricular function.

This article shows that amrinone may be the first drug that we have in our armamentarium to specifically improve diastolic ventricular function. Now the questions are, What do we do with it? For what kinds of clinical conditions would we use it in the operating room?

It may be that the reason amrinone seems to work better in combination with epinephrine in many patients has to do with its improvement of diastolic ventricular function while epinephrine is working on the systolic side. This is just speculation, but I think we will be hearing more about amrinone in the future.—J.H. Tinker, M.D.

Amrinone Attenuates Airway Constriction During Halothane Anesthesia
Lenox WC, Hirshman CA (Johns Hopkins Univ, Baltimore, Md)
Anesthesiology 79:789–794, 1993   101-95-5-29

Introduction.—By inhibiting the enzymes that metabolize and inactivate cyclic adenosine monophospate (cAMP) and cyclic guanosine monophosphate in airway smooth muscle, cyclic nucleotide phosphodiesterase (PDE) inhibitors may be useful agents for managing patients with cardiac and reactive airway disease during anesthesia. The effects of amrinone, a PDE inhibitor, on airway reactivity to methacholine challenge and on the release of endogenous catecholamine were studied in dogs undergoing anesthesia with thiopental/fentanyl and with halothane.

Methods.—Five dogs were studied in 4 randomly ordered anesthetic conditions that were separated by at least 1 week. The 4 anesthetic protocols were thiopental/fentanyl anesthesia, thiopental/fentanyl anesthesia with amrinone infusion, halothane anesthesia, and halothane anesthesia with amrinone infusion. Lung resistance and dynamic compliance were evaluated during inhalation challenge with increasing doses of methacholine aerosol. Venous blood was drawn immediately after induction of anesthesia and before and after methacholine challenge to measure plasma epinephrine and norepinephrine concentrations.

Results.—Without amrinone infusion, lung resistance increased and dynamic compliance decreased in a dose-related fashion during methacholine challenge with both thiopental/fentanyl and halothane anesthesia. With amrinone infusion, the changes both in lung resistance and dynamic compliance were significantly reduced at all doses of methacholine challenge in dogs under thiopental/fentanyl anesthesia, whereas the increases in lung resistance at the 3 highest doses of methacholine challenge were significantly attenuated in dogs under halothane anesthesia. Pulmonary responses to methacholine were similar with both anesthetic agents. Amrinone infusion did not induce increased plasma epinephrine and plasma norepinephrine concentrations.

Discussion.—Amrinone attenuated airway responses to methacholine, even during halothane anesthesia, by direct effect, rather than indirectly through catecholamine release. Amrinone may have positive effects on both the airways and the cardiovascular system during anesthesia. Therefore, it may have therapeutic usefulness in managing perioperative bronchospasm during inhalational anesthesia.

▶ I selected this article to poke a bit of fun at it. The authors have a well-established dog model of airway constriction in which they have previously shown that halothane is a little better than isolfurane in terms of attenuating airway constriction in response to a methacholine challenge. This article, which "plugs" amrinone into this model, reads like the authors might be reaching a bit for all sorts of drugs to test with their model. Of course, amrinone is a special kind of cAMP inhibitor, and, in that respect, it is related to theophylline. It probably ought to be a reasonable bronchodilator.—J.H. Tinker, M.D.

Intraoperative Octreotide for Refractory Carcinoid-Induced Bronchospasm

Quinlivan JK, Roberts WA (Strong Mem Hosp, Rochester, NY)
Anesth Analg 78:400–402, 1994   101-95-5–30

Introduction.—Carcinoid syndrome occurs in only 18% of patients with carcinoid tumors. Various symptoms can occur, including bronchospasm, which may resist interventions. Octreotide, a long-acting somatostatin analogue, has been used to medically manage patients with carcinoid tumors because it prevents the release of tumor products. Octreotide was used intraoperatively in a patient with carcinoid syndrome associated with a metastatic carcinoid tumor.

Case Report.—Woman, 53, had undergone primary resection of a carcinoid tumor of the terminal ileum and chemotherapy, which did not control hepatic metastasis. She was treated with octreotide for 1 year before she was readmitted with fever and right-sided pelvic pain. She was prepared for exploratory laparotomy and an expected evacuation of a pelvic abscess. Preoperative subcutaneous administration of 150 µg of octreotide preceded induction of anesthesia. After endotracheal intubation, respiration stopped and could not be induced with aerosolized albuterol or isoflurane. The patient became cyanotic and bradycardia and hypotension developed. Octreotide, 200 µg, was administered intravenously, the bronchospasm decreased, and ventilation began within 15 seconds. The hypoxia and bradycardia resolved within 3 minutes. Surgery revealed a metastatic carcinoid tumor of the adnexa and omentum, which was confirmed histologically. The patient was given an additional subcutaneous dose of octreotide before extubation and had no postoperative respiratory complications.

Discussion.—Octreotide should be available during anesthesia induction of all patients with carcinoid tumors. Subcutaneous octreotide therapy also should be maintained perioperatively. A prophylactic supplemental dose of octreotide administered immediately before anesthesia induction might prevent bronchospasm, but this requires more study.

▶ A previous case report (Abstract 101-95-2–4) described the use of octreotide during removal of an insulinoma, but it is important to understand that octreotide is now a mainstay of therapy in the long-term management of malignant carcinoid syndrome, and it is very effective in the management of life-threatening symptoms in the operating room. In this case report, octreotide was rapidly effective in the therapeutic management of refractory carcinoid-induced bronchospasm that occurred at the time of anesthesia induction.

It is important to remember that a common clinical feature of carcinoid syndrome is cutaneous flushing, which may be provoked by many agents, including epinephrine. Thus, hypotensive episodes should not be treated with β-agonists because, by stimulating the release of vasoactive substances from the tumor, they can exaggerate and prolong the cardiovascular disturbance. Therefore, octreotide, rather than albuterol, should be administered to manage bronchospasm.—M. Wood, M.D.

Flumazenil in Cirrhotic Patients in Hepatic Coma: A Randomized Double-Blind Placebo-Controlled Crossover Trial
Pomier-Layrargues G, Giguère JF, Lavoie J, Perney P, Gagnon S, D'Amour M, Wells J, Butterworth RF (Université de Montréal; Northern Regional Forensic Lab, Sault Ste-Marie, Ont, Canada)
Hepatology 19:32–37, 1994   101-95-5–31

Objective.—Patients with biopsy specimen–proven hepatic cirrhosis were examined to determine whether benzodiazepines contributed to neural inhibition in hepatic encephalopathy. Flumazenil specifically antagonized benzodiazepine receptors in the brain.

Design.—Seventy-seven cirrhotic patients, 18 to 70 years of age, in stage 4 hepatic encephalopathy were considered for the prospective, double-blind, crossover trial. After excluding 56 patients who had multiorgan failure or in whom coma had been precipitated by benzodiazepine use, the remaining 21 patients were randomized to receive 2 mg of IV flumazenil or placebo. Two observers evaluated the patients blindly at 15-minute intervals for 6 hours using a modified Glasgow scale, and electroencephalograms were read blindly by 2 independent observers.

Results.—Allowing for the crossover of patients who remained in grade 4 encephalopathy, 13 flumazenil and 15 placebo periods were available for analysis. Encephalopathy improved from grade 4 to grade 2 in 4 flumazenil-treated patients. Two of these patients never returned to

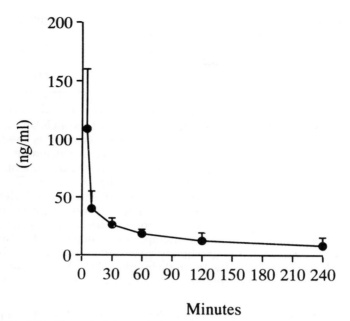

Minutes

Fig 5–12.—Mean (± standard deviation) plasma concentration time profiles of flumazenil in cirrhotic patients in hepatic coma. (Courtesy of Pomier-Layrargues G, Giguère JF, Lavoie J, et al: *Hepatology* 19:32–37, 1994.)

their baseline level of consciousness. Electroencephalographic improvement was observed in 4 actively treated patients and in 2 placebo recipients. The drug was rapidly eliminated from the circulation (Fig 5–12).

Conclusion.—Flumazenil may lessen the severity of neurologic symptoms without causing serious side effects in some patients with cirrhosis who are in a hepatic coma.

▶ Flumazenil has potential benefits other than specifically reversing benzodiazepine-induced respiratory or neurologic depression. As a specific competitive antagonist of only synthetic benzodiazepines, flumazenil is both therapeutic and diagnostic when used in the emergency department to care for comatose patients who are suspected of benzodiazepine overdose. The rationale for flumazenil's use in the treatment of hepatic encephalopathy (HE) is based on the so-called benzodiazepine hypothesis of the pathogenesis of HE. Flumazenil may simply displace endogenous benzodiazepine-like compounds from their γ-aminobutyric acid–like receptors and improve HE.—D.M. Rothenberg, M.D.

Methylprednisolone Increases Sensitivity to β-Adrenergic Agonists Within 48 Hours in Basenji Greyhounds

Sauder RA, Lenox WC, Tobias JD, Hirshman CA (Johns Hopkins Univ, Baltimore, Md)
Anesthesiology 79:1278–1283, 1993   101-95-5–32

Introduction.—Use of the combination of corticosteroids with bronchodilators is more effective in the treatment of bronchospasm than combining a placebo with bronchodilators. Corticosteroids modify β-adrenergic function by changing the rates of receptor degradation and synthesis. As a result, they seem to increase the protective benefits of β-adrenergic agonists against the bronchostimulator stimuli. The time course of this combination therapy is of interest when considering preoperative preparation of patients with reactive airway disease. The Basenji greyhound is less sensitive to albuterol, a β-adrenergic agonist, than control dogs, whereas long-term therapy with methylprednisolone, a corticosteroid, increases the greyhound's sensitivity to albuterol. Basenji greyhounds were pretreated with methylprednisolone for 1, 2, or 7 days to see whether albuterol protected them against methacholine-induced airway constriction.

Methods.—Nine adult greyhounds were studied over a 3-week period before and after daily subcutaneous injections of methylprednisolone under 5 conditions: no pretreatment; pretreatment with IV albuterol, 1μg/kg; and pretreatment with IV albuterol 1, 2, and 7 days after the start of daily corticosteroid, 2mg/kg/day. Anesthesia was introduced, the trachea was intubated, and the dogs were ventilated with 100% oxygen while supported in a standing position. End-tidal carbon dioxide was continuously monitored. Airflow by pneumotachograph, pleural pressure by esophageal balloon, airway opening pressure by airway needle, transpulmonary pressure (difference between pleural pressure and opening pressure), and tidal volume were determined. All channels were connected to a dedicated microprocessor to determine lung resistance and dynamic compliance averaged over 6 breaths. Gas samples were determined at the point of maximal expiratory flow. Thirty minutes after anesthesia, 5 concentrations of methacholine, ranging from .03 to 3 mg/mL, were administered by aerosol until lung resistance increased 200% and compliance decreased to 65% of control levels. Baseline resistance and compliance responses from methacholine challenge were determined when the dogs were untreated, after albuterol pretreatment, and before methylprednisolone treatment.

Results.—Baseline resistance and compliance measures were constant across the conditions. These measures were not changed by administration of methylprednisolone or albuterol before or after the 1-, 2-, and 7-day corticosteroid treatment period. All conditions showed methacholine-induced increases in resistance and decreases in compliance. Albuterol did not alter responses before methylprednisolone treatment to the challenge in control tests. Methylprednisolone did not change airway responses to methacholine in dogs that were pretreated with albuterol after 1 day; however, responsiveness was decreased after 2 days and after 1 week of corticosteroid treatment.

Conclusion.—Sensitivity to the β-adrenergic agonist albuterol within 2 days of treatment is increased with daily methylprednisolone treatment. Whereas the data may not be directly applicable to humans who are asthmatic, 48 hours of corticosteroids before surgery may be beneficial for patients who need intraoperative β-adrenergic agonists.

▶ Hirshman and co-workers have made exciting advances in the management of restrictive airway disease during anesthesia using the Basenji greyhound model. I think it was interesting that a short period of steroid therapy itself had no effect on baseline airway tone but instead increased the effect of β-adrenergic agonists. In asthmatic patients, careful preoperative preparation is the key to avoiding intraoperative problems, and a short period of preoperative steroid therapy can be beneficial for patients who might require a β-adrenergic agonist, such as albuterol.—M. Wood, M.D.

The Competitive NMDA Antagonist MDL-100,453 Reduces Infarct Size After Experimental Stroke
Hasegawa Y, Fisher M, Baron BM, Metcalf G (Medical Ctr of Central Massachusetts-Memorial, Worcester; Univ of Massachusetts, Worcester; Marion Merrell Dow Research Inst, Cincinnati, Ohio)
Stroke 25:1241–1246, 1994   101-95-5–33

Background.—Levels of excitatory amino acids such as glutamate and aspartate increase after an ischemic/hypoxic insult and may stimulate postsynaptic receptors to an excessive degree. Activation of N-methyl-D-aspartate (NMDA) receptors during acute ischemia promotes the entry of calcium ions into neurons and leads to progressive and irreversible neuronal damage. A new competitive antagonist of glutamate, MDL-100,453, acts at the level of the NMDA receptor complex.

Objective.—The neuroprotective efficacy of MDL-100,453 was examined in rats that were subjected to a focal ischemic insult through occlusion of the proximal anterior cerebral artery, distal internal carotid artery, middle cerebral artery, and the origin of the posterior communicating artery on one side.

Methods.—Groups of rats were assigned to receive an IV bolus of MDL-100,453, 100 mg/kg, followed by saline for 24 hours (M-S); isotonic saline as a bolus, followed by the antagonist, 100 mg/kg, over 24 hours (S-M); active drug at both times (M-M); or saline at both times (S-S). An osmotic minipump was attached to the jugular vein. Infarct volume was estimated by 2,3,5-triphenyltetrazolium chloride staining after 24 hours of vascular occlusion.

Results.—Animals that were given a bolus of MDL-100,453 followed by an infusion of the antagonist had significantly smaller infarcts than control animals. Infusion of the antagonist without a bolus injection also reduced the infarct size. The infarct volume correlated inversely with the blood levels of MDL-100,453 at 1 and 2 hours after injection.

Conclusion.—An NMDA antagonist substantially reduced the volume of cerebral infarction after arterial occlusion in this rat model.

▶ The competitive NMDAs are another class of agents that may offer protection from cerebral ischemia. The intriguing aspects of this particular agent are its rapid action (as soon as 2 minutes after an IV dose) and its resultant ability to be used *after* the onset of stroke.—D.M. Rothenberg, M.D.

Aprotinin Could Promote Arterial Thrombosis in Pigs: A Prospective Randomized, Blind Study

Samama CM, Mazoyer E, Bruneval P, Ciostek P, Bonnin P, Bonneau M, Roussi J, Bailliart O, Pignaud G, Viars P, Caen JP, Drouet LO (Hôpital Pitié, Paris; Institut des Vaisseaux et du Sang, Paris; Hôpital Broussais, Paris; et al)
Thromb Haemost 71:663–669, 1994   101-95-5–34

Introduction.—Aprotinin is a polypeptide that inhibits serine protease and has potent antifibrinolytic effects; therefore, it may increase the risk for thrombosis.

Study Plan.—A blinded, randomized study was done in pigs to assess the thrombogenicity of aprotinin. Blood flow was measured by a pulsed Doppler unit, and bleeding times were estimated by the ear immersion technique before and after the femoral arteries had successfully stenosed for 30-minute periods. After a bolus of saline or aprotinin and an ongoing infusion, stenosis was reapplied to the arteries. Aprotinin was given in a bolus of 4 million kallikrein inactivator units (KIU), followed by 1 million KIU/hr^{-1}.

Results.—Six of 8 arteries that were exposed to aprotinin developed partial thrombosis or showed a cyclical-flow reduction or a permanent cessation of blood flow. Only 2 of 19 control vessels were affected. Morphologic studies showed thrombosis in 4 of 7 aprotinin-exposed arteries and in 1 of 9 control arteries. Bleeding times did not differ significantly, and there were no differences in activated partial thromboplastin time, prothrombin time, or fibrinogen concentration.

Implications.—Administration of aprotinin to a patient with severe arterial stenosis may increase the risk of thrombosis.

▶ Can drugs reduce perioperative surgical blood loss? Two classes of drugs have recently undergone investigation—lysine analogues such as tranexamic acid and aminocaproic acid and the serine protease inhibitors, of which aprotinin is an example. Desmopressin is now rarely used on a routine basis during cardiac surgery, except in patients with uremia, but we are still searching for ways to reduce bleeding and transfusion requirements, especially in coronary artery bypass surgery.

Aprotinin is a polypeptide protease inhibitor that has several effects on the coagulation system. It inhibits plasmin and kallikrein and is therefore a potent antifibrinolytic compound. What of concerns about safety (1)? Are drugs that reduce bleeding associated with a higher mortality or morbidity because of excess coagulation or clot formation? Is there evidence of a higher incidence of postoperative myocardial ischemia in patients who are treated with aprotinin? Also at issue is dosage, and large multicenter trials that compare dosage are considered essential. This particular study does not resolve these concerns, but as the authors point out, it does highlight a warning about the use of aprotinin in patients with severely stenosed arteries.—M. Wood, M.D.

Reference

1. Roysten D: *Lancet* 341:1629, 1993.

DNA Single-Strand Breaks in Peripheral Lymphocytes of Clinical Personnel With Occupational Exposure to Volatile Inhalational Anesthetics

Reitz M, Coen R, Lanz E (Univ of Mainz, Germany)
Environ Res 65:12–21, 1994

101-95-5–35

Background.—Rooms in which anesthesia is administered show traces of volatile anesthetics, resulting in chronic exposure of anesthesia personnel. Although there is no consistent evidence of increased cancer rates or other health hazards among anesthesia personnel, there is some evidence that volatile inhalational anesthetics may have genotoxic effects. Very sensitive tests are available to detect possible DNA damage by these agents. Increased rates of DNA single-strand breaks, which are normally reversible, would suggest an increased rate of failure of DNA repair. The rates of DNA single-strand breaks in peripheral lymphocytes were assessed in anesthetic personnel and controls.

Methods.—Forty-one practitioners who administered anesthesia on a daily basis and 44 controls who had no exposure to volatile inhalational anesthetics were included; comparable numbers of the 2 groups were cigarette smokers. Single-strand DNA breaks in peripheral lymphocytes were assessed by nucleoid sedimentation.

Results.—Nonsmoking anesthesia personnel had a higher rate of DNA single-strand breaks than nonsmoking controls. Strand break rates were also increased among smokers in both the anesthetic and control groups. The rate of damage was slightly higher for nonsmoking nurse-anesthetists than for nonsmoking anesthesiologists.

Conclusion.—Chronic exposure to traces of volatile inhalational anesthetics is associated with increased rates of DNA single-strand breaks in nonsmoking anesthetic personnel compared with nonsmoking controls. Smokers have increased damage rates regardless of anesthetic exposure. Single-strand breaks may reflect damage that is detected before the start of the DNA repair process; as a result, these breaks may be reversible. However, not all DNA repairs are perfect, so the increased rates of DNA single-strand breaks in anesthetic personnel could potentially lead to irreversible DNA damage.

▶ Occupational exposure to volatile inhalational anesthetics has been of concern for many years. This article may be one of the most important in a long time in this area. The authors reported that DNA damage in peripheral lymphocytes may be detectable in anesthesia personnel at a considerably higher rate than in controls. They were very careful not to overspeculate, but it is nonetheless tempting to worry that this may be a mechanism involved in carcinogenesis.

Although the authors directly measured the DNA only in lymphocytes, it would be wrong to limit this speculation to the lymphomas. On the other hand, our modern-day scavenged operating rooms are probably much safer places to work, in the aggregate, than many places to which American workers report daily.—J.H. Tinker, M.D.

A Comparison of the Efficacy and Toxic Effects of Sustained- vs Immediate-Release Niacin in Hypercholesterolemic Patients
McKenney JM, Proctor JD, Harris S, Chinchili VM (Virginia Commonwealth Univ, Richmond; Baptist Med Ctr, Little Rock, Ark; Pennsylvania State Univ, Hershey)
JAMA 271:672–677, 1994   101-95-5–36

Background.—Nicotinic acid has a number of salutary effects when it is used to treat hypercholesterolemia, but it is generally not well tolerated because of its vasodilatory side effects, especially when it is given in immediate-release (IR) form. Sustained-release (SR) forms have been proposed, but they are more likely to produce gastrointestinal side effects.

Objective and Methods.—Increasing doses of IR and SR niacin were compared in 46 adult patients whose levels of low-density lipoprotein (LDL) cholesterol remained higher than 160 mg/dL after 1 month on a step 1 National Cholesterol Education program diet. Using a randomized, double-blind, parallel-group design, the patients received sequential daily doses of 500, 1,000, 1,500, 2,000 and 3,000 mg of niacin in IR and SR dosage forms, each for a 6-week period.

Efficacy.—At daily doses of 1,500 mg and greater, SR niacin reduced levels of LDL cholesterol significantly more than IR niacin. Levels of high-density lipoprotein cholesterol increased significantly more with IR niacin at all dose levels. Triglyceride levels were reduced to a similar degree by both dose forms.

Adverse Effects.—About half the patients who took IR niacin in doses of 500 or 1,000 mg daily were bothered by vasodilatory symptoms, particularly flushing. Such symptoms were not increased over baseline in those who used SR niacin. Gastrointestinal symptoms were more prevalent in patients who took 3,000 mg of SR niacin daily. Fatigue was reported with both formulations. Patients who took SR niacin had substantial increases in liver enzymes. Thirty-nine percent of patients who were given IR niacin and 78% of those assigned to SR niacin were withdrawn from the study before completing it.

Conclusion.—Because of its hepatotoxic effects, the use of SR niacin should be restricted, pending further safety studies. Even SR niacin should be given only when patients will be closely followed by experienced health professionals.

▶ This article was included to educate us about niacin and the role of the Food and Drug Administration (FDA). In this article, the new SR preparations of niacin that are available over the counter in many nutritional supplement stores are shown to have great potential for injuring the liver. The slow-release form of niacin was hepatotoxic for at least 50% of patients who took it when they got into the therapeutic dose of 3 g or more per day.

As a result, niacin, which seems like a nice inexpensive treatment for hypercholesterolemia, ends up being a very expensive treatment because of the toxicity it causes and the probability that more than 30% of patients who take the IR form, 50% of patients who take the slow-release form, and 75% of patients who take the SR form will stop taking it.

It also appears that hepatotoxicity may be insidious and not associated with taking this drug. Therefore, in educating ourselves about niacin, we should be cautioned not only about the flushing side effect (which I knew about beforehand) and the other vasodilatory effects, but also about the gastrointestinal symptoms of nausea, gas, heartburn, and diarrhea, the fatigue symptoms, and the potential to reactivate ulcer disease and cause hepatotoxicity.

Because niacin is a vitamin, all the SR dosage forms are available as nonprescription drugs for the treatment of nicotinic acid deficiency, and they are not regulated by the FDA. Clearly, the authors emphasize that niacin should be regulated, and therefore there is a rationale for supporting the FDA in this endeavor.—M.F. Roizen, M.D.

6 Neuromuscular Blocking Agent Pharmacology and Toxicology

Comparison of Rocuronium, Succinylcholine, and Vecuronium for Rapid-Sequence Induction of Anesthesia in Adult Patients
Magorian T, Flannery KB, Miller RD (Univ of Calif, San Francisco)
Anesthesiology 79:913–918, 1993   101-95-6–1

Objective.—Succinylcholine is generally given in clinical conditions involving the need for emergency airway protection during rapid-sequence induction of anesthesia. An alternative in this situation might be rocuronium, a new nondepolarizing muscle relaxant that has a brief onset of action but lacks the adverse reactions associated with succinylcholine. Rocuronium, succinylcholine, and vecuronium were compared for rapid-sequence induction of anesthesia in a randomized study.

Methods.—The study included 50 adult patients in American Society of Anesthesiologists physical status I–III. After premedication with midazolam and fentanyl, the patients received their assigned muscle relaxant: rocuronium, .6, .9, or 1.2 mg/kg; vecuronium, .1 mg/kg; or succinylcholine, 1 mg/kg. Sixty seconds later, tracheal intubation was attempted by a clinician who was unaware of the patient's medication assignment. Neuromuscular monitoring began before administration of the muscle relaxant and continued through complete ablation of T1 and recovery of T1 to 25%.

Findings.—Onset times, i.e., times to complete ablation of T1, were similar for patients receiving the 2 higher doses of rocuronium and those receiving succinylcholine: 50–75 seconds. Significantly longer times were noted with the low dose of rocuronium and with vecuronium, 89 and 144 seconds, respectively. The highest dose of rocuronium had the longest clinical duration of action, 73 minutes, and succinylcholine had the shortest duration of action, 9 minutes. Intermediate values of 37–53 minutes were noted in the other 3 groups. There were no differences between groups in intubating conditions; only patients in the succinylcholine group had fasciculations.

Conclusion.—In patients treated with rocuronium, the onset time increased along with the dose. At the 2 higher doses, rocuronium had a similar onset time to succinylcholine but a significantly longer duration of action. At doses of .9–1.2 mg/kg, the brief onset time of rocuronium makes it a viable alternative to succinylcholine for rapid-sequence induction of anesthesia. Rocuronium has a long duration of action, which could be a disadvantage, especially in patients undergoing short surgeries.

▶ The new muscle relaxant rocuronium has a very brief onset of action. A nondepolarizing muscle relaxant with an onset time as short as that of succinylcholine would be a considerable advance for rapid-sequence induction of anesthesia. The onset time of rocuronium for rapid-sequence intubation is fast enough only at higher doses, so it is achieved at a cost—prolonged duration of effect. I do not predict the disappearance of succinylcholine.—M. Wood, M.D.

Determination of the Hemodynamics and Histamine Release of Rocuronium (Org 9426) When Administered in Increased Doses Under N₂O/O₂-Sufentanil Anesthesia

Levy JH, Davis GK, Duggan J, Szlam F (Emory Univ, Atlanta, Ga)
Anesth Analg 78:318–321, 1994   101-95-6–2

Introduction.—Rocuronium is a steroidal nondepolarizing neuromuscular-blocking agent that resembles vecuronium electrophysiologically except for a more rapid onset of action. Its duration of action is about half as long as that of vecuronium in animal studies. Hypersensitivity reactions to rocuronium have not been reported.

Objective.—The histamine-releasing potential of rocuronium was studied using a new, sensitive radioimmunoassay for histamine in 45 American Society of Anesthesiologists physical status I–III adults who were to undergo general elective surgery.

Methods.—The patients were randomly assigned to receive 1 of 3 intubating doses of rocuronium, 600, 900, or 1,200 μg/kg (2, 3, and 4 times the effective dose for 95% (ED_{95}), in preparation for endotracheal intubation. The maintenance dose was rocuronium, 150 μg/kg. The patients received diazepam before induction as well as IV midazolam, followed by IV sufentanil as needed. Rocuronium was injected as a bolus 2 minutes after induction. Anesthesia was maintained with nitrous oxide in oxygen and sufentanil.

Results.—Plasma histamine levels did not vary significantly with the dose of rocuronium. There were no signs of histamine release. The clinical effects of the rocuronium 600-, 900-, and 1,200-μg/kg doses lasted 45, 66, and 85 minutes, respectively.

Conclusion.—There is no appreciable risk of substantial histamine release or hemodynamic abnormality when rocuronium is given in a wide range of doses up to 4 times the ED_{95} dose.

▶ I certainly hope that most practicing anesthesiologists can do a better job than I can in keeping information straight on the steady influx of new neuro-muscular-blocking agents. I cannot remember which ones are long-acting, which ones are short-acting, or the appropriate doses. I think I understand that if the drug name ends in the suffix "onium," it probably doesn't have his-tamine-releasing potential, whereas if it ends in the suffix "curium," the company that manufactures it is very defensive about the possibility of histamine. I have no idea what all that means, either.

This article from an investigative group I respect indicates that perhaps this drug will "catch on," big time. I hope one of these drugs takes hold soon in a big way, so that I can memorize the dosage and not have to worry about all the others!—J.H. Tinker, M.D.

Pharmacokinetics and Pharmacodynamics of Rocuronium (Org 9426) in Elderly Surgical Patients
Matteo RS, Ornstein E, Schwartz AE, Ostapkovich N, Stone JG (Columbia Univ, New York; Presbyterian Hosp, New York)
Anesth Analg 77:1193–1197, 1993   101-95-6–3

Introduction.—Rocuronium (Org 9426) is a newly synthesized steroi-dal muscle relaxant designed to have a speed of onset approaching that of succinylcholine but without a markedly prolonged duration of action or unwanted side effects. It is chemically related to vecuronium, which has shown a prolonged duration of action in the elderly. The pharmaco-kinetics and pharmacodynamics of rocuronium in the elderly were stud-ied.

Methods.—Twenty elderly and 20 younger—older than 70 years and younger than 60 years, respectively—patients had surgery with nitrous oxide/oxygen, fentanyl anesthesia. The patients' responses to an IV bo-lus of rocuronium, 600 µg/kg, which was given after induction of anes-thesia, were studied.

Results.—The onset times were the same in the 2 groups, but the el-derly patients had a significantly prolonged duration of action of rocuronium. Plasma clearance was significantly decreased in the elderly patients—3.67 vs. 5.03 mL/kg^{-1}/min^{-1}—as was the volume of distribu-tion—399 vs. 553 mL/kg. During recovery, the 2 groups showed no sig-nificant difference in the log plasma concentration vs. twitch tension re-sponse relationship between 20% and 80% paralysis.

Conclusion.—Elderly and younger patients experienced significant dif-ferences in the action of rocuronium, which were explained by variations in the distribution and elimination of the drug. These pharmacokinetic differences were probably the result of the decreased total body water and decreased liver mass of the elderly.

▶ Many drugs have been shown to have altered pharmacokinetics when they are given to elderly patients, and this includes the new steroid muscle relaxant, rocuronium. The duration of action of rocuronium can be expected to be longer in this age group.—M. Wood, M.D.

The Pharmacokinetics and Pharmacodynamics of the Stereoisomers of Mivacurium in Patients Receiving Nitrous Oxide/Opioid/Barbiturate Anesthesia

Lien CA, Schmith VD, Embree PB, Belmont MR, Wargin WA, Savarese JJ (New York Hosp–Cornell Univ Med Ctr, New York; Burroughs Wellcome Co, Research Triangle Park, NC)
Anesthesiology 80:1296–1302, 1994   101-95-6–4

Background.—Mivacurium chloride is a short-acting, nondepolarizing neuromuscular-blocking agent that consists of a mixture of 3 stereoisomers: 34% to 40% *cis-trans,* 52% to 60% *trans-trans,* and 4% to 8% *cis-cis.* In terms of neuromuscular blocking potency, the *trans-trans* and *cis-trans* isomers are equipotent, whereas the *cis-cis* isomer is only one thirteenth as potent.

Objective.—Studies were done in 18 American Society of Anesthesiologists physical status I or II men between the ages of 33 and 55 years to ascertain the pharmacokinetic properties of the stereoisomers of mivacurium and the dose proportionality of the more potent isomers.

Methods.—The patients were scheduled to undergo lengthy but minor elective operations under fentanyl/nitrous oxide/oxygen anesthesia. Neuromuscular function was monitored by a mechanomyograph as the ulnar nerve was stimulated at the wrist at a frequency of .15 Hz. Mivacurium, 5 and 10 µg/kg/min, was infused for 1 hour each. The plasma levels of each isomer were estimated using a stereospecific high-performance liquid chromatographic technique. Pharmacokinetic parameters were determined by noncompartmental analysis.

Results.—An 83% neuromuscular block was produced by the lower infusion rate, and a 99% block occurred at the higher rate. After withdrawal of the infusion, 25% of baseline muscle strength was achieved in 9.3 minutes on average. The respective volumes of distribution of the *cis-trans, trans-trans,* and *cis-cis* isomers were .29, .15, and .34, and their respective elimination half-lives were 1.8, 1.9, and 53 minutes. The clearance of the *cis-trans* and *trans-trans* isomers did not vary with the infusion rate. However, the plasma clearance of these isomers was highly dependent on the plasma cholinesterase activity (Fig 6–1).

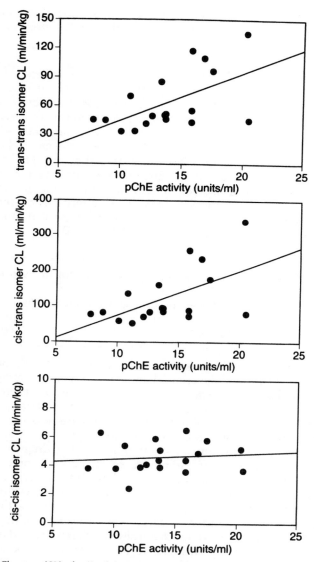

Fig 6–1.—Clearance (CL) of each of the isomers as a function of plasma cholinesterase (pChE) activity. Although the CL of the *cis-trans* and *trans-trans* isomers is dependent on plasma cholinesterase activity (r^2 is .323 and .326, respectively; $P < .05$), there is no relationship between the CL of the *cis-cis* isomer and plasma cholinesterase activity ($r^2 = .016$, $P = .62$). (Courtesy of Lien CA, Schmith VD, Embree PB, et al: *Anesthesiology* 80:1296–1302, 1994.)

Conclusion.—The high metabolic clearances and short elimination half-lives of the potent isomers of mivacurium are consistent with its short duration of action.

▶ Many drugs (e.g., ketamine, bupivacaine, and propranolol) are actually mixtures of isomers. Assays usually measure the total concentration, and stereospecific assays are required to determine plasma concentrations of each isomer. Mivacurium consists of 3 stereoisomers; 2 of the isomers (*cis-trans* and *trans-trans*) that make up most of mivacurium have a very short elimination half-life, whereas the *cis-cis* isomer (only 4% to 8% of the mixture) is less potent, but it has an elimination half-life similar to that of vecuronium. The *cis-cis* isomer is excreted by the kidney and might accumulate in renal failure. Isomers can have varying degrees of activity, but they can also inhibit the clearance of the other isomer; so giving drugs as mixtures of isomers can make life very complicated. Some pharmacologists think that drugs should be administered only as a single isomer.—M. Wood, M.D.

Prolonged Weakness After Infusion of Atracurium in Two Intensive Care Unit Patients
Meyer KC, Prielipp RC, Grossman JE, Coursin DB (Univ of Wisconsin, Madison; Clinical Science Ctr, Madison, Wis)
Anesth Analg 78:772–774, 1994   101-95-6-5

Background.—The ICU patient has ventilation facilitated, intracranial hypertension controlled, shivering eliminated, oxygen consumption decreased, and diagnostic procedures eased by neuromuscular-blocking drugs, usually vecuronium and pancuronium. Unfortunately, weakness can persist for days after prolonged use. When weakness is reported, 3 features seem to be common: lack of peripheral nerve twitch monitoring when a blocking agent is infused continuously; other drugs, particularly high-dose corticosteroids, are administered at the same time; and dysfunction of an end organ, such as renal failure. When receiving corticosteroids, use of a nonsteroidal-blocking agent such as atracurium is considered. Ester hydrolysis yields metabolites that are inactive at the neuromuscular junction and are cleared despite liver or kidney dysfunction. Two patients, who were mechanically ventilated, treated with corticosteroids and atracurium, and had no history of liver or kidney problems, experienced severe muscular weakness.

Case 1.—Man, 38, with history of testicular cancer 3 years earlier, was evaluated for skeletal pain and found to be pancytopenic. A bone marrow examination showed acute myelocytic leukemia. Transretinoic acid, 100 mg/day, and dexamethasone, 2 mg every 6 hours, were begun. Fever and rigors were experienced on the fourth hospital day, and ticarcillin and tobramycin were begun. The fever subsided after vancomycin and amphotericin B were administered. By the eighth day, increasing respiratory distress resulted in the patient's transfer to the

ICU, where he was intubated and ventilation was begun on the 10th day. Infusion of atracurium, 10 μg/kg/min, followed a 50-mg bolus. Peripheral nerve monitoring was checked every 2–4 hours. A total of 13,958 mg of atracurium were given over 8 days. The patient had profuse muscular weakness and could not lift his arms or legs. The weakness was still evident despite withdrawal of tobramycin, reduction of dexamethasone, and infusion of calcium gluconate. Extubation occurred on the 36th day. Electromyographic tests showed myopathic changes, without fasciculations, and regeneration. Nerve conduction studies showed demyelinating motor neuropathy. Although the patient's strength slowly improved, he still could not ambulate when discharged on the 60th day.

Case 2.—Woman, 28, was referred 1 week after having hemoptysis and hematuria. Methylprednisolone, cyclophosphamide, and plasmapheresis were begun 3 days before a diagnosis of Goodpasture's syndrome was made. The patient was transferred to the ICU because of massive alveolar hemorrhage, where she was intubated and ventilated. Etomidate, midazolam, and vecuronium were given when she was intubated. Atracurium, 7–14 μg/kg/min, was infused for a total of 6,572 mg over 6 days. After atracurium was discontinued, some spontaneous movement and the cough reflex returned within hours. Muscle wasting was obvious, with prominent proximal weakness and diffuse tremor. Electromyographic study showed normal conduction velocities, no fasciculations, and evidence of early reinnveration after neuropathic processes. With normal creatine kinase and aldolase, the test results were consistent with postparalysis syndrome, as confirmed by neurologic consultation. The patient was extubated on the 37th day, discharged from the ICU on the 40th day, and released from the hospital on the 58th day for several weeks of physical therapy to regain normal strength.

Comment.—Clinical weakness and myopathy, despite no muscle biopsies, appeared to be caused by an interaction of atracurium and corticosteroids. Although there are reports of myopathy when either of these drugs is used alone, the bulk of reports of muscle weakness are the result of combining the drugs. Despite monitoring peripheral nerve stimulation, prolonged muscle weakness has been demonstrated in patients who are receiving corticosteroids and atracurium infusion. This weakness is similar to that seen with the aminosteroids, vecuronium and pancuronium. Caution is urged in the use of neuromuscular-blocking agents, especially when corticosteroids are also being administered. Current methods of nerve stimulation monitoring may not be able to stop this complication. If sedatives and analgesics can facilitate ventilation, neuromuscular blocks can be avoided.

▶ This article and another similar report (1) exemplify what I concluded some time ago was simply a matter of time: With an increase in ICU use of atracurium, prolonged muscle weakness would eventually occur. The shift toward benzylisoquinolinium neuromuscular-blocking (NMB) agents in the ICU and away from the more traditionally used aminosteroid NMB agents is based primarily on reports of prolonged weakness after discontinuation of drugs such as vecuronium or pancuronium, often in association with concomitant corticosteroid use and/or renal failure. However, these 2 cases warn against such a practice.

This article also validates the concern of a number of previously reported studies that indicate NMB agents should be given only to patients in whom proper sedation (amnesia) and analgesia have been ensured. Indeed, in the first of the 2 cases reported, there was no mention of simultaneous sedative/analgesic therapy during atracurium infusion, thereby raising concern for unrecognized patient distress and recall.

The authors also note that routine train-of-4 monitoring failed to detect or prevent prolonged muscle weakness. This finding, along with a similar conclusion reached in a previous report (2), suggests that other methods of preventing this syndrome could be considered. Serum levels of both drug and metabolite, as well as periods of drug cessation to assess motor strength, may be warranted.

A multicenter trial is currently evaluating which NMB agent is safest for use in critically ill patients. Until then, it is best to use NMB agents only in extreme circumstances and even then with great caution.—D.M. Rothenberg, M.D.

References

1. Branney SW, et al: *Crit Care Med* 22:1699, 1994.
2. Segredo V, et al: *N Engl J Med* 327:524, 1992.

Studies on the Interaction of Steroidal Neuromuscular Blocking Drugs With Cardiac Muscarinic Receptors

Appadu BL, Lambert DG (Leicester Royal Infirmary, England)
Br J Anaesth 72:86–88, 1994
101-95-6-6

Background.—Older nondepolarizing neuromuscular-blocking drugs such as pancuronium produce tachycardia and increase arterial blood pressure. Newer agents such as vecuronium, pipecuronium, and rocuronium reportedly have minimal cardiovascular effects, but bradyarrhythmia has been described in a few instances. Pipecuronium and pancuronium have bisquaternary structures, whereas vecuronium and rocuronium are monoquaternary compounds.

Objective.—How various steroidal neuromuscular-blocking agents interact with muscarinic receptors in the rat heart was examined in vitro using a tritiated N-methyl hyoscine binding assay. The drugs examined included pancuronium, pipecuronium, rocuronium, and vecuronium.

Results.—Of the drugs studied, pancuronium interacted most closely with cardiac muscarinic receptors, followed in order by vecuronium, pipecuronium, and rocuronium. All the drugs other than pipecuronium exhibited complex binding characteristics, with a "Hill coefficient" less than unity.

Conclusion.—The hemodynamic consequences of neuromuscular-blocking agents may reflect the way in which they interact with cardiac M_2 muscarinic receptors.

▶ New muscle relaxants have been developed in an attempt to provide drugs that do not have cardiac muscarinic effects. This study shows that vecuronium, pipecuronium, and rocuronium do not bind to rat cardiac muscarinic receptors with as great of an affinity as pancuronium, which is a possible explanation for the difference in cardiovascular effects in clinical practice.—M. Wood, M.D.

Call Mosby Document Express at **1 (800) 55-MOSBY** to obtain copies of the original source documents of articles featured or referenced in the YEAR BOOK series.

7 Malignant Hyperthermia: Diagnosis and Therapy

A Clinical Grading Scale to Predict Malignant Hyperthermia Susceptibility

Larach MG, Localio AR, Allen GC, Denborough MA, Ellis FR, Gronert GA, Kaplan RF, Muldoon SM, Nelson TE, Ørding H, Rosenberg H, Waud BE, Wedel DJ (Pennsylvania State Univ College of Medicine, Philadelphia; Australian Natl Univ, Canberra; Univ of Leeds, England; et al)
Anesthesiology 80:771–779, 1994   101-95-7–1

Background.—Because the nature of acute malignant hyperthermia reaction is nonspecific and the incidence of many of its clinical signs and laboratory findings is variable, diagnosing this condition by clinical criteria can be difficult. The availability of a standardized tool for estimating the qualitative likelihood of malignant hyperthermia in a given patient without specialized diagnostic testing would facilitate management of and research into this disease.

Methods.—A multifactorial malignant hyperthermia clinical grading scale comprised of standardized clinical diagnostic criteria was developed. The Delphi method was used, and an international panel of 11 experts on the disease was involved in the grading scale's development. The scale was designed for classification of existing records and application to new patients.

Findings.—The scale ranked the qualitative likelihood that an adverse anesthetic event represents malignant hyperthermia and, with further exploration of family history, the likelihood that an individual will be thought of as being susceptible to malignant hyperthermia. The assigned rank indicated the lower boundary on the likelihood of malignant hyperthermia. On the clinical grading scale, the anesthesiologist had to judge whether specific clinical signs were appropriate for the patient's medical condition, anesthetic method, and surgical procedure.

Conclusion.—The malignant hyperthermia clinical grading scale can be used to more objectively define this disease. It provides a new, comprehensive clinical case definition for the malignant hyperthermia syndrome.

▶ The authors are to be congratulated for a major start in understanding clinical malignant hyperthermia. They have graded this phenomenon into 6 processes: rigidity, muscle breakdown, respiratory acidosis, temperature increases, cardiac involvement, and family history. We should all read this interesting article to broaden our knowledge of malignant hyperthermia.—M.F. Roizen, M.D.

Masseter Muscle Rigidity and Malignant Hyperthermia Susceptibility in Pediatric Patients: An Update on Management and Diagnosis
O'Flynn RP, Shutack JG, Rosenberg H, Fletcher JE (Hahnemann Univ, Philadelphia)
Anesthesiology 80:1228–1233, 1994   101-95-7-2

Objective.—There is ongoing debate about the definition of masseter muscle rigidity (MMR) and anesthetic management subsequent to it. A strong association between MMR and malignant hyperthermia susceptibility (MHS) has been demonstrated, leading some investigators to recommend that anesthesia be discontinued after trismus. Current anesthetic management after MMR was reported, along with the estimated incidence of clinical malignant hyperthermia (MH) and MHS in patients with MMR.

Methods.—Pediatric patients with evidence of MMR after succinylcholine were referred by practicing anesthesiologists for biopsy. The clinical findings were classified as MMR alone or MMR followed by signs of MH. These included an arterial carbon dioxide tension of greater than 50 mm Hg, an arterial pH of 7.25 or less, and a base deficit of greater than 8. Caffeine-halothane muscle contracture testing was done to assess MHS.

Results.—The patients were 50 boys and 20 girls; the anesthetics involved were halothane-succinylcholine in 83% of the cases. The anesthetic was discontinued in 68% of cases and continued with a nontriggering agent in 11% and with a triggering agent in 13%. In 59% of the patients, MHS was diagnosed by muscle biopsy. Clinical MH developed within 10 minutes of MMR in 7% of patients.

Conclusion.—Using the current protocol of the North American Malignant Hyperthermia Group, a 59% incidence was found for MHS associated with MMR. The incidence of clinical MH is 7% in patients with MMR. Most anesthesiologists discontinue anesthesia when the patient has MMR. Given the high concordance between MMR and MHS, this appears to be the most prudent course. If the surgery is urgent, continuing the anesthesia with a nontriggering anesthetic and appropriate monitoring would be an acceptable option.

▶ Although some diehards still dispute the putative connection between MMR and MHS, this article is convincing, at least to me, that the occurrence of MMR should constitute an immediate "cease and desist" order to an anesthesiologist if that is at all possible. If it is not possible, MMR should probably constitute a major emergent situation in which all triggering anesthetics are stopped and a "purged" machine with new tubing is put into use as soon as possible.

This article is an example of the kind of definitive work that can be done with national registries. I have long advocated the formation of a "national anesthesia risk registry" that would combine risk data from many sources and in all sorts of directions. Protecting such data from medicolegal discovery is a major stumbling block to such a registry.—J.H. Tinker, M.D.

Jaw Relaxation After a Halothane/Succinylcholine Sequence in Children

Hannallah RS, Kaplan RF (Children's Natl Med Ctr, Wash, DC; George Washington Univ, Wash, DC)
Anesthesiology 81:99–103, 1994   101-95-7–3

Background.—Previous reports have described failure of complete jaw relaxation in patients who receive a halothane-succinylcholine sequence. However, most of these studies have been retrospective, and they disagree about the magnitude and incidence of the problem. These issues were studied prospectively in 500 consecutive unmedicated children who received IV succinylcholine during halothane anesthesia.

Methods.—All patients received at least a 2-mg dose of IV succinylcholine per kg after induction of anesthesia with halothane. Forty-five to 60 seconds later, a single observer assessed the degree of jaw relaxation using a standardized clinical scale. Relationships among the degree of relaxation, the type of surgical procedure, and the presence and intensity of fasciculations were sought.

Results.—Ninety-five percent of patients had complete relaxation, which was defined as full and easy mouth-opening. Another 4% had incomplete relaxation, with firm manual separation required to open the mouth fully. One patient had masseter muscle rigidity, in which the mouth could not be fully opened but intubation was still possible. None of the patients had trismus, in which the teeth clamped shut. There was no correlation among the incidence of incomplete relaxation or masseter muscle rigidity, the presence or degree of fasciculations, or the type of surgical procedure. None of the patients showed any signs of hypermetabolism or myoglobinuria.

Conclusion.—The 4% incidence of incomplete jaw relaxation in children who received a halothane-succinylcholine sequence should be considered a normal response. Although masseter muscle rigidity and trismus are rare, until proven otherwise, they should be considered indicators of malignant hyperthermia.

▶ This article attempts to divide "incomplete relaxation" of the jaw after succinylcholine from "masseter muscle rigidity or trismus." The latter, which is rare, clearly indicates the very real possibility of malignant hyperthermia in the future. According to this article, the anesthesiologist is supposed to be able to decide whether a given patient is a "2," a "3," or a "4." Because the consequences of this clinical decision are enormous, i.e., cancel the case, if it is elective, and get everybody all worried about MH, on the one hand, or go blithely ahead and assume that things are fine, on the other hand, I hope that this kind of an arbitrary grading scale does not get accepted. Perhaps the best thing we can do is simply get rid of succinylcholine. I can't believe I actually said that, because it is has been an old friend for many years, but maybe it is true.—J.H. Tinker, M.D.

Viability Criterion of Muscle Bundles Used in the *In Vitro* Contracture Test in Patients With Neuromuscular Diseases
Adnet PJ, Krivosic-Horber RM, Krivosic I, Haudecoeur G, Reyford HG, Adamantidis MM, Medahoui H (Centre Hospitalier Régional Universitaire, Lille, France)
Br J Anaesth 72:93–97, 1994   101-95-7-4

Background.—The in vitro contracture test for susceptibility to malignant hyperthermia (MH) examines the sensitivity of cut muscle fibers to halothane or caffeine. Variable test results are obtained in most patients with neuromuscular disease; only those with central core disease exhibit a good correlation between clinical MH and the in vitro test findings.

Objective and Methods.—The contractile and electrophysiologic properties of muscle fiber segments were compared in 28 patients who had various neuromuscular disorders (NMDs) and 93 MH-related family patients. Bundles of muscle fiber segments were dissected from the vastus lateralis muscle or in 7 patients with NMD from the deltoid muscle. Muscle strips 15–20 mm in length and 2–3 mm in diameter were used for in vitro testing. Halothane was used in concentrations of .5, 1, 2, and 3 volume%, and caffeine was used in concentrations ranging from .5 to 32 mmol/L.

Results.—Only 1 of the 28 patients with NMD had a positive test result; 6 others had equivocal findings, and 21 had negative results. The muscle bundles had significantly smaller resting membrane potentials and smaller predrug twitch tension amplitudes than those from MH-related family patients. No fiber segments in the MH family member group had resting potentials less than −60 mV. Eight of 180 fiber segments had a maximum predrug twitch tension amplitude of less than 1 g. Some muscle specimens from the patients with NMD were from muscles that were damaged or rapidly deteriorating. None of the patients with NMD or their relatives were known to have had an anesthetic event that clearly represented MH.

Conclusion.—A positive in vitro contracture test result in a patient with myopathic disease does not prove that the patient is really susceptible to MH.

▶ This article dramatically points out problems with the in vitro contracture test, which is still our "gold standard" for the prediction of MH. I think it is important for anesthesiologists to realize that this test, although it is accepted as a gold standard, is really very complex and difficult to perform well, let alone interpret. This article should scare anyone who lives in an area populated by MH families.—J.H. Tinker, M.D.

8 Monitoring

The Pulse Oximeter: Applications and Limitations—An Analysis of 2000 Incident Reports
Runciman WB, Webb RK, Barker L, Currie M (Univ of Adelaide, Australia;- Prince of Wales Hosp, Sydney, Australia)
Anaesth Intensive Care 21:543–550, 1993   101-95-8–1

Objective.—Pulse oximetry represents a major advance in patient monitoring. If blood supply to a finger is being maintained well enough to register a waveform, it is usually safe to assume that there is adequate blood supply to the heart and brain as well. However, pulse oximeters have disadvantages, including unreliability in certain circumstances and a fairly high rate of "false alarms." The Australian and New Zealand College of Anaesthetists recommended that a pulse oximeter be available by the beginning of 1990 for each patient undergoing anesthesia. The first 2,000 incidents reported to the Australian Incident Monitoring Study were analyzed to help define the applications and limitations of pulse oximetry in clinical anesthetic practice.

Findings.—Pulse oximetry initially detected 9% of these incidents, and desaturation was recorded in another 9%. General anesthesia was involved in 1,256 of the 2,000 incidents, 48% of which were classified as "human detected" and 52% as "monitor detected." Twenty-seven percent of the monitor-detected incidents were discovered by pulse oximetry. If a pulse oximeter had always been used—and if its modulated pulse tone had been used instead of the "bleep" of the ECG—this figure would have increased to more than 40%. In 87% of the 76 cases in which it was used, the pulse oximeter detected the common occurrence of endobronchial intubation, for which it was the "frontline" monitor. Pulse oximetry was also an invaluable backup monitor in 40 life-threatening situations in which commonly used frontline monitors were not in use or failed.

Other situations that were detected by pulse oximetry included circuit disconnection, circuit leak, severe shunt, esophageal intubation, aspiration or regurgitation, pulmonary edema, endotracheal tube obstruction, severe hypotension, failure of oxygen delivery, hypoxic gas mixture, hypoventilation, anaphylaxis, air embolism, bronchospasm, malignant hyperthermia, and tension pneumothorax. Pulse oximeter "failure" was reported in 15 cases; in most of these incidents, the model in use had no modulated tone or alarm or was working adequately. A theoretical analysis suggested that use of pulse oximetry on its own would have detected

82% of incidents related to general anesthesia, had they been allowed to progress. Sixty percent of the incidents would have been detected before any organ damage occurred.

Conclusion.—The growing recommendations for pulse oximetry monitoring during anesthesia were supported. An appropriate pulse oximeter should be used to monitor all patients from the time they arrive in the induction room until their protective reflexes return and they show adequate saturation while breathing room air. It is an invaluable frontline monitor in some situations and a backup monitor in others; it detects many serious problems that are not reliably detected initially by any particular monitor.

▶ I included this article because after the enormously rapid and wide acceptance of the pulse oximeter as a monitor for just about everything, many anesthesiologists put it on a mental shelf labeled "important, well understood." However, the pulse oximeter, like all other devices of importance, has its problems and pitfalls, such as overuse, misuse, and underuse.

This article is an excellent compilation of some of the advantages and pitfalls noted over the past several years by a nationwide registry in Australia. I think it is an outstanding summary.—J.H. Tinker, M.D.

Congenital Methaemoglobinaemia Detected by Preoperative Pulse Oximetry
Chisholm DG, Stuart H (St Helier Hosp, Surrey, England; Hosp for Sick Children, London)
Can J Anaesth 41:519–522, 1994   101-95-8–2

Objective.—Because congenital or acquired methemoglobinemia is an unusual cause of cyanosis that may not be immediately apparent, appropriate treatment may be delayed. A patient with asymptomatic cyanosis resulting from congenital methemoglobinemia was reported.

Case Report.—Woman, 24, was being evaluated for evacuation of retained products of conception. Pulse oximetry performed before induction of anesthesia gave a reading of 82%. With the benefit of this finding, cyanosis was detected on clinical examination. The patient had no medical history relevant to cyanosis and was not taking any medications. On arterial blood gas analysis with the patient breathing room air, the arterial oxygen partial pressure was 90 mm Hg, the arterial carbon dioxide partial pressure was 33 mm Hg, and the arterial oxygen saturation was 97%. On co-oximeter analysis of the same sample, the methemoglobin content was 13%. The surgery was performed successfully; anesthesia was induced and maintained with incremental doses of propofol and fentanyl, along with a spontaneous breathing technique using oxygen in nitrous oxide. The patient received no specific treatment for methemoglobinemia. On later evaluation in the hematology clinic, a diagnosis of congenital methemoglobin reductase deficiency was made. One of the patient's 4 siblings subsequently was found to have a low methemoglobin concentration as well.

Discussion.—The widespread use of perioperative pulse oximetry sometimes yields surprising abnormalities, as in this case of congenital methemoglobinemia resulting in asymptomatic cyanosis. Unexpected results of pulse oximetry should be accepted critically, because their interpretation requires a working knowledge of the principles of this monitoring technique. When dyshemoglobins are present, arterial blood gas analysis should be used in conjunction with co-oximeter readings.

▶ The article indicates the important thing: Preoperative pulse oximetry is one of the major advances in patient monitoring in recent years, but unexpected results should not be accepted uncritically. I think that unexpected results on anything, including all our monitoring tools, should not be accepted uncritically. Such observations can lead to valuable insights and the prevention of disease. In this instance, the evaluation process clearly led to a new diagnosis, and although knowledge of it did not change preoperative care considerably, for the rest of her life it will be important for this patient to know that certain drugs such as prilocaine (in EMLA cream), sulfonamides, and certain antimalarials, antileprosy, and antiseizure medications also should be avoided.—M.F. Roizen, M.D.

A Modified Sensor for Pulse Oximetry in Children

Howell SJ, Blogg CE, Ashby MW (John Radcliffe Hosp, Oxford, England; Radcliffe Infirmary, Oxford, England; St Bartholomew's Hosp, London)
Anaesthesia 48:1083–1085, 1993   101-95-8-3

Objective.—A modification of the semidisposable "Oxiband" sensor for pulse oximetry has been developed for use in children. The standard Oxiband probe (model OX1-A/N) may be difficult to attach to a child who is uncooperative.

Methods.—Using this modification, the probe was mounted around the barrel of a 5-mL syringe that had been cut approximately halfway along its length. The optical components were placed opposite each other, and the probe was secured to the syringe barrel with adhesive tape, enabling it to be slipped onto the child's finger so that the diodes transmitted through the fingertip. The modified sensor was assessed in 27 children aged 1–7 years who were receiving anesthesia for elective plastic surgery. Saturation readings were obtained for each child using both the modified probe and a conventional probe. The probes were placed on adjacent fingers and alternated for monitoring after induction.

Results.—A total of 113 pairs of observations were collected. The modified probe produced consistent results, although it tended to be underread by approximately 1.6%. However, the error introduced by the modification was less than the error reported in the data sheet as being innate to the Oxiband probe. As a result, the degree of inaccuracy of the modified probe was acceptable for clinical purposes. The probe accurately indicated when peripheral oxygen saturation had declined to 90% or less.

Conclusion.—This modified probe is inexpensive and easy to use. Because the modification may reduce the wear and tear involved in applying and removing the Oxiband probe, its useful life may be extended. The probe should not be forced onto a finger for which it is too small, and movement artifacts may be a problem in the child who is awake.

▶ I think this is an important technique, because it is inexpensive, it extends the life of the sensor, and it is probably faster to apply and more comfortable for children. However, the authors cautioned that only 1 probe and 1 brand of syringe were used, and they could not comment on the range of variation between different probes and syringes or ascertain whether different syringes would absorb the light of the wavelengths of 660 and 940 differently and therefore cast doubt on the oximetry reading. The Oxiband Nellcor sensor and the B-D Plastipak 5-mL syringe appear to be appropriate and available.—M.F. Roizen, M.D.

The Capnograph: Applications and Limitations—An Analysis of 2000 Incident Reports

Williamson JA, Webb RK, Cockings J, Morgan C (Univ of Adelaide, Australia; Royal Victorian Eye and Ear Hosp, East Melbourne, Australia)
Anaesth Intensive Care 21:551–557, 1993   101-95-8-4

Purpose.—The clinical value of capnography has long been recognized, although until recently its use has been limited by cost. Recently, the Australian and New Zealand College of Anaesthetists recommended that a carbon dioxide monitor be available for every patient who was intubated and/or ventilated. The first 2,000 incidents of capnography reported to the Australian Incident Monitoring Study were analyzed for uses and limitations.

Findings.—Of these 2,000 incidents, 8% were initially detected by capnography. In another 1%, the capnograph played a contributory role in detection. A total of 1,256 incidents were associated with general anesthesia, 48% of which were classified as "human detected" and 52% as "monitor detected." Twenty-four percent of the latter group were detected by capnography; if a correctly checked and calibrated capnograph had been used in every case, this figure would have increased to nearly 30%. Capnography was the frontline monitor for problems of esophageal intubation, failure of ventilation, anesthetic circuit faults, gas embolism, sudden circulatory collapse, and malignant hyperthermia. It was also a valuable backup monitor when other monitors were not used or failed; failures included circuit leaks, overpressure of the breathing circuit, bronchospasm, leakage of the ventilator-driving gas into the patient circuit, aspiration and/or regurgitation, and hypoventilation.

Failure of the capnograph was reported in 20 cases, more than two thirds of which could have been prevented by appropriate checking and calibration. Gas-sampling problems led to 7 of these problems and apnea alarm failure to 6. Capnography failed to detect 2 circuit leaks and 2 faulty unidirectional valves. In other cases, problems were related to power failure, calibration problems, or misinterpretation of an alarm. If used on its own, capnography would have detected 55% of general anesthesia-related incidents if they had been permitted to evolve. Forty-three percent would have been detected before any organ damage occurred.

Conclusion.—An appropriate, correctly checked and calibrated capnograph should be used in all patients who are intubated and ventilated. Capnographic monitoring should start at the moment of intubation and continue until extubation. For patients who are breathing spontaneously with a mask, capnography is useful in the apnea detection mode.

▶ Capnography has come to be accepted and is also stored on our mental shelf labeled "well understood." There are even more pitfalls, problems, and difficulties associated with capnometry than with pulse oximetry. This is an excellent summary of a large experience with outcomes that are related to capnometry in one way or another.—J.H. Tinker, M.D.

Continuous Intra-Arterial Blood Gas and pH Monitoring in Critically Ill Patients With Severe Respiratory Failure: A Prospective, Criterion Standard Study
Haller M, Kilger E, Briegel J, Forst H, Peter K (Ludwig-Maximilians-Univ of Munich)
Crit Care Med 22:580–587, 1994   101-95-8-5

Introduction.—Critically ill patients and those undergoing anesthesia for major surgery often experience acute changes in arterial blood gas values and therefore require frequent blood gas analysis. A continuous intra-arterial blood gas monitoring system has been developed that has a larger sensor composed of 2 fluorescent dyes immobilized around the external surface of a length of the fiber. The 2 dyes emit signals at different wavelengths, and 1 does not emit a signal in the presence of oxygen. The accuracy and clinical usefulness of the device were evaluated.

Methods.—The intra-arterial blood gas monitoring system was used in 13 patients who were critically ill and mechanically ventilated. The sensor, which consisted of 3 optical fibers and a thermistor, was inserted. A Y-piece at the insertion site enabled blood withdrawal and arterial blood pressure monitoring. The sensors were calibrated with tonometry before insertion. Two other conventional blood gas analyzers were used periodically, and the results were compared with the results of the continuous

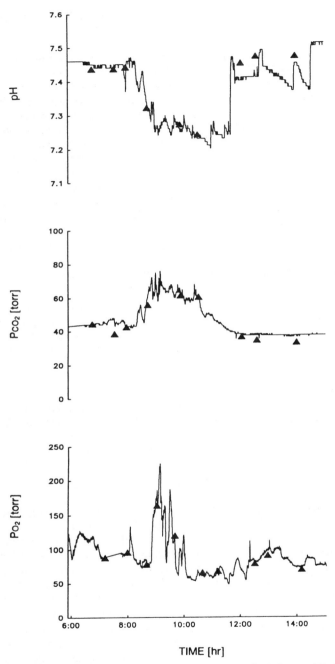

Fig 8–1.—Online recording of intra-arterial blood gas monitoring of pH, P_{CO_2}, and P_{O_2} before, during (8:20 to 10:25 hours), and after bronchoscopy including several biopsies in a single-lung transplant recipient. *Triangles* indicate conventional blood gas analysis values. (Courtesy of Haller M, Kilger E, Briegel J, et al: *Crit Care Med* 22:580–587, 1994.)

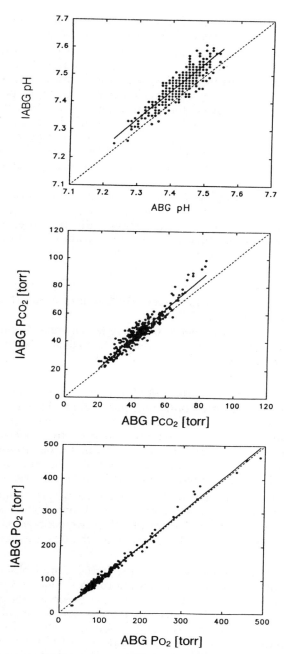

Fig 8–2.—Scatterplots of the intra-arterial blood gas monitoring (*IABG*) pH, partial pressure of carbon dioxide (*P*co$_2$) and of oxygen (*P*o$_2$) with conventional blood gas analysis values (*ABG*). *Solid lines* indicate regression lines; *dashed lines*, the lines of identity (1 mm Hg = .133 kPa). (Courtesy of Haller M, Kilger E, Briegel J, et al: *Crit Care Med* 22:580–587, 1994.)

monitoring system (Fig 8–1). The ability to trace blood pressure and withdraw blood using the system's Y-piece was assessed.

Results.—Insertion was uncomplicated in all patients, and the system was used for 7.7–170.1 hours. Comparisons of the blood gas values obtained by the continuous monitoring system with those obtained by the conventional blood gas analyzers revealed that measures of partial pressure of oxygen (PO_2) showed the greatest agreement, followed by the partial pressure of carbon dioxide (PCO_2), and pH (Fig 8–2). The agreement between methods was greatest in the clinically important range of values and when detecting sudden changes. The sensor did not significantly change the quality of blood pressure tracings or hamper blood withdrawal.

Discussion.—This continuous intravascular blood gas monitoring system measured pH, PCO_2, PO_2, and presumed temperature with reasonable accuracy for at least 72 hours without affecting arterial pressure monitoring or blood withdrawal. It was simple to insert and operate and functioned consistently under clinical conditions.

Performance of a Patient-Dedicated, On-Demand Blood Gas Monitor in Medical ICU Patients

Kees Mahutte C, Sasse SA, Chen PA, Holody M (Veterans Affairs Med Ctr, Long Beach, Calif; Univ of California, Irvine; 3M Healthcare, Tustin, Calif)
Am J Respir Crit Care Med 150:865–869, 1994   101-95-8-6

Background.—A patient-dedicated blood gas monitor, the CDI 2000, which consists of a cassette containing fluorescent pH, partial pressure of carbon dioxide (PCO_2), and partial pressure of oxygen (PO_2) sensors was recently introduced. After calibration in vitro, the cassette is placed in the arterial line tubing and blood gases can be determined on demand, as often as desired, by drawing blood through the cassette. Results are available within 2 minutes, and the blood is then reinjected.

Objective.—The performance of the CDI 2000 was compared with that of 6 models of blood gas analyzers from 3 manufacturers in a multicenter study. A total of 683 pairs of values were obtained using the monitor and a conventional blood gas analyzer in 50 medical ICU patients.

Results.—Ex vivo calibration, using the initial paired blood samples, yielded biases of .02 for pH, −.1 mm Hg for PCO_2, and 4.3 mm Hg for PO_2. For all paired samples, the respective biases were .004 pH unit, .6 mm Hg, and 2.7 mm Hg. The bias for PO_2 was greater as the values increased. Standard deviations for both blood gas values also increased with the magnitude of the variables. The degree of pH bias was not affected by the serum sodium concentration. Daily drift of the 3 sensors was negligible.

Conclusion.—This new on-demand blood gas monitor performs as well as conventional blood gas analyzers.

▶ The preceding 2 articles (Abstracts 101-95-8–4 and 101-95-8–5) are offered as follow-up references from last year's review by Shapiro and associates in the 1994 YEAR BOOK OF ANESTHESIOLOGY AND PAIN MANAGEMENT (p 142). These studies compared conventional arterial blood gas analyzers with continuous blood gas monitors that used intra-arterial sensory technology and on-demand fluorescent optode systems, respectively. Both monitors compared favorably in regard to the accuracy of pH, P_{CO_2}, and P_{O_2} determinations that were derived from standard methods, and they provided clinically useful information rapidly and reliably.

These innovative technologies appear to offer accurate data, while minimizing patient blood loss. Whether either system proves to be cost-effective has yet to be determined. However, the continuous monitor may prove to be too cumbersome because of the need for a separate freestanding system.—D.M. Rothenberg, M.D.

Anesthetic Depth Defined Using Multiple Noxious Stimuli During Isoflurane/Oxygen Anesthesia: I. Motor Reactions

Zbinden AM, Maggiorini M, Petersen-Felix S, Lauber R, Thomson DA, Minder CE (Univ of Bern, Switzerland)
Anesthesiology 80:253–260, 1994

101-95-8–7

Introduction.—The minimal alveolar concentration (MAC) required to prevent movement in 50% of patients in response to a skin incision ($MAC_{skin\ incision}$) is the standard measure of anesthetic potency. However, because a skin incision is usually a single event, potency determinations cannot be repeated in an individual patient. The traditional $MAC_{skin\ incision}$ also cannot predict patient responses to other noxious stimuli. The effects of other noxious stimulation patterns were investigated and then compared with that of the $MAC_{skin\ incision}$ by measuring the end-tidal concentrations of isoflurane and the corresponding arterial concentrations.

Methods.—Twenty-six adult patients scheduled for elective abdominal surgery received isoflurane anesthesia. During various noxious stimuli, the end-tidal and arterial concentrations of isoflurane necessary to suppress response in 50% of patients were measured. The responses and stimuli were eye-opening in response to a verbal command and the motor response to a trapezius squeeze, 50 Hz of electric tetanic stimulation, laryngoscopy, skin incision, and tracheal intubation.

Results.—The end-tidal concentrations of isoflurane required to suppress responses in 50% of patients were .37 vol% for vocal command, .84 for trapezius squeeze, 1 for laryngoscopy, 1.03 for tetanic stimulation, 1.16 for skin incision, and 1.76 for intubation. The corresponding equivalent arterial values, adjusted to sea level, were .36 vol% for vocal command, .65 for trapezius squeeze, .78 for laryngoscopy, .8 for tetanic stimulation, .97 for skin incision, and 1.32 for intubation. Very high concentrations of isoflurane were needed to suppress responses to intubation, and, even then, excessive reactions were noted.

Conclusion.—The suppression of motor responses to different noxious stimuli requires different concentrations of isoflurane. The stimuli of tetanic stimulation and, to a lesser extent, trapezius squeeze can be useful alternatives to skin incision for the evaluation of anesthetic potency. Unlike skin incisions, these stimuli are simple to perform, noninvasive, reproducible, and repeatable.

▶ I included this article largely to criticize it. In Eger et al.'s (1) original work on anesthetic potency, they carefully pointed out that, for a legitimate end point of MAC, a "supramaximal" stimulus had to be delivered. It has long been known that responses to so-called submaximal stimuli are not suppressed at the same concentrations of anesthetics; that is, the "worse" the stimulus, the more anesthetic is needed to suppress it. This makes sense and is well known, so I just don't see why the journal gave the article such prominence, including publication of an editorial about it. In addition, I think that in the very near future we will be much more sophisticated in our ability to assess anesthetic "depth" using sophisticated computer-driven neurophysiologic techniques, including cortical-evoked potential.—J.H. Tinker, M.D.

Reference

1. Eger EI, et al: *Anesthesiology* 26:756, 1965.

Motor Signs of Wakefulness During General Anaesthesia With Propofol, Isoflurane and Flunitrazepam/Fentanyl and Midlatency Auditory Evoked Potentials

Schwender D, Faber-Züllig E, Klasing S, Pöppel E, Peter K (Univ of Munich)
Anaesthesia 49:476–484, 1994   101-95-8–8

Introduction.—Previous studies have used auditory evoked potentials (AEPs) as an indicator of patient awareness during anesthesia. In patients who received combined general and local anesthesia, it may be difficult to assess the adequacy of suppression of wakefulness using autonomic signs. Motor signs of intraoperative wakefulness, cardiovascular variables, and midlatency AEPs were assessed in patients who received epidural analgesia combined with 3 different general anesthetic regimens.

Methods.—Thirty patients undergoing elective laparotomy received continuous epidural analgesia to block pain to the T5 level. General anesthesia was induced and maintained with 3 different regimens in groups of 10 patients each: propofol, 2.5 mg/kg^{-1}, followed by propofol, 3–5 mg/kg^{-1}; thiopental, 5 mg/kg^{-1}, followed by isoflurane, .4–.8 vol%; or etomidate, .3 mg/kg^{-1}, followed by flunitrazepam and fentanyl, .005

mg/kg^{-1}, by bolus injection every 20–30 seconds. Continuous recordings of heart rate and arterial pressure were made, and purposeful limb movements, eye-opening, coughing, and other movements were recorded as motor signs of intraoperative wakefulness. Before anesthesia and during induction and maintenance, AEPs were recorded as well.

Results.—Patients in the flunitrazepam-fentanyl group showed significantly more frequent motor signs of intraoperative wakefulness than those in the propofol or isoflurane groups. Wakefulness did not correlate with the cardiocirculatory measurements. While awake, the patients' midlatency AEPs demonstrated high peak-to-peak amplitudes and a periodic waveform. After all 3 induction regimens and during maintenance with propofol and isoflurane, the midlatency AEPs were severely attenuated or abolished. During maintenance with flunitrazepam-fentanyl, high peak-to-peak amplitudes were reestablished. Persistent midlatency AEPs occurred coincident with a high incidence of wakeful motor signs.

Conclusion.—For patients who are receiving combined regional and general anesthesia, the use of isoflurane or propofol appears to yield better suppression of motor signs of wakefulness than intermittent bolus injections of flunitrazepam-fentanyl. The midlatency AEP may be a useful indicator of the cortical excitability and the functional state of the brain during general anesthesia. Further studies are needed to relate the midlatency AEP to intraoperative recall and to assess its ability to measure the "depth of anesthesia."

▶ This is an example of an important recent concern accompanying the rising popularity of propofol. To put it mildly, some anesthetics with propofol tend to be "light." The idea of adapting the routine use of AEPs to help ensure blockage of awareness during anesthesia is nicely explored in this article.—J.H. Tinker, M.D.

Effects of Adenosine Triphosphate (ATP) on Somatosensory Evoked Potentials in Humans Anesthetized With Isoflurane and Nitrous Oxide
Andoh T, Ohtsuka T, Okazaki K, Okutsu Y, Okumura F (Yokohama City Univ, Japan)
Acta Anaesthesiol Scand 37:590–593, 1993   101-95-8-9

Background.—Adenosine triphosphate (ATP) reduces the need for inhalational anesthetic in humans. Patients who receive a low-dose anesthetic combined with ATP infusion rapidly emerge from anesthesia. Adenosine triphosphate may be a useful adjuvant to anesthesia for patients undergoing spinal surgery, in which rapid postoperative emergence from anesthesia is required for neurologic examination immediately after surgery. Such surgeries are often monitored by somatosensory evoked potentials (SSEPs); however, no previous studies have examined the effect of ATP on SSEPs. Eight patients who were under anesthesia with isoflurane and nitrous oxide were studied.

Methods.—The patients were studied while undergoing tibial or femoral osteotomy for osteoarthritis. Each underwent recordings of SSEP while anesthesia was maintained with a .5% end-tidal concentration of isoflurane in 60% nitrous oxide, after addition of ATP infusion at rates of 100 and 200 $\mu g/kg^{-1}/min^{-1}$, and when the isoflurane concentration was increased to 1.5% after cessation of ATP infusion.

Results.—An intraoperative blood pressure increase was effectively inhibited by ATP infusion combined with .5% isoflurane and 60% nitrous oxide. Administration of 1.5% isoflurane reduced the amplitude of the cortical component of SSEP as it increased the cortical and spinal latencies and the central conduction time (CCT). Neither rate of ATP infusion significantly altered latencies, amplitude, or CCT.

Conclusion.—Adjuvant ATP that is given with .5% isoflurane in 60% nitrous oxide may be a useful form of anesthesia for patients undergoing operations with intraoperative SSEP monitoring. With this technique, adequate depth of anesthesia can be maintained with a low concentration of anesthetics without further suppression of SSEPs. Use of ATP during spinal surgery appears to be safe.

▶ Adenosine was released for acute IV use for an obscure and uncommon indication—treatment of acute supraventricular tachydysrhythmias. The drug company knew very well that this drug might have considerably wider potential use. Adenosine triphosphate is much more water-soluble than adenosine, but it is probably broken down to adenosine immediately. Whether and why it might reduce anesthetic requirements are unknown.

These authors report that ATP can be used to lower the requirement for volatile anesthetics so that SSEPs can be used with less likelihood of awareness. This article falls in the "too good to be true" category. I always say "beware of enthusiastic early reports of success," an adage that I think applies here. Nonetheless, if this finding is confirmed, it will be an interesting development.—J.H. Tinker, M.D.

Isoflurane Compared With Nitrous Oxide Anaesthesia for Intra-Operative Monitoring of Somatosensory-Evoked Potentials

Lam AM, Sharar SR, Mayberg TS, Eng CC (Univ of Washington, Seattle)
Can J Anaesth 41:295–300, 1994   101-95-8–10

Introduction.—It is common practice to monitor somatosensory evoked potentials (SSEPs) intraoperatively when the CNS is at risk. Potent inhalational anesthetics depress the cortical response in a dose-related manner, but with low doses it is generally possible to record potentials. Nitrous oxide and inhaled anesthetics have an additive depressant effect on the amplitude of the cortical response. The optimal anesthetic regimen for use when recording SSEPs was defined by comparing the effects of .6 minimum alveolar concentration (MAC) of nitrous oxide with those of an equipotent dose of isoflurane. Eight American Society of Anesthesiologists physical status I or II patients whose mean age was 35 years participated in the study.

Methods.—Somatosensory evoked potentials were recorded from an electrode over the right parietal cortex in response to electric stimulation of the contralateral median nerve. Patients were premedicated with midazolam, and anesthesia was induced with thiopental and fentanyl. The SSEPs were recorded during the delivery of .6 MAC isoflurane alone, isoflurane plus .6 MAC of nitrous oxide, and nitrous oxide alone, all in equipotent concentrations. Patients received 38% inspired oxygen throughout the monitoring period.

Results.—The combination of isoflurane and nitrous oxide had the most marked depressant effect on cortical amplitude, reducing it by 67% on average. Nitrous oxide alone decreased the amplitude of cortical potentials more than an equipotent dose of isoflurane. Latency increased slightly during anesthesia with isoflurane or both isoflurane and nitrous oxide, but it was unchanged with nitrous oxide alone.

Conclusion.—It appears feasible to monitor SSEPs during anesthesia with nitrous oxide or isoflurane or when both agents are used together, but cortical potentials are best preserved with isoflurane alone. Anesthesia with both agents has less than an additive effect on the amplitude of cortical potentials.

▶ This article tends to debunk the long-held dogma that volatile anesthetics are somehow contraindicated when intraoperative monitoring involving SSEPs is used. It indicates that modest doses of isoflurane are better, if anything, than similar potency levels of nitrous oxide. The article also contains the intriguing concept that nitrous oxide and isoflurane, at least with respect to suppression of these evoked potentials, are *not* additive. There really isn't any reason why they should be additive, simply because they are additive with respect to suppression of tail clamping, that is, MAC determinations. I would argue that this might prove to be a most intriguing finding, especially if (I think when) we go in the direction of building machines that actually control anesthesia. We will almost certainly want to control anesthesia using some sort of cortical evoked potentials. If the anesthetics in their "MAC ratios" are not additive, then these machines of the future will either have to use only 1 agent or will have to be programmed in a more complex manner than would be envisioned by the use of MAC alone.

As an aside, who would operate an "anesthesia controller" of the future? Science has a way of getting political in a big hurry.—J.H. Tinker, M.D.

Use of the Electrospinogram for Predicting Harmful Spinal Cord Ischemia During Repair of Thoracic or Thoracoabdominal Aortic Aneurysms

Stühmeier K-D, Grabitz K, Mainzer B, Sandmann W, Tarnow J (Heinrich-Heine-Universität, Düsseldorf, Germany)

Anesthesiology 79:1170–1176, 1993   101-95-8–11

Introduction.—Paraparesis and paraplegia are serious but somewhat unpredictable complications of repairing aneurysms of the thoracic and thoracoabdominal aorta. Monitoring the epidural somatosensory evoked potentials (ESEPs), which are elicited by stimulating the posterior tibial nerve repeatedly, yields many false positive responses. An alternative is to epidurally stimulate the ESEPs below the spinal segment and record them above the spinal segment at risk in the form of the electrospinogram.

Methods.—Real-time epidural ESEPs were recorded from the T3–4 level of the cord after epidural stimulation of the lumbar cord at the L2–3 level. Recordings were made in 100 consecutive patients who had aortic aneurysms resected. The time from cross-clamping to disappearance of the ESEPs was recorded, as well as the duration of complete potential loss and the time to recovery after declamping. The neurologist was unaware of the ESEP recordings.

Results.—Thirty-one of the 100 patients had no loss of ESEPs and exhibited no neurologic deficit. Of 29 patients in whom ESEPs were lost more than 15 minutes after cross-clamping of the aorta, 2 (7%) had a deficit (Fig 8–3). When ESEPs were lost earlier, 12 of 40 patients (30%) had a neurologic deficit. A total ESEP loss exceeding 40 minutes was 100% sensitive and 68% specific for neurologic deficit. A recovery time of more than 20 minutes after declamping was 93% sensitive and 86% specific.

Conclusion.—The electrospinogram is a reliable means of monitoring spinal cord function during operations that require cross-clamping of the aorta.

▶ I thought that this was a very interesting article. Spinal cord ischemia that leads to damage during repairs of thoracic and thoracoabdominal aortic aneurysms is a dreaded complication. A variety of measures, such as prophylactic drug therapy, CSF drainage, hypothermia, shunting, and partial cardiopulmonary bypass, have all been attempted without any clear benefit. It would be a tremendous advance to have a monitoring tool that warned of potential poor neurologic outcome so we could take steps to prevent harm. These authors have not shown that use of the electrospinogram changed the outcome, but the stage is now set for prospective studies that compare the use of such a technique with that of other therapeutic strategies.—M. Wood, M.D.

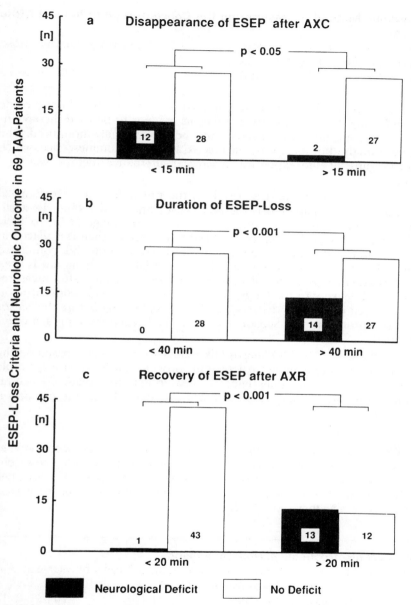

Fig 8–3.—Relations between intraoperative epidural somatosensory evoked potentials (*ESEPs*) findings and postoperative neurologic outcome of 69 consecutive patients with intraoperative ESEP loss during thoracic or thoracoabdominal aortic aneurysm repair. Three criteria were separated: **a,** disappearance of ESEP (within 15 minutes) after aortic cross-clamping (*AXC*); **b,** duration of total ESEP loss; and **c,** recovery time after aortic declamping (*AXR*; P values refer to chi-square test comparing the proportion of patients with neurologic deficits according to the time criteria shown in **a** through **c.** (Courtesy of Stühmeier K-D, Grabitz K, Mainzer B, et al: *Anesthesiology* 79:1170–1176, 1993.)

A Simple Method for Monitoring the Concentration of Inhaled Nitric Oxide

Petros AJ, Cox P, Bohn D (Royal Liverpool Children's Hosp, England; Hosp for Sick Children, Toronto)

Anaesthesia 49:317–319, 1994   101-95-8-12

Background.—Interest in the potential benefits of inhaled nitric oxide is increasing. However, if inhaled nitrous oxide is to be used therapeutically, the concentration delivered must be very carefully monitored. The current method of measuring nitrous oxide is chemiluminescence, which can be difficult and expensive. A simpler alternative method was presented.

Methods.—The method is based on the principle of electrochemical detection. The equipment is the NO Sensor Stik model 4586. Its accuracy depends on the calibrating gas, which is in the range of 5% to 10%. The Sensor Stik is allowed to stabilize for 1–2 hours, then it is placed in the breathing system just before the catheter mount and connected through a T-piece and a slip-on collar. A special catheter mount is used to decrease nitrous oxide absorption over a short distance after measurement and delivery to the lungs. Because the nitrous oxide concentration is measured just before delivery, any loss from binding before the sensor is not a problem. The Sensor Stik is checked regularly using a transfer standard.

Conclusion.—The NO Sensor Stik model 4586, which is based on the principle of electrochemical detection, provides an inexpensive, simple alternative to chemiluminescence for measuring nitrous oxide concentration. With this technique, most ICUs can use inhaled nitric oxide if needed.

▶ If nitric oxide becomes a commonly used potent pulmonary vasodilator, as most anesthesiologists believe it will, some method of controlling and monitoring its dosage is needed. The electrochemical detection system described here and the other 3 alluded to in the article seem to provide relatively accurate ($\pm$ 5%) monitors.—M.F. Roizen, M.D.

A Novel Electrochemical Heparin Sensor

Yang VC, Ma S-C, Liu D, Brown RB, Meyerhoff ME (Univ of Michigan, Ann Arbor; Nova Biomedical Corp, Waltham, Mass)

ASAIO J 39:195M–201M, 1993   101-95-8-13

Objective.—Although heparin is one of the most commonly used anticoagulant drugs, too much can cause serious hemorrhage. A quaternary ammonium salt–based polymer membrane electrode that can monitor heparin levels during extracorporeal therapy was studied.

Methods.—Polymer membranes were prepared, their responses were evaluated, and the solution was deposited onto the surface of a silicon chip. During open heart surgeries, blood samples were drawn before and after heparin administration and after the administration of a heparin antagonist. Heparin levels were determined by the polymer membrane electrode and by blood activated clotting time measurement.

Results.—The electrode appeared to be adequately sensitive and to yield a linear potentiometric response to macromolecular heparin in both plasma and saline solutions. The high sulfate content and polymeric structure of heparin and its analogues appear to be necessary to elicit electrode response. Sensitivity increases with molecular weight and sulfate content. The electrode can be regenerated with 1–2 molar sodium chloride or else produced as a disposable device.

Conclusion.—Tridodecylmethylammonium chloride directly and selectively detects heparin in whole blood samples. It can be designed as an inline detection device or as a disposable measuring unit, which is equally effective before and after administration of heparin antagonists.

▶ This article describes the development of a method of measuring heparin in blood. It probably can be made online or inline; for example, in extracorporeal circulation systems. Is it the pharmacokinetics of heparin that we seek? I thought we sought to give the drug for its pharmacodynamic effects. Doesn't simply measuring the concentration of the product and not the effect of heparin that we seek move us farther away from helping prevent morbidity?—M.F. Roizen, M.D.

9 Risk, Outcome, and Cost Studies

Epidural Morphine Reduces the Risk of Post-Operative Myocardial Ischaemia in Patients With Cardiac Risk Factors
Beattie WS, Buckley DN, Forrest JB (McMaster Univ, Hamilton, Ont, Canada)
Can J Anaesth 40:532–541, 1993   101-95-9-1

Introduction.—The stressful perioperative period is characterized by neural, hormonal, and physiologic alterations. The sympathetic activation has been linked to myocardial ischemia, an important cause of perioperative myocardial infarction (PMI). Perioperative myocardial infarction is an important cause of surgical mortality and morbidity. The sympathetic response to pain can be attenuated by the use of epidural opiates. The effects of intraoperative and postoperative epidural analgesia were compared with the effects of parenteral morphine sulfate in patients with multiple risk factors for myocardial ischemia. Patients were observed for 24 hours after surgery.

Methods.—Patients with at least 2 cardiac risk factors who were scheduled for major elective surgery (e.g., intra-abdominal, vascular, or orthopedic total joint surgery) were studied. The decision to use epidural anesthesia was made by the anesthesiologist. After placement of the catheter, morphine, .1 mg/kg, was administered followed by 2% lidocaine, .1–.3 mg/kg, before induction. Routine intraoperative variables were monitored. Intravenous narcotics were avoided in the epidural group, because the interaction is associated with respiratory depression. The parenteral group received sufentanil, 1 μg/kg, or the equivalent of an opioid. The epidural analgesia was maintained for pain control throughout the postoperative period. Epidural morphine, .1 mg/kg, was begun every 12 hours and adjusted to maintain a pain rating of 2 or less on a 10-point visual analogue scale. Patients receiving parenteral morphine also had their medication adjusted to achieve a pain rating of 2 on the same 10-point scale; unfortunately, equipotent analgesia between groups was not achieved. These patients had higher pain scores and balanced pain against side effects. Electrocardiograms, for determination of ischemia and arrhythmias, were obtained with Holter monitors. Major events included chest pain, shortness of breath, tachyarrhythmia, congestive heart failure, MI, or death.

Results.—Fifty-five patients were studied, with 29 receiving epidural analgesia. All ischemic events were silent. Significantly fewer patients who received epidural analgesia had ischemic events and tachyarrhythmias, with an overall fourfold reduction in the relative risk for either complication. The 5 major events occurred in patients with perioperative ischemia. Ischemic events typically occurred at 1–4, 9–12, or 22–24 hours after surgery. One third occurred in the first 4 hours after surgery and lasted for 1–31 minutes. Forty-two percent of ischemic episodes happened when the heart rate was 20% greater than baseline or greater than 100 beats/min.

Conclusion.—That postoperative ischemia was silent, regardless of the method of analgesia was of concern. Patients who received epidural analgesia had fewer episodes of ischemia. However, the small number of patients studied rules out concluding that this analgesic method reduces major postoperative morbidity. The results suggest that the most serious perioperative ischemia could be "nonhemodynamically mediated."

▶ These patients were placed in the epidural or parenteral morphine groups partly on the basis of the "modified Goldman" scale, as modified by Detsky. If you take that at face value, the groups look fairly even with respect to their "cardiovascular risk." Unfortunately, the Goldman "point scale" of cardiovascular risk has not survived validation tests that were done subsequent to its original publication in 1977. Why we keep using it, I can't imagine; it simply isn't valid. Because these patients were divided into 2 groups on the basis of an invalid "risk classification," I do not see why these results are valid.

Another problem with this study is that the authors believe the study was blinded, because the observers did not know the analysis of the occurrence of ischemia. They conveniently forgot that the anesthetists were not blinded. It's very hard to blind whether you are putting in an epidural. What is the significance of this? It means that there is an enormous possibility of the introduction of bias. I mentioned this earlier in my comments regarding the "Porsche syndrome," where person A buys a Porsche, coddles it, puts it up on blocks in the winter, never parks it near another car, and so on. Person B buys a Plymouth and hardly ever cleans it out inside let alone washes it (that's me). Guess what? The Porsche lasts longer than the Plymouth, but the 2 cars were not exactly treated the same way; they didn't exactly cost the same either. My message is not that I am "anti" epidural analgesia vs. IV analgesia; it is simply "beware of results that move in the direction of your biases and those that move in the direction of complexity or making more money for anesthetists." I *hope* these results will stand the test of time, but I won't hold my breath.—J.H. Tinker, M.D.

Perioperative Myocardial Ischemia: Its Relation to Anatomic Pattern of Coronary Artery Stenosis
Hogue CW Jr, Herbst TJ, Pond C, Apostolidou I, Lappas DG (Washington Univ, St Louis, Mo)
Anesthesiology 79:514–524, 1993   101-95-9–2

Introduction.—An association between intraoperative myocardial ischemia and postoperative myocardial infarction has been established in patients who undergo coronary artery bypass surgery (CABG). Relationships between preoperative and intraoperative myocardial ischemic episodes have also been noted, suggesting that both are caused by an aspect of coronary artery disease. The relationship between the anatomical location of coronary artery stenosis and perioperative myocardial ischemia was examined.

Methods.—Coronary angiographic findings determined the group assignment of 100 adult patients scheduled for CABG surgery. Group 1 (40 patients) had steal-prone coronary anatomy. Group 2 (17 patients) had either left main coronary artery stenosis or left main equivalent stenosis. Group 3 (43 patients) had at least a 70% stenosis in at least 2 major coronary arteries. Continuous ECG monitoring was performed in the preoperative, intraoperative, and postoperative periods, and the frequency and duration of ischemic episodes were recorded for each patient.

Results.—Fifty-nine of the 100 patients experienced 335 ischemic episodes. Almost all were asymptomatic. Perioperative ischemic episodes occurred in 29 of 40 patients in group 1, 9 of 17 patients in group 2, and 21 of 43 patients in group 3. Group 1 had significantly more frequent and longer preoperative ischemia episodes than did group 3; there were no significant differences between groups 1 and 2 or groups 2 and 3 in either frequency or duration of ischemic episodes in the preoperative period. There were no significant differences between groups in the duration or frequency of ischemic episodes in the intraoperative or postoperative periods. The probability of experiencing an ischemic episode was twice as high in group 1 as in group 3 during the preoperative period, but there were no differences in the relative risk among the groups during the perioperative period. Ischemic episodes were most frequent in the preoperative period, and they decreased both in the intraoperative and postoperative periods.

Discussion.—Patients who require CABG have frequent, mostly asymptomatic ischemic episodes before surgery. Patients with steal-prone coronary artery stenosis (group 1) are more likely to have preoperative myocardial ischemic episodes, but they have a risk of intraoperative and postoperative ischemic episodes similar to that of patients with other anatomical patterns of coronary artery stenosis.

▶ This article gives me a chance to ventilate about one of my pet peeves against "buzzwords," such as "coronary steal," "stress-free anesthesia," and more recently "steal-prone anatomy." They are similar in many ways to political slogans, because they convey a small amount of information or a sentiment, but they just don't work (or help).

The authors have shown that patients with steal-prone anatomy had more *preoperative* ischemia and that it lasts longer in each episode; despite this, the patients did no worse perioperatively. Steal-prone anatomy always seemed to me to be problematic for another reason. I don't think very many anesthesiologists (including me) really know what it is supposed to be! How many of us can determine from a preoperative angiogram, if one is available, whether a patient has it or not?—J.H. Tinker, M.D.

ECG and Cardiac Enzymes After Glycine Absorption in Transurethral Prostatic Resection

Hahn RG, Essén P (Huddinge Univ, Sweden)
Acta Anaesthesiol Scand 38:550–556, 1994   101-95-9-3

Introduction.—Patients having transurethral prostatic resections are about 25% more likely than those having open prostatectomies or other operations to die within 5 years, primarily of myocardial infarction. One possible cause is absorption of the glycine solution that is used to irrigate the bladder during surgery.

Study Plan.—Electrocardiographic changes and serum enzyme levels were monitored in a prospective series of 22 men, aged 55 to 89 years, who had transurethral resection of the prostate. Half of them absorbed more than 1 L of irrigating fluid during the operation, as determined by the detection of alcohol in the expired breath. The fluid consisted of 1.5% glycine and 1% ethanol. The 2 patient groups were similar in age, American Society of Anesthesiologists physical status, arterial pressure during surgery, operating time, and extent of resection.

Findings.—No patient had myocardial infarction, but 9 of the 11 who absorbed more than 1 L of irrigating fluid had ECG changes, primarily T-wave flattening. Only 1 of the other patients had an ECG abnormality. On multiple regression analysis, only the volume of fluid absorbed correlated significantly with the appearance and degree of new ECG changes. In 5 patients in the high-absorption group, all of whom had clear ECG changes, the serum levels of creatine kinase and aspartate transaminase increased after surgery. In 85% of samples with increased creatine kinase activity, the creatine kinase-MB isoenzyme was present.

Conclusion.—Absorption of a large amount of irrigating solution during transurethral prostatic resection may adversely affect cardiac function.

Changes in Haemodynamic Variables During Transurethral Resection of the Prostate: Comparison of General and Spinal Anaesthesia

Dobson PMS, Caldicott LD, Gerrish SP, Cole JR, Channer KS (Royal Hallamshire Hosp, Sheffield, England)
Br J Anaesth 72:267–271, 1994   101-95-9-4

Objective and Methods.—Hemodynamic status was examined by transcutaneous Doppler aortovelography in 22 patients who had transurethral resection of the prostate on an elective basis under either spinal or general anesthesia. The patients were randomly assigned to receive subarachnoid anesthesia with .5% hyperbaric bupivacaine or to receive general anesthesia with enflurane and nitrous oxide in oxygen. Patients in both groups received 500 mL of Hartmann's solution for 10 minutes after the induction of anesthesia.

Results.—Cardiac output decreased significantly from 4.6 to 3.1 L/min^{-1} after induction of general anesthesia. The mean arterial pressure and heart rate both decreased, and the systemic vascular resistance increased by 41%. The cardiac output increased toward baseline as resection proceeded. Spinal anesthesia was accompanied by a significant decrease in the mean arterial pressure and an initial reduction in cardiac output, but the heart rate and vascular resistance did not change. The extent of resection was similar in the 2 groups, but the operations were shorter and less irrigation fluid was used in the spinal group.

Conclusion.—Hemodynamic function remains more stable during spinal anesthesia for transurethral prostatic resection than during general anesthesia.

▶ Transurethral resection of the prostate (TURP) has in many instances replaced open prostatectomy for surgical management of benign prostatic hyperplasia. However, it is still important to note that there are complications associated with TURP, such as hemorrhage and intravascular absorption of the irrigating fluid that can lead to glycine toxicity manifested as nausea, dilutional hyponatremia, and cerebral edema. In 1989, Roos and associates, in a somewhat surprising retrospective study, reported that TURP may result in a higher long-term mortality when compared with open prostatectomy for benign hyperplasia (1).

Most of the morbidity associated with TURP appears to be related to the cardiovascular system, probably because many of these patients are older and constitute a relatively high-risk population. We know that systemic absorption of irrigating fluid can occur and in some cases lead to hypervolemia, pulmonary edema, hypertension, and the precipitation of congestive cardiac failure. A recent study in a small number of patients undergoing enflurane anesthesia showed hemodynamic evidence of cardiac stress during TURP; important hemodynamic disturbances were noted during TURP but not during control procedures (2).

The preceding 2 articles (Abstracts 101-95-9–3 and 101-95-9–4) addressed the issue of cardiovascular morbidity after TURP. Dobson and co-workers reported a descriptive randomized study of a small number of patients and showed that hemodynamic changes were greater during general than spinal anesthesia. It is important to note that the researchers measured a surrogate end point and not the outcome. The study by Hahn and Essén showed an association between glycine absorption and ECG changes. Follow this story.—M. Wood, M.D.

References

1. Roos NP, et al: N *Engl J Med* 320:1120, 1989.
2. Evans J, et al: *BMJ* 304:666, 1992.

Myocardial Ischaemia and Spinal Analgesia in Patients With Angina Pectoris

Christensen EF, Søgaard P, Egebo K, Bach LF, Riis J (Skejby Sygehus, Denmark)

Br J Anaesth 71:472–475, 1993
101-95-9-5

Introduction.—Conflicting findings have been reported regarding the effects of spinal and extradural analgesia in patients with myocardial ischemia. Myocardial ischemia can be monitored noninvasively with continuous ECG Holter monitoring and ST-segment analysis. Patients were monitored to assess myocardial ischemia on a normal day and on a day when they underwent minor surgery with spinal analgesia. The findings were compared to assess the effects of spinal anesthesia on ischemia.

Methods.—Fourteen patients with stable angina pectoris received 24-hour Holter monitoring on a normal day and on the day of surgery. The data collected included the number of ischemic events, their length and onset, the greatest ST-segment change, and the highest heart rate at the onset.

Results.—On the day of normal activities, 7 of the 14 patients had 27 ischemic events, whereas on the day of surgery, 10 of 14 patients had 70 ischemic events. The total duration of the ischemic events and the mean maximum decrease in ST-segment were highly significantly greater on the day of surgery compared with on the reference day. There were no significant differences between the 2 days in the mean heart rate, but the mean heart rate during the first ischemic event on the day of surgery was significantly higher than the mean heart rate during all ischemic events (103 vs. 92). No ischemic events occurred immediately after the induction of spinal analgesia, although the mean arterial pressure declined shortly after induction; the first event occurred a mean of 338 minutes after induction. The duration of the first ischemic event was 45% of the total duration of all ischemic events on the day of surgery.

Discussion.—These patients with stable angina pectoris experienced longer, more frequent, and more severe ischemic events after the administration of spinal analgesia while undergoing minor surgery than on days of normal activity. The initial ischemic event was not associated with induction of spinal analgesia, the decline in the mean arterial pressure after induction, or the administration of ephedrine.

▶ The use of spinal and epidural anesthesia in patients with ischemic heart disease has always been controversial, because a decrease in arterial pressure might reduce coronary blood flow and worsen or even induce ischemia, whereas by contrast, a reduction in preload and afterload secondary to sympathetic blockade might decrease cardiac work and reduce myocardial oxygen demand. It may also be true that perioperative fluid administration is greater in patients who are receiving regional anesthesia, beecause many anesthesiologists routinely volume-load in this clinical setting.

This study describes only a small number of patients (14) and reports "more frequent, longer and more severe silent ischaemic events after spinal analgesia for minor surgery in patients with stable angina pectoris compared with a reference day of normal daily activities."

I found it fascinating that myocardial ischemia occurred late and was not necessarily associated with a decrease in blood pressure, the onset of spinal analgesia, or ephedrine administration, but rather it was related to cessation of the block. Why? We can speculate that this may possibly be the result of reduced sympathetic blockade and relative volume overload.

Detailed descriptive studies in a small number of patients were carried out about 20 years ago to describe hemodynamic events in untreated hypertensive patients who were undergoing anesthesia and surgery. However, to determine the correct therapeutic regimen (i.e., should antihypertensive medications be discontinued or maintained until the time of surgery?), large, prospective, randomized, rigidly controlled clinical trials were necessary. Rigorous prospective clinical studies in a large number of patients are now required to evaluate the risks and benefits of regional anesthesia for a specific operation.—M. Wood, M.D.

Oesophageal Intubation: An Analysis of 2000 Incident Reports
Holland R, Webb RK, Runciman WB (Univ of Newcastle, Australia; Univ of Adelaide, Australia)
Anaesth Intens Care 21:608–610, 1993   101-95-9–6

Purpose.—Unrecognized esophageal intubation of a patient who is paralyzed is a catastrophic occurrence in anesthetic practice. Even with a wide range of methods available to detect this complication, its incidence has not decreased. Cases of esophageal intubation reported to the Australian Incident Monitoring Study (AIMS) were reviewed to determine the efficacy of various methods for detecting this complication and the circumstances under which these methods failed.

Methods and Results.—The AIMS consisted of voluntary anonymous reports of any unintended incident that reduced or had the potential to reduce the margin of safety for a patient. Of the first 2,000 such incidents reported, 35 involved esophageal intubation. In 8 cases, the esophageal intubation was classified as "obvious" to the reporting physicians. The number of reports of esophageal intubation decreased during the 4 years of the study, from 13 in the first year to 6 in the fourth year. Esophageal intubations occurred in the hands of both anesthetic specialists and trainees; auscultation was not a reliable test of its occurrence.

Capnography was used alone or with oximetry in 16 cases, with no false positives. There was 1 false negative, which could have been avoided if the appropriate machine check had been performed. Complications occurred in 9 cases, including death in 1, postponement of the operation in 4, and aspiration in 3.

Conclusion.—The use of monitors, especially capnography, to detect esophageal intubation has increased. Because capnography can detect esophageal intubation at an early stage, many anesthetists may no longer regard it as a "critical" incident. Capnography should continue to be available in the operating room, with capnographic confirmation of the expected concentration of carbon dioxide in expired gas immediately after the placement or replacement of any endotracheal tube.

▶ I must step back and comment for the record about Dr. Ross Holland. He is a giant, no other word seems to suffice, in the area of understanding the real risks associated with anesthesia. His name is not well known to American anesthesiologists, but it should be. Dr. Holland has been carefully reporting various risks and outcomes associated with anesthesia for more than 30 years. Taken together, his reports are by far the most comprehensive and consistent over time and are probably the best-analyzed long series of studies on this important subject that has ever been done.

Dr. Holland has managed to keep the medicolegal "hounds" at bay in Australia and to convince Australian anesthesiologists to trust his competent use of these sensitive incidents and data. I want to take this opportunity to pay a heartfelt tribute to Dr. Holland and his colleagues for these enormously important efforts. Think about it. Could "an analysis of 2,000 incident reports" related to anesthesia have ever been compiled in the American medicolegal climate?

I know what you are about to say: "Wait a minute. What about the American Society of Anesthesiologists (ASA) closed claims study?" The ASA closed-claims study is another enormous and important undertaking to be sure, but by its nature, it can only study incidents and outcomes that have been brought to the medicolegal system. These do not get brought to the medicolegal system by doctors but by plaintiffs and their lawyers. Plaintiffs' lawyers prefer cases that are likely to achieve major financial recovery, because they operate on a contingent-fee basis. The ASA closed-claim study necessarily "discriminates" against various outcomes and/or kinds of patients. For example, in the latter group, elderly patients are not likely to be appropriately represented. When they die or get injured, it is difficult to "prove" that their lives were "worth" large amounts of money. I do not want to take anything whatsoever away from the ASA study, but I think American anesthesiologists should also be aware of the truly wonderful work that Dr. Holland and his colleagues have been patiently doing for more than 30 years in Australia. Dr. Holland, I salute you.—J.H. Tinker, M.D.

Risk of Aspiration With the Laryngeal Mask

Akhtar TM, Street MK (King's College, London; Royal Sussex County Hosp, Brighton, England)
Br J Anaesth 72:447–450, 1994

101-95-9–7

Introduction.—The laryngeal mask airway (LMA) is better tolerated than tracheal intubation. However, it covers both the laryngeal inlet and the esophagus, and there is concern that the risk of gastric regurgitation and aspiration may be increased with the use of the LMA in patients who are mechanically ventilated. The incidence of aspiration using the LMA was compared in patients under general anesthesia with either mechanical or spontaneous ventilation.

Methods.—Fifty patients undergoing routine surgery were randomly assigned to receive anesthesia by either mechanical or spontaneous ventilation using the LMA. Ten minutes before the induction of anesthesia, patients swallowed a capsule containing methylene blue powder to turn their gastric contents blue. After surgery, the presence of dye was noted by direct laryngoscopy.

Results.—Those in the 2 groups were comparable in age, weight, and male-to-female ratio. After surgery, 1 patient in each group had methylene blue dye in the pharynx. The patient in the mechanical ventilation group was a woman undergoing diagnostic laparoscopy who was placed in the lithotomy position with her head tilted down 15 degrees. She had extensive blue-dye staining of her pharynx, larynx, and tracheal lumen, although she experienced no postoperative respiratory complications. The patient in the spontaneous ventilation group was a man undergoing varicose vein surgery in the supine position. He had blue-dye staining of his LMA and pharynx but none in his larynx.

Discussion.—There was an overall 4% incidence of regurgitation into the pharynx, which is higher than is desirable. Although there was no difference in the incidence of regurgitation, the dye was present in the trachea in the mechanically ventilated patient, suggesting that mechanical ventilation with an LMA may increase the risk of aspiration.

▶ The LMA was introduced more than 10 years ago by Brain (1), and it has taken a long time to become popular in the United States. It is a very useful device, and as anesthesiologists become more comfortable with it, its application in difficult clinical situations is increasing.

This study emphasizes that although the LMA is a useful device, it does not protect the patient's airway from aspiration of gastric contents. Does silent pulmonary aspiration occur more frequently than spontaneous ventilation in patients who require mechanical ventilation? Many anesthesiologists now routinely use mechanical ventilation with the LMA. Although the incidence of aspiration was the same in both groups, that is, whether they underwent mechanical or spontaneous ventilation, the authors did study a small number of patients and found that good anesthetic technique and skill were always important.

It is noteworthy that the investigators were very careful to control airway pressure generated during ventilation to less than 25 cm H_2O. The incidence of aspiration in this study was more than 4%, which is much smaller than that reported in other studies, and it may be as high as 23%.

The usual warning that a conventional LMA should not be used in patients with a full stomach who require emergency anesthesia still applies. A new esophageal vent–laryngeal mask, which is a combination of a hollow esophageal tube that prevents regurgitation (like an esophageal obturator) and a laryngeal mask, has recently been described (2). An esophageal balloon may be inflated through a nonreturn valve.—M. Wood, M.D.

References

1. Brain AIJ: *Br J Anaesth* 55:801, 1983.
2. Akhtar TM: *Br J Anaesth* 72:52, 1994.

Seroprevalence of HIV in Orthopaedic Patients in Zimbabwe
Cohen B, Piscioneri F, Candido FJ, Rankin KC (Mpilo Hosp, Bulawayo, Zimbabwe)
J Bone Joint Surg (Br) 76B:477–479, 1994   101-95-9–8

Introduction.—Because HIV can be transmittted by blood and other body fluids, surgeons and their assistants are at risk when operating on patients who are HIV-positive. Orthopedic surgeons are at particular risk because of the increased likelihood of glove and skin puncture by sharp bone spicules and of blood aerosols. The prevalence of asymptomatic HIV infection in Zimbabwe is unknown. The feasibility of a screening program was determined by assessing the incidence of HIV-positive patients undergoing orthopedic procedures.

Methods.—Enzyme-linked immunosorbent assays for HIV-1 and HIV-2 were used to screen blood samples from all patients having elective orthopedic surgery at 2 hospitals in Zimbabwe within a 3-month period. The patients were examined for signs of HIV infection.

Results.—Fifty-six men and 20 women were tested; 10 men (18%) and 2 women (10%) were found to be HIV-positive. Only 2 of the HIV-positive patients had clinical signs of HIV infection; the others were completely asymptomatic.

Discussion.—This group of patients had a high incidence of HIV seropositivity. The finding that 10 of the 12 HIV-positive patients were completely asymptomatic indicated the inadequacy of clinical screening to identify at-risk patients preoperatively. If there had been no serologic testing, surgery on 10 of the infected patients would have been performed without the additional infection control precautions of double-gloving, eye protection, and waterproof garments.

▶ It appears that East Africa has a real epidemic of HIV-positivity, because more than 15% of patients who agreed to be tested were positive for the disease. The setting of this hospital isn't clear, that is, is it a hospital that serves groups that are at high risk for HIV? Also, what percentage of patients at this hospital refused screening?—M.F. Roizen, M.D.

Nocturnal Orthopaedic Operating: Can We Let Sleeping Orthopaedic Surgeons Lie?

Yeatman M, Kingsmill Moore JM, Cameron-Smith A (Ashford Hosp, Middlesex, England)
Ann R Coll Surg Engl 76:90–94, 1994   101-95-9–9

Introduction.—Recent studies have questioned the wisdom of nocturnal surgery that is performed by less experienced surgeons and have instead proposed a classification system to reduce this practice. The system assesses the nature and severity of injury and designates emergency, urgent, scheduled, and elective status, thereby identifying patients for whom surgery can be delayed until daytime. The extent of nocturnal surgery and the degree to which it could be reduced in orthopedic surgery cases were reviewed retrospectively.

Methods.—The records of all patients undergoing emergency orthopedic surgery at 1 hospital within a 1-year period were reviewed. Data were derived that documented each patient's age and sex, the nature, time, and duration of each emergency surgical procedure, and the time the patient was seen to determine the extent of nocturnal surgery. The case notes were examined, and each patient was classified as being an emergency, urgent, or scheduled case to determine the need for immediate surgery.

Results.—Of the 1,534 patients who were admitted for orthopedic treatment, 272 (17.7%) underwent emergency surgery. Hip joint surgery accounted for the largest group of emergency procedures (37.6%), followed by femoral neck fractures (34.7%). Most (66.2%) of the emergency procedures were performed outside the normal working day. These procedures accounted for 62.5% of the total surgical hours. However, most of the patients (58.8%) were seen during the normal working day. Classification of the injury severity revealed that only 1 patient should have been classified as an emergency case; 32 procedures were urgent, and 149 (81.9%) could have been scheduled cases.

Discussion.—Although most of the patients arrived in the emergency department during normal working hours, most of the surgical procedures were performed outside normal working hours. Deferring surgery for patients in the scheduled category until the next morning would have reduced nocturnal surgical procedures by 81.2%.

▶ It is clear from the studies by the University of South Florida that closer observation results in less morbidity. Apparently, in the British system, closer observation is only available during daytime hours when consultants are at work. This article reveals that 81% of the patients who had orthopedic operations during nocturnal hours could have had surgery as a scheduled case the next day. Such scheduling of cases could lead to increased operating room efficiency and decreased operating room use at hours when personnel are less efficient, when times are longer, and when operating room nursing is more expensive. Furthermore, by decreasing complication rates, the product would be better and inherently less costly because the complications would not have to be treated or dealt with, and treating complications is always much more expensive than doing surgery right the first time.—M.F. Roizen, M.D.

A Twenty-Five Year Survey of a Solo Practice in Rural Surgical Care
Callaghan J (Winneshiek County Mem Hosp, Decorah, Iowa)
J Am Coll Surg 178:459–465, 1994   101-95-9–10

Introduction.—About 25% of the United States population lives in a rural area. However, there is very little information published that documents the activities of rural surgeons. The 25-year experience of a single surgeon practicing in a 50-bed rural hospital in northeastern Iowa was described.

Methods.—A total of 13,793 surgical procedures performed between 1967 and 1991 were reviewed from a personal log book, which documented the patient, pathologic findings, procedure, and outcome.

Results.—During the 25-year period, 5 patients sustained cardiac arrests during surgery or recovery; 4 were successfully resuscitated. Two patients experienced complete wound dehiscences. The procedures performed included 1,410 groin hernia repairs, with 1 death and 6 wound infections. Groin hernia repair accounted for the largest number of surgical procedures, followed by gallbladder operations, appendectomies, tonsillectomies and adenoidectomies, colorectal resections, anorectal operations, mastectomy, ventral herniorrhaphy, gastroduodenal operations, release of bowel obstruction, varicose vein operations, and skin grafting. Of the 1,052 gallbladder operations, there were 2 deaths in patients with gangrenous cholecystitis, 3 deaths from cardiovascular complications, and 4 cases of retained common duct stones. Instrumentation for laparoscopic cholecystectomy became available at the hospital in 1991, and it has since become the procedure of choice for patients with chronic cholecystitis. Of the 863 appendectomies performed, 103 were performed in patients who received an incorrect diagnosis. Since 1979, the use of diagnostic laparoscopy has reduced diagnostic inaccuracy.

Other procedures that have only been performed more recently include upper gastrointestinal endoscopy, colonoscopy, therapeutic laparoscopy, and colposcopy.

Discussion.—The experience of this surgeon reveals that the range of surgical procedures performed is greater than that generally performed by a surgeon in a metropolitan hospital. As a result, surgeons who practice in a rural area should get adequate training for the great variety of situations they face.

▶ This is a remarkable series, but is it true? There is no audit trail, but the authoritarian nature of the article seems to indicate that it may well be. This one surgeon performed endoscopies, orthopedic hip pinning and hip replacement, esophageal resections, colon resections, and parathyroidectomies, all with mortality and morbidity rates that approach the best in the literature and all without the aid of postoperative ventilatory support, invasive hemodynamic monitoring, or modern pain control methods. Either the people of rural Iowa are of heartier stock, the operations were minor events in the patients' lives and they weren't sick to begin with, this is a remarkable surgeon, or the data I derived from the literature aren't the best. All the operations were performed with the surgeon supervising a nurse-anesthetist, and all occurred within 60–70 miles of a major metropolitan center. Is this true today? Do patients prefer to have surgery locally when only 1 to 1½ hours away they can get the best medical care in the country by other standards? Is this just 1 remarkable human being who has done this in this 1 community, or do all 55 million Americans who live 60 miles or more from a major center, which is approximately 20% to 25% of the nation's total population, prefer surgery performed in small hospitals by the local physician who cares? I don't know whether this is a rare result, but it is certainly one that opened my eyes.—M.F. Roizen, M.D.

A National Audit of Antimicrobial Prophylaxis in Vascular Surgery

Winslet MC, Obeid ML (Royal Free Hosp, London; Dudley Road Hosp, Birmingham, England)
Eur J Vasc Surg 7:638–641, 1993   101-95-9–11

Background.—Patients undergoing vascular reconstructive surgery have a 1% to 5% incidence of wound infection. Graft infection, which occurs in about 2.5% of patients, is a major source of morbidity. The incidence of these infectious complications can be reduced by perioperative antimicrobial prophylaxis and meticulous technique, although debate continues about the type and duration of prophylaxis. British vascular surgeons were surveyed to determine their antimicrobial prescribing practices.

Methods.—The study questionnaire, which addressed antimicrobial prophylaxis for elective and emergency vascular surgery, was sent to 262 practicing vascular surgeons. The response rate was 68%.

Findings.—Sixty-one percent of the respondents used a cephalosporin-based antimicrobial regimen; 39% used penicillin and 6.5% used an aminoglycoside. Sixteen percent used more than 1 antibiotic, and 19% routinely used a specific antianaerobic cover. All the surgeons used prophylaxis for patients who received a prosthetic graft, compared with 76% for cases of an autogenous vein graft. A 3-dose regimen was the most popular overall; a single-dose regimen was more often used for an autogenous vein graft than for an umbilical vein or synthetic graft, 14% vs. 4.5%, respectively. About 3% of the respondents used a different regimen for suprainguinal vs. infrainguinal surgery; 4.5% used a modified regimen in emergency cases.

Conclusion.—British vascular surgeons usually prescribe a 3-dose cephalosporin regimen, without an antianaerobic cover, for antimicrobial prophylaxis. Although this regimen has theoretical limitations, it represents a standard against which future trials of prophylaxis should be compared. Choices of antibiotic prophylaxis should be based on local sensitivity patterns.

▶ The similarity in antibiotic choices across the United Kingdom is remarkable. The lack of a rationale based on sensitivity patterns is also amazing. A 3-dose cephalosporin regimen without an antianaerobic cover seems to be a prescribing standard in the United Kingdom, which must have less virulent anaerobes than are found in the United States.—M.F. Roizen, M.D.

Outcome After Day-Care Surgery in a Major Teaching Hospital
Osborne GA, Rudkin GE (Royal Adelaide Hosp, South Australia)
Anaesth Intensive Care 21:822–827, 1993   101-95-9-12

Objective.—Because of cutbacks in health care spending, the number of operations performed on an ambulatory basis is increasing. Few studies have evaluated the outcome of such surgery. The outcome of ambulatory surgery in the first 6,000 patients treated in a major Australian teaching hospital was measured prospectively.

Methods.—Outcome was evaluated in terms of unanticipated hospital admissions, complications, morbidity, recovery time, patient satisfaction, and community support needs.

Results.—Most of the 6,000 patients were female, aged 20–29 years. More than 90% were followed up by telephone. The most common surgical procedures were oral, gynecologic, ophthalmologic, and orthopedic. Most of the 1.34% of unanticipated hospital admissions were related to surgery. Most of the .5% of major complications were related to surgery or anesthesia. Anesthesia complications were more common with general anesthesia than with local or regional anesthesia, and recovery times were concomitantly longer. Postoperative discomfort consisted primarily of pain, nausea, and vomiting. Recovery times were significantly longer for patients who received general anesthesia for laparoscopic gynecologic procedures than for other procedures. There was no correlation between recovery time and age. As a result of ambulatory surgery, 4% of patients visited a physician and 3.1% visited the hospital emergency department. Most patients were satisfied with the results of the ambulatory surgery and the service provided.

Conclusion.—Ambulatory surgery provides an acceptable standard of care for patients.

▶ Patient satisfaction was assessed by postoperative telephone follow-up of these patients. Although a little over 7% saw a physician in either an emergency department or a local physician for problems related to their perioperative care, this seems to be a very satisfactory outcome for day surgery that was started in a university hospital. Ninety-eight percent of the patients expressed satisfaction, and only 5% of patients expressed feelings of undue pain afterward. The unanticipated hospital admission rate of 1.34% seems to be about what others are experiencing in hospital-based ambulatory surgery units.—M.F. Roizen, M.D.

Call Mosby Document Express at **1 (800) 55-MOSBY** to obtain copies of the original source documents of articles featured or referenced in the YEAR BOOK series.

10 Operating Room Environment: Safety Issues; Exposure Issues

Impairment of Anesthesia Task Performance by Laser Protection Goggles
Boucek C, Freeman JA, Bircher NG, Tullock W (Univ of Pittsburgh, Pa)
Anesth Analg 77:1232–1237, 1993   101-95-10-1

Background.—All operating room personnel are advised to wear goggles during the performance of laser surgery so that eye injury can be prevented. The effect of these goggles on the ability of anesthesia personnel to accurately perform their tasks has not been reported. The influence of wearing tinted goggles on the identification and sorting of medications and on manual dexterity under lighting conditions that approximated the operating room was examined.

Methods.—Thirty volunteer anesthesia providers were randomly assigned to 1 of 2 study groups that were evaluated as they performed the Stromberg Dexterity Test and the Medication Sorting Task, an investigator-designed test, twice. Those in group 1 wore tinted goggles during the first performance of the tests only, and those in group 2 wore tinted goggles during the second performance of the tests only. All volunteers were first screened for color-blindness. Testing was performed under standardized lighting conditions that simulated operating room lighting during laser surgery.

Results.—When no tinted goggles were used on the first performance of the Stromberg Dexterity Test, the second attempt using goggles was an average of 4.53 seconds slower than the first. When goggles were used first in performing the Stromberg test and removed for the second performance, the second attempt averaged 12.2 seconds faster than the first. When no goggles were used in the first performance of the Medication Sorting Task, the second performance was 14 seconds slower on average than the first. When goggles were used first and then removed for the second performance of the Medication Sorting Task, the second sorting was 88 seconds faster, a significant increase. Major medication sorting errors occurred 12 times when colored goggles were being worn and 5 times when they were not being worn. The association between wearing goggles and medication errors was significant. Minor errors occurred 6 times when goggles were worn and 8 times when they were not worn. Goggle-wearing and minor medication errors were not significantly associated.

Conclusion.—The pressure to meet time constraints during the administration of anesthesia, combined with the wearing of tinted goggles and decreased room lighting during laser surgery, may reduce patient safety. The development of user-friendly eyewear should be encouraged. Allotment of more time to the performance of anesthesia tasks under the working conditions required when laser surgery is performed would enhance patient safety.

▶ This important study illustrates how the environment around us can change and cause decrements in our performance. Although this effect may be obvious to some, the subtle change to wearing goggles may have major consequences. The authors are to be congratulated, not only for doing a superb job in performing the study, but for discussing its implications. Although the time difference was small, the major errors occurred 12 times when goggles were worn and 5 times when no goggles were worn during these 30 trials. Thus, the authors have shown a significant effect and something of which we all must be aware in our daily practice.—M.F. Roizen, M.D.

Blood Contact and Exposures Among Operating Room Personnel: A Multicenter Study
White MC, Lynch P (Univ of California, San Francisco; Univ of Washington, Seattle)
Am J Infect Control 21:243–248, 1993   101-95-10–2

Background.—Exposure to blood is recognized as being a risk for infection by agents such as hepatitis and HIV. Several categories of health care workers have higher rates of hepatitis B than other populations. Definitions of blood exposure in the operating room and research methods have varied from study to study. A multicenter study investigated all blood contacts in the operating room.

Methods.—Nine community and university hospitals participated. The definition of cutaneous exposure was visible blood on the skin and that of parenteral exposure was visible blood on nonintact skin or mucous membranes or when a puncture or cut occurred with a used sharp. During 8,502 surgical procedures, circulating nurses asked surgical staff about blood exposures and filled out data collection forms.

Results.—Blood contact occurred in 864 procedures in 1,054 individuals. The rate of parenteral exposure was 2.2% and the rate of cutaneous exposure was 10.2%. Among surgeons, about 21% of blood contacts were parenteral compared with 11% among nonsurgeons. The face and neck accounted for 24.2% of blood contacts. Of parenteral exposures, 36.2% occurred during suturing, and 27% occurred during surgically related cutting activities. Of cutaneous exposures, 46.9% occurred from unknown sources or surprise spatters. Parenteral exposures occurred 2.2 times more often in a university hospital than a community hospital.

Discussion.—Many individuals in the operating room did not wear gloves, long sleeves, or leg or foot coverings and did not always cover their faces and necks during surgeries in which a blood spatter could have been anticipated. Blood contact during surgery was frequent, but many exposures could have been prevented by changes in practice and the use of protective clothing.

▶ This study confirms the high rate of nonparenteral exposure to blood in the operating room. Nine hospitals participated; 7 community hospitals and 2 university hospitals. Among the cutaneous exposures of interest, most were surprise spatters, whereas among parenteral exposures, most were from needlestick injuries. Although they did not have a high degree of the total contacts, anesthesia personnel did have a large number of cutaneous exposures to intact skin.—M.F. Roizen, M.D.

Accidental Skin Punctures During Ophthalmic Surgery
Callanan DG, Borup MD, Newton J, Smiddy WE (Univ of Miami, Fla)
Ophthalmology 100:1846–1850, 1993   101-95-10–3

Introduction.—The incidence of skin puncture—which carries the risk of hepatitis B and HIV transmission—during ophthalmic surgery was determined. Although several studies have examined the problem in general surgical procedures, there is a lack of data on accidental skin punctures in ophthalmic procedures.

Methods.—All incident reports of skin punctures in the Bascom Palmer Eye Institute operating rooms that occurred between January 1990 and November 1991 were reviewed. The evaluation continued prospectively from December 1991 through May 1992. All known patient sources were tested once for hepatitis A and B and HIV serology in incidents involving a possibly contaminated instrument. Employees of the institute were offered a hepatitis B vaccination at the time of employment.

Results.—During the period of the retrospective review, 37 sharp injuries occurred during 14,878 ophthalmic operations, for an incidence of .25%; the incidence was .28% for the prospective period. Overall, a total of 49 injuries in 19,124 operations yielded an incidence of .26%. Twenty-five (51%) incidents involved the scrub nurse, and the surgeon or circulating nurse was injured in 7 incidents (14%) each. Instruments most commonly involved were a needle with a lumen (43%), a microsurgical blade (31%), and a suture needle (10%). The instrument was known to be contaminated with the patient's fluids in 63% of the cases; the contamination status was unknown in 22%, and instruments were uncontaminated in 14%. Therefore, health care workers were at risk of possible bloodborne infection in 86% of the incidents. One of the patients involved in an incident was known to be HIV-positive. All employees were tested, and none is known to have seroconverted for either HIV or hepatitis.

Conclusion.—Although the incidence of accidental skin puncture was low in ophthalmic procedures, the potential risk to personnel involved justifies precautions to decrease these events. Although HIV seroconversion is a prominent concern, health care workers are at greater risk of acquiring hepatitis B infection. Approximately 200 health care workers are estimated to die each year of occupationally acquired infection. In addition to the usually recommended precautions, it is suggested that the surgical assistant be placed on the side opposite the scrub nurse to decrease congestion in the "traffic" flow area of instruments.

▶ This study probably has artificially low skin puncture data. Because of the way it was reported, only when physicians or operating room personnel reported actual skin punctures were they then pursued. Because between 50% and 90% of skin punctures go unrecognized, the rate is apparently too low by a factor of between 2 and 9. The anesthesiologist was involved in 6% of the reported injuries, whereas the scrub nurse was involved in 51% of the reported injuries. This relative risk is probably related to reporting, I would presume, rather than actual incidents of injuries, although it is not clear from this study. Nevertheless, this study indicates that, even during ophthalmic surgery, there is a risk of occupational disease transmission.—M.F. Roizen, M.D.

Permeability of Latex and Thermoplastic Elastomer Gloves to the Bacteriophage ϕX174
Hamann CP, Nelson JR (SmartPractice, Phoenix, Ariz; Nelson Labs, Salt Lake City, Utah)
Am J Infect Control 21:289–296, 1993   101-95-10-4

Background.—Studies that have evaluated the permeability of gloves used by health care workers have concentrated on latex and vinyl gloves. Many individuals have allergies develop to various elements in latex gloves, and the durability of vinyl has been questioned. An alternative glove material has been developed that is a nonlatex, nonvinyl, thermoplastic elastomer with a tensile strength equal or superior to that of latex. The protective barriers of 2 brands of latex gloves and thermoplastic elastomer gloves were compared against that of the bacteriophage ϕX174.

Methods.—Gloves were filled with phosphate-buffered saline solution and exposed to ϕX174 in a flask that was shaken for 180 minutes at 37°C. At baseline and at 30, 60, 120, and 180 minutes, a 5-mL sample was collected from each glove. After 180 minutes, the remaining fluid was also collected. Contents of the gloves were screened for ϕX174 by a standard plaque assay and an extremely sensitive qualitative assay.

Results.—With the standard plaque assay, ϕX174 was detected in 30% of brand 1 latex gloves, 80% of brand 2 latex gloves, and none of the thermoplastic elastomer gloves. With the more sensitive qualitative assay, virus was detected in 70% of brand 1 latex gloves, 100% of brand 2 gloves, and 30% of the thermoplastic elastomer gloves.

Discussion.—The deterioration of latex may affect the shelf life of gloves that are bought in bulk and stored for long periods. Thermoplastic elastomer gloves are impermeable to antineoplastic drugs, offer a more microscopically complete barrier than latex gloves, and are free of latex allergens.

▶ This article presents a great review of the permeability of latex and thermoplastic gloves. The authors reveal that the glove manufacturer is perhaps more important than the actual substance when dealing with latex gloves, because the failure rate of 4 brands of latex examination gloves ranged from 3% to 20%, and nonsterile examination gloves, whether latex or vinyl, tended to leak more often than sterile surgical gloves. Furthermore, hours of use weaken the vinyl gloves dramatically and also weaken latex gloves. Washing latex gloves with detergent increases the size of micropores, whereas latex deteriorates because the unsaturated carbon bond that holds the latex together is weakened by stretching, humidity, ultraviolet light, and other things.

Although those of us in clinical settings have attributed the breakdown of effectiveness of the barrier gloves provide against punctures from needles or sharps to manufacturing defects, these findings imply that simply wearing gloves for long periods of time and exposure to heat, humidity, and other things cause them to wear down.

This article prompted me to try to determine where we can obtain thermoplastic elastomer gloves. If you believe in universal precautions, these gloves appear to be significantly better at protecting individuals than the usual vinyl or latex examination gloves we use in our practice. For those who seek another implication in this study, it is that your hospital probably should be alerted that the difference in the manufacture and quality of gloves is very important and that quality is not necessarily reflected by price differences.—M.F. Roizen, M.D.

Efficacy of BCG Vaccine in the Prevention of Tuberculosis: Meta-Analysis of the Published Literature

Colditz GA, Brewer TF, Berkey CS, Wilson ME, Burdick E, Fineberg HV, Mosteller F (Harvard School of Public Health, Boston; Massachusetts Gen Hosp, Boston; Mount Auburn Hosp, Cambridge, Mass)

JAMA 271:698–702, 1994   101-95-10–5

Background.—The current increase in the number of tuberculosis (TB) cases in the United States has been accompanied by an increase in multiple drug–resistant TB. Five health care workers or prison guards have died as the result of multiple drug–resistant TB from institutional spread. Such developments have prompted a reconsideration of the broadened use of bacille Calmette-Guérin (BCG) vaccine in the United States, although the efficacy of this vaccine has been debated. The hypothesis that rates of TB are different in BCG-vaccinated and nonvaccinated control populations was tested using meta-analysis.

Methods.—Clinical trials of BCG vaccine efficacy were identified through MEDLINE, using the index terms BCG vaccine, tuberculosis, and human, and by scanning references of these reports and contacting experts in the field. A total of 1,264 articles or abstracts were reviewed, and 70 were examined in depth. Eligible trials randomly established concurrent comparison groups that received and did not receive BCG vaccine and provided equal surveillance and follow-up for these groups. Fourteen prospective trials and 12 case-control studies were selected for the meta-analysis. The relative risk (RR) or odds ratio (OR) of TB provided the measure of vaccine efficacy, and the protective effect was then computed by 1-RR or 1-OR.

Results.—The trials showed the RR of TB to be .49 for vaccine recipients compared with nonrecipients, for a protective effect of 51% for BCG vaccine. Seven trials that reported tuberculous deaths yielded a protective effect of 71% from the vaccine; 5 studies that reported on meningitis demonstrated a protective effect from BCG vaccine of 64%. In the trials, the efficacy of BCG vaccination increased with greater distance from the equator and with higher study validity. The data validity score was the only variable that explained a substantial amount (36%) of the heterogeneity among the case-control studies. Different strains of BCG were not consistently associated with more or less favorable results in the trials.

Conclusion.—The BCG vaccine significantly reduces the risk of active TB cases and deaths across many populations, study designs, and forms of TB. Overall, its protective effect against TB infections was 50%. The age at vaccination did not predict the efficacy of the vaccine.

▶ Meta-analysis has enjoyed a resurgence in popularity because of its usefulness in evaluating studies that have a comparable study design and seemingly controversial results. The authors use the more compelling confidence interval reporting of their meta-analysis and reveal that BCG vaccination is recommended for tuberculin-negative infants and children who have continuing exposure to isoniazid- and rifampin-resistant active TB and cannot take isoniazid but have ongoing exposure to infectious TB or who belong to groups with rates of new tuberculosis infection that exceed 1% per year. Thus, the question not only for children but for health care workers who are exposed to TB patients is: Should they receive BCG prophylaxis? A drawback to BCG prophylaxis is that it voids the ability to do tuberculin skin testing to find the presence of TB or of conversion resulting from infection with TB.

The results of this analysis are impressive. The vaccine is only about 50% effective (confidence intervals, 39% to 64%), but the efficacy increases with greater distance from the equator and with better study data, meaning that the studies that show greater efficacy are those that appear to have been done in a more valid fashion. The slightly higher rates of protection against severe forms of TB, such as disseminated disease, meningitis, and death, may in fact not reflect better protection, but rather better data on these inputs. The authors conclude that, in general, they think the results of the meta-analysis add weight and confidence to the arguments that favor use of BCG vaccine, at least in the populations indicated by the Centers for Disease Control and Prevention.—M.F. Roizen, M.D.

Influence of Abuse of Nicotine and Alcohol on Postoperative Bacterial Infection

Stopinski J, Staib I, Weissbach M (Cliniques de la ville de Darmstadt, Germany)
J Chir 130:422–425, 1993   101-95-10–6

Introduction.—Postoperative bacterial infection (PBI) slows the wound-healing process and prolongs hospitalization. The use of prophylactic antibiotics has markedly reduced the PBI rate in patients undergoing colon surgery; however, the PBI rate in other areas has remained relatively constant within the past 10 years. The impact of alcohol and nicotine abuse on the PBI rate was assessed.

Patients.—The sample consisted of 213 patients, of whom 57 underwent inguinal hernia repair, 80 had cholecystectomy or choledochotomy, and 76 underwent colon cancer operations. Alcohol abuse was defined as a daily alcohol intake of more than 60 g. Patients were classified as nonsmokers, moderate smokers (1–19 cigarettes per day), or heavy smokers (more than 20 cigarettes per day). The PBIs included in the analysis were pneumonia, urinary infection, and delayed wound-healing.

Results.—The PBI rate was 3.5% for patients who underwent hernia repairs, 18.75% for those who underwent cholecystectomy or choledochotomy, and 31.6% for those who had colon cancer surgery. Fifteen patients (7.1%) were alcohol abusers and 60% of those had PBIs. By contrast, the PBI rate among nonabusers was only 15.8%, a statistically significant difference. Thirty-three patients were heavy smokers and 29 were moderate smokers. The PBI rate was 22.5% for smokers and 16.7% for nonsmokers. This difference was not statistically significant. However, the PBI rate among heavy smokers was 33.3%, almost twice that of nonsmokers.

Conclusion.—The risk of PBI for heavy smokers is twice as high as that for nonsmokers or moderate smokers. Consumption of more than 60 g of alcohol per day increases the risk of PBI by a factor of 4.

Effects of a Protective Foam on Scrubbing and Gloving

Larson E, Anderson JK, Baxendale L, Bobo L (Georgetown Univ, Washington, DC; Johns Hopkins Univ, Baltimore, Md)
Am J Infect Control 21:297–301, 1993   101-95-10–7

Background.—Neither gloves nor chemical barriers are impermeable to potentially infectious microbes. Protective skin creams, lotions, and foams have been developed as adjuncts to gloving. There is concern about the effect of the protectants on the surgical scrub. The effects of a foam protectant on the microbial counts on hands were examined, as were the effects of the foam on glove leakage.

Methods.—On 3 days, 49 participants performed a standard surgical scrub using 1 of 4 cleansing products. A protective foam was applied after the scrub on day 1 and before the scrub on day 3. Foam was not used on day 2. The participants wore sterile gloves for 2 hours after all 3 scrubs.

Results.—There were significantly lower bacterial counts in the research subjects who scrubbed with alcohol and 4% chlorhexidine gluconate than in those who scrubbed with 7.5% povidone-iodine or plain soap. There were no significant differences between the microbial counts on hands with or without foam, and there were no differences in glove leakage associated with foam.

Discussion.—The foam did not affect the efficacy of the scrub or the permeability of the gloves. The participants put on gloves after the protectant was dry; the results may have been different if the protectant had been wet or if gloves had been worn for more than several hours. Foams used to reduce allergy and minimize skin dryness may be useful adjuncts to hand hygiene.

▶ This article presents several important findings. Alcohol or chlorhexidine gluconate is significantly better than povidone-iodine for bacterial protection and decreasing bacterial counts. I wonder how we got away from alcohol and went to chlorhexidine gluconate or povidone-iodine at our institution. Also, glove leakage is extremely common; approximately 1½% of unworn gloves and 12.7% of gloves worn for 2 hours leaked, rates that appear to increase considerably with time simply because of the stretching of the latex of the gloves.

The authors found that the protectants now in use to either reduce the desiccating effects of frequent surgical scrubbing of the hands or to protect them from latex allergy do not affect leakage rates. Clearly, the application of the protectant may have been important in this trial if the subjects had waited until the foam was completely dry before donning gloves. How often this occurred in the rush of the operating room environment is open to question, because drying took several minutes. The authors did not study the effects of foam on glove leakage when the gloves were applied before the lotion dried or were worn for more than several hours.—M.F. Roizen, M.D.

The Use of a Visual Aid to Check Anaesthetic Machines: Is Performance Improved?
Groves J, Edwards N, Carr B (Northern Gen Hosp, Sheffield, England; Univ of Sheffield, England)
Anaesthesia 49:122–125, 1994   101-95-10–8

Introduction.—Failure to check equipment adequately is a frequent cause of "critical incidents" that occur during anesthesia. A checklist was produced by the Association of Anaesthetists of Great Britain and Ireland (AAGBI) to improve safety. The use of a pictorial checklist based on recommended procedures of the AAGBI was examined.

Methods.—Three BOC Boyle International Mk 2 machines were set up that had 10 faults of varying seriousness, 9 of which were of major significance. Twenty anesthetists and 7 operating department assistants (ODAs) were asked to check the machines according to their normal practice. Their performance was recorded and the tests were repeated 2 weeks later. At the time of the second test, the anesthetists and assistants used a visual aid and completed a questionnaire about the test. The faults were similar in the second test, but they had been placed in different machines.

Results.—Even with the visual aid, none of the participants detected all the faults, and no individual fault was detected by all participants on either occasion. They identified 58% of the faults using their own technique and 68% using the AAGBI visual checklist, a statistically significant difference. The visual aid was most helpful in increasing the detection rate of machine leaks. However, the detection rate was not improved for the empty vaporizer, the empty oxygen cylinder, and disconnected suction. Only 5 of 20 anesthetists always checked their machines before use, but all ODAs regularly checked their machines. Two thirds of the study participants thought that a checklist should be used, and 59% thought that the visual aid was helpful.

Conclusion.—Of the 10 faults that were incorporated in the machines, 5 were detected more frequently with the visual aid, 3 had the same detection rate on both occasions, and 2 were detected less often. The overall results are a cause for concern because at least one third of the problems were not caught at the time of either test. Clearly, there is a need for improved methods of detecting anesthetic machine faults.

▶ Ergonomics is an important subject: It tells us how to design anesthesia machines with complex monitoring systems so that they are foolproof in use. This article shows that, even with a visual checklist but without a mandatory checkoff procedure, 32% of the faults were missed. Therefore, this article argues for a guideline-based checklist to be used routinely before administering anesthesia.—M.F. Roizen, M.D.

The Risk From Radiation Exposure During Operative X-Ray Screening in Hand Surgery
Arnstein PM, Richards AM, Putney R (Queen Victoria Hosp, East Grinstead, England)
J Hand Surg (Br) 19B:393–396, 1994   101-95-10–9

Introduction.—Within the last decade, legislation has delineated protective guidelines for the use of ionizing radiation. Radiographic screening in hand surgery was investigated to quantify the amount of radiation exposure in the operating theater.

Methods.—A fresh cadaveric adult male hand was x-rayed with the image intensifier's diaphragms open and the antiscatter grid in place, with the diaphragms coned down enough to reduce the field by half and the antiscatter grid in place, and with the diaphragms open and the antiscatter grid removed. The levels of scattered radiation produced by the hand were measured in each case at radial distances of 15, 30, and 50 cm to reproduce the probable distances from the patient's hand to the surgeon's hands and eyes.

Results.—The scattered radiation measurements were reasonably uniform at any angle from the primary x-ray beam. Closing the image intensifier's diaphragms to lessen the field size reduced radiation scatter proportionally. Removing the antiscatter grid reduced scattered radiation by 63%. Combining reduction of the field size with removal of the antiscatter grid reduced scattered radiation by 82%.

Discussion.—Using careful radiologic practice, a surgeon could screen 19,000 patients without exceeding the annual radiation dose limit for the fingers and 21,000 patients without exceeding the annual dose limit for the eyes. However, the annual dose limit would be exceeded within 13 hours of work if the surgeon's hands were within the primary x-ray beam. The following measures were recommended to ensure safe radiologic practice in hand surgery: Cone down the image to reduce the field size by 50%; remove the antiscatter grid if possible; avoid the primary beam; and use a remote positioning device if possible.

▶ The authors of this fascinating study looked at the average time for hand surgery and studied radiation exposure for a typical image intensifier with the diaphragms open and the antiscatter grid in place, with the diaphragms coned and the antiscatter grid in place, and with the diaphragms open and the antiscatter grid removed.

The antiscatter grid improves the quality of the image by rejecting scattered radiation that would otherwise reach the intensifier. However, the power of the primary beam must be increased with this grid in place to maintain the image; thus, an increased level of scatter occurs when antiscatter grids are in place. On the other hand, when you cone a device, you decrease scatter.

The authors looked at the amounts of radiation from 15 cm, 30 cm, and 50 cm away, the last being the closest the anesthesiologist would probably get to the typical x-ray beam. Reducing the field size by closing the diaphragms produced a directly proportional reduction in scatter. Halving the x-ray beam area reduced the scattered radiation by an average of 52%. Removing the antiscatter grid reduced the average scattered radiation by 63%. Combining the 2 reduced the total scattered radiation by 82%, thereby reducing the amount of radiation that is likely to substantially affect surgeons. All else being equal and if the time for exposure is the same, it would be in our best interest to advocate that a coned field without an antiscatter grid be used in operating rooms. The general measures for minimizing radiation exposure and wearing correct protective clothing, including glasses, are definitely important.

This report was generated because of a radiographer who had cancer develop because he frequently held the patient's hand for radiographs. The overall message is that general measures, such as wearing protective lenses and protective garments, are most important, as is avoiding the primary beam, not using the antiscatter grid, and coning the primary source.—M.F. Roizen, M.D.

11 Cardiopulmonary Resuscitation and Prehospital Care

The Syringe Aspiration Technique to Verify Endotracheal Tube Position
Jenkins WA, Verdile VP, Paris PM (Westmoreland Regional Hosp, Greensburg, Pa; Albany Med College, NY; Univ of Pittsburgh, Pa)
Am J Emerg Med 12:413–416, 1994   101-95-11-1

Background.—Prehospital endotracheal intubation in patients who are acutely ill or injured is often performed by physician extenders. These physician extenders have demonstrated a 9% rate of endotracheal tube misplacement. The syringe aspiration technique (SAT) has been used with 100% accuracy in animals and patients in the operating room. The accuracy of the use of SAT by emergency department and prehospital personnel was tested to verify correct placement of endotracheal tubes.

Methods.—Ninety consecutive patients required urgent intubation in the emergency department or before hospitalization. After intubation, a 60-mL syringe connected to a straight anesthesia circuit adapter was attached to the end of the endotracheal tube after the cuff was inflated (Fig 11-1). The syringe plunger was withdrawn or aspirated with 60 mL of air. The ability to withdraw air into the syringe without resistance and without syringe plunger rebound was considered evidence of tracheal intubation; resistance or rebound of the syringe plunger indicated esophageal intubation.

Results.—In 88 patients, aspiration occurred without resistance or syringe plunger rebound. Standard detection methods confirmed tracheal placement in all these patients. Both remaining patients had resistance with aspiration and syringe plunger rebound. Direct laryngoscopy revealed inadequate esophageal intubation. These endotracheal tubes had been placed by paramedics, with auscultation as the only means of detection. The SAT did not directly cause any negative complications or endotracheal tube movement.

Conclusion.—The SAT is a safe, effective device for verifying endotracheal tube position in patients who require urgent airway control. The

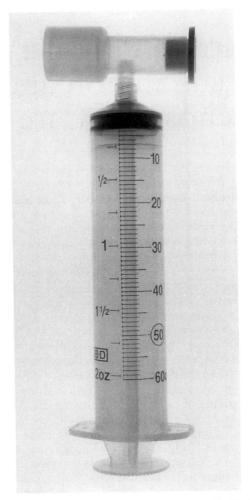

Fig 11–1.—Syringe aspiration device. (Courtesy of Jenkins WA, Verdile VP, Paris PM: *Am J Emerg Med* 12:413–416, 1994.)

use of the SAT by prehospital care providers should be the next phase of study.

▶ This is a simple and inexpensive method to assist in verifying endotracheal tube position during respiratory or cardiopulmonary arrest in the field or the emergency room or on the general ward, where end-tidal carbon dioxide monitoring is often absent.—D.M. Rothenberg, M.D.

Intubation Techniques in the Helicopter

Vilke GM, Hoyt DB, Epperson M, Fortlage D, Hutton KC, Rosen P (Univ of California, San Diego; Life Flight of San Diego, Calif)
J Emerg Med 12:217–224, 1994

101-95-11–2

Introduction.—Advanced helicopter medical evacuation programs offer active airway intervention and management of trauma victims. Intubation can be achieved by rapid-sequence induction (RSI) orotracheal, non–rapid-sequence induction (NRSI) orotracheal, blind nasotracheal (NT), and cricothyrotomy. Although there is extensive literature on each of these methods, the optimal procedure is unclear.

Methods.—Nasotracheal intubation, RSI, and NRSI were compared in an analysis of 630 field intubations of trauma patients by personnel of the San Diego Life Flight program. The 3 techniques were compared for the success of intubation, complications, and overall outcome. The patients were treated within a 4-year period.

Results.—An airway was established in 538 patients: 44% by NT, 27% by NRSI, 26% by RSI, and 3% by cricothyrotomy. Ninety percent of RSI attempts, 84% of NRSI attempts, and 75% of NT attempts were successful (Table 1). Non–rapid-sequence induction was initially successful in 90% of patients in whom it was attempted, RSI in 88%, and NT in 74%. Complications occurred in 23% of NT, 88% of NRSI, and 9% of RSI patients (Table 2). Patients who were intubated by the RSI technique were more likely to be discharged home and spent less time in the hospital than the other 2 groups.

Conclusion.—Rapid-sequence induction orotracheal intubation is associated with a higher success rate, fewer complications, and better patient outcomes that either the NRSI or NT techniques. The RSI technique should be the standard in prehospital airway management for trauma patients.

TABLE 1.—Success Rate for Each Technique Overall

N

Airway Type	Total Attempts	Total Patients Attempted	Total Successes	% Successful
Nasal	455	315	237	75
NRSI	220	170	143	84
RSI	226	156	140	90

Note: More than 1 technique may have been used for a single patient.
Abbreviation: NRSI, non–rapid-sequence induction.
(Courtesy of Vilke GM, Hoyt DB, Epperson M, et al: *J Emerg Med* 12:217–224, 1994.)

TABLE 2.—Complications Noted in the Field or Trauma Resuscitation: Comparison of Methods

Complication	N (%)			P-value*	P-value†
	Nasal (n = 237)	NRSI Oral (n = 143)	RSI Oral (n = 140)		
Esophageal intubation-unrecognized	0 (0)	0 (0)	0 (0)		
Esophageal intubation-recognized	8 (3)	28 (20)	5 (4)	=	‡
Mainstem intubation-recognized	5 (2)	2 (1)	1 (1)		
Mainstem intubation-unrecognized	7 (3)	11 (8)	0 (0)	=	
Stricture encountered	1 (0.5)	2 (1)	0 (0)		
Tube used was too large	7 (3)	7 (5)	2 (1)		
Cuff torn or leaky	2 (1)	7 (5)	0 (0)	§	
Equipment problem	3 (1)	7 (5)	0 (0)	§	
Laryngospasm	4 (2)	7 (5)	0 (0)	‡	
Dysrhythmias	0 (0)	5 (4)	1 (1)	§	
Vomiting	2 (1)	21 (15)	0 (0)	=	
Unable to visualize	0 (0)	24 (17)	3 (2)	=	
Extubated in transit	2 (1)	1 (1)	0 (0)		
Epistaxis	3 (1)	2 (1)	0 (0)		
Broken teeth	0 (0)	2 (1)	0 (0)		
Tracheal perforation	1 (0.5)	0 (0)	0 (0)		
Total	55	126	12	=	‡

* Comparison across all 3 groups.
† Comparison between nasal and rapid-sequence induction (RSI) oral.
‡ P < .05.
§ P < .01.
|| P < .001.
Abbreviation: NRSI, non-rapid-sequence induction.
(Courtesy of Vilke GM, Hoyt DB, Epperson M, et al: J Emerg Med 12:217–224, 1994.)

▶ The title of this article fascinated me, because I anticipated learning about the difficulties of managing the airway during an emergency "chopper" flight. Unfortunately, all intubations apparently took place in the field and on the ground. We are left with a retrospective, biased study that promotes the use of RSI with fentanyl and succinylcholine for the comatose or nearly comatose trauma victim. The authors conclude that RSI is associated with improved survival, and therefore they recommend this technique as "standard" for the trauma victim in the field; I could just as easily reach the conclusion that succinylcholine decreases mortality. I hope that our emergency physician colleagues will question the methodology of this study before they wholeheartedly embrace the results.—D.M. Rothenberg, M.D.

Hemodynamic Responses to Shock in Young Trauma Patients: Need for Invasive Monitoring
Abou-Khalil B, Scalea TM, Trooskin SZ, Henry SM, Hitchcock R (State Univ of New York, Brooklyn; Kings County Hosp Ctr, Brooklyn, NY)
Crit Care Med 22:633–639, 1994   101-95-11–3

Introduction.—Whether early invasive monitoring is necessary in young trauma patients was determined. It has been axiomatic that young patients without any history of cardiovascular disease have enough reserve to respond to substantial blood loss injuries. However, studies of elderly patients have shown an inadequate cardiovascular response to trauma.

Methods.—Thirty-nine male patients (mean age, 26 years) with penetrating thoracic and/or abdominal trauma caused by gunshot or stab wounds were treated within a 5-month period. All patients received more than 6 units of blood during exploration and surgery (thoracotomy in 11 patients, sternotomy in 2, laparotomy in 26, and neck exploration in 2), and invasive hemodynamic monitoring with percutaneous insertion of arterial and pulmonary artery catheters was performed as early as possible. The usual vital signs, laboratory values, and hemodynamic and oxygen transport values were compared at 1, 8, and 24 hours after surgery. Oxygen delivery was increased until a state of non–flow-dependent oxygen consumption and a normal serum lactate concentration were achieved. Blood transfusion was continued until the hematocrit reached 35% to 40%.

Results.—Despite normal blood pressure, heart rate, and urine output, only 5 (15%) patients achieved an optimized state 1 hour after surgery. Two patients achieved an optimized state with volume infusion alone; 32 patients (82%) required inotropes. Seven patients (18%) died; 5 patients never reached the target level of hemodynamic performance and died within 3 days; 2 patients optimized early but became septic and died within 10 days. Between survivors and nonsurvivors, there was no difference in temperature, mean arterial pressure, central venous pressure, pulmonary artery occlusion pressure, heart rate, or cardiac index (table). Survivors had a significantly lower pulmonary vascular resistance and serum lactate concentration and significantly higher oxygen delivery and mixed venous oxygen saturation.

Conclusion.—Young trauma patients have substantial but clinically occult myocardial depression after shock, and inotropes are required to optimize and clear circulating lactate. The adequacy of the cardiac re-

Hemodynamic Data for Survivors and Nonsurvivors in 39 Patients

	At 1 Hr			At 24 Hrs		
	Survivor	Nonsurvivor	p Value	Survivor	Nonsurvivor	p Value
MAP (mm Hg)	106 ± 3.6*	105 ± 4.5	NS	102 ± 2.8	101 ± 3.5	NS
HR (beats/min)	104 ± 8.3	105 ± 7.2	NS	104 ± 9.1	105 ± 11.1	NS
CVP (mm Hg)	12 ± 1	11 ± 1.4	NS	13 ± 0.83	12 ± 1.4	NS
PAOP (mm Hg)	11 ± 0.9	13 ± 0.99	NS	11 ± 0.7	13 ± 1.7	NS
Hct (%)	38 ± 2.3	36 ± 3.1	NS	34 ± 2.1	35 ± 1.2	NS
CI (L/min/m^2)	3.2 ± 0.18	3 ± 0.62	NS	5.7 ± 0.15	5.2 ± 0.46	NS
SVRI (dyne·sec/cm^5·m^2)	3010 ± 266	3202 ± 308	NS	1531 ± 53.9	1358 ± 58.1	NS
PVRI (dyne·sec/cm^5·m^2)	301 ± 18.4	532 ± 36.1	.001	105 ± 14.3	165 ± 12.2	.02
Ḋo$_2$I (mL/min/m^2)	519 ± 55.1	428 ± 80.1	.02	1098 ± 76.1	895 ± 78.2	.02
V̇o$_2$I (mL/min/m^2)	129 ± 8.8	127 ± 10	NS	278 ± 14.1	168 ± 20.1	NS
Lactate (mg/dL) (mmol/L)	4.1 ± 0.62	7.7 ± 1.2	.001	1.9 ± 0.19	4.2 ± 0.72	.001
Svo$_2$ (%)	73 ± 3.3	63 ± 4.1	.03	81 ± 4.2	78 ± 3.1	NS

* Mean ± standard error of the mean.

Abbreviations: MAP, mean arterial pressure; HR, heart rate; CVP, central venous pressure; PAOP, pulmonary artery occlusion pressure; Hct, hematocrit; CI, cardiac index; SVRI, systemic vascular resistance index; PVRI, pulmonary vascular resistance index; Ḋo$_2$I, oxygen delivery index; V̇o$_2$I, oxygen consumption index; Svo$_2$, mixed venous oxygen saturation.

(Courtesy of Abou-Khalil B, Scalea TM, Trooskin SZ, et al: *Crit Care Med* 22:633–639, 1994.)

sponse can be defined by early invasive monitoring. Patients in shock, based on oxygen transport parameters, should not be allowed to become anemic, and blood should be given as the initial volume expander. Controversy about the ideal resuscitation fluid remains, and transfusion should be continued, until patients achieve a state of non–flow-dependent oxygen consumption.

▶ This nonrandomized study suggests that early volume and inotropic resuscitation improve occult oxygen deficits and survival in young patients who experience penetrating trauma. Although it is considerably smaller, the study is presented as a contrast to the Bickell study (Abstract 101-95-21–10). The reader is left to determine whether early or delayed resuscitation is best.—D.M. Rothenberg, M.D.

Bystander Cardiopulmonary Resuscitation: Is Ventilation Necessary?
Berg RA, Kern KB, Sanders AB, Otto CW, Hilwig RW, Ewy GA (Univ of Arizona, Tucson)
Circulation 88:1907–1915, 1993   101-95-11–4

Background.—The basic life support recommendations advocated by the American Heart Association include mouth-to-mouth ventilation combined with chest compressions. This complex psychomotor task is not easy to remember or perform. Moreover, some bystanders may be reluctant to carry out mouth-to-mouth resuscitation because of the perceived risks of contracting infectious diseases. Preliminary experimental data suggest that chest compressions alone result in physiologic benefits comparable to chest compressions combined with ventilation. Whether the initial treatment of cardiac arrest by chest compressions with or without ventilation results in comparable rates of survival and good neurologic outcome was investigated.

Method.—Thirty seconds after ventricular fibrillation, swine were randomly assigned to either 12 minutes of chest compressions combined with mechanical ventilation, chest compressions only, or no CPR. Standard cardiac life support was then provided. The animals that were successfully resuscitated were supported for 2 hours in intensive care and observed for an additional 24 hours.

Results.—In all 16 swine that received chest compressions with mechanical ventilation (group A) or chest compressions only (group B), spontaneous circulation was restored and the animals survived for 24 hours and were neurologically normal. By contrast, the 8 swine that had no CPR had restoration of spontaneous circulation, but only 2 survived for 24 hours and only 1 was neurologically normal. The 95% confidence interval for 24-hour survival was 79% to 100% in groups A and B but only .3% to 53% in group C.

Conclusion.—In this swine model of basic life support after cardiac arrest, no significant differences in survival and neurologic outcome were seen when life support included chest compressions plus ventilation or chest compressions alone. If these results can be confirmed by additional studies, the use of prompt chest compression alone during initial resuscitation for human cardiac arrests may provide a simpler and more appealing method of basic life support in the setting of single-rescuer bystander CPR.

▶ The fear of contracting a virally mediated disease such as hepatitis or AIDS or a bacterially mediated disease such as tuberculosis often precludes even CPR instructors from initiating mouth-to-mouth resuscitation (MMR) during a witnessed cardiac arrest. Recognizing that this fear exists, the American Heart Association recommends in its *Guidelines for Advanced Cardiac Life Support* that closed-chest cardiac massage be initiated, even if MMR is avoided. This article and others suggest that early ventilation is less important than early chest compressions in the setting of a cardiac arrest, with MMR potentially contributing to hypercarbic acidosis and an adverse outcome during CPR (1).

Although in this study all animals in the treated group survived to be "eating, drinking, alert, active, observant, distrusting swine that were rooting around and difficult to catch," it is hard to extrapolate these results to patients with preexisting coronary artery disease. Therefore, the data presented should not be used to validate that MMR is not necessary, but rather to emphasize that survival correlates best with adequate coronary artery perfusion.—D.M. Rothenberg, M.D.

Reference

1. Wenzel V, et al: *Chest* 106:1806, 1994.

Developing Strategies to Prevent Inhospital Cardiac Arrest: Analyzing Responses of Physicians and Nurses in the Hours Before the Event

Franklin C, Mathew J (Cook County Hosp, Chicago; The Chicago Med School)
Crit Care Med 22:244–247, 1994   101-95-11–5

Background.—Cardiac arrest might be prevented or its consequences diminished if premonitory signs or symptoms are quickly recognized, monitored, and treated. The rate of warning signs or symptoms within 6 hours before a cardiac arrest and the reactions to them by nurses and physicians were evaluated.

Methods.—The medical records were reviewed for every patient who had a cardiac arrest while admitted to the internal medicine/family prac-

TABLE 1.—Outcome of 150 Consecutive Inhospital
Cardiac Arrests

Immediate deaths	104 (69)	Successful resuscitations	46 (31)
Hospital deaths	137 (91)	Hospital survivors	13 (9)
Neurologic damage	143 (95)	No damage	7 (5)

Note: Numbers in parentheses represent percentages expressed as conditional
percentage of patients in each subgroup calculated for successful outcome.
(Courtesy of Franklin C, Mathew J: *Crit Care Med* 22:244–247, 1994.)

tice services of a 1,000-bed urban hospital during a 20-month period
from 1990 to 1991. In all, there were 150 cardiac arrests.

Results.—The cardiac arrest rate was 7 arrests per 1,000 patients on
the internal medicine/family practice services. Table 1 depicts the outcome of patients who had a cardiac arrest. The immediate mortality was
69% and the total hospital mortality was 91%. Only 4.7% of the patients
who had a cardiac arrest were discharged from the hospital with their
baseline cognitive and motor functions intact. Patients who had been
discharged from the ICU during that admission had a cardiac arrest rate
that was significantly higher than that of the other patients (14.7 per
1,000 patients). According to the clinical signs or symptoms, 66% of the
arrests could have been anticipated. Table 2 indicates that of the 99 arrests in which a physician or nurse had documented a deterioration in
the patient's condition within 6 hours before the arrest, a nurse did not
notify a physician in 25 cases. In 42 cases, the house officer did not notify an ICU triage officer; an arterial blood gas sample was not obtained
in 30 cases; and in 22 of 32 cases, the ICU fellow did not sufficiently stabilize the patient before transferring him or her to the ICU.

Conclusion.—Warning signs or symptoms were commonly present
before cardiac arrests on the general wards of the hospital. More train-

TABLE 2.—Analysis of 99 Cardiac Arrests With
Clinical Antecedents

1. Nurse documents abnormalities, does not inform physician	25	(25%)
2. Abnormal mental status	19/25	
3. Physician sees patient, no ICU notification	42	(43%)
4. Abnormal or no arterial blood gas measurement	38/42	
5. ICU triage error	32	(32%)
6. Poorly stabilized before MICU transfer	22/32	

Abbreviation: MICU, medical ICU.
(Courtesy of Franklin C, Mathew J: *Crit Care Med* 22:244–247, 1994.)

ing of nurses and physicians would probably decrease the rate of these cardiac arrests.

▶ For survival rates to improve for patients who suffer inhospital cardiac arrest, 3 areas must be addressed: First, prevention "strategies," as described in this article, must be followed. The nurse who restrains an agitated patient, the intern who at 2 A.M. orders haloperidol for a confused patient and rolls over and goes back to sleep, and the ICU resident who misinterprets the signs of muscle fatigue on an arterial blood gas and fails to intubate a patient before transfer to the ICU are all examples of improper recognition and treatment of the hypercarbic, hypoxemic patient. It will be interesting to see whether the authors will now use a proactive approach to better educate or reeducate nursing and medical staff to improve the survival rates of inhospital arrests.

Second, research involving brain protection, both in the form of pharmacologic agents and rapid techniques to restore circulation, must consistently show improvement in neurologic outcome and survival to discharge.

Finally, CPR protocols should be applied only to those patients in whom the arrest is not a natural progression of the underlying disease (i.e., CPR should not be applied in futile situations, and do-not-resuscitate orders should be initiated in a more timely fashion; see reference 1.—D.M. Rothenberg, M.D.

Reference

1. 1994 Year Book of Anesthesiology and Pain Management, pp 184–185.

Correction of Intramyocardial Hypercarbic Acidosis With Sodium Bicarbonate
Sonett J, Pagani FD, Baker LS, Honeyman T, Hsi C, Knox M, Cronin C, Landow L, Visner MS (Univ of Massachusetts, Worcester)
Circ Shock 42:163–173, 1994   101-95-11–6

Introduction.—Animal studies suggest that sodium bicarbonate fails to correct intramyocardial acidosis during CPR when hypoperfusion and ischemia persist, partly because the carbon dioxide (CO_2) that is generated promotes hypercarbic acidosis. It is not clear whether the resultant myocardial dysfunction is caused by an increased partial pressure of carbon dioxide (pCO_2) or from hydration and a reduction in myocardial pH.

Methods.—Anesthetized dogs received sodium bicarbonate by the intracoronary route when they were eucapneic and after the production of systemic hypercabia, as the interstitial pH, regional coronary venous pCO_2, and regional myocardial stroke work were monitored. An 8.4% preparation of sodium bicarbonate was infused to deliver a total dose of 30 mEq. An equiosmolar solution of 5% sodium chloride was infused to

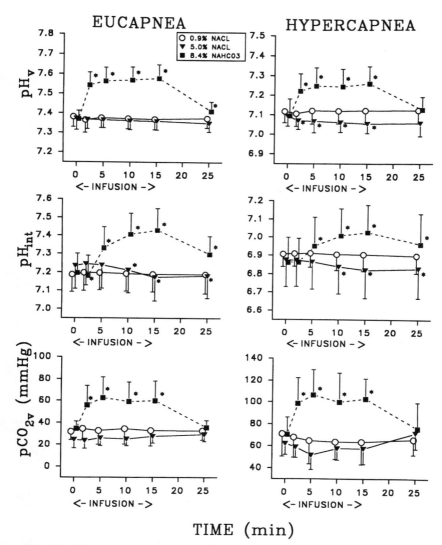

Fig 11–2.—Changes in coronary venous pH (pH_v), interstitial pH (pH_{int}), and coronary venous partial pressure of carbon dioxide (pCO_{2v}) during left anterior descending artery infusions of sodium chloride (NACL) and sodium bicarbonate (NAHCO₃) solutions. * P < .05 compared with baseline. (Courtesy of Sonett J, Pagani FD, Baker LS, et al: *Circ Shock* 42:163–173, 1994.)

control for the hypertonicity and sodium load of the bicarbonate solution, and physiologic saline was used as an isotonic control. Hypercapnia and acidosis were induced by hypoventilation to an arterial pCO_2 of 60–80 mm Hg. The vena cava was transiently occluded to assess the ef-

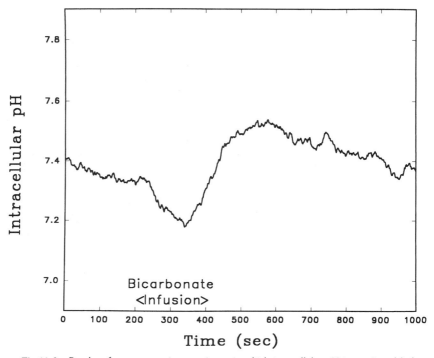

Fig 11–3.—Results of a representative experiment in which intracellular pH is monitored before, during, and after the infusion of sodium bicarbonate into the perfusate bathing a guinea pig papillary muscle. (Courtesy of Sonett J, Pagani FD, Baker LS, et al: *Circ Shock* 42:163–173, 1994.)

fects of hypoventilation on intrinsic myocardial contractility. Interstitial pH was recorded fluorometrically.

Results.—Left ventricular end-diastolic pressure increased after bicarbonate administration under both eucapnic and hypercapnic conditions. The regional coronary venous pH and pCO_2 increased significantly when bicarbonate was delivered (Fig 11-2). The interstitial pH increased significantly, whether eucapnic or hypercapnic conditions prevailed. Regional stroke work decreased significantly after intracoronary bicarbonate but recovered within 5 minutes. In a study of the guinea pig papillary muscle, exposure of the muscle to sodium bicarbonate led to a rapid decline in intracellular pH (Fig 11-3).

Conclusion.—Intracoronary delivery of sodium bicarbonate has the effect of alkalinizing the intramyocardial pH under conditions of preexisting eucapnia or hypercarbic acidosis. The intracellular pCO_2 increases, but contractile function is only transiently compromised.

▶ The battle continues to rage over the use of sodium bicarbonate as a buffer during periods of lactic acidosis. This study shows that perhaps the ineffectiveness of sodium bicarbonate during CPR relates to its inability to deliver the buffer to the myocardium where it may be most effective.—D.M. Rothenberg, M.D.

Call Mosby Document Express at **1 (800) 55-MOSBY** to obtain copies of the original source documents of articles featured or referenced in the YEAR BOOK series.

12 Cardiac Anesthesia

Comparison of Desflurane and Fentanyl-Based Anaesthetic Techniques for Coronary Artery Bypass Surgery
Parsons RS, Jones RM, Wrigley SR, MacLeod KGA, Platt MW (UMDS, London; Imperial College of Science, Technology and Medicine, London)
Br J Anaesth 72:430–438, 1994   101-95-12-1

Background.—To preserve myocardial function during anesthesia, systemic arterial pressure and cardiac rhythm must be predictably controlled. New anesthesia agents should be able to do this before they are accepted. Earlier work has shown that in a dose-dependent response, desflurane decreases arterial pressure and vascular resistance with no change in heart rate or cardiac index. Preliminary investigations indicate that desflurane would be a useful anesthetic for patients with coronary artery disease because of its ability to rapidly control circulatory responses with limited myocardial stress and ischemia. An inhaled anesthetic based on desflurane was compared with an anesthetic based on fentanyl in patients undergoing coronary artery bypass surgery.

Methods.—After screening patients for exclusion criteria (e.g., age, weight, neurologic disease, women of childbearing age, patients receiving CNS drugs), a total of 51 patients, American Society of Anesthesiologists physical status II and III, participated. While the patient inhaled 100% oxygen, fentanyl, 50 μg/kg, was induced over a period of 5–10 minutes, or desflurane, 10 μg/kg, was induced over a period of 5 minutes. The inspired mixture of desflurane was 6% (1 minimum alveolar concentration [MAC]) in oxygen. Additional doses of the anesthetic were administered at the discretion of the anesthesiologist. The lungs were ventilated to maintain a partial pressure of carbon dioxide ($PaCO_2$) of 4.6–5.3 kPa. End-tidal carbon dioxide (CO_2) was monitored continually, except during cardiopulmonary bypass. The pressures monitored included systolic, diastolic, mean, pulmonary artery, central venous, and pulmonary wedge. Also monitored were heart rate, ECG (leads II and V_5), cardiac output, end-tidal CO_2, arterial and venous blood gases, nasopharyngeal temperature, and desflurane concentration. These data were recorded at baseline, after insertion of all cannulas and catheters, after induction, after intubation, during skin preparation, after skin incision, after sternotomy, 15 minutes after cardiopulmonary bypass, and at the end of surgery. Cardiac index, stroke volume, and stroke work, as well as systemic and pulmonary vascular resistance, were computed.

Results.—Systemic arterial pressure was maintained at awake levels during sternotomy and incision by desflurane, but it was decreased at all other times. With fentanyl, the pressure was increased at sternotomy (+ 20 mm Hg vs. desflurane) and incision. Before bypass, the heart rate was maintained at 60–67 beats per minute with desflurane. This was typically 5–15 beats less than with fentanyl. The cardiac index was greater in the fentanyl group at induction, laryngoscopy, and during skin preparation, but it was lower before aortic cannulation. Vasodilators and glyceryl trinitrate were more commonly used in the patients who received fentanyl. There were no deaths.

Conclusion.—Desflurane, when complemented by low-dose fentanyl, is an appropriate anesthetic for patients undergoing coronary artery bypass surgery. The hemodynamic state was well controlled in these patients who were at risk for myocardial ischemia.

Pure Opioid Versus Opioid-Volatile Anesthesia for Coronary Artery Bypass Graft Surgery: A Prospective, Randomized, Double-Blind Study
Ramsay JG, DeLima LGR, Wynands JE, O'Connor JP, Ralley FE, Robbins GR
(McGill Univ, Montreal; Emory Univ, Atlanta, Ga; Univ of Ottawa Heart Inst, Ont, Canada)
Anesth Analg 78:867–875, 1994   101-95-12–2

Background.—Patients with coronary artery disease (CAD) are subject to a greater degree of stress and a higher incidence of dysrhythmias and myocardial ischemia in the perioperative period than are those without CAD. Results of previous studies of the effects of different anesthetic techniques on hemodynamic stability and the incidence of myocardial ischemia have been inconsistent. Incidence of prebypass ischemia, perioperative myocardial infarction, and hemodynamic stability were determined in patients receiving opioid vs. opioid-volatile anesthesia during coronary artery bypass surgery.

Methods.—Anesthesia was induced with sufentanil, 5 μg/kg, and pancuronium after standard premedication in 75 patients who were undergoing elective coronary artery bypass grafting (CABG). Anesthesia was maintained with isoflurane, enflurane, or sufentanil increments. Blood pressure was monitored continuously during surgery. Myocardial ischemia was assessed intraoperatively by ECG and Holter monitoring. Postoperative myocardial infarction was assessed by myocardial creatinine phosphokinase determination and ECG on 3 occasions within 2 days after surgery.

Results.—Hypertension was treated in about 50% of patients. Those receiving isoflurane or enflurane were successfully treated by adjustment of the vaporizer setting with or without additional sufentanil. Hypertension in most patients in the sufentanil-only group lasted longer and could not be controlled without nitroglycerin infusion. Intraoperative β-blockade was required for control of tachycardia more often in the sufentanil-only and enflurane groups, but this requirement was not associated with ischemia or myocardial infarction. The incidence of myocardial ischemia and myocardial infarction was not significantly different among the 3 groups.

Conclusion.—Isoflurane or enflurane provides better hemodynamic control during CABG after induction with sufentanil than sufentanil increments alone. No significant differences were noted in incidence of myocardial ischemia or infarction among the 3 anesthetic protocols used.

A Comparison of the Perioperative Neurologic Effects of Hypothermic Circulatory Arrest Versus Low-Flow Cardiopulmonary Bypass in Infant Heart Surgery

Newburger JW, Jonas RA, Wernovsky G, Wypij D, Hickey PR, Kuban KCK, Farrell DM, Holmes GL, Helmers SL, Constantinou J, Carrazana E, Barlow JK, Walsh AZ, Lucius KC, Share JC, Wessel DL, Hanley FL, Mayer JE Jr, Castaneda AR, Ware JH (Children's Hosp, Boston; Harvard Med School, Boston; Harvard School of Public Health, Boston)
N Engl J Med 329:1057–1064, 1993   101-95-12–3

Introduction.—Hypothermic circulatory arrest is widely used during cardiac surgery in infants, but its effects on neurologic function remain uncertain. An alternative approach is low-flow cardiopulmonary bypass, which maintains continuous cerebral circulation but may expose the brain to pump-related sources of injury, such as embolism and inadequate perfusion.

Objective.—The risk of perioperative brain injury was examined in 171 infants with D-transposition of the great arteries who underwent an arterial switch operation. Surgery was done under deep hypothermia, with a mean tympanic membrane temperature of 32.7°C at the start of bypass. Total circulatory arrest was used in 87 infants, and 84 were assigned to low-flow cardiopulmonary bypass. Twenty-one infants in each group had a ventricular septal defect. Total support and cross-clamp times were comparable in the 2 groups.

Results.—Infants in the 2 groups had similar operative mortality and hospital courses. Clinical seizures were more frequent in the circulatory arrest group, and they also correlated with longer periods of total circulatory arrest. These infants also tended to have more epileptiform activity on electroencephalographic monitoring in the first 48 hours after surgery. Both circulatory arrest and longer arrest times were associated with a greater release of creatine kinase BB isoenzyme. The clinical neurologic findings were similar in the 2 groups.

Conclusion.—When transposition of the great arteries was corrected under deep hypothermia, total circulatory arrest was associated with more neurologic perturbation in the early postoperative period than was low-flow cardiopulmonary bypass.

▶ Clinical studies that investigate outcome are always very difficult to perform correctly, because it is difficult to exclude the many variables that may occur during the perioperative period, and it is often not possible to study an adequate size sample to give findings sufficient statistical power. However, this investigation is important. It was a randomized single-center study, and the criteria for eligibility were carefully controlled. It appears that total circulatory arrest with profound hypothermia compared with low-flow cardiopulmonary bypass results in greater neurologic changes during the early postoperative period in infants who undergo cardiac surgery in the first 3 months of life. Although this article does not have direct relevance to many anesthesiologists in clinical practice, it may change or cause a reevaluation of the current cardiopulmonary perfusion practice at many university institutions.—M. Wood, M.D.

Effects of Aprotinin on Anticoagulant Monitoring: Implications in Cardiovascular Surgery
Najman DM, Walenga JM, Fareed J, Pifarré R (Loyola Univ, Maywood, Ill)
Ann Thorac Surg 55:662–666, 1993   101-95-12–4

Introduction.—Aprotinin has been used to improve hemostasis during cardiopulmonary bypass (CPB). The reduced blood loss achieved with aprotinin has been attributed to preservation of platelet adhesive capacity, although other mechanisms may be operative as well. Recent reports have suggested an increased rate of thrombosis after cardiac operations using aprotinin. A series of in vitro experiments was done to assess the effect of aprotinin on heparin dosage monitoring during cardiac operations as well as the mechanisms of interaction between platelets and aprotinin.

Methods and Results.—Aprotinin was added to heparinized whole blood at a concentration of 30 μg/mL, which is equal to that used during CPB operations. Aprotinin concentrations of 2 and 4 times this level were assessed as well. The activated clotting time (ACT) with heparin alone was 384 seconds; the addition of aprotinin synergistically elevated the ACT to 536 seconds at 30 μg/mL, 651 seconds at twice that level, and 787 seconds at 4 times that level. The addition of protamine to the heparin-aprotinin mixtures did not completely neutralize the heparin, with ACT values of 131 seconds vs. 98 seconds. On specific testing, aprotinin's effects on ACT were not equal to heparin's anticoagulant effects. Supplementation of normal platelets with aprotinin significantly inhibited their aggregation; however, this was not the case for platelets from postoperative patients.

Conclusion.—For optimal safety and efficacy during CPB operations, the effects of aprotinin on the hemostatic system and drug interactions must be considered. When aprotinin is used with ACT monitoring, there is a risk of underheparinization. The protamine doses used to reverse heparin should be based on the heparin concentration, not on ACT. Aprotinin may interact more favorably with the nonactivated platelet surface than with activated platelets in reducing or inhibiting receptor expression.

▶ Aprotinin is an old drug. It reminds me of steroids in some ways. For years, various people tried to prove that massive doses of steroids did something valuable in shock, in head trauma, or whatever. Aprotinin is another drug that has a loyal group of supporters who continuously advocate its use.

I am always wary of strongly positive results for a drug in which the mechanism is as obscure as it is with aprotinin. In the first paragraph of this article, 10 separate references are used to show that aprotinin does practically everything but cure flat feet! I am always wary of panaceas. Aprotinin currently has legions of true believers, most of them surgeons. I hope, but doubt, that aprotinin is this great.—J.H. Tinker, M.D.

Cardiac Surgery in a Patient Taking Monoamine Oxidase Inhibitors: An Adverse Fentanyl Reaction
Insler SR, Kraenzler EJ, Licina MG, Savage RM, Starr NJ (Cleveland Clinic Found, Ohio)
Anesth Analg 78:593–597, 1994   101-95-12-5

Background.—Monoamine oxidase inhibitors (MAOIs) have been reported to interact with drugs, predominantly opioids, to produce a syndrome of hyperpyrexia, hypertension, tachycardia, and coma; hepatotoxicity has also been described. Twelve cases in the world literature implicate the combination of meperidine and an MAOI as being potentially fatal.

Case Report.—Woman, 62, with insulin-dependent diabetes, had a history of chronic obstructive lung disease, congestive heart failure, and depression. She was admitted 1 week after myocardial infarction for coronary bypass graft surgery and repair of the regurgitant mitral valve. In addition to nitroglycerin, diltiazem, captopril, and a diuretic, the patient was taking 15 mg of phenelzine twice daily. Anesthesia was induced with fentanyl and vecuronium and maintained with fentanyl and midazolam. The maintenance dose was fentanyl, 15 μg/kg/hr. The patient required significant amounts of nitroprusside to support the blood pressure during cardiopulmonary bypass. After an increase in the doses of fentanyl and midazolam, she became hypertensive and a supraventricular tachycardia developed. Fentanyl and midazolam were withdrawn after respective doses of 78 and 190 μg/kg had been delivered. The hyperdynamic state soon began to resolve, and the patient remained stable. Propofol was used for sedation before the trachea was extubated.

Implications.—Opioids, especially those in the same class as meperidine, should be avoided if possible in patients who are receiving an MAOI and undergo cardiac surgery. These drugs include fentanyl, sufentanil, and alfentanil. If ventricular function is markedly impaired, it may be best to discontinue MAOI treatment 2 weeks or more before surgery.

▶ This article is an excellent example of the pendulum swinging in medicine. Taking patients off MAOIs as long as 2 weeks before surgery was de rigeur not that many years ago. Then the pendulum swung in the direction of pure iconoclasm, namely, "Don't take your patients off MAOIs at all if they need the drug for depression." Sure enough, maybe the old physicians weren't totally wrong. Monoamine oxidase inhibitors, if they are on board, should still raise significant red flags.

Mark Twain said something to the effect that when he was 18 he thought his father was the stupidest man around, but by the time he was 25, he was amazed at how much his father had learned in 7 years!—J.H. Tinker, M.D.

Desmopressin Does Not Decrease Bleeding After Cardiac Operation in Young Children
Reynolds LM, Nicolson SC, Jobes DR, Steven JM, Norwood WI, McGonigle ME, Manno CS (Univ of Pennsylvania, Philadelphia)
J Thorac Cardiovasc Surg 106:954–958, 1993   101-95-12–6

Objective.—Young children who undergo complex cardiac operations tend to lose more blood after cardiopulmonary bypass than older patients. Whether desmopressin limits blood loss in this setting was studied.

Study Plan.—One hundred twelve patients from 1 day to 16 years of age were scheduled for cardiac surgery. The patients were randomly assigned to receive either desmopressin or saline by IV infusion over a 15-minute period, starting 5 minutes after a protamine sulfate bolus, 4 mg/kg, was administered. Desmopressin, .3 μg/kg, was given, and heparin was added to the bypass pump prime in an age-related dose.

Results.—The desmopressin-treated patients and controls had similar amounts of blood loss over 24 hours, and their hematocrit values were identical 24 hours postoperatively. Their coagulation profiles were similar before surgery and at 30 minutes and 3 hours afterward.

Conclusion.—Preoperative infusion of desmopressin does not reduce blood loss in children who are undergoing cardiopulmonary bypass for cardiac surgery.

▶ Desmopressin swept onto the cardiac surgical scene a few years ago, perhaps because of its demonstrated efficacy in treating mild-to-moderate bleeding episodes in hemophiliacs. As seems to happen relatively often in cardiac surgery, I think it was uncritically accepted. Studies like this one, which was well done, are now emerging to indicate that desmopressin probably doesn't do much good.—J.H. Tinker, M.D.

Inhaled Nitric Oxide in Patients With Normal and Increased Pulmonary Vascular Resistance After Cardiac Surgery
Snow DJ, Gray SJ, Ghosh S, Foubert L, Oduro A, Higenbottam TW, Wells FC, Latimer RD (Papworth Hosp, Cambridge, England)
Br J Anaesth 72:185–189, 1994   101-95-12–7

Background.—Nitric oxide (NO), the active element of endothelium-derived relaxation factor, is a potent vasodilator. Adding NO to inhalational anesthetics selectively reduces pulmonary vascular resistance and the mean pulmonary artery pressure in patients with adult respiratory distress syndrome or secondary pulmonary hypertension. In volunteers who inhaled hypoxic gas mixtures, NO counteracted hypoxic pulmonary vasoconstriction.

Objective and Methods.—The hemodynamic effects of inhaling 40 ppm of NO were examined in 12 patients who had elective repair or replacement of the mitral valve and 10 others who had coronary bypass graft surgery on an elective basis. All the patients had good left ventricular function. Studies were done within 2 hours after surgery while sedation was maintained with propofol. Nitric oxide was given by the ventilator for 20 minutes. Only 2 patients received nitroprusside during the study.

Results.—Patients undergoing mitral valve replacement had significant reductions in pulmonary vascular resistance of about 20% to 30% and an insignificant decrease in systemic vascular resistance. The decline in pulmonary vascular resistance correlated with significant reductions in diastolic and mean pulmonary artery pressures. No significant hemodynamic changes were noted in patients who had coronary bypass graft surgery.

Conclusion.—Inhaled NO in a concentration of 40 ppm acts as a selective pulmonary vasodilator in patients with preexisting pulmonary hypertension.

▶ Nitric oxide, as most readers know, has been "sweeping the world" since the discovery that it indeed was the famous "endothelial relaxant factor." Carefully administered NO does decrease dilate pulmonary vasculature, and it has been used successfully in infants who would otherwise have died. It is logical that NO would be tried in patients who have problems with increased pulmonary vascular resistance after cardiac surgery. Experience with NO clearly shows that methemoglobin levels must be monitored and that NO administration in extraordinarily low doses (e.g., 20–50 ppm) must be carefully monitored. To my knowledge, we have no other drugs that are administered at this dose level; therefore, a new apparatus must be built and we must learn how to use it. I also believe that sooner or later we ought to be able to learn how to "deliver" NO in some form to the systemic arterial side of the circulation. Right now, we have only 1 drug capable of doing that, namely nitroprusside, which unfortunately has cyanide liability. I included this article because I think that NO therapy for various diseases in a variety of pharmacologic forms is coming soon and will be a welcome addition to our armamentarium.—J.H. Tinker, M.D.

Suspected Protamine Allergy: Diagnosis and Management for Coronary Artery Surgery
Pharo GH, Horrow J, Van Riper DF, Levy JH (Hahnemann Univ, Philadelphia; Emory Univ, Atlanta, Ga)
Anesth Analg 78:181–184, 1994   101-95-12–8

Introduction.—A wide range of drugs that are used during anesthesia has been associated with anaphylactic reactions, but protamine allergy has rarely been documented.

Case Report.—Man, 56, with a history of reactive airway disease and a "silent" myocardial infarction 2 years earlier underwent cardiac catheterization. After catheterization by the femoral route, the patient was given IV protamine, 15 mg, to neutralize heparin. Marked hypotension and bradycardia developed within 15 minutes, and the patient described itching and dyspnea. Wheezing was noted bilaterally along with diffuse urticaria. Diphenhydramine, hydrocortisone, and ranitidine were given for 2 days, at which point coronary bypass surgery was necessary on an urgent basis. The patient reported having had a vasectomy. An intradermal test with protamine was negative, and no antiprotamine antibody was demonstrated. After bypass surgery, protamine was infused in a stepwise manner after a 1-mg test dose. A full neutralizing dose of 400 mg was administered uneventfully.

Discussion.—This patient probably had an anaphylactoid reaction to IV contrast medium. Graded exposure to protamine will minimize allergen exposure. Preoperative desensitization is another possible approach.

▶ I don't usually include case reports, but I think cardiac anesthesiologists might benefit from reading this thorough and careful analysis of suspected protamine allergy. The other reason I included this article was to vent one of my pet peeves, namely, that as cardiac anesthesiologists, we are forced to depend so heavily for our patients' lives and our livelihoods on a drug that is derived from fish sperm! It would seem that we could do better in this age of the molecular biology–derived "magic bullet," which always seems to be "just around the corner" and has been for years and years and billions of dollars. I would like to think that our molecular biologists could come up with something to replace such a product. It's time for the people who brought us such breakthroughs as the "growth hormone" and erythropoietin to work on this problem.—J.H. Tinker, M.D.

The Misplaced Intraaortic Balloon Pump
Coffin SA (Univ of Iowa, Iowa City)
Anesth Analg 78:1182–1183, 1994
101-95-12–9

Introduction.—Reports have appeared of an intra-aortic balloon pump (IABP) being incorrectly placed within the left ventricle, the subclavian artery, and the renal artery. A patient was reported who was the first one known to have an IABP in the contralateral femoral artery.

Case Report.—Man, 78, was admitted 13 months after a coronary bypass operation with congestive heart failure. Iron-deficiency anemia and chronic renal insufficiency also were present. Catheterization showed all 3 vein grafts to be stenosed. Apical akinesia was confirmed, with a left ventricular ejection fraction of 35%. Recurrent heart failure prompted a decision to repeat the bypass graft procedure and replace the mitral valve. When an attempt failed to separate the patient from cardiopulmonary bypass, an IABP was placed through the right femoral artery using the Seldinger technique. Peak pressures of 70–100 mg Hg were recorded from the balloon catheter tip, but pressure in the right radial artery was only 30 mm Hg and the waveform was damped. Transesophageal echocardiography failed to demonstrate the balloon in the descending thoracic aorta. The pulsating balloon was palpated in the contralateral groin and immediately removed. The balloon then was advanced through a right femoral cannula under ultrasound guidance and positioned 2–3 cm below the aortic arch. The patient was removed from bypass, but he required repair of a small hole at the superior vena caval cannulation site. The IABP was removed on the second postoperative day. Thoracentesis was necessitated by a large pleural effusion, but the patient was discharged 11 days postoperatively.

Discussion.—Had a transesophageal ultrasound transducer not been in place, this patient might have died of cerebral and myocardial hypotension. It is wise to routinely note the insertion length of an IABP from surface landmarks and to confirm correct positioning by a chest radiograph in the surgical ICU.

▶ When the echo first was touted, some of us old cardiovascular hands tended to discount its utility and emphasize its tremendous cost. The truth is that the device has validity and utility despite its cost. This unique case resulted in the saving of a life, nothing less.—J.H. Tinker, M.D.

A Potential Mechanism of Vasodilation After Warm Heart Surgery: The Temperature-Dependent Release of Cytokines

Menasché P, Haydar S, Peynet J, Du Buit C, Merval R, Bloch G, Piwnica A, Tedgui A (Hôpital Lariboisière, Paris)
J Thorac Cardiovasc Surg 107:293–299, 1994   101-95-12–10

Introduction.—One of the clinical concerns that arises with warm heart surgery is the development of peripheral vasodilation, because when the vasodilation is sufficient to require vasopressors, the blood flow through new arterial and venous bypass grafts may be compromised. Temperature-mediated cytokines have been implicated in the development of peripheral vasodilation. The effect of temperature on the production of cytokines was examined in a 2-part study, including both animal data and a prospective clinical trial.

Methods.—In the first part of the study, peritoneal macrophages were obtained from rabbits and incubated for 1, 2, 3, 4, 6, or 9 hours at 30°C or 37°C with lipopolysaccharide. Tumor necrosis factor (TNF) activity in the supernatant was measured by a bioassay. In the second part of the study, 30 consecutive patients who were undergoing valve or coronary artery bypass surgery were assigned to have either a cold or warm bypass. Arterial blood was obtained after the induction of anesthesia but before sternotomy and at 2, 4, 10, and 24 hours after cardiopulmonary bypass (CPB) was instituted. The levels of TNF-α, interleukin-1β (IL-1β), and IL-6 were assayed.

Results.—The release of TNF by the endotoxin-activated rabbit macrophages increased to higher levels at 37°C than at 30°C. The levels of TNF stayed relatively low for 3 hours and increased thereafter in the group that was incubated at 30°C, whereas the levels of TNF increased steeply between 1 and 6 hours and then plateaued in the group that was incubated at 37°C. In the clinical study, the normothermic group had consistently higher levels of cytokines. The levels of TNF-α were similar in both groups until 2 hours after CPB; by 4 hours, the levels of TNF-α had declined almost to baseline in the hypothermic group. Similar patterns occurred in the production of IL-1β and IL-6, but the peaks occurred at 4 hours. Six patients in the normothermic group and 3 in the hypothermic group required vasoactive therapy. These patients had significantly higher levels of cytokines than those who did not require pressor therapy.

Discussion.—Both the experimental and clinical findings indicate that the production of cytokines is temperature-dependent. The association between high levels of cytokines and the need for pressor support indicates that cytokines have vasodilatory effects. Allowing the core temperature to drift during bypass may decrease the vasodilatory response while it maintains myocardial aerobiosis.

▶ The modern trend toward "warm heart surgery" has replaced an earlier set of problems with a new set of problems, one of which is massive vasodilation. These authors have attributed at least some of this to elevated cytokines. Unfortunately, many other things are "elevated" during and after CPB.

I am skeptical about whether any particular group of "out of whack" hormones can be definitively nailed down with current technology as the culprit. Nonetheless, the authors make a pretty good case for at least modest hypothermia. Although they did not study neurologic dysfunction, others have and found it to be worse during warm CPB. When you do mine, I would just as soon have a reasonable degree of hypothermia, based on my current understanding of the literature.—J.H. Tinker, M.D.

Administration of Vancomycin During Cardiopulmonary Bypass
Baraka A, Taha S, Bijjani A, Arab W, Meshefedjian G (American Univ of Beirut, Lebanon)
Anaesthesia 47:1086–1087, 1994   101-95-12–11

Background.—Vancomycin prophylaxis is recommended for selected patients who are undergoing open heart surgery. However, serious anaphylactoid reactions have been reported after vancomycin infusion; these complications may be potentially life-threatening in the period before cardiopulmonary bypass (CPB). The cardiovascular changes associated with giving vancomycin after the initiation of CPB were assessed.

Methods and Results.—Twelve anesthetized patients undergoing open heart surgery received vancomycin during CPB. The antibiotic was given in a dose of 1 g within 60 seconds through the venous inlet of the oxygenator. Vancomycin administration resulted in a moderate and transient decrease in the mean arterial pressure, from 76 to 53 mm Hg. These values returned to control levels after 6 minutes. Within 10 minutes after vancomycin was administered, the mean reservoir volume gradually decreased from 2.37 to 1.82.

Conclusion.—Vancomycin can be safely administered after the initiation of CPB. The minimal arterial pressure reaction in this study appears to have resulted from dilution of vancomycin by the extracorporeal circuit volume; from bypass of the lungs, which are an important storage site of vasoactive substances; and from the maintenance of adequate perfusion flow during CPB. Giving vancomycin after the initiation of CPB may decrease the incidence of adverse hemodynamic reactions.

▶ I included this article for 2 reasons. First, I *hate* vancomycin! I have seen major grief (i.e., cardiovascular collapse) with this antibiotic when it was apparently injected too fast. Giving it over a period of about a month makes sense to me, although that might not fit surgery in a nonacademic center. These authors administered it after initiation of circulatory support CPB. This concept makes sense from the standpoint of protection against hemodynamic disaster, although I do not know that the authors have shown that it makes sense from the standpoint of antibiotic prophylaxis.

I chose this article also because it comes from someone I greatly admire, Dr. Anis Baraka, who has maintained an excellent anesthesiology training program for many years under the most difficult circumstances imaginable, during a war and in one of the most troubled regions on the planet—Beirut, Lebanon. Not only does he manage to train superb anesthesiologists, he also performs clinical studies and writes them up in a scholarly fashion. Dr. Baraka, I salute you.—J.H. Tinker, M.D.

Call Mosby Document Express at **1 (800) 55-MOSBY** to obtain copies of the original source documents of articles featured or referenced in the YEAR BOOK series.

---

13 Cardiopulmonary Bypass

ACE-Inhibitors, Calcium Antagonists and Low Systemic Vascular Resistance Following Cardiopulmonary Bypass: A Case-Control Study
Myles PS, Olenikov I, Bujor MA, Davis BB (Alfred Hosp, Prahran, Australia)
Med J Aust 158:675–677, 1993   101-95-13-1

Introduction.—No specific cause has been identified to explain an increased incidence of low systemic vascular resistance (SVR) after cardiopulmonary bypass (CPB). The incidence of SVR was investigated after cardiac surgery and CPB to determine whether it is more common in patients who received angiotensin-converting enzyme (ACE) inhibitors or calcium antagonists, drugs used to treat hypertension, myocardial ischemia, and cardiac failure.

Methods.—The exposure to ACE inhibitors or calcium antagonists was determined in 42 patients in an ICU who had low SVR syndrome and received CPB, had valve surgery, or both in 1991. These patients were matched with 84 controls.

Results.—No association was seen between therapy with ACE inhibitors (adjusted odds ratio [OR], 1.33) or calcium antagonists (adjusted OR, .49) and the low SVR syndrome after CPB. The incidence of low SVR syndrome was 7.4%. Patients with low SVR syndrome were more likely to spend more time in the cardiothoracic ICU and to be treated with norepinephrine, epinephrine, and dopamine.

Conclusion.—After CPB, the low SVR syndrome was not associated with preoperative therapy with ACE inhibitors or calcium antagonists. Despite an apparent increase in the incidence of low SVR syndrome, that coincided with the increased popularity of these drugs, the association would appear to be spurious. A well-designed prospective study with more extensive documentation may produce more information.

▶ Many investigators have been trying to understand why so many patients these days have such a vasodilated state after bypass. This article debunks the common notion that it might be related to ACE inhibitors. It must be cytokines (whatever *they* are).—J.H. Tinker, M.D.

Cerebral Hemodynamics During Cardiopulmonary Bypass in Children Using Near-Infrared Spectroscopy

Fallon P, Roberts I, Kirkham FJ, Elliott MJ, Lloyd-Thomas A, Maynard R, Edwards AD (Hosp for Sick Children, London; Royal Postgraduate Med School, London)
Ann Thorac Surg 56:1473–1477, 1993   101-95-13–2

Introduction.—Because the effects of cardiopulmonary bypass on cerebrovascular regulation can contribute to the neurologic impairment seen in some children, the method of near-infrared spectroscopy was used to monitor cerebrovascular function perioperatively in 28 children 15 days to 7½ years of age who underwent bypass for the repair of congenital heart defects.

Methods.—Cardiopulmonary bypass was performed using a nonpulsatile roller pump and membrane oxygenator. Cerebral blood flow and cerebral blood volume were measured after steady-state conditions were achieved using standardized anesthesia. The change in cerebral blood volume with changing carbon dioxide tension (CBVR) also was measured. Measurements were made using a commercial spectrophotometer and light at 4 wavelengths; it was applied to the frontoparietal region by a flexible fiberoptic bundle.

Findings.—Cerebral blood flow ranged from 16 to 53.5 mL/100 g/min. Cerebral blood volumes ranged from 4.3 to 8 mL/100 g during bypass at full pump flow of 2.4 L/min^{-1}/m^{-2} and increased to 14.7 mL/100 g during bypass at half flow. The CBVR was .12 mL/100 g/kPa preoperatively and was independent of the mean arterial pressure. During hypothermic bypass at 25°C, the CBVR declined significantly to .05 mL/100 g/kPa, and negative pressures were recorded at 3 points when the mean arterial pressure was less than 40 mm Hg.

Application.—Using near-infrared spectroscopy, it was possible to quantify cerebral blood flow, volume, and CBVR during cardiopulmonary bypass. This approach may prove useful as a noninvasive means of assessing cerebral hemodynamics during that procedure.

▶ I included this article because I think it is long overdue that we develop noninvasive hemodynamic monitoring techniques. As many have heard me say ad nauseam, we have a tube that is 1 in. in diameter that contains blood moving at 5 L/min complete with iron-containing particles located only a few inches under the sternum and we cannot measure the flow in it! We should be exploring things such as "near-infrared spectroscopy."—J.H. Tinker, M.D.

Elevation of Cytokines During Open Heart Surgery With Cardiopulmonary Bypass: Participation of Interleukin 8 and 6 in Reperfusion Injury

Kawamura T, Wakusawa R, Okada K, Inada S (Iwate Med Univ, Uchimaru,

Morioka, Japan)
Can J Anaesth 40:1016–1021, 1993   101-95-13–3

Introduction.—Myocardial ischemia is a major cause of low cardiac output in patients who have open heart surgery. Myocardial damage associated with ischemia and reperfusion has been attributed in part to the actions of neutrophils, their interaction with vascular endothelial cells, and the effects of various cytokines.

Objective and Methods.—Myocardial cell injury was related to concentrations of the putative neutrophil activators interleukin-6 (IL-6) and IL-8 in 11 patients who had open heart surgery under cardiopulmonary bypass. Anesthesia was induced with fentanyl and maintained with high-dose fentanyl and oxygen. Neutrophil counts were made serially, along with estimations of granulocyte elastase (GEL), IL-6, IL-8, tumor necrosis factor-α (TNF-α), creatine phosphokinase (CK), and the CK-MB fraction.

Findings.—Serum values of CK and CK-MB increased 1 hour after the aorta was declamped, as did counts of polymorphonuclear leukocytes. The plasma GEL was increased 1 hour after declamping; a high level persisted at 3 hours. Serum levels of both IL-6 and IL-8 also increased. The level of IL-8 for as long as 3 hours after declamping exceeded that observed at 1 hour after aortic occlusion. The TNF-α level was decreased 1 hour after aortic occlusion.

Conclusion.—Circulating levels of IL-6 and IL-8 increase as a result of myocardial ischemia. These cytokines may play a part in reperfusion injury by activating neutrophils.

▶ This paper represents one of the current studies of cardiopulmonary bypass in which it is gradually being recognized that cardiopulmonary bypass is extraordinarily complex in its physiologic trespass. I also think this article sheds light on the mechanism of reperfusion injury, which is a problem not only for the heart but also for the brain.—J.H. Tinker, M.D.

Effect of Cardiopulmonary Bypass on Gastrointestinal Perfusion and Function

Gaer JAR, Shaw ADS, Wild R, Swift RI, Munsch CM, Smith PLC, Taylor KM (Hammersmith Hosp, London)
Ann Thorac Surg 57:371–375, 1994   101-95-13–4

Introduction.—Gastrointestinal complications may not be unduly frequent after open heart surgery, but they produce considerable morbidity and mortality and require more hospital time. The nature of these complications and their precise causes remain uncertain.

Objective.—Tonometric measurements were made in the gastric mucosa to assess the adequacy of gastrointestinal perfusion in 10 patients who had elective coronary revascularization. The patients, who were all younger than 80 years of age, were prospectively randomized to receive either pulsatile or nonpulsatile flow during the time the aorta was cross-clamped.

Methods.—The gastric mucosal pH was measured by an indirect tonometric method based on the Tonomitor. Monitoring began before the start of bypass and continued at 30-minute intervals for 4 hours and then hourly for 12 hours. Patients received standardized anesthesia with fentanyl. Blood gases were managed by an alpha-state regimen. The myocardium was protected by antegrade cold blood cardioplegia at 4°C along with topical cooling.

Results.—None of the 10 patients had gastrointestinal complications postoperatively. The total bypass times averaged 86 minutes in the pulsatile group and 72 minutes for the nonpulsatile group. In all cases, the gastric mucosal pH declined during bypass, reflecting reduced mucosal perfusion. The change occurred independent of changes in arterial pH. The mucosal pH decreased significantly more when nonpulsatile flow was used.

Conclusion.—Gastric mucosal blood flow is reduced during cardiopulmonary bypass in patients who have open heart surgery, especially when nonpulsatile flow is used. Gastric mucosal acidosis may predispose them to gastrointestinal complications postoperatively.

▶ This article once again comes under the category of "at last." Finally, after 40 years and hundreds and hundreds of thousands of patients, it really focuses on the "physiologic trespass" of cardiopulmonary bypass. The breakdown of the gastric mucosal barrier is probably also associated with the breakdown of other intestinal barriers, which in turn presents intriguing possibilities for the release of all sorts of evil humors contained in those organs.—J.H. Tinker, M.D.

Computer Simulation of Brain Cooling During Cardiopulmonary Bypass

Dexter F, Hindman BJ (Univ of Iowa, Iowa City)
Ann Thorac Surg 57:1171–1179, 1994   101-95-13–5

Objective.—During cardiopulmonary bypass (CPB), cerebral hypothermia is the principal means by which neurologic protection is achieved. However, recent studies have raised important questions about the optimal use of cerebral hypothermia and highlighted the need for a more complete understanding of the rate at which brain cooling occurs and the final brain temperature is achieved. The effects of convection, metabolism, and conduction on these parameters during CPB were evaluated using a mathematical model of heat transport.

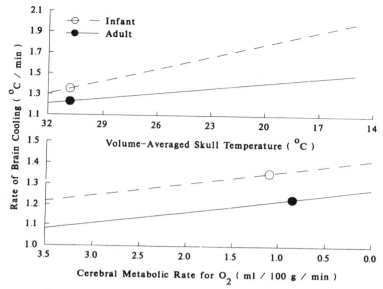

Fig 13–1.—Effect of heat conduction and brain metabolism on the rate of brain cooling. The volume-averaged skull temperature appropriate for a brain temperature of 32°C (reference value, 30.8°C) is used in **bottom** and is represented by *circles* in **top.** When the brain temperature equals 32°C and the head is packed in ice, the skull temperature may be as low as 15°C for adults and 15.2°C for infants. The cerebral metabolic rate for a brain temperature of 32°C (reference values, .85 and 1.1 mL oxygen [O$_2$]/100 g^{-1}/min^{-1} for adults and infants, respectively) is used in **top** and represented by *circles* in **bottom.** The blood temperature is kept fixed at its reference value (27°C). The cerebral blood flow is kept fixed at reference values appropriate for a brain temperature of 32°C. (Courtesy of Dexter F, Hindman BJ: *Ann Thorac Surg* 57:1171–1179, 1994.)

Methods.—Heat transport within the brain of adults and infants was predicted using a standard bioheat transport model. The effects of variations in these parameters were assessed across a clinically relevant range, with all other variables being held at fixed values.

Findings.—The most important measure of the rate of brain cooling was convection, which is a function of the cerebral blood flow and arterial blood temperature. The final temperature was determined almost entirely by the arterial blood temperature. Conduction, or head surface cooling, was of little importance to the rate of brain cooling or final brain temperature in adults, although it may have some moderate influence in infants. In neither age group did the metabolic production of heat by the brain have any significant direct effects (Fig 13–1).

In a simulation of convective cooling of the adult brain to 27°C using routine perfusion techniques, brain temperature equilibration occurred rapidly, within 16 minutes. Only small brain-blood temperature gradients were achieved. In a simulation of cooling of the infant brain to 17°C, brain temperature equilibration took 22–26 minutes; this longer cooling time was needed to avoid excessive brain-blood temperature gradients.

Conclusion.—Convection was by far the most important process in determining the rate of brain cooling. The only significant determinant of final brain temperature was the arterial blood temperature. Prearrest cooling times of at least 20 minutes were needed to ensure adequate brain temperature equilibration in infants. With shorter durations, nasopharyngeal or tympanic temperatures are likely to underestimate brain temperature and result in a false impression of brain temperature equilibration.

▶ I included this article from my own department because it is, in my biased opinion, an excellent example of how mathematical and computer modeling can be used to get us to think about common problems. The animal rights activists are constantly railing at us to do studies of this type instead of studies on animals. Studies of this type will never replace animal studies, but they might enable us to direct precious resources more effectively. My advice to clinical anesthesiologists would be to read this article, not for its mathematics (which I most certainly don't understand very well), but for its potential.—J.H. Tinker, M.D.

14 Anesthesia for Vascular Procedures

Perioperative Morbidity in Patients Randomized to Epidural or General Anesthesia for Lower Extremity Vascular Surgery
Christopherson R, Beattie C, Frank SM, Norris EJ, Meinert CL, Gottlieb SO, Yates H, Rock P, Parker SD, Perler BA, Williams GM, Perioperative Ischemia Randomized Anesthesia Trial Study Group (Johns Hopkins Med Institutions, Baltimore, Md; Johns Hopkins Univ, Baltimore, Md; VA Med Ctr, Portland, Ore)
Anesthesiology 79:422–434, 1993   101-95-14–1

Background.—Studies comparing postoperative mortality and morbidity of regional and general anesthesia have been conducted in different populations with varying results. In a randomized, prospective study, epidural (EA) and general (GA) anesthesia/analgesic regimens were compared in patients undergoing lower extremity revascularization for atherosclerotic peripheral vascular disease.

Methods.—One hundred patients received either EA followed by epidural analgesia or GA with subsequent IV patient-controlled analgesia. Monitoring included continuous electrocardiography from the day before surgery through the first 3 postoperative days, followed by serial ECGs and cardiac enzyme determination. Additional morbidity was determined at hospital discharge and at 1 and 6 months.

Results.—The mortality and major cardiac morbidity rates did not differ between the treatment groups. Cardiac ischemia occurred in 35% of patients after EA and in 45% after GA. Perioperative cardiac ischemia was a significant predictor of major cardiac morbidity: 7 of the 40 patients with ischemia had major morbidity compared with only 1 of 60 without ischemia. Significantly more GA patients than EA patients required regrafting or embolectomy before discharge. A similar, nonsignificant trend was observed for amputations of the foot or leg. Regression analysis revealed GA as the only risk factor that was significantly related to regrafting or embolectomy.

Discussion.—A clinical recommendation regarding use of EA vs. GA is not possible because major cardiac morbidity occurred equally in both groups. The higher prevalence of graft occlusion with GA may be related to depression. Epidural anesthesia preserves cardiac output and also enhances arterial inflow and venous emptying in the lower extremities.

Conclusion.—In this population, carefully managed regimens of EA followed by epidural analgesia or GA followed by IV patient-controlled analgesia did not cause a difference in the overall mortality, major cardiac morbidity, or myocardial ischemia. Any difference between the anesthetics was most pronounced immediately after surgery. Inadequate tissue perfusion was more prevalent with GA and often necessitated early repeat surgery.

▶ This article caused a considerable stir this past year. The authors found that EA was associated with less reoperation than general anesthesia for inadequate perfusion in these vascular cases. I think many anesthesiologists believe this. Historically, various surgical trials of complete lumbar surgical sympathectomies to try to keep these operations open have *not* proved effective. So if surgical sympathectomy doesn't work, why does EA? Maybe there is something we are missing, or perhaps there is more bias in this study than meets the eye. Because it is virtually impossible to "double blind" a study in which EA and GA are being compared, maybe what we have here is a variation of what I call the "Porsche syndrome." Your neighbor buys a Porsche, drives it only on weekends, washes it every week, parks it way out on the end of the line in the shopping center so no one will ding it, puts it up on blocks in the winter so that it won't be damaged by salt or road sludge, and then, at cocktail parties, loudly proclaims that it is lasting much longer than his Chevy. Perhaps the morbidity reflects the effort. Who knows? As the reader can tell, I remain unconvinced.—J.H. Tinker, M.D.

A Randomized Double-Blind Comparison of Epidural Sufentanil Versus Intravenous Sufentanil or Epidural Fentanyl Analgesia After Major Abdominal Surgery

Geller E, Chrubasik J, Graf R, Chrubasik S, Schulte-Mönting J (Univ of Bern, Switzerland)
Anesth Analg 76:1243–1250, 1993   101-95-14–2

Introduction.—Epidural administration of opiates is an established method of alleviating postoperative pain. In a randomized, double-blind study, the equianalgesic dosage ratios of epidural sufentanil (S_{EPI}), IV sufentanil (S_{IV}), and epidural fentanyl (F_{EPI}) were compared. During treatment, the serum concentrations of sufentanil and fentanyl were measured.

Methods.—Forty-five patients were studied after major abdominal surgery: 15 received S_{EPI}, 15 received S_{IV}, and 15 were given F_{EPI}. The S_{IV} group was given a 15-μg bolus and then a 5-μg/hr infusion, the S_{EPI} group was given the same dose epidurally, and the F_{EPI} group was given a 60-μg bolus and 20-μg/hr infusion. Patient-controlled supplementary boluses were tailored continuously to individual needs, with supplements of 3.1 μg of sufentanil or 12.5 μg of fentanyl, or by a 50% reduction in the opiate infusion rate at predetermined intervals.

Results.—The pain scores, respiratory rate, and circulatory variables did not differ among the groups. To maintain analgesia for 24 hours, the mean opiate dosage requirements were 202 μg of S_{IV}, 149 of S_{EPI}, and 627 of F_{EPI}. The relative analgesic potencies (APs) calculated from the equianalgesic dose requirement ratios were 1.4 for IV AP-S_{EPI} and 4.2 for AP-epidural fentanyl/sufentanil. The S_{IV} group needed more supplementary boluses than the S_{EPI} group, was more sedated during the entire treatment, had a higher arterial carbon dioxide pressure, and had higher serum concentrations of sulfentanil within the first 3 hours of treatment. Soon after the start of treatment, 4 patients in the S_{IV} group had severe respiratory depression despite serum concentrations of sufentanil of less than .3 ng/mL. Sedation was slightly more intense with sufentanil than with fentanyl, even though the 2 epidural groups required a similar number of supplementary boluses and had similar serum concentrations and blood gas results.

Conclusion.—Because of the risk of respiratory depression, IV administration of an equipotent initial dose is hazardous, even though S_{IV} and S_{EPI} are almost equipotent. However, slower administration or a smaller S_{IV} bolus might have avoided the extent of this life-threatening side effect. Epidural administration is favored because of the higher degree of sedation observed with S_{IV} during the entire treatment. In pain treatment after abdominal operations, the equianalgesic dose of S_{EPI} was about 4 times less than the F_{EPI} dose, but only slightly less than that of S_{IV}.

▶ Whether adequate analgesia after major abdominal surgery, especially vascular surgery, makes any difference in outcome or not, its administration is clearly a humanitarian act. This study is interesting because it comes up with yet a different ratio for the relative potencies of fentanyl vs. sufentanil. Is it 10 to 1, 5 to 1, or down to 4 to 1, as noted in this study? I wonder why we can't nail this down. I don't think we really understand the advantages, if any, of sufentanil vs. fentanyl in any given clinical circumstance.—J.H. Tinker, M.D.

Combined Epidural and General Anaesthesia Versus General Anaesthesia for Abdominal Aortic Surgery: A Prospective Randomised Trial
Davies MJ, Silbert BS, Mooney PJ, Dysart RH, Meads AC (St Vincent's Hosp, Melbourne, Australia)
Anaesth Intensive Care 21:790–794, 1993   101-95-14–3

Background.—Conflicting results have been reported for studies designed to examine the effect of regional anesthesia on the outcome after vascular surgery. The outcome of general anesthesia and postoperative IV morphine analgesia was compared with the results of combined epidural and general anesthesia and postoperative epidural analgesia in cases of abdominal aortic surgery.

Methods.—Fifty consecutive patients who were scheduled for elective abdominal aortic surgery were randomly assigned to receive either general anesthesia and postoperative IV morphine analgesia or combined epidural and general anesthesia with postoperative epidural analgesia. Anesthesia was given using routine standardized methods.

Results.—Intraoperative vasopressors were used significantly more often in the combined group compared with the general anesthesia group. The intraoperative use of glyceryl trinitrate on the other hand was significantly increased in the general anesthesia group. The estimated blood losses or volume replacement did not differ between groups. In the immediate postoperative period, 2 patients from the combined anesthesia group died. Four patients in the general anesthesia group were not extubated immediately after surgery compared with 1 in the combined anesthesia group, but this difference was not statistically significant. One patient in each group required ventilation for longer than 24 hours. There were no significant differences between groups in the predefined criteria of postoperative morbidity, with 17 complications occurring in 14 patients in the combined anesthesia group compared with 13 complications in 11 patients in the general anesthesia group. There were no statistical differences between the groups in the length of stay in the ICU or in the hospital.

Conclusion.—The use of combined epidural and general anesthesia in abdominal aortic surgery is associated with different intraoperative cardiovascular management than that used with general anesthesia alone. The clinical advantages of combined anesthesia compared with general anesthesia in terms of outcome require further investigation.

▶ The authors do not indicate the power of their study before doing it or even why they attempted to test their hypothesis with only 50 patients. I think this study did not involve enough patients to find a difference, if there was one.—M.F. Roizen, M.D.

Effect of Sodium Nitroprusside on Paraplegia During Cross-Clamping of the Thoracic Aorta

Cernaianu AC, Olah A, Cilley JH Jr, Gaprindashvili T, Gallucci JG, DelRossi AJ (Univ of Medicine and Dentisty of New Jersey, Camden)
Ann Thorac Surg 56:1035–1038, 1993   101-95-14–4

Introduction.—Surgical repair of the thoracic aorta is associated with a 5% to 7% incidence of postoperative paraplegia as a result of spinal cord ischemia. Vasodilators such as sodium nitroprusside (SNP), which is used to control excessive proximal pressure after aortic cross-clamping, may exacerbate spinal cord ischemia. The effects of SNP on circulatory dynamics, somatosensory evoked potentials (SSEPs), and neurologic outcome after cross-clamping of the thoracic aorta were evaluated in a canine model of thoracic occlusion.

Methods.—Ten anesthetized adult mongrel dogs underwent a left thoracotomy and 45 minutes of cross-clamping of the aorta distal to the left subclavian artery. Five animals were randomized to receive saline solution, and in the other 5 the systolic blood pressure was controlled with SNP, 50 mg/kg in 250 mL of 5% dextrose in saline solution. The neurologic status was evaluated 24 hours after surgery using Tarlov's criteria.

Results.—At baseline, the control and SNP-treated groups did not differ significantly in proximal and distal mean arterial pressure (MAP). However, after surgery, the groups showed a statistically significant difference in hemodynamics and a significant difference in the amount of time required for SSEPs to return and in the 24-hour postoperative neurologic outcome. Four of 5 SNP-treated animals exhibited paraplegia, and 1 was unable to stand. Four controls had a completely normal neurologic outcome, and 1 could stand but could not walk normally.

Conclusion.—There is currently no clinical evidence for the superiority of any method for protection against paraplegia after cross-clamping of the thoracic aorta. The use of SNP for controlling blood pressure may produce a statistically significant decrease in proximal MAP and a statistically significant reduction in distal MAP, leading to a poor neurologic outcome. Caution must be used when SNP is used in this situation. Other drugs for the control of blood pressure may prove to be safer during operations on the thoracic aorta.

▶ This important article indicates that preservation of cardiac function by lowering proximal blood pressure during cross-clamping of the thoracic aorta may be bad for CNS spinal cord function. There has always been a CNS-heart dichotomy, so I suppose it would be no different, but the degree of change, 15 minutes vs. 44 minutes, is so striking that if the human is like the dog in terms of spinal cord blood flow arrangements, we must be even more judicious in lowering proximal pressure, and we need more monitoring systems (e.g., echocardiography, read online for segment function) to ensure that the heart is viable than we have used in the past. The balancing of cardiac well-being and neurologic function is always difficult, and the use of both echocardiography for the heart and SSEPs for the spinal cord may have to become routine if we want to preserve myocardium and CNS tissue better than we can now.—M.F. Roizen, M.D.

Regional Deep Hypothermia of the Spinal Cord Protects Against Ischemic Injury During Thoracic Aortic Cross-Clamping
Salzano RP Jr, Ellison LH, Altonji PF, Richter J, Deckers PJ (Hartford Hosp, Conn)
Ann Thorac Surg 57:65–71, 1994   101-95-14–5

Background.—Operations on the thoracic aorta carry a risk of neurologic complications, including paraplegia. The mechanism of injury appears to be end-organ spinal cord ischemia. The incidence of paraplegia is thought to greatly increase when a certain time period for aortic clamping is exceeded. The effects of selective CSF cooling on the spinal cord and systemic temperatures were examined as well as whether selective spinal cord hypothermia protects against ischemic injury during thoracic aortic cross-clamping.

Methods.—Adult pigs weighing 17–26 kg were used. Eight control animals underwent aortic cross-clamping at the distal aortic arch just above the diaphragm for 30 minutes. The 8 experimental animals had 2 subarachnoid perfusion catheters placed through laminectomies at T4 and the lower lumbar region. A normal saline solution at 6°C was used to perfuse the subarachnoid space. Infusion rates were adjusted to maintain cord temperatures at less than 20°C. The infusion was stopped after 30 minutes of aortic cross-clamping, and the cord was allowed to warm to body temperature.

Results.—All 8 control animals had complete limb paralysis (Tarlov grade 0) after recovery from anesthesia. In the experimental group, only 1 animal had complete limb paralysis; the remaining 7 had preservation of motor function with spontaneous hind-limb movement. However, none could stand on its hind limbs. The lumbar cords of control animals showed changes typical of acute ischemic necrosis. Ischemic changes were much less severe in the experimental group, which showed a predominance of preserved normal histology in anterior horn motor cells.

Conclusion.—Regional deep hypothermia of the spinal cord in pigs provided some protection against ischemic injury during aortic cross-clamping. This technique may be useful as an adjunct to other methods for protection against spinal cord ischemic injury. In humans, the spinal cord could be cooled through percutaneously placed thoracic subarachnoid catheters, and the subarachnoid space could be drained through percutaneously placed lumbar catheters.

▶ The pig appears to be an appropriate model for this study, although I understand that the anatomy of the rabbit spinal cord is closer to that of the human than that of the pig. Nevertheless, this study is well done, and it shows that a simple measure such as inducing hypothermia of the spinal cord is important for preserving thoracic spinal cord function during thoracic aortic cross-clamping.

I believe that the major deficit of this important article is its lack of a dose-response curve for the time of ischemia. The worst results we ever had with aortic cross-clamping occurred when warming a patient by using a heated mattress that was directly under the spinal cord of the experimental animals while studying the effects of glucose and narcotics on preserving spinal cord function; in other words, maintaining core body temperature is okay if it is done from the top down, but it is bad if it is done from the spinal cord in. Thus, I believe there may be real value in preserving spinal cord function by decreasing spinal cord temperature.—M.F. Roizen, M.D.

Influence of Renal Artery Blood Flow on Renal Function During Aortic Surgery

Welch M, Knight DG, Carr HMH, Smyth JV, Walker MG (Manchester Royal Infirmary, England)
Surgery 115:46–51, 1994   101-95-14-6

Introduction.—The frequency of renal functional impairment and how it relates to intraoperative fluctuations in renal artery flow and cardiac output were prospectively studied in 19 patients undergoing elective surgery on the infrarenal aorta.

Methods.—Eleven patients were operated on for an aortic aneurysm, and 8 were operated on for occlusive aortoiliac disease. Creatinine clearance was measured 2 days before and 2 and 3 days after surgery, and renal arterial blood flow (RABF) was measured using an electromagnetic flow probe. All operations were done under general halothane anesthesia.

Findings.—Estimates of an index of renal function based on the change in creatinine clearance showed postoperative renal impairment in 12 patients (63%), 3 of whom had overt renal failure; no patient required dialysis. The patients with and without renal impairment had similar values for left ventricular stroke work. A sustained decline in RABF was noted at the time of cross-clamp placement in patients with renal functional impairment, whereas flow increased slightly in those in whom renal function remained intact.

Conclusion.—Patients who have decreased RABF during aortic cross-clamping for surgery on the infrarenal aorta are at risk of renal functional impairment.

▶ I wonder how much the placement of the electromagnetic flowmeter actually disturbed renal blood flow, and how much surgical technique contributed to impaired renal function postoperatively. Perhaps more modern techniques such as ultrasonography with contrast agents could be used to validate these findings.

Apparently data show that preservation of renal function with prophylactic measures confers no greater clinical benefit when mannitol or dopamine is used compared with normalization of intervascular volume (1, 2).—M.F. Roizen, M.D.

References

1. Alpert RA: *Surgery* 95:707, 1984.
2. Paul MD, et al: *Am J Nephrol* 6:427, 1986.

Hypothermia and Bleeding During Abdominal Aortic Aneurysm Repair

Kahn HA, Faust GR, Richard R, Tedesco R, Cohen JR (Long Island Jewish Med Ctr, New Hyde Park, NY; Albert Einstein College of Medicine, New York)

Ann Vasc Surg 8:6–9, 1994   101-95-14–7

Background.—Bleeding during and after surgery is a significant complication of abdominal aortic aneurysm repair. Patients undergoing such surgery also routinely have substantial decreases in core body temperature, and hypothermia has been shown to interfere with coagulation. Intraoperative and postoperative bleeding times of patients undergoing aneurysmal repair were measured to determine the effect of body temperature on platelet function.

Materials.—Bleeding times were measured hourly in 10 patients undergoing abdominal aortic aneurysm repair until the core body temperature returned to 37°C. The patients had had anti-inflammatory medication stopped 10 days before surgery, and their preoperative coagulation profiles were normal. Heparin, 100 units/kg, was administered during surgery and was subsequently reversed with protamine sulfate, 1 mg/100 units.

Results.—The mean starting core body temperature was 36.5°C, and the mean lowest temperature was 34.8°C. The mean surgical duration was 139.5 minutes. Bleeding time and core body temperature were highly and negatively correlated. In 7 of the 10 patients, the greatest increase in bleeding time occurred when the core temperature was lowest, not when heparin was administered.

Conclusion.—Bleeding times of patients undergoing surgery are extended by hypothermia. Further research is needed to describe the mechanism by which this occurs as well as the threshold temperature at which significant coagulation interference becomes detectable.

▶ At first I was skeptical of this article, but the data appear solid. Even in a temperature range of 34°C to 37°C, there appears to be a correlation between inhibition of platelet function and temperature. Although I wish that more data were provided (for instance, there are no standard error and standard deviation bars in a figure, and we don't know the clinical significance of a change in bleeding time of 3½ minutes, which is probably still within the control range), this article points out that hypothermia can cause a bleeding diathesis. On the other hand, there are certain advantages to hypothermia, such as preservation of cardiac and CNS tissue and probably renal and hepatic tissue as well, so the benefits and the risks of hypothermia must be balanced. I await further study of this problem and data on the relative benefits and risks of hypothermia.—M.F. Roizen, M.D.

Incidence of Diagnosis, Operation and Death From Abdominal Aortic Aneurysms in Danish Hospitals: Results From a Nation-Wide Survey, 1977–1990

Eickhoff JH (Gentofte County Hosp, Hellerup, Denmark)

Eur J Surg 159:619–623, 1993

101-95-14-8

Background.—Considerable resources have been allocated to vascular surgery during recent decades, and vascular surgeons have devoted much of their work to the detection and treatment of abdominal aneurysm. The age- and sex-specific incidence rates of hospital admission, operation, and hospital death for abdominal aortic aneurysm during a 14-year period were examined, using data from an entire country. Particular attention was given to whether the increase in vascular surgical activity has had an influence on mortality.

Methods.—A retrospective evaluation was made of a computerized data base covering all admissions to Danish hospitals from 1977 to 1990.

Results.—Admissions during which abdominal aortic aneurysm was diagnosed increased significantly from 362 in 1977 to 1,317 in 1990 (incidence rate, 7.1–25.8 admissions per 100,000). Men represented three fourths of all cases throughout the study, and the incidence increased in both sexes and all age groups gradually throughout the period. The incidence peaked for both sexes during the eighth decade of life. Yearly admissions for abdominal aortic aneurysm that resulted in surgery increased significantly from 66 in 1977 to 307 in 1990. Deaths in the hospital increased gradually and significantly from 119 in 1978 to 200 in 1990. However, if mortality data from the last 3 years are considered separately, there was a significant reduction.

Conclusion.—The incidence of abdominal aortic aneurysm was 2–5 times higher in men than women. The number of patients with abdominal aortic aneurysms who reach the hospital is increasing over time. The decrease in mortality in the 1988–1990 period corresponds to similar reports from the United States during the last decade, and they may reflect vascular surgery's increased effectiveness in preventing deaths from abdominal aortic aneurysm.

▶ From this fascinating case-control study, it appears that the incidence of aortic aneurysms and life-threatening aortic aneurysms is increasing. The author implies that an elective operation can decrease the mortality rate for an entire country. I have trouble believing that there has been such a rapid increase in the disease and its death rate in so short a period, but maybe there are factors among the Danish people that could account for such a rapid increase in the incidence of this disease.—M.F. Roizen, M.D.

Plasma Catecholamine Concentrations During Abdominal Aortic Aneurysm Surgery: The Link to Perioperative Myocardial Ischemia

Riles TS, Fisher FS, Schaefer S, Pasternack PF, Baumann FG (New York Univ)
Ann Vasc Surg 7:213–219, 1993   101-95-14-9

Background.—Myocardial infarction is the chief cause of morbidity and death in patients undergoing reconstructive surgery of the aorta. Such patients frequently have coronary artery disease, but other factors probably are responsible for precipitating myocardial ischemia perioperatively. That β-adrenergic blockade prevents ischemia in patients undergoing vascular surgery resulted in a study of catecholamine levels in patients who were having an abdominal aortic aneurysm repaired.

Study Plan.—Plasma catecholamine concentrations were estimated serially in 18 patients who were having elective resection of an abdominal aortic aneurysm, beginning 2 hours preoperatively and continuing for 24 hours after surgery. No vasopressors were given, apart from the epinephrine that accompanied epidural analgesia.

Results.—Plasma epinephrine levels increased before induction of anesthesia and increased to higher levels after aortic cross-clamping. The peak level of 510 pg/mL was reached 1 hour postoperatively; at 24 hours, it had declined to 112 pg/mL. All patients had an increase in plasma epinephrine to greater than normal levels, and 12 of the 18 patients had at least a fivefold increase. Plasma norepinephrine levels increased from 420 pg/mL preoperatively to 795 pg/mL 1 hour postoperatively. Only 1 patient had evidence of acute myocardial injury.

Implications.—An abnormal increase in plasma epinephrine is seen in all patients who undergo surgery on the abdominal aorta, suggesting that catecholamines may be responsible for myocardial injury in this setting. If it can be confirmed by further studies, then it may be possible to pharmacologically prevent the production or effects of catecholamines.

▶ One of my "pet" theories about perioperative myocardial infarction and other thrombotic events is that there must be subgroups of postoperative patients who have 1 or more pathways leading to hypercoagulability, or perhaps there might simply be protracted periods of decreased critical vascular diameter in one bed or another.

We have spent many years studying blood vessels. Now perhaps it is time to focus on what happens to the blood in those vessels. There must be subgroups of patients in which abnormalities occur that are perhaps triggered by the elevated catecholamines that were so well demonstrated in this study.

This study does not shed light on why, despite the uniform elevation of patients' catecholamines, only 1 patient had a perioperative myocardial infarction; nonetheless, this is 1 in 18 patients, an unacceptably high incidence.

We carefully titrate diabetes postoperatively, watching blood sugar levels and using sliding scales. However, we don't titrate β-blockers, anticoagulants, fibrinolytic agents, or any other such agents when we detect elevations in preclotting factors; maybe we should. Perhaps we should concentrate more on these hormonal changes postoperatively.—J.H. Tinker, M.D.

Adjuncts to Reduce the Incidence of Embolic Brain Injury During Operations on the Aortic Arch
Kouchoukos NT (Washington Univ, St Louis, Mo)
Ann Thorac Surg 57:243–245, 1994   101-95-14-10

Introduction.—The most commonly used technique for protection of the brain during operations that involve the aortic arch is hypothermic circulatory arrest, which can cause diffuse injury that is manifested by confusion, lethargy, choreoathetosis, and focal injury, producing a discrete neurologic deficit. Two adjunctive techniques—retrograde perfusion of cold oxygenated blood through the superior vena cava and establishment of antegrade aortic flow after hypothermic circulatory arrest—should reduce or eliminate the embolization of air and particulate matter into the cerebral circulation and could reduce the incidence of brain injury.

Technique.—Two vena caval cannulas and a cannula in the common femoral artery for arterial return are used to establish flow. The shunt connecting arterial and venous lines is clamped. During retrograde perfusion of cold oxygenated blood through the superior caval cannula, the shunt between the venous and arterial lines is opened, and the arterial and inferior vena caval cannulas are clamped. Air is evacuated from the brachiocephalic arteries and the distal aorta. An 8-mm collagen-impregnated Dacron graft for arterial return is used for cardiopulmonary bypass reestablishment. The shunt is occluded and the femoral arterial cannula is removed. Arterial flow is established in the antegrade direction.

Results.—These techniques have been used in 35 patients who had resection and graft replacement of the aortic arch alone or in combination with procedures on the ascending aorta and the heart. One patient died of low cardiac outut; another patient who had a left-sided stroke before surgery had accentuation of the neurologic deficit postoperatively. No focal neurologic deficits were detected in the remaining patients. Four patients experienced agitation and confusion in the early postoperative period, but these symptoms cleared completely within 4 days in all patients. Twenty-one patients (60%) were extubated in the first 24 hours after surgery.

Conclusion.—Patients who have retrograde cerebral perfusion awaken earlier than patients who do not have this procedure. These adjunctive techniques are safe and easy to apply, and they potentially reduce embolization of air and artheromatous debris. They do not increase the duration of circulatory arrest. The 8-mm Dacron graft for antegrade perfusion is more flexible than the rigid cannula, because it allows greater exposure for the remainder of the procedure.

▶ This is a fascinating article because of the low incidence of complications here after such a serious operation. Dr. Kouchoukos and the anesthesiologists who work with him should be congratulated.

There is 1 additional statement in this article that the casual reader may overlook which is very interesting: "It is our impression, and that of others, that patients in whom retrograde cerebral perfusion is used awaken earlier than patients in whom it is not used." Should we all be doing some of this for many other types of operations, including coronary artery bypass surgery?—M.F. Roizen, M.D.

A Comparison of Systolic Blood Pressure Variations and Echocardiographic Estimates of End-Diastolic Left Ventricular Size in Patients After Aortic Surgery
Coriat P, Vrillon M, Perel A, Baron JF, Le Bret F, Saada M, Viars P (Paris VI Univ)
Anesth Analg 78:46–53, 1994   101-95-14–11

Introduction.—Left ventricular preload is usually assessed by measuring the pulmonary artery occlusion pressure, but this technique has many limitations. Animal studies have shown that a fair indicator of left ventricular preload is the systolic pressure variation (SPV), that is, the difference between maximum and minimum values of systolic blood pressure after a single positive-pressure breath. The ability of the SPV to reflect preload status was assessed by using the left ventricular filling estimated by a transesophageal echocardiogram.

Methods.—The SPV was measured in 21 patients, aged 49–75 years, who had abdominal aortic surgery and whose lungs were mechanically ventilated after the procedure. The preoperative radionuclide ejection fraction was greater than 45%. After surgery, the mechanical ventilatory patterns were the same for all patients. The left ventricular dimensions at end diastole correlated well with the SPV ($r = .8$) and its delta downcomponent, that is, the degree by which systolic pressure decreases with each mechanical breath ($r = .83$). In all but 3 patients, volume loading was performed twice with 250 mL of human albumin 5%.

Results.—Each volume-loading step caused a significant increase in the mean end-diastolic area index and cardiac index and a significant decrease in the mean SPV and its delta down-component. In response to the infusion of 500 mL of colloid solution, the initial preinfusion delta down values showed a significant linear correlation to the increase in end-diastolic area ($r = .63$) and cardiac index ($r = .55$). The higher the initial delta down, the greater was the change in the cardiac index and end-diastolic area after volume-loading. By contrast, no significant linear relationship was found between the initial indexed end-diastolic area and the initial pulmonary artery occlusion pressure.

Conclusion.—The results of animal experiments have been confirmed in this study, which demonstrated the usefulness of SPV in estimating the filling of the left ventricle. After vascular noncardiac surgery in patients who are mechanically ventilated, pressure waveform analysis may provide reliable information concerning the response to left ventricular volume loading and preload estimation. The limitations of the pulmonary artery catheter in reliably reflecting hypovolemia were confirmed.

▶ This is the latest iteration of the old Homer Warner idea that, somehow, it should be possible to assess hemodynamics from the pulse contour. Systolic pressure variation may indeed be a reasonable indication of ventricular preload. This kind of new measure requires testing with respect to outcomes.—J.H. Tinker, M.D.

15 Anesthesia for Thoracic Surgery

Anaesthesia for Thoracoscopic Pulmonary Lobectomy
Lamb JD (Saskatoon City Hosp, Saskatchewan, Canada)
Can J Anaesth 40:1073–1075, 1993   101-95-15–1

Background.—Traditional open surgical methods can be accomplished using minimally invasive surgery techniques. The advantages include less postoperative pain, less interference with pulmonary function, and earlier recovery and discharge.

Case Report.—Woman, 76, had a 3-cm lesion in the right middle lobe of her lung confirmed by CT scanning. Pulmonary function was normal and bronchoscopy was negative. A CT-guided biopsy was ruled out and surgery was scheduled. Anesthesia was induced with 70 mg of lidocaine, 200 mg of fentanyl, and 300 mg of thiopental. A left-sided double-lumen tracheal tube was inserted after 70 mg of succinylcholine was administered. Intra-arterial blood pressure, pulse oximetery, and capnography were monitored. A trocar was inserted in the right lateral hemithorax so a thoracoscope could visualize lung decompression. With multiple trocars, the upper and middle lobes were divided and secured. The lobes were placed in a plastic bag and removed through an enlarged trocar site. Bronchial integrity was confirmed by the absence of bubbles in a saline-flooded surgical field after the tracheal lumen had been unclamped. The total time was 7 hours, 40 minutes. About 500 mL of blood was lost during the procedure, and single-lung ventilation was well tolerated. An adenocarcinoma was identified in the resected tissue. The patient was ventilated overnight, and the trachea was extubated 14 hours after surgery. Patient-controlled analgesia with morphine continued for 60 hours. Her recovery was uneventful.

Commentary.—The percentage of an anesthesiologist's practice that involves minimally invasive surgery is increasing. Numerous procedures that were previously performed in an open manner can now be done thoracoscopically, which presents some unique challenges for the anesthesiologist. First, patient safety is a primary concern. Many patients must have optimized preoperative pulmonary function. However, loss of control of hilar vascular structures may result in hemorrhage and death, and current instruments may not be able to deal with such an event. Good vascular access and the rapid availability of blood products are necessary for the anesthesiologist to deal with the patient's deteriorating condition. Second, the lengthy operating time makes temperature regulation, hydration, and positioning to avoid brachial plexus injury worthy of particular attention. Hypoxia from fluid in the dependent lung during differential lung ventilation can occur intraoperatively. Third, surgical visualization and tissue removal require a collapsed lung. The ability to position, perform, and maintain differential lung ventilation is a requirement for lobectomy. Finally, although undocumented, the postoperative analgesic requirement seems to be less in minimally invasive surgery because there is neither a long intercostal incision nor a spreading of the ribs. Analgesia controlled by the patient is satisfactory; neuraxial analgesia through an epidural catheter may be an alternative. Pulmonary function can be compromised after open thoracotomy, but it may show better function after minimally invasive surgery. As tools and techniques improve, the number of minimally invasive surgeries will increase, providing many, mostly unsubstantiated, advantages.

▶ Anesthesia for minimally invasive surgery is now the norm, and I am told by my surgical colleagues that robotic surgery will be the next step forward! To some extent, the development of new short-acting anesthetic agents has been part of this advance.

I selected this article because of the increased use of thoracoscopic endoscopy for pulmonary procedures. This case report highlights that major pulmonary resections are now being done using this technique. Differential lung ventilation (which must be perfect I might add or the surgeon can't operate!) is required. At our institution, we are placing more double-lumen tubes than ever before. Thoracoscopic endoscopy for minor pulmonary procedures is so routine now that I wonder whether the mandatory use of intra-arterial blood pressure and central venous pressure monitoring that is inherent in double-lumen tube placement should still apply to healthy patients undergoing minor procedures, such as biopsy, when we have pulse oximetry and capnography readily available. As a postscript, the total operating room time was 7 hours, 40 minutes, indicating that this was not a short procedure.—M. Wood, M.D.

16 Anesthesia for Outpatient Procedures

Propofol Depresses the Hypoxic Ventilatory Response During Conscious Sedation and Isohypercapnia
Blouin RT, Seifert HA, Babenco HD, Conard PF, Gross JB (Univ of Connecticut, Farmington)
Anesthesiology 79:1177–1182, 1993

101-95-16-1

Purpose.—Conscious sedation can be reliably obtained by subanesthetic doses of propofol. However, the ventilatory effects of propofol at sedative doses have not been determined. The effects of propofol sedation on the hypoxic ventilatory response were examined.

Methods.—Eight healthy young men received a dose of propofol, 1 mg/kg^{-1}, followed by a propofol infusion to maintain a constant level of subanesthetic sedation. An isocapnic rebreathing technique was used to measure a hypoxic ventilatory response. End-tidal pressure of carbon dioxide was kept constant at about 6 mm Hg above baseline; continuous recordings of minute ventilation and tidal volume were made as oxygen saturation (SpO_2) declined from 98% to 70%. Before, during, and after propofol infusion, hypoxic response determinations were made.

Results.—Propofol sedation was associated with a decrease in the mean slope of the hypoxic ventilatory response curve from .88 to .17 L/min^{-1}/% SpO_2. The slope returned to presedation values 30 minutes after cessation of propofol infusion. At an SpO_2 of 90%, the minute ventilation declined from 16 to 9 L/min^{-1}, with a similar decline in the tidal volume from 1,099 to 523 mL. These measures also returned to presedation values 30 minutes after cessation of propofol infusion.

Conclusion.—Patients receiving propofol infusion for conscious sedation show a significantly decreased slope and a downward shift of the hypoxic ventilatory response curve during isohypercapnia. Because of the effect of propofol on the hypercarbic ventilatory response, this situation may further predispose patients to hypoxia during propofol sedation. Appropriate monitoring and airway support are essential for patients receiving propofol for conscious sedation.

▶ Propofol is a very useful agent for providing "conscious sedation," and I have used this technique when I knew that the procedure might take some time. However, this study, which shows that subanesthetic doses of propofol depress the hypoxic ventilatory response, clearly indicates that only person-nel who are skilled in airway management should use this technique. These findings also have implications for care in the postanesthetic recovery room when subanesthetic doses of propofol are present and other drugs that can potentially cause respiratory depression may be concomitantly adminis-tered.—M. Wood, M.D.

Guidelines for Sedation by Nonanesthesiologists During Diagnostic and Therapeutic Procedures
Holzman RS, Cullen DJ, Eichhorn JH, Philip JH (Harvard Med School, Boston; Univ of Mississippi, Jackson)
J Clin Anesth 6:265–276, 1994   101-95-16–2

Objective.—In 1992, the Executive Committee of the Department of Anesthesia at Harvard Medical School accepted a set of guidelines for the safe administration of sedation and analgesia by staff who are not anesthesiologists. Sedatives are increasingly being used to make patients more comfortable during diagnostic and therapeutic procedures.

Personnel and Training.—At a minimum, the person doing the proce-dure and an assistant who monitors the patient's physiologic state must be present from the time the sedative medication is given until recovery is judged to be adequate or other personnel take over. The director of the service or care unit must certify that all those who give sedatives have been appropriately trained in their safe use as well as in airway manage-ment. The anesthesia department should help to educate hospital staff in how to safely use sedative medications and monitor patients.

Equipment and Monitoring.—A self-inflating positive-pressure oxygen delivery system must be available, as should a source of suction and an emergency cart or kit. A pulse oximeter should be used continuously, whether the patient is conscious or deeply sedated. Continuous observa-tion is necessary for patients who are deeply sedated. The heart rate, res-piratory rate, head position, skin color, and oxygen saturation must all be watched.

Consent and Documentation.—The patient or guardian must know the risks of sedation and that there are alternatives available. All aspects of care must be documented in writing, preferably using a standardized form. The vital signs, adequacy of oxygenation, medications given, dis-charge plan, and instructions for the patient should all be noted.

▶ This is a very important issue, and readers who are in charge of depart-mental quality assurance programs will recognize the problems. Many anes-thesiology departments are being asked to provide sedation for increasing numbers of patients outside the operating room, such as in radiology suites and electrophysiologic laboratories, and they find that in these days of cost reduction, they do not have the staff to provide anesthesia services throughout the hospital. It is important to recognize that a reduced standard of care is not acceptable in areas outside the operating room and that adequate monitoring and resuscitative facilities, including pulse oximetry, should be available. More and more nonanesthesiologists are providing "conscious sedation." Often, the hospital administration has little knowledge of the circumstances and qualifications of the individuals who provide sedation, which raises considerable liability and credentialling issues.—M. Wood, M.D.

True Patient-Controlled Sedation

Cook LB, Lockwood GG, Moore CM, Whitwam JG (Royal Postgraduate Med School, London)
Anaesthesia 48:1039–1044, 1994   101-95-16–3

Objective.—A patient-controlled pump is now available that allows patients to completely control the use of drugs to relieve anxiety and provide sedation on the basis of their subjective perceptions. The system permits the repeated, rapid administration of small doses of drug with no lockout and no maximum allowable dose.

Methods.—A standard patient-controlled analgesia pump was modified to eliminate the lockout interval and to double the infusion rate to 200 mL/hr (3.3 mL/min). A .3-mL bolus dose was infused in slightly more than 5 seconds. The pump was loaded with either 300 mg of propofol or 10 mg of midazolam, each in 30 mL of saline. Each demand led to the delivery of 3 mg of propofol or .1 mg of midazolam. As many as 11 doses could be delivered each minute, for a total of 33 mg of propofol and 1.1 mg of midazolam.

Evaluation.—Study participants were 47 women scheduled to have transvaginal, ultrasound-guided oocyte retrieval on an outpatient basis as a prelude to in vitro fertilization. Twenty-five of them received propofol and 22 received midazolam.

Results.—Cardiovascular function remained stable in all patients, and oxygen saturation never decreased to less than 96%. All patients could transfer themselves to a trolley at the end of the procedure, could eat and drink within 20 minutes, and were ready to leave within 1 hour. The 2 drugs yielded similar results. Patients who were given propofol often had pain at the infusion site. Sedation began more rapidly in the propofol group. The number of demands for drugs was similar in the 2 groups except in the first 5 minutes, when patients treated with midazolam made more demands. Psychometric test performance after 30 minutes was more impaired in patients receiving midazolam.

Conclusion.—This system of patient-controlled sedation was safe and convenient. None of these patients were dangerously oversedated.

▶ This study enabled patients to have complete control over their sedation. Further studies are needed, but patient-controlled systems to provide sedation during surgery may be preferred by patients.

Will a system such as this reduce the supervision by a clinician? I have always thought that good sedation in the operating room is fraught with hazards, that it is not a simple anesthetic, and that it requires skill and experience. Although patient-controlled analgesia has become well established, safety issues for sedation must be addressed.—M. Wood, M.D.

Intra-Operative Patient-Controlled Sedation and Patient Attitude to Control: A Crossover Comparison of Patient Preference for Patient-Controlled Propofol and Propofol by Continuous Infusion
Osborne GA, Rudkin GE, Jarvis DA, Young IG, Barlow J, Leppard PI (Royal Adelaide Hosp, South Australia; Univ of Adelaide, South Australia)
Anaesthesia 49:287–292, 1994   101-95-16-4

Background.—Patient-controlled sedation (PCS) with propofol has been found to compare favorably with standard methods using midazolam and fentanyl during extraction of third molar teeth. Although the effect of propofol on mood may contribute to increased patient satisfaction during PCS, recent research suggests that patients may prefer the method itself. The nature and extent of the specific advantages of PCS were further investigated.

Methods.—Thirty-eight American Society of Anesthesiologists physical status I or II day surgery patients undergoing 2-stage bilateral extraction of third molar teeth under local anesthesia were enrolled in the randomized, crossover trial. Intraoperative PCS with propofol at a bolus dose of 18 mg over 5.4 seconds, with a lockout period of 1 minute, was compared with continuously infused propofol, 3.6 mg/kg^{-1}/hr^{-1}. A 20-mg bolus of propofol was given when the infusion was begun to speed induction of sedation, with further 10-mg doses being given every minute

TABLE 1.—Sedation Scale

Grade	Description
1	Fully awake.
2	Drowsy.
3	Eyes closed, but rousable to command.
4	Eyes closed, but rousable to mild physical stimulation.
5	Eyes closed and unrousable to mild physical stimulation.

(Courtesy of Osborne GA, Rudkin GE, Jarvis DA, et al: *Anaesthesia* 49:287–292, 1994.)

TABLE 2.—Scoring System for Patient Cooperation

Score	Description
1	No cooperation. Procedure abandoned.
2	Minimal cooperation. Continuous movement requiring continual physical restraint.
3	Minimal cooperation. Intermittent movement requiring intermittent restraint.
4	Good cooperation with occasional movement requiring no restraint.
5	Full cooperation.

(Courtesy of Osborne GA, Rudkin GE, Jarvis DA, et al: *Anaesthesia* 49:287–292, 1994.)

until patients reached grade 3 sedation (Table 1). Seventy-six procedures were done. Patient cooperation was scored on a 5-point scale (Table 2).

Findings.—The mean propofol used was less with PCS than with infusion, although the difference was nonsignificant (Table 3). The differences between the methods on postoperative recovery of cognitive function were minor, and there were no differences between patient cooperation and surgeon satisfaction with sedation. Nineteen patients preferred PCS, 10 preferred continuous infusion, and 9 had no preference. Preferences, which were recorded as mild, moderate, or strong, were significantly stronger for PCS (Fig 16–1). In all 76 procedures, sedation was no deeper than eyelid closure with command response. This level of sedation was achieved in all patients who were given infusion but in only 26 of the 38 patients given PCS. Twelve patients in the latter group remained less sedated (Fig 16–2).

TABLE 3.—Mean Standard Deviation Summary Data for Dose of Propofol and Measures of Sedation Outcome for Procedures Carried Out Under Patient-Controlled Sedation (PCS) and Continuous Infusion Using a Crossover Design

	PCS ($n = 38$)		Infusion ($n = 38$)	
Total propofol dose; mg.kg	2.39	(1.28)	2.58	(0.84)
Patient intra-operative feeling	8.1	(1.8)	8.1	(2.4)
Patient cooperation	4.6	(0.7)	4.4	(0.9)
Surgeon's satisfaction	8.6	(2.2)	8.2	(2.7)
Recovery time to sit; min	40.3	(9.2)	40.3	(10.3)
Recovery time to discharge; min	124.9	(32.7)	122.9	(29.8)

(Courtesy of Osborne GA, Rudkin GE, Jarvis DA, et al: *Anaesthesia* 49:287–292, 1994.)

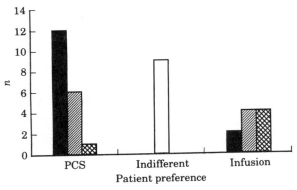

Fig 16–1.—Distribution of patient preference for sedation method, between patient-controlled sedation (PCS) with propofol and continuous propofol infusion. *Solid bar*, strong preference; *hatched bar*, moderate preference; *cross-hatched bar*, slight preference. (Courtesy of Osborne GA, Rudkin GE, Jarvis DA, et al: *Anaesthesia* 49:287–292, 1994.)

Conclusion.—No significant differences were found between sedation methods in many of the objective measures of outcome. Sedation with PCS was safely and strongly preferred over infusion by a large percentage of the patients.

▶ The idea of patient-controlled postoperative analgesia is well established, so it is not surprising that the next step is PCS. Well-informed patients have always liked to participate in their health care, and this technique gives them the opportunity.—M. Wood, M.D.

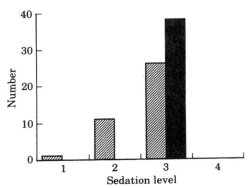

Fig 16–2.—Distribution of maximum sedation grades reached by patients during patient-controlled sedation (*hatched bars*) with propofol and continuous propofol infusion (*solid bar*) in a crossover study of 38 patients. (Courtesy of Osborne GA, Rudkin GE, Jarvis DA, et al: *Anaesthesia* 49:287–292, 1994.)

17 Anesthesia for Transplant, General Surgery, and Orthopedics

Combined Veno-Venous Bypass and High Volume Hemofiltration During Orthotopic Liver Transplantation
Bellomo R, Harris C, Kang Y, Daniel E, Fung JJ, Bronsther O (Presbyterian Univ, Pittsburgh, Pa)
ASAIO J 39:954–956, 1993

101-95-17-1

Background.—Orthotopic liver transplantation, which is now an established treatment for end-stage liver disease, may require the administration of large amounts of blood, blood products, and colloid and crystalloid solutions to compensate for ongoing blood losses and extravascular fluid shifts. Continuous high-volume venovenous hemofiltration has recently been developed for removing fluids and replacing renal function. To maximize the advantages and minimize the complexity of this technique, high-volume hemofiltration was incorporated into the bypass procedure by creating a parallel circuit to that of the bypass pump. An experience in a patient with low-pressure pulmonary edema and anuric renal failure who was undergoing liver transplantation was reported.

Methods and Findings.—The patient was a man, 51 years of age, hospitalized for progressive liver failure caused by ethanol-induced cirrhosis. When a donor liver became available, orthotopic liver transplantation was begun. A venovenous bypass circuit that incorporated a parallel continuous venovenous hemofiltration side-circuit was attached to the bypass pump console. Blood moved from the inferior vena cava and portal vein to the bypass pump and then was driven back into the left axillary vein from the venous outlet of the pump. Isotonic fluid, 4 L, was removed over a 1-minute period with no evidence of hemodynamic instability. Blood urea nitrogen levels declined from 70 mg/dL to 45 mg/dL during the procedure. Overall, 11 units of whole blood, 10 units of platelets, and 5 L of normal saline was transfused.

Conclusion.—Combined high-volume venovenous hemofiltration and venovenous bypass is effective and easy to perform. The procedure does not require additional anticoagulation, and significant fluid removal can be achieved within a short time.

▶ This report illustrates the feasibility and safety of high-volume hemofiltration using venovenous bypass during liver transplantation. It is probably the first time that these 2 extracorporeal techniques have been combined. Why is this needed or beneficial?

The authors cite evidence that hemofiltration results in the removal of middle-sized molecules in patients with acute liver failure and that these molecules may participate in the induction of hepatic encephalopathy. In addition, continuous hemofiltration has been shown to lower intracranial pressure in oliguric patients with severe hepatic encephalopathy. Thus, although liver transplantation has gradually become safer and safer, with fewer complications and at much less cost than it was only 4 years ago on a cost-of-resources basis, if use of the technique of liver transplantation is routinely resumed in patients with severe hepatic encephalopathy, perhaps it will become commonplace.—M.F. Roizen, M.D.

Preoperative Fasting Improves Survival After 90% Hepatectomy

Sarac TP, Sax HC, Doerr R, Yuksel U, Pulli R, Caruana J (Univ of Rochester, New York; State Univ of New York, Buffalo; Texas College of Osteopathic Medicine, Dallas)
Arch Surg 129:729–733, 1994 101-95-17–2

Purpose.—Compared with two thirds hepatectomy, 90% hepatectomy in rats markedly decreases successful liver regeneration and host survival. Partial hepatectomy appears to result in increased fat oxidation and a shift in glucose metabolism toward glucogenesis. Stimulation of these 2 pathways, which is most easily achieved by a 24-hour fast, might enhance liver regeneration and survival. Rats were used to determine whether these fasting-induced alterations affected liver regeneration and survival after 90% hepatectomy.

Methods.—The randomized, controlled trial included 157 female Wistar rats. One group fasted for 24 hours before 90% hepatectomy, and the other was permitted to feed ad libitum until the time of surgery. Postoperatively, the 2 groups were further randomized to receive either 20% glucose or tap water ad libitum. Survival was compared among the groups. Serial measurements of DNA synthesis in the hepatic remnant, glucokinase activity and glycogen content, serum ketone bodies, free fatty acid, and ad libitum glucose consumption were also made.

Results.—Survival at 49 hours was 95% in fasting animals that were allowed glucose postoperatively compared with 52% in those that fed preoperatively and received glucose postoperatively. The peak rate of DNA synthesis was also higher in the fasted/glucose group than in the fed/glucose group at 550 vs. 275 disintegrations/min/.001 mg of DNA.

For rats that were given only tap water after hepatectomy, survival was only 12% to 31%. The fasted/glucose group had a higher glucose consumption 1 hour after hepatectomy than the fed/glucose group, but their glucokinase activity was suppressed. Both free fatty acid and serum ketone bodies were increased by preoperative fasting and postoperative glucose consumption. The fasted/glucose group maintained normal glucose, whereas the fed/glucose group had decreased glucose at 8 hours postoperatively.

Conclusion.—In rats undergoing 90% hepatectomy, preoperative fasting shifts energy use to fat oxidation and gluconeogenesis, apparently ameliorating postoperative liver failure. Prehepatectomy fasting appears to promote optimal regeneration of the liver remnant, thereby permitting a "normal" regeneration response and increased survival. Studies to define the biomechanical mechanisms that occcur after extended hepatectomy in humans are being conducted.

▶ The mechanism by which preoperative fasting improves survival is not clear to me. Perhaps it is the ability of the fasted group to maintain fat oxidation in glucose levels throughout the period. The data that support enhanced fat oxidation and possibly gluconeogenesis in the fasted group permit the switch to fat oxidation as a fuel source. Although this explanation is plausible, it is by no means proved by the article. I urge young researchers to read this article, because it may stimulate an entire area of investigation, and they could discover the reason why fasting is better for the liver.—M.F. Roizen, M.D.

High-Dose Aprotinin Reduces Blood Loss in Patients Undergoing Total Hip Replacement Surgery

Janssens M, Joris J, David JL, Lemaire R, Lamy M (Univ Hosp of Liège, Belgium)
Anesthesiology 80:23–29, 1994   101-95-17–3

Introduction.—Hip replacement surgery is often associated with massive blood loss that requires transfusion. Blood loss in cardiac surgery has been reduced with the use of high doses of aprotinin, although the mechanisms involved are not fully understood. The effect of aprotinin on blood loss during total hip replacement surgery was assessed in a controlled, randomized, double-blind study.

Methods.—Forty patients undergoing primary elective total hip replacement surgery were randomly assigned to receive IV injections of either aprotinin or normal saline throughout the procedure. All the procedures were performed by the same surgeon and anesthesiologist, who used standardized techniques and were blinded to the group assignments. Perioperative bleeding was evaluated by the surgeon. Postoperative bleeding was measured for the first 2 days, and the need for transfusion was recorded. Blood samples were obtained before and immediately after surgery, and at 5 hours and 1, 4, and 7 days after surgery to assess the effects of aprotinin on fibrinolysis, prothrombin time, coagulation pathways, and platelet function. Liver and renal function indices were assessed. Clinical signs of deep venous thrombosis were monitored.

Results.—The patients who received aprotinin experienced total blood loss reductions of 26%, with reductions both perioperatively and postoperatively. The aprotinin group required 1.8 blood transfusion units, whereas the control group required 3.4 units. The control group experienced nonsignificantly more increases in D-dimers. The intrinsic coagulation pathway demonstrated early postoperative inhibition in the aprotinin group, whereas the extrinsic coagulation pathway was not affected. There were no differences between the 2 groups in platelet counts or function or in activation of the coagulation system, and there were no significant differences in the incidence of deep venous thrombosis. Aprotinin caused no side effects; renal and hepatic function were normal in both groups.

Discussion.—High perioperative doses of aprotinin reduce the bleeding experienced during total hip replacement surgery and reduce the need for blood transfusion without adverse side effects. There was no evidence that the mechanisms involved in the hemostatic effect included an antifibrinolytic effect, activation of the coagulation system, or altered platelet function. Further study is required to idenify the mechanisms governing aprotinin's hemostatic effect.

▶ Aprotinin is a proteinase inhibitor that decreases activation of plasminogen and thereby inhibits the breakdown of clots. Epsilon–aminocaproic acid is a much cheaper version, but it hasn't been studied as well. When it was used, it was associated anecdotally with sudden coronary thromboses postoperatively.

This study was biased to find a difference. Normally, the type of anesthesia used here would not be given for total hip replacement; even if general anesthesia is used, there is a tendency to do intentional hypotension with it to decrease perioperative blood loss. In this case, general anesthesia was used, and routine deep venous thrombosis prophylaxis with heparin, antistasis stockings, and mobilization were used postoperatively. Importantly, there was no difference in the clinical detection of deep venous thrombosis postoperatively. Thus, it appears that aprotinin may be a valuable adjunct to operations in which considerable blood loss can be expected when other anesthetic techniques or means to decrease blood loss are not possible.—M.F. Roizen, M.D.

18 Neuroanesthesia

Sevoflurane and Halothane Reduce Focal Ischemic Brain Damage in the Rat: Possible Influence on Thermoregulation
Warner DS, McFarlane C, Todd MM, Ludwig P, McAllister AM (Univ of Iowa, Iowa City)
Anesthesiology 79:985–992, 1993   101-95-18–1

Introduction.—Anesthetics often are given to patients who undergo neurosurgical procedures as well as to laboratory animals that are subjected to focal cerebral ischemia. Few systematic studies have examined the comparative effects of anesthesia and the waking state on the outcome of cerebral ischemia. Neurologic function and infarct volume were monitored in rats that were subjected to a temporary focal ischemic insult. Some animals were maintained in the unanesthetized state, whereas others were anesthetized with either sevoflurane or halothane.

Methods.—All animals were anesthetized with halothane and prepared for filament occlusion of the middle cerebral artery. Some animals remained anesthetized with approximately a 1.4 minimum alveolar concentration (MAC) of halothane. Others had sevoflurane substituted for halothane to the point where electroencephalographic (EEG) burst suppression was evident at approximately 1.4 MAC. A final group of rats was allowed to awaken just after the onset of ischemia, which lasted 90 minutes in all groups. In another study, rats that were anesthetized with halothane underwent focal ischemia as their pericranial temperature was maintained at 38°C or 39.2°C.

Results.—Compared with in awake animals, the mean cortical infarct volume was reduced 85% in the halothane group and by 69% in animals anesthetized with sevoflurane. Subcortical infarct volumes exhibited a similar pattern. Substantially fewer anesthetized animals had severe hemiparesis develop. Hyperthermic animals had poorer neurologic scores 96 hours after ischemia. Subcortical and total infarct volumes were greater in hyperthermic than in normothermic animals, and the total infarct volume correlated with the neurologic score.

Implications.—Anesthetized rats that were subjected to focal cerebral ischemia for 90 minutes had a better outcome than those that were not anesthetized. Because awake animals may be mildly hyperthermic, and even a small increase in pericranial temperature appears to influence ischemic outcome, further study is needed to determine whether the benefits of anesthesia can be ascribed to a temperature effect.

▶ I included this article not because it comes from my institution, although I am very proud of that, but because it describes what I consider to be an elegant model for studying focal cerebral ischemia without a massively invasive procedure, and it does it in an animal that is small enough so as to be economical. Although passing this fine filament up to the middle cerebral artery is not easy, it produces a superior model for these experiments. Because this filament can be removed, it allows genuine outcome studies to be done in these animals. Sure enough, both halothane and sevoflurane reduced cerebral ischemic damage.—J.H. Tinker, M.D.

Call Mosby Document Express at **1 (800) 55-MOSBY** to obtain copies of the original source documents of articles featured or referenced in the YEAR BOOK series.

19 Obstetric Anesthesia

Maternal Positioning Affects Fetal Heart Rate Changes After Epidural Analgesia for Labour

Preston R, Crosby ET, Kotarba D, Dudas H, Elliott RD (Univ of Ottawa, Ont, Canada)

Can J Anaesth 40:1136–1141, 1993

101-95-19-1

Rationale.—Fetal heart rate (FHR) changes suggesting fetal hypoxia are seen in 16% to 27% of parturients during initiation of an epidural block for analgesia in labor. It is possible that the wedged supine position in which women in labor are traditionally nursed does not reliably prevent compression of the aorta and vena cava and that uterine blood flow and fetal oxygenation may be impaired as a result.

Study Plan.—Whether nursing patients in the full lateral position prevents aortocaval compression was studied in a series of 88 American Society of Anesthesiologists physical status I and II term parturients with uncomplicated singleton pregnancies. Labor began spontaneously and was not augmented, and the fetal heart pattern was initially normal. The patients were nursed in either the wedged supine position (group I) or the full lateral position (group II) when an epidural block was initiated.

Results.—Similar peak sensory levels were reached in the 35 assessable group I patients and the 35 group II women. Thirteen women in group I and 7 in group II exhibited FHR changes. Decelerations, the most common change, were similarly frequent in the 2 groups. Most abnormalities occurred 10–25 minutes after delivery of the full analgesic dose of bupivacaine. Severe decelerations occurred in 15% of group I women but in none of those in group II; in no instance did they coincide with maternal hypotension. There were no adverse fetomaternal outcomes.

Conclusion.—Nursing parturients in the full lateral position rather than the wedged supine position when epidural analgesia is initiated will help prevent aortocaval compression and consequent severe FHR decelerations. This is especially important for parturients who are at high risk of placental insufficiency.

▶ I wholeheartedly endorse the authors' conclusion that the full lateral position is the preferred one during and after administration of epidural analgesia during labor. Posture has little effect on the symmetric onset of epidural analgesia. Unilateral sensory blockade is more likely to result from malpositioning of the epidural catheter than assumption of the lateral position. It is unnecessary—and hazardous—for pregnant women to assume the supine position in an effort to achieve bilateral sensory blockade. Assumption and maintenance of the full lateral position probably will decrease the incidence of FHR abnormalities during and after administration of epidural analgesia during labor.—D.H. Chestnut, M.D.

Epidural Test Dose: Lidocaine 100 mg, Not Chloroprocaine, Is a Symptomatic Marker of *IV* Injection in Labouring Parturients

Colonna-Romano P, Lingaraju N, Braitman LE (Hahnemann Univ Hosp, Philadelphia)
Can J Anaesth 40:714–717, 1993   101-95-19–2

Background.—Local anesthetics that are intended to be injected epidurally may be accidentally injected intravascularly, which can result in seizures and cardiac arrest. The epidural test dose has been developed to avoid this complication. The value of lidocaine, 100 mg, and chloroprocaine, 100 mg, in detecting intravascular injection in laboring patients was investigated.

Methods.—Forty-eight unmedicated laboring parturients were enrolled in the prospective, double-blind, randomized study. A lumbar epidural catheter was placed in all patients, who then received 5 mL of IV normal saline; IV lidocaine (LD), 100 mg; or IV 2-chloroprocaine (CH), 100 mg. All agents were injected during uterine diastole. The patients' perceptions of the presence of a metallic or a funny taste, dizziness, and tinnitus over the next 1–2 minutes were recorded.

Findings.—In the LD and CH groups, no symptom alone reached clinically acceptable levels of sensitivity. In the LD group, tinnitus plus taste and dizziness plus taste reached a sensivity of 100%, with specificities of 81% and 69%, respectively. The negative predictive value was 100% for both pairs of symptoms, but the positive predictive value was only 42% for tinnitus plus taste and 30% for dizziness plus taste.

Conclusion.—Lidocaine, 100 mg, is a sensitive marker for intravascular injection in laboring parturients. Tinnitus plus taste is the most reliable indicator of IV injection.

▶ The administration of 100 mg of lidocaine as a marker of IV injection mandates the earlier exclusion of unintentional subarachnoid injection of local anesthetic. The anesthesia care provider should first administer 40–50 mg of lidocaine using the epidural catheter to exclude unintentional subarachnoid placement of the epidural needle or catheter. Three to 5 minutes later, the anesthesia care provider can administer 100 mg of lidocaine to exclude unintentional IV placement of the needle or catheter. The anesthesia care provider should inject the test dose immediately after a uterine contraction to increase the likelihood that the patient will report subjective symptoms of IV injection of local anesthetic.—D.H. Chestnut, M.D.

Patient-Controlled Epidural Analgesia in Labour: Varying Bolus Dose and Lockout Interval

Gambling DR, Huber CJ, Berkowitz J, Howell P, Swenerton JE, Ross PLE, Crochetière CT, Pavy TJG (Univ of British Columbia, Vancouver, Canada; Grace Hosp, Vancouver, BC, Canada)

Can J Anaesth 40:211–217, 1993

101-95-19-3

Introduction.—Patient-controlled epidural analgesia (PCEA) is a safe and effective technique that reduces local anesthetic requirements compared with continuous-infusion epidural anesthesia (CIEA). So far, the dosing variables for PCEA have been arbitrarily chosen. The optimal initial combination of bolus dose and lockout interval (LI) during PCEA in the first stage of labor were assessed in a randomized, double-blind, prospective study; in addition, bolus-only PCEA was compared with CIEA.

Methods.—The analysis included 68 patients with uncomplicated singleton pregnancies who were in established labor and requested epidural analgesia. All patients self-administered .125% bupivacaine with 1:400,000 epinephrine and fentanyl, 2.5 $\mu g/mL^{-1}$, using patient-controlled analgesia pumps. The patients were assigned to 5 groups with different pump programming: group A received a 2-mL bolus with a 10-minute LI; group B received a 3-mL bolus with a 15-minute LI; group C received a 4-mL bolus with a 20-minute LI; group D received a 6-mL bolus with a 30-minute LI; and group E received a continuous infusion at 8 mL/hr^{-1}. The latter infusion was delivered through a patient-controlled analgesia pump with an inactive demand button. Pain and patient satisfaction scores, sensory and motor block, and bupivacaine and fentanyl consumption were assessed hourly. At birth, maternal and fetal fentanyl concentrations were measured.

Results.—Excellent analgesia was obtained in most patients in all groups, with no differences in the number of patients requesting epidural supplements (Fig 19–1). Bupivacaine and fentanyl consumption were greater in group E than in the 4 groups receiving PCEA. The mean bupivacaine consumption was 9.4 mg/hr^{-1} in group E compared with 5.2 mg/hr^{-1} in groups A–D; corresponding figures for fentanyl were 19.6 and 12.6 $\mu g/hr^{-1}$. Only minimal motor block was noted. At 3 and 4 hours, groups D and E had higher sensory levels than groups A–C. All plasma fentanyl measurements were less than .5 ng/mL^{-1}. Mild pruritus was reported, but there were no serious sequelae of fentanyl.

Conclusion.—At all initial dose variables used, bolus-only PCEA using bupivicaine, epinephrine, and fentanyl was a safe and effective alternative to CIEA for women in the first stage of labor. Pain relief was similar to that achieved with CIEA, but PCEA reduced bupivacaine and fentanyl

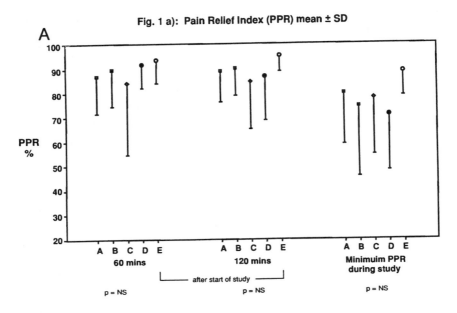

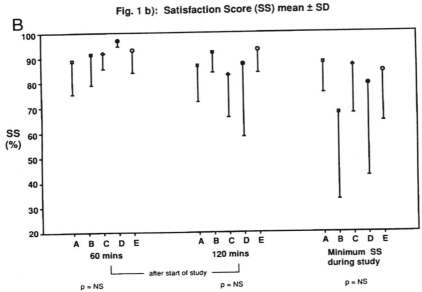

Fig 19–1.—**A,** pain relief index. **B,** satisfaction score. (Courtesy of Gambling DR, Huber CJ, Berkowtiz J, et al: *Can J Anaesth* 40:211–217, 1993.)

consumption. The PCEA regimen should ensure that hourly maximum doses are not exceeded and that minimum hourly doses are met.

▶ There is no doubt that PCEA works well in selected laboring women. Two questions remain: Does use of this technology result in improved obstetric outcome, and what patients are best suited for use of this technique? This study suggests that PCEA does not result in greater maternal satisfaction when compared with CIEA alone.—D.H. Chestnut, M.D.

Effect of Epidural Analgesia for Labor on the Cesarean Delivery Rate
Morton SC, Williams MS, Keeler EB, Gambone JC, Kahn KL (RAND, Santa Monica, Calif; Univ of California, Los Angeles; Health Devices Research Inst, Redwood City, Calif)
Obstet Gynecol 83:1045–1052, 1994   101-95-19–4

Background.—The use of epidural analgesia for labor and delivery has increased dramatically both in the United States and the United Kingdom. The possible effects of epidural analgesia on cesarean delivery rate were examined in a meta-analysis.

Methods.—The English-language literature from 1981 to 1992 was searched to identify articles about epidural anesthesia, cesarean section, and primiparous women. A total of 230 articles were reviewed in detail, including articles with data on women who had standard obstetric risk and on cesarean delivery rates for a group receiving epidural analgesia and a concurrent group not receiving epidural analgesia. Six studies were identified for primary analysis and 2 more for secondary analysis. The sample size of the epidural and nonepidural groups and the number of cesarean deliveries in each group were extracted. Tests of homogeneity were done, and the pooled risk for cesarean delivery as a result of epidural analgesia was estimated.

Results.—When all 6 studies with control groups that did not receive epidural analgesia were combined, the pooled cesarean delivery rate was 16% in the epidural group and 6.2% in the nonepidural group. When all studies or only the randomized studies were pooled, a greater than 9% increase in cesarean deliveries for dystocia was seen in the epidural group.

Conclusion.—Epidural analgesia was shown to be associated with an increased cesarean delivery rate. However, the available data cannot explain this association. The findings can be considered when a physician assesses the risks and benefits of the individual patient's situation. The balance between analgesia provided by epidurals and the postpartum morbidity and costs associated with cesarean delivery should be studied further.

▶ A meta-analysis is only as strong as the size and quality of the studies examined. This meta-analysis looked at only 6 studies that included a control group of patients who did not receive epidural analgesia. Only 2 of those studies randomized patients to receive either epidural analgesia or an alternative method of pain relief during labor. Clearly, this review does not prove that epidural analgesia results in an increased incidence of cesarean section. I was pleased the authors acknowledged that "the increased risk [of cesarean section] may be justified given the value of an epidural in relieving pain." —D.H. Chestnut, M.D.

Respiratory Depression After Intrathecal Sufentanil During Labor

Hays RL, Palmer CM (Univ of Arizona, Tucson)
Anesthesiology 81:511–512, 1994

101-95-19-5

Background. —The use of intrathecal opioids in labor is gaining acceptance both for the profound pain relief it provides and for the absence of motor block and hemodynamic changes that are seen with local anesthetics. Intrathecal sufentanil has been shown to be highly effective during labor, despite the occasional incidence of nausea and pruritus. There have been few cases of respiratory depression. In 1 patient with respiratory depression, intrathecal sufentanil was the only analgesic used.

Case Report. —Woman, 21, was seen with labor pains and a history of routine pregnancy. Shortly after admission to the labor suite, she requested analgesia, and intrathecal sufentanil in combination with epidural local anesthetics was planned. The patient received 15 μg of sufentanil diluted to a volume of 2 mL with preservative-free saline. The epidural catheter was then inserted without incident. Within 5 minutes after administration of sufentanil, the patient reported complete relief of labor pains as well as a mild pruritus. Ten minutes later, the patient's respiratory rate became irregular and her respiration appeared to be labored. She was somnolent with a partial upper airway obstruction and indicated that she felt sleepy. Other than the respiratory rate, her vital signs were normal. With stimulation, her low hemoglobin oxygen saturation was elevated but she returned to sleep, and it declined again to 89%. One hour after the injection, her respiratory rate returned to normal while she was sleeping. The patient remained drowsy, but 2 hours and 50 minutes after the injection, she entered the second stage of labor and delivered a 3,905-g boy. Both mother and infant did well. Despite receiving no further analgesics, the woman reported good pain relief during both stages of labor.

Conclusion. —This case of early respiratory depression after the intrathecal injection of sufentanil in a patient in labor has caused changes in the protocol for the use of intrathecal sufentanil in labor. The dose of sufentanil has been reduced to 10 μg, 1-on-1 nursing is provided to monitor each patient receiving intrathecal opioids, and the respiratory rate is checked every 15 minutes for the first hour after injection and every 30 minutes for the next 2 hours. The onset of drowsiness or somnolence may be an important warning sign of impending respiratory depression.

▶ Intrathecal administration of sufentanil during labor has its risks. This patient received 15 μg of sufentanil, which is a slightly larger dose than the one I typically administer when using the combined spinal-epidural technique. (I usually give 7.5 μg or 10 μg of sufentanil when using this technique.) However, I am convinced that the potential for early respiratory depression exists, even when giving 7.5–10 μg of sufentanil intrathecally in laboring women. Intrathecal opioid administration mandates careful monitoring of the maternal circulation and respiration.—D.H. Chestnut, M.D.

Can Parturients Distinguish Between Intravenous and Epidural Fentanyl?

Morris GF, Gore-Hickman W, Lang SA, Yip RW (Univ of Saskatchewan, Saskatoon, Canada)
Can J Anaesth 41:667–672, 1994   101-95-19–6

Introduction.—Unintentional intravascular placement of an epidural catheter occurs in 2% to 9% of patients. Generally, a test dose should precede epidural anesthesia to ensure that a bolus of anesthetic solution will not be deposited either intravenously or intrathecally. It is hypothe-

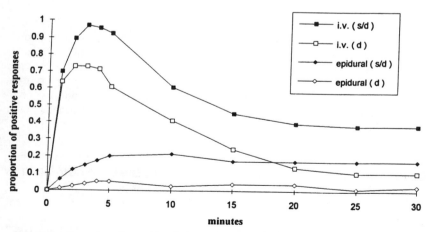

Fig 19–2.—Proportion of parturients declaring symptoms of sedation or dizziness (s/d) in response to fentanyl administration in contrast to those patients assessed for dizziness alone (d). (Courtesy of Morris GF, Gore-Hickman W, Lang SA, et al: *Can J Anaesth* 41:667–672, 1994.)

sized that the sedative, euphoric, and analgesic effects of IV fentanyl would distinguish IV from epidural administration.

Methods.—One hundred American Society of Anesthesiologists physical status I and II parturients in labor participated in a prospective, double-blind, randomized, crossover trial. One group received fentanyl, 100 μg IV, and saline through an epidural catheter, and the other received IV saline and fentanyl, 100 μg, through the epidural catheter. Subjective symptoms, such as sedation, dizziness or lightheadedness, euphoria, and analgesia were monitored. In addition, 19 anesthetists, including 8 staff and 11 residents, recorded a "guess" as to whether the patient had received IV fentanyl.

Results.—The anesthetists correctly guessed the route of administration of fentanyl in 61 of 66 IV doses and in 69 of 75 epidural doses, for a sensitivity of 92.4%, a specificity of 92%, a positive predictive value of 91%, and a negative predictive value of 93.2%. Forty-one patients were crossed over to receive fentanyl by the alternate route, and 38 (92.7%) detected a difference between the routes of administration. Most patients experienced prompt, definite, short-lived symptoms of sedation, dizziness, or lightheadedness. Dizziness was the most distinct discriminator for IV fentanyl, and its presence within the first 5 minutes was strongly indicative of IV fentanyl, whereas observations made later markedly lost their sensitivity (Fig 19–2). There were no clinically significant differences in the fetal heart rate pattern or in maternal desaturation between groups.

Conclusion.—Subjective symptoms can accurately distinguish IV from epidural fentanyl administration in laboring parturients. Fentanyl should be a safe and reliable test dose for intravascular placement of an epidural catheter for obstetric anesthesia.

▶ Anesthesia care providers continue to search for the "perfect" epidural test dose. In my opinion, there is no perfect test dose. Some patients experience euphoria and/or sedation after epidural administration of 100 μg of fentanyl. By contrast, administration of 3 mL of 1.5% lidocaine with 1:200,000 epinephrine enables an objective assessment of either unintentional intrathecal or IV injection. There also is very little downside to the unintentional intrathecal or IV administration of 3 mL of 1.5% lidocaine with 1:200,000 epinephrine.—D.H. Chestnut, M.D.

Comparison of the Addition of Three Different Doses of Sufentanil to 0.125% Bupivacaine Given Epidurally During Labour

Vertommen JD, Lemmens E, Van Aken H (Katholieke Universiteit Leuven, Belgium)
Anaesthesia 49:678–681, 1994   101-95-19-7

Background.—The addition of incremental doses of sufentanil, 10 μg, to a maximum of 30 μg, to .125% bupivacaine with epinephrine has been shown to reduce the incidence of instrumental deliveries while it improves the quality and duration of analgesia without depressing the neurobehavioral status of the infant. However, the 10 μg-dose was chosen arbitrarily, and a real dose-response study has not been done. The effectiveness of the addition of different doses of sufentanil to bupivacaine with epinephrine was evaluated to establish the lowest optimal dose.

Methods.—A total of 150 pregnant women who requested epidural analgesia for labor were randomly assigned to 1 of 3 equal groups receiving intermittent injections of 10 mL of .125% bupivacaine with epinephrine, along with sufentanil in a dose of 5, 7.5, or 10 μg. The onset and duration of analgesia were recorded, and women were asked to rate its effects on a 4-point scale at 10 and 20 minutes after each injection and after episiotomy, delivery, and suturing.

Results.—The spread of analgesia and its onset and duration did not differ greatly among those in the 3 groups, nor was there any difference in the quality of analgesia provided after the first injection. However, at 10 and 20 minutes after the second injection, more women rated the quality of analgesia as good or excellent when either 7.5 or 10 μg of sufentanil was added to the local anesthetic. However, there was no significant difference in the quality of analgesia during episiotomy, delivery, and suturing. Respectively, 88%, 85%, and 79% of the women rated the quality of analgesia during the second stage of labor as being good or excellent after receiving 5, 7.5, or 10 μg of sufentanil. No significant differences in the duration of either stage of labor were seen in the 3 groups.

Conclusion.—There were no significant differences in onset, duration, and quality of analgesia when 7.5 μg of sufentanil instead of 10 μg was added to .125% bupivacaine with epinephrine. However, a lower dose of 5 μg does not appear to provide the same quality of analgesia as the higher doses. Therefore, it can be concluded that 7.5 μg is the optimal dose of sufentanil to add to intermittent epidural injections of 10 mL of .125% bupivacaine with epinephrine to enhance the quality of analgesia during labor.

▶ This is the authors' second study of the effects of adding sufentanil to 10-mL bolus injections of .125% bupivacaine. In both studies, the authors evaluated the intermittent bolus injections of epidural bupivacaine with sufentanil. Furthermore, the authors administered sufentanil only with the first three 10-mL bolus injections of .125% bupivacaine with 1:800,000 epinephrine. Thereafter, they gave .125% bupivacaine with 1:800,000 epinephrine, *without* opioid. Limiting the dose of opioid should decrease the likelihood of neonatal respiratory depression.—D.H. Chestnut, M.D.

Epidural Anesthesia in Early Compared With Advanced Labor

Ohel G, Harats H (Hadassah Univ Hosp, Ein Karem, Israel)

Int J Gynaecol Obstet 45:217–219, 1994   101-95-19-8

Background.—The use and safety of continuous lumbar epidural analgesia for labor and delivery are well documented. However, its effect on the course of labor and type of delivery is still a subject of debate, and little has been reported about the effect of its timing in relation to the outcome of labor. The outcome of vaginal deliveries when epidural analgesia was given in early labor was compared with the outcome after administration in advanced labor.

Methods.—A retrospective study was conducted of 563 consecutive cephalic vaginal deliveries in which epidural analgesia was given for pain relief in the course of labor at term. Relevant clinical information obtained included extent of cervical dilatation and position of the fetal head at the time the epidural analgesia was initiated, parity, gestational age, presence of meconium and premature rupture of membrane, use of oxytocin and meperidine, weight of the newborns, and type of vaginal delivery. The type of delivery was compared in 2 groups: those in which epidural analgesia was initiated at a cervical dilatation of 3 cm or less (group 1) and those who received epidural analgesia at a cervical dilatation of greater than 3 cm (group 2).

Results.—Eighty-four women in group 1 received epidural blocks early in labor, and 479 women in group 2 received late epidural blocks. The rate of instrumental deliveries was significantly higher in primiparous than in multiparous women. However, it was not affected by the timing of the epidural analgesia. The position of the fetal head above or below the ischial spine at the time of initiation of analgesia did not correlate with the type of delivery, nor were there differences in newborn birth weights between the 2 groups. The incidence of premature rupture of membranes, meconium staining of the amniotic fluid, and administration of oxytocin and meperidine was also similar between the 2 groups.

Conclusion.—An equal incidence of instrumental vaginal delivery was noted, regardless of the stage of delivery at which epidural analgesia was started. The practice of withholding epidural analgesia from women in early labor was not supported.

▶ It is disappointing that the authors limited their analysis to 563 consecutive patients who received epidural analgesia and subsequently underwent *vaginal* delivery. It would have been interesting had the authors assessed obstetric outcome for *all* patients who received epidural analgesia during labor, and had they assessed whether the early administration of epidural analgesia affected the cesarean section rate.—D.H. Chestnut, M.D.

Combined Spinal-Epidural Analgesia in Advanced Labour

Abouleish A, Abouleish E, Camann W (Harvard Medical School, Boston; Univ of Texas, Houston)
Can J Anaesth 41:575–578, 1994   101-95-19–9

Introduction.—Spinal opioid analgesia alone may be less than optimal for patients in advanced labor; the onset of epidural analgesia may be too slow to be effective in relieving severe labor pain. The effectiveness of combining sufentanil with a local anesthetic in a low dosage was studied in 38 women in advanced labor who requested regional anesthesia.

Study Plan.—The participants—3 primiparae and 35 multiparae—all had an uncomplicated medical and obstetric history and normal results on electronic fetal heart monitoring. Patients were given 2.5 mg of isobaric bupivacaine without dextrose along with 10 μg of sufentanil in a total volume of 3 mL. The drugs were injected into the subarachnoid space, and the spinal needle was then replaced by an epidural catheter in the event additional analgesia was requested. Patients received incremental 3-mL doses of .25% bupivacaine or 3% 2-chloroprocaine until satisfactory analgesia was achieved.

Results.—All patients had satisfactory analgesia within 5 minutes of drug injection. Fifteen of the 38 women required supplemental local anesthetic. The overall mean interval from spinal drug injection to delivery was slightly more than 2 hours. All the newborn infants were vigorous. Two patients were treated for moderate pruritus. One had mild lower-limb weakness and 1 had a mild, transient decline in blood pressure. None reported a postdural puncture headache. The patients and those attending them were satisfied with the quality of spinal analgesia.

Conclusion.—Combining intrathecal opioid with a low dose of local anesthetic is a safe, effective, and possibly less expensive way of relieving pain during advanced active labor.

▶ These authors gave both sufentanil, 10 μg, and bupivacaine, 2.5 mg, intrathecally before introducing a catheter into the epidural space. I find it unnecessary to give both intrathecal sufentanil and bupivacaine during administration of combined spinal-epidural analgesia in laboring women. Instead, when using the combined spinal-epidural technique, I give sufentanil, 10 μg, before placing the epidural catheter. For patients in early labor, I delay the epidural administration of local anesthetic (with or without an opioid) until the onset of recurrent pain. For patients in advanced labor, I immediately begin an epidural infusion of .125% bupivacaine, which typically results in satisfactory epidural analgesia before the effect of the intrathecal sufentanil subsides.—D.H. Chestnut, M.D.

Repeat Epidural Analgesia and Unilateral Block

Withington DE, Weeks SK (Royal Victoria Hosp, Montreal; McGill Univ, Montreal)
Can J Anaesth 41:568–571, 1994   101-95-19–10

Introduction.—At many centers, epidural analgesia is now the preferred method of relieving labor pain. A number of women who are in their second or third pregnancy request repeat epidural analgesia, but the effect of previous epidural injection on the outcome of any subsequent procedures is not clear. Unilateral blockade may occur more often in women who are given a second epidural.

Objective.—The outcome of first and second epidural analgesias was examined in a prospective series of 221 women, including 150 who were receiving their first epidural injection and 71 who had received epidural analgesia or anesthesia in a previous pregnancy. The multiparae were older and had greater cervical dilatation at the time of catheter placement.

Methods.—Three 4-mL increments of .25% plain bupivacaine were administered at 5-minute intervals. Pain was quantified using a visual analogue scale.

Results.—Ten primiparae (6.7%) and 13 multiparae (18.3%) exhibited unilateral block. The 2 groups did not differ in the frequency of persistent unilateral block where pain was not relieved by further bupivacaine, fentanyl, or adjustment of the epidural catheter. Five of the 13 affected multiparae had received a previous unilateral block. The dura was not entered in any case.

Conclusion.—Women who have received epidural analgesia previously are at an increased risk of unilateral block when they are given a second epidural during labor. Additional local anesthesia and/or catheter adjustment was effective in most instances.

▶ I have not observed an increased incidence of unilateral epidural analgesia in parous women. In this study, the authors did not describe the mechanism responsible for the increased incidence of unilateral block in parous women. Interestingly, all the parous patients had received epidural analgesia during a previous pregnancy. The results would have been interesting had the authors studied a third group of parous women who had not previously received epidural analgesia.—D.H. Chestnut, M.D.

Does Early Administration of Epidural Analgesia Affect Obstetric Outcome in Nulliparous Women Who Are in Spontaneous Labor?

Chestnut DH, McGrath JM, Vincent RD Jr, Penning DH, Choi WW, Bates JN, McFarlane C (Univ of Iowa, Iowa City)
Anesthesiology 80:1201–1208, 1994   101-95-19–11

	Method of Delivery		
	Early (n = 172)	Late (n = 162)	P
Spontaneous vaginal	92 (53%)	80 (49%)	NS
Instrumental vaginal	63 (37%)	69 (43%)	
Cesarean section	17 (10%)	13 (8%)	
Indication for instrumental vaginal delivery			
Elective	27 (16%)	21 (13%)	NS
Nonreassuring FHR tracing	22 (13%)	35 (22%)	
Prolonged second stage (≥ 3 h)	14 (8%)	13 (8%)	
Indication for cesarean section			
Dystocia	14 (8%)	8 (5%)	NS
Nonreassuring FHR tracing	3 (2%)	5 (3%)	

Abbreviation: FHR, fetal heart rate.
(Courtesy of Chestnut DH, McGrath JM, Vicent RD Jr, et al: *Anesthesiology* 80:1201–1208, 1994.)

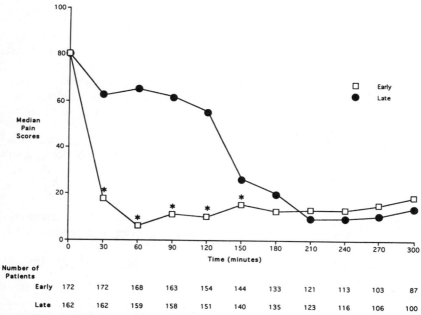

Fig 19–3.—Median pain scores over time. Patients in the early group had significantly lower scores at 30, 60, 90, 120, and 150 minutes after randomization ($P < .005$). Pain score assessments are discontinued when a patient achieved complete cervical dilation. Thus, the *x-axis* lists the number of patients who had not achieved complete dilation at each period of assessment. (Courtesy of Chestnut DH, McGrath JM, Vincent RD Jr, et al: *Anesthesiology* 80:1201–1208, 1994.)

Background.—Epidural analgesia may prolong labor and increase the incidence of cesarean delivery, especially if it is given before 5 cm of cervical dilatation is achieved. The effects of early epidural analgesia on obstetric outcome in nulliparous women in spontaneous labor were investigated.

Methods.—Three hundred forty-four healthy, nulliparous women with singleton fetuses in a vertex presentation were enrolled in the study. All had requested epidural analgesia during spontaneous labor at 36 weeks' gestation or later. By random assignment, patients received either early or late epidural analgesia. In the early group, epidural bupivacaine analgesia was given immediately; in the late group, 10 mg of IV nalbuphine was administered after cervical dilatation was at least 5 cm or after at least 1 hour had passed after a second dose of nalbuphine.

Findings.—Early epidural analgesia administration did not increase the incidence of oxytocin augmentation, extend the interval between randomization and the diagnosis of complete cervical dilatation, or increase the incidence of malposition of the vertex at delivery. The early administration of epidural analgesia did not increase the incidence of cesarean or instrumental vaginal delivery; 10% of the women in the early group and 8% of those in the late group had cesarean section (table). Those in the early group had lower pain scores 30–150 minutes after randomization (Fig 19–3). Infants born to women in the late group had lower umbilical arterial and venous blood pH and greater umbilical venous blood carbon dioxide tension values at delivery.

Conclusion.—In this series of nulliparous women in spontaneous labor at term, the early administration of epidural analgesia did not prolong labor or increase the incidence of oxytocin augmentation or of cesarean delivery when compared with IV nalbuphine followed by late administration of epidural analgesia. Early epidural bupivacaine administration was clearly more effective than IV nalbuphine in providing analgesia.

Does Early Administration of Epidural Analgesia Affect Obstetric Outcome in Nulliparous Women Who Are Receiving Intravenous Oxytocin?

Chestnut DH, Vincent RD Jr, McGrath JM, Choi WW, Bates JN (Univ of Iowa, Iowa City)
Anesthesiology 80:1193–1200, 1994   101-95-19–12

Background.—Although epidural analgesia during labor has been associated with an inceased risk of prolonged labor and surgical delivery, there is still controversy as to whether the association is causal. Some women, especially those receiving IV oxytocin for labor induction or augmentation, have severe pain during early labor. The effects of early

	Method of Delivery		
	Early (n = 74)	Late (n = 75)	*P*
Spontaneous vaginal	29 (39%)	24 (32%)	NS
Instrumental vaginal	32 (43%)	37 (49%)	NS
Cesarean section	13 (18%)	14 (19%)	NS
Indication for instrumental vaginal delivery			
Elective	19 (26%)	17 (23%)	NS
Nonreassuring FHR tracing	8 (11%)	15 (20%)	
Prolonged second stage (≥ 3 h)	5 (7%)	5 (7%)	
Indication for cesarean section			
Dystocia	9 (12%)	12 (16%)	NS
Nonreassuring FHR tracing	4 (5%)	2 (3%)	

Abbreviation: FHR, fetal heart rate.
(Courtesy of Chestnut DH, Vincent RD Jr, McGrath JM, et al: *Anesthesiology* 80:1193–1200, 1994.)

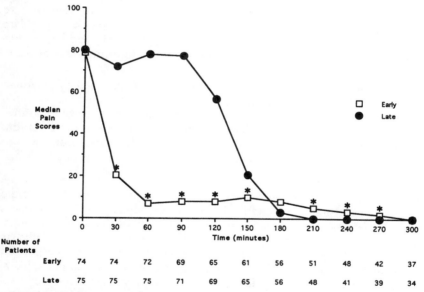

Fig 19–4.—Median pain scores over time. Patients in the early group had significantly lower pain scores at 30, 60, 90, and 120 minutes after randomization ($P < .005$). Patients in the late group had significantly lower pain scores at 210, 240, and 270 minutes after randomization ($P < .005$). Pain score assessments were discontinued when a patient achieved complete cervical dilation. Thus, the *x-axis* lists the number of patients who had not achieved complete cervical dilation at each period of assessment. (Courtesy of Chestnut DH, Vincent RD Jr, McGrath JM, et al: *Anesthesiology* 80:1193–1200, 1994.)

epidural analgesia administration on obstetric outcome in nulliparous women who received IV oxytocin were studied.

Methods.—The participants were healthy nulliparous women with a singleton fetus in vertex presentation who requested epidural analgesia while receiving IV oxytocin at 36 weeks' gestation or later. By random assignment, women received either early or late epidural analgesia. Women in the early group immediately received epidural bupivacaine analgesia, and those in the late group received 10 mg of IV nalbuphine. Patients in the late group did not receive epidural analgesia until their cervical dilatation was 5 cm or greater or until 1 hour or more had passed after a second nalbuphine dose.

Findings.—Early epidural analgesia administration did not extend the interval between randomization and the diagnosis of complete cervical dilatation. In addition, it did not increase the incidence of malposition of the vertex at delivery. Early administration did not increase the incidence of cesarean section or instrumental vaginal delivery; 18% of the 74 women in the early group and 19% of the 75 women in the late group had cesarean delivery (table). Women in the early group had lower pain scores 30–120 minutes after randomization and were more likely to have transient hypotension (Fig 19-4). Infants born to women in the late group had lower umbilical arterial and venous blood pH and higher umbilical arterial and venous blood carbon dioxide tension values at delivery.

Conclusion.—In these nulliparous women who received IV oxytocin for labor induction or augmentation, the early administration of epidural analgesia did not prolong labor or increase the incidence of operative delivery compared with IV nalbuphine and late administration of epidural analgesia. Clinicians do not have to wait until the cervix is dilatated to 5 cm before administering epidural analgesia in this patient population.

▶ Do these 2 studies (Abstracts 101-95-19–11 and 101-95-19–12) refute the randomized trial published by Thorp and colleagues (1)? The answer is both no and yes. The answer is no because in both of these studies, all patients ultimately received epidural analgesia. The answer is yes because Thorp and colleagues concluded that the increased rate of cesarean section associated with epidural analgesia "may be limited by delaying the epidural placement to a cervical dilatation of ≥5 cm." The 2 studies suggest that administration of epidural analgesia between 3 and 5 cm of cervical dilatation does not increase the incidence of cesarean section when compared with IV nalbuphine followed by late administration of epidural analgesia in nulliparous women who are either in spontaneous labor or are receiving IV oxytocin at term.—D.H. Chestnut, M.D.

Reference

1. Thorp JA, et al: *Am J Obstet Gynecol* 169:851, 1993.

Subarachnoid Labor Analgesia: Fentanyl and Morphine Versus Sufentanil and Morphine

Arkoosh VA, Sharkey SJ Jr, Norris MC, Isaacson W, Honet JE, Leighton BL
(Thomas Jefferson Univ, Philadelphia)
Reg Anesth 19:243–246, 1994   101-95-19–13

Objective.—A prospective, randomized, double-blind study was conducted to compare the duration of pain relief and the incidence of side effects using 2 subarachnoid-administered drug combinations for labor analgesia.

Treatment.—Thirty healthy primigravid patients with a cervical dilatation of 5 cm or less received either fentanyl, 25 μg, with morphine, .25 mg, or sufentanil, 10 μg, with morphine, .25 mg, subarachnoid with simultaneous epidural catheter placement using a double-needle technique. Blood pressure and patient assessment of pain, nausea, and pruritus on 10-cm visual analogue scales were assessed at 0, 5, 10, 15, 20, 25, 30, and every 30 minutes therafter until the patient requested additional analgesia. Patients were followed up for 24–48 hours after delivery.

Results.—The onset of analgesia was rapid in both groups. Pain visual analogue scores tended to be lower in the sufentanil and morphine group, but the duration of anesthesia was similar in both groups: 114 minutes in the fentanyl and morphine group and 134 minutes in the sufentanil and morphine group. Both groups experienced pruritus, but the sufentanil and morphine group experienced significantly more severe pruritus. All patients in both groups requested additional epidural analgesia.

Conclusion.—Subarachnoid fentanyl, 25 μg, and subarachnoid sufentanil, 10 μg, both in combination with morphine, 25 mg, provided adequate first-stage labor analgesia, but neither reliably provided adequate analgesia for the duration of labor. Sufentanil was associated with more severe pruritus than fentanyl, because of its higher binding affinity for the opioid receptor site.

▶ In this study, intrathecal administration of 10 μg of sufentanil resulted in analgesic efficacy similar to that provided by intrathecal administration of 25 μg of fentanyl. The authors hypothesized that "this decrease in relative potency of subarachnoid sufentanil illustrates the lack of correlation between systemic and subarachnoid potency ratios." Interestingly, the addition of .25 mg of morphine to either fentanyl or sufentanil appeared to produce little benefit. Others have observed that intrathecal admnistration of 10 μg of sufentanil alone—without morphine—results in approximately 2 hours of analgesia during labor.—D.H. Chestnut, M.D.

Intrathecal Sufentanil Compared to Epidural Bupivacaine for Labor Analgesia

D'Angelo R, Anderson MT, Phillip J, Eisenach JC (Wake Forest Univ, Winston-Salem, NC)

Anesthesiology 80:1209–1215, 1994   101-95-19-14

Background.—When delivered epidurally, bupivacaine provides adequate analgesia for the first stage of labor; however, it may lead to maternal hypotension, compromise uterine perfusion, and produce motor blockade that can interfere with expulsion of the fetus. Intrathecal sufentanil reportedly provides excellent analgesia for as long as 3 hours without producing motor blockade or hemodynamic depression.

Study Plan.—Fifty American Society of Anesthesiologists physical status I or II parturient women with singleton pregnancies who were in active labor had both an epidural catheter and a spinal needle inserted. They randomly received either 10 µg of intrathecal sufentanil or 30 mg

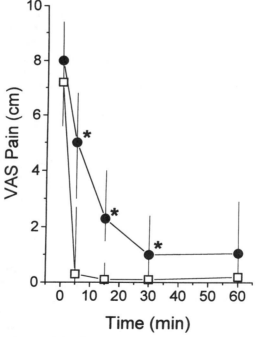

Fig 19–5.—Visual analogue scale (VAS) pain scores after injection of intrathecal sufentanil (*squares*) or epidural bupivacaine (*circles*). Time 0 is the time of the initial epidural injection. Sufentanil was injected at −2 minutes, and the total epidural dose was completed at +3 minutes. Each point represents the median ± 25th and 75th percentiles of 25 patients. All time points beyond baseline differ from their respective baseline values. *P < .05 vs. sufentanil. (Courtesy of D'Angelo R, Anderson MT, Phillip J, et al: *Anesthesiology* 80:1209–1215, 1994.)

of epidural bupivacaine. The alternative route was used to deliver a saline placebo. The 2 groups were comparable demographically and obstetrically.

Results.—Patients who were given sufentanil had significantly lower pain scores, as recorded on a visual analogue scale, for up to 30 minutes, but similar scores were recorded at 1 hour (Fig 19–5). The mean duration of analgesia was 68 minutes in bupivacaine recipients and 123 minutes in women given sufentanil. The duration of labor and methods of delivery were similar in the 2 groups. Significantly more sufentanil-treated patients had pruritus, whereas those given bupivacaine more often experienced subjective motor blockade. Five patients in the sufentanil group had a sensory block more cephalad than T4. Blood pressure reductions were comparable in the 2 groups.

Conclusion.—Intrathecal sufentanil provides more rapid analgesia in early labor than epidural bupivacaine, and it does not produce motor blockade. However, sensory blockade may spread rapidly to the upper thoracic region, dictating caution when using this approach as well as the need to monitor blood pressure and respiration.

▶ These authors made 2 important observations. First, they noted the occurrence of hypotension with equal frequency in women who received intrathecal sufentanil and in those who received epidural bupivacaine. Second, they observed a rapid onset of sensory blockade of the upper thoracic dermatomes after intrathecal administration of sufentanil, suggesting that intrathecal sufentanil administration is followed by a rapid cephalad distribution of drug within the CSF and that early-onset respiratory depression may occur. Both of these observations clearly indicate that intrathecal administration of sufentanil requires careful monitoring of maternal circulation and respiration.—D.H. Chestnut, M.D.

Pharmacokinetic Profile of Morphine in Parturients Following Intravenous or Epidural Administration

Zakowski MI, Ramanathan S, Sutin KM, Grant GJ, Turndorf H (New York Univ; Univ of Pittsburgh, Pa)
Reg Anesth 19:119–125, 1994   101-95-19–15

Background.—A plasma level of morphine greater than 16 ng/mL is associated with systemic analgesia that is mediated primarily by brain opioid receptors. Morphine is readily absorbed from the richly vascular epidural space, suggesting that the analgesic effect of epidural morphine may not be solely mediated by opioid receptors in the spinal cord. Morphine plasma levels during the first 24 hours after epidural administration were reported.

Methods.—Sixteen healthy parturient patients who were scheduled for elective cesarean delivery were studied. They received lumbar spine epidural anesthesia to a T4 sensory level using lidocaine 2% with epinephrine 1:200,000. One hour after the last dose, the patients were randomly assigned to receive 5 mg of morphine intravenously or epidurally. Venous blood and urine samples were obtained periodically to determine morphine levels.

Findings.—Plasma levels of unconjugated morphine were similar in the 2 groups after 15 minutes. At .033, .067, .1, and .184 hours, the mean plasma concentrations of unconjugated morphine were greater in the IV group; thereafter, the mean plasma concentrations did not differ significantly between groups. Maximum plasma levels of unconjugated morphine were noted at or before the first sample at .033 hours in the IV group and at .5 hours in the epidural group. Morphine conjugates quickly appeared in both groups. The maximum concentration was seen at 1 hour in the IV group and at 2 hours in the epidural group. In the IV group, the plasma level decay curves followed a triexponential pattern. A distinct absorption phase occurred in the epidural group that was followed by a biexponential decay. The IV group had greater urinary morphine concentrations and total 24-hour excretion of unconjugated and total morphine.

Conclusion.—Compared with epidural morphine, IV administration results in greater plasma morphine levels in the first 15 minutes but in a shorter duration of postcesarean analgesia. The urinary elimination of unconjugated and total morphine in the first day was higher in women who were given IV morphine compared with in those who were given epidural morphine.

▶ Recently, I visited one of my employees who had undergone a cesarean section at another hospital. She vividly described 18 hours of severe nausea, pruritus, and dysphoria after receiving 5 mg of epidural morphine for postcesarean analgesia. The early reports of epidural morphine for postcesarean analgesia described 5 mg as the usual dose. I am amazed that many investigators and practitioners continue to administer this large of a dose. In my experience, epidural administration of 3–3.5 mg of preservative-free morphine provides analgesia of similar efficacy, with a decreased incidence of side effects, when compared with epidural administration of 5 mg of morphine.—D.H. Chestnut, M.D.

The Role of Continuous Background Infusions in Patient-Controlled Epidural Analgesia for Labor and Delivery
Ferrante FM, Rosinia FA, Gordon C, Datta S (Harvard Med School, Boston)
Anesth Analg 79:80–84, 1994   101-95-19-16

Introduction.—When a background infusion is used with IV patient-controlled analgesia, more drug is consumed without augmenting analgesia. It is not clear whether a background infusion is advantageous for

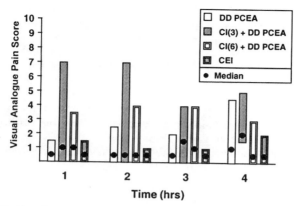

Fig 19–6.—Visual analogue pain scores. Each *bar* represents median and range, respectively, for 7–15 patients. There is no statistical difference in pain scores over the study period (Friedman's χ^2_r). *Abbreviations:* DD PCEA, demand-dose, patient-controlled epidural analgesia; CI, continuous infusion (*numbers* in *parentheses* represent continuous background infusion rate); CEI, continuous epidural infusion. (Courtesy of Ferrante FM, Rosinia FA, Gordon C, et al: *Anesth Analg* 79:80–84, 1994.)

women in labor who receive patient-controlled epidural analgesia (PCEA).

Objective.—Sixty women with American Society of Anesthesiologists physical status I or II in the early stage of labor were studied to determine whether a background infusion is advantageous.

Methods.—The women were randomized to receive a demand dose of 3 mL of .125% bupivacaine with 2 µg of fentanyl per mL with a lockout interval of 10 minutes; demand-dose PCEA plus continuous infusion of either 3 or 6 mL/hr; or a fixed-rate continuous epidural infusion (CEI) of 12 mL/hr. A double-blind, placebo-controlled design was used. Visual analogue pain scores were recorded at 30-minute intervals, and pinprick analgesia and motor strength were assessed by a blinded observer.

Results.—Those in the 3 groups did not differ significantly with regard to pain scores (Fig 19–6), the cephalad extent of sensory analgesia, or the degree of motor block. The cumulative hourly use of anesthetic was comparable in all groups that were given PCEA, but patients in the CEI group required 35% more bupivacaine. The need for a physician to administer supplemental anesthetic in the first stage of labor was least among PCEA patients who received the higher-rate background infusion. These patients received one third of their maximum hourly demand dose as a background infusion.

Conclusion.—A background infusion is not necessary to achieve adequate analgesia for labor and delivery using the PCEA technique, but it does reduce the need for physician-administered supplemental analgesia.

▶ In theory, PCEA is attractive for use in laboring women. Intuitively, it seems that this technique might result in the administration of a decreased total dose of local anesthetic. It might obviate the tendency to give an excessive dose of local anesthetic to some patients, which is often done to reduce the need for intermittent bolus injections of local anesthetic. In clinical practice, I am not convinced that the more complex PCEA technique offers a clear advantage when compared with the CEI of local anesthetic, with or without an opioid.—D.H. Chestnut, M.D.

Spinal Anaesthesia for Caesarean Section Following Epidural Analgesia in Labour: A Relative Contraindication
Gupta A, Enlund G, Bengtsson M, Sjöberg F (Univ Hosp, Linköping, Sweden)
Int J Obstet Anesth 3:153–156, 1994   101-95-19–17

Introduction.—Total spinal anesthesia has been reported after the administration of spinal anesthesia in patients who underwent failed epidural blocks for cesarean section. This complication also occurred in 3 patients who underwent cesarean section and received spinal administration of anesthesia after epidural analgesic infusions during labor.

Patients.—Three pregnant women were admitted for vaginal deliveries: an obese primigravida 21 years of age; a healthy primigravida 24 years of age; and a multigravida 27 years of age. Epidural bupivacaine was used for pain control during labor. In all 3 cases, labor did not progress, and a decision was made to perform a cesarean section using spinal administration of 10–15 mg of hyperbaric bupivacaine. Immediately after injection, the patients were positioned on their backs with the beds tilted to the left. Within 1 minute of injection, the anesthesia had extended to T4. Within 2–5 minutes, each patient had difficulty in breathing and apnea developed. General anesthesia with tracheal intubation and ventilation enabled cesarean delivery of healthy infants. All 3 patients began spontaneously breathing toward the end of surgery and could be extubated. Postoperative recovery was uneventful, and the patients did not complain of adverse effects of the anesthesia.

Discussion.—Total spinal anesthesia may be caused by an excessive dose of local anesthetic, by patient placement in the Trendelenburg position, or by the use of plain bupivacaine. However, none of these was a factor in these 3 patients. Possible causes of total spinal block in these patients include absorption of a higher-than-expected amount of bupivicaine into the CSF, making the spinal dose too high, reduced volume of CSF caused by elevated epidural pressure that compressed the spinal dura, and a higher spread of anesthetic associated with fine-needle injection. Because the complication can be at least partly attributed to a previous epidural block, spinal administration after functioning epidural analgesia during labor is relatively contraindicated.

▶ Others have observed this complication after the administration of spinal anesthesia in patients who had a failed epidural block for cesarean section. The authors concluded that a preexisting epidural block is a "relative contra-indication to administration of spinal anesthesia." I agree that extension of preexisting epidural analgesia is preferable to single-shot spinal anesthesia in patients who require an emergency cesarean section. If a decision is made to administer single-shot spinal anesthesia despite the presence of preexisting epidural analgesia, it seems prudent to administer a reduced dose of a local anesthetic. Of course, an unanswered question remains: How does one decide what dose to give in those circumstances?—D.H. Chestnut, M.D.

Patient-Controlled Analgesia After Cesarean Delivery: Epidural Sufentanil Versus Intravenous Morphine

Grass JA, Zuckerman RL, Sakima NT, Harris AP (Johns Hopkins Hosp, Baltimore, Md)
Reg Anesth 19:90–97, 1994   101-95-19–18

Introduction.—For patients who have had a cesarean section, patient-controlled epidural analgesia (PCEA) can potentially combine the superior pain relief of epidural morphine with the increased satisfaction of IV patient-controlled analgesia (IV-PCA). With its faster onset of analgesia, epidural sufentanil may be better suited for PCEA than epidural morphine. Sufentanil PCEA was compared with morphine IV-PCA for postoperative analgesia after cesarean delivery.

Methods.—Fifty patients who had had cesarean delivery under epidural anesthesia were randomly assigned to receive either sufentanil, 30 μg as a bolus injection, followed by PCEA that featured an initial demand dose of 8 μg, a lockout interval of 10 minutes, and a basal rate of 6 μg/hr, or morphine IV-PCA, with an initial bolus of 5 mg, a demand dose of 5 mg, a lockout interval of 5 minutes, and a basal rate of 1 mg/hr. Pain was assessed on a 100-mm visual analogue scale through 4 P.M. on the day after delivery; sedation, side effects, recovery times, and patient satisfaction were also evaluated.

Results.—The 2 groups had similar analgesia. The only differences were noted after the initial loading dose: Pain was significantly less in the PCEA group at 30 minutes (6 mm compared with 38 mm) and at 2 hours (7 mm compared with 27 mm). Sedation at 2 hours was lower in the PCEA group, but there was no significant difference in the incidence of nausea and vomiting. Fifty-seven percent of patients in the PCEA group required treatment for pruritus compared with 12% of the IV-PCA group. The length of hospitalization or patient satisfaction did not significantly differ.

Conclusion.—In women who underwent cesarean delivery, sufentanil PCEA provided satisfactory and sustained postoperative analgesia. However, after the initial physician-administered loading dose, sufentanil PCEA offered no clear advantages over morphine IV-PCA. The use of opioid PCEA may reduce the incidence of dose-dependent adverse effects associated with continuous epidural infusion of opioids.

▶ The future of postoperative PCEA is cloudy. It is likely that third-party payers will reimburse for this modality only in those patients for whom there is evidence that it offers a clear advantage over simpler, less expensive techniques or there is clear documentation of a benefit in other outcome measures. In this study, after the initial physician-administered loading dose, PCEA provided no clear advantage over patient-controlled IV morphine analgesia after cesarean section. There was no difference between the 2 groups in measures of postoperative recovery.—D.H. Chestnut, M.D.

The Effects of Regional Anaesthesia for Caesarean Section on Maternal and Fetal Blood Flow Velocities Measured by Doppler Ultrasound
Valli J, Pirhonen J, Aantaa R, Erkkola R, Kanto J (Turku Univ, Finland)
Acta Anaesthesiol Scand 38:165–169, 1994   101-95-19–19

Background.—Although regional anesthesia for cesarean deliveries has several advantages over general anesthesia, its impact on placental and fetal hemodynamics is not fully understood. The effects of spinal, epidural, and combined spinal and epidural anesthesia on maternal, placental, and fetal blood flow velocities were investigated.

Methods.—Twenty-four healthy parturients with uncomplicated singleton pregnancies were studied using the Doppler technique. Before anesthesia was induced, the women were prehydrated with a balanced electrolyte solution, 15 mL/kg^{-1}, over a 15-minute period. After induction, the systolic blood pressure was maintained within 15% of the limits of the preoperative values using a prophylactic etilefrine infusion in the patients undergoing spinal and combined anesthesia. Before and after prehydration, and after the onset of T7 analgesia and determination of pulsatility indices (PIs), Doppler ultrasound was used to record the flow velocity waveforms of the maternal femoral artery, the main branch of the uterine artery, and the fetal umbilical and middle cerebral arteries.

Findings.—Rapid IV prehydration did not affect uteroplacental or fetal circulation, as evidenced by unchanged uterine, umbilical, and fetal middle cerebral artery PIs. After the onset of T7 analgesia, the uterine artery PI was increased in the group that had spinal anesthesia, indicating greater uterine vascular resistance; there were no changes in the other 2 groups. None of the neonates in any group was adversely affected, as determined by their Apgar score and acid-base status.

Conclusion.—All the methods of regional anesthesia tested were safe in cesarean delivery. However, these findings cannot be extrapolated to women who have pregnancies complicated by compromised uteroplacental blood flow. Further research on the effects of regional anesthesia in such cases is needed.

▶ The authors noted that "in recent years, Doppler studies and flow velocity waveform analysis have become important tools in clinical as well as investigative obstetrics." I disagree. Although Doppler velocimetry has been used for a large number of provocative clinical studies, it is unclear that this technique is useful in clinical practice.

This study provides an example of the limitations of this technique. The authors observed a significant increase in the uterine artery PI after the onset of the T7 sensory level in the spinal group but not in the epidural or the combined spinal-epidural group; however, there was no difference between the 2 groups in neonatal outcome, as assessed by Apgar scores and umbilical arterial and venous blood gas and pH measurements. The authors concluded that "all the described methods of regional anaesthesia proved safe in connection with caesarean section." This information is not new. There is probably little difference in neonatal outcome among these 3 techniques when they are administered to healthy parturients at term.—D.H. Chestnut, M.D.

Overpressure Isoflurane at Caesarean Section: A Study of Arterial Isoflurane Concentrations

McCrirrick A, Evans GH, Thomas TA (Bristol Royal Infirmary, England; St Michaels Hosp, Bristol, England)
Br J Anaesth 72:122–124, 1994   101-95-19–20

Introduction.—General anesthesia during cesarean section should eliminate patient awareness and recall without a detriment to mother or infant. A recent review of 3,000 patients who had cesarean section found that .4% to 1.3% of them experienced awareness under general anesthesia. Two patterns of isoflurane administration were evaluated to determine whether an "overpressure" technique could reduce patient awareness.

Methods.—Eighteen women were scheduled for elective cesarean section under general anesthesia. Nine were randomized to receive 1% isoflurane throughout the operation and 9 to receive 2% isoflurane for the first 5 minutes, 1.5% for the next 5 minutes, and .8% thereafter. Arterial blood samples were obtained before induction of anesthesia and at periods ranging from 1 to 30 minutes after induction. Arterial pressure, end-tidal isoflurane concentration, and arterial oxygen saturation were recorded at the same time.

Results.—The 2 groups were comparable in age, weight, and blood loss during surgery. Infants from the 2 groups had similar Apgar scores. However, arterial isoflurane concentrations were significantly higher in the second group, with the greatest differences occurring from 1 to 4 minutes and at 8 minutes; the scatter of results was marked in both groups. No clear correlation was found between end-tidal isoflurane measurements and arterial isoflurane concentrations. When questioned the next day by an anesthetist, none of the women reported awareness or recall.

Conclusion.—The "overpressure" technique used in the second group of patients rapidly produced a large mean arterial concentration of isoflurane, which may have reduced the risk of awareness during general anesthesia for cesarean section. Increasing the initial inspired concentration of isoflurane did not cause greater blood loss or adversely affect fetal well-being.

▶ Both groups of patients here received a higher inspired concentration of isoflurane than I typically administer for general anesthesia in cesarean section. In most patients, I give IV sodium thiopental, 4–5 mg/kg, followed by administration of 50% nitrous oxide and approximately .6% to .7% isoflurane until delivery. In my practice, I am unaware of any cases of maternal awareness with the use of this technique.

The authors reported no differences between groups in estimated blood loss, and no information was given regarding the incidence of uterine atony, the requirement for ecbolic drugs other than oxytocin, or perioperative changes in hematocrit. I know of no reason to give 1% isoflurane for 30 minutes or 1.5% to 2% isoflurane for 10 minutes during routine administration of general anesthesia in healthy patients undergoing cesarean section.—D.H. Chestnut, M.D.

Low Dose of Intrathecal Hyperbaric Bupivacaine Combined With Epidural Lidocaine for Cesarean Section: A Balance Block Technique
Fan S-Z, Susetio L, Wang Y-P, Cheng Y-J, Liu C-C (Natl Taiwan Univ, Taipei, Republic of China)
Anesth Analg 78:474–477, 1994   101-95-19–21

Introduction.—Both spinal and epidural anesthesia offer advantages over general anesthesia for cesarean section. The combination of these 2 techniques should be beneficial if the incidence of complications remains low. Most studies of this issue have used relatively large doses of intrathecal anesthetics, with epidural agents added as a supplement or for postoperative pain control. Thus, most of the complications were caused by spinal block. An attempt was made to balance the 2 components of a spinal-epidural anesthetic technique for patients undergoing cesarean section.

Methods.—Different doses of hyperbaric bupivacaine combined with epidural lidocaine were injected using a single-level, needle-through-needle technique in patients undergoing elective cesarean section. The goals were to find the lowest dose of intrathecal bupivacaine that was capable of blocking the somatosensory area of the surgical field and to abolish visceral sensation slowly through the use of lidocaine for a lumbar epidural block that extended to the high thoracic level. Eighty healthy term parturients were randomly assigned to 1 of 4 anesthesia groups. The intrathecal .5% hyperbaric bupivacaine dose was 2.5 mg in group A, 5 mg in group B, 7.5 mg in group C, and 10 mg in group D. Fifteen minutes later, the level of anesthesia was increased to T4 with epidural injections of 2% lidocaine, 3 mL, which were repeated every 5 minutes as needed. Outcome evaluations included the degree of muscle relaxation and perioperative comfort.

Results.—The mean lidocaine doses were 22 mL in group A, 10 mL in group B, and 1 mL or less in groups C and D. The group A regimen failed to provide sufficient muscle relaxation. The group B regimen provided satisfactory analgesia with a rapid onset and minimal side effects. In groups C and D, anesthesia brought about mainly by spinal block resulted in complications that included hypotension, nausea, and dyspnea.

Conclusion.—A successful balance block technique of spinal-epidural anesthesia for cesarean section was presented. Intrathecal bupivacaine, 5 mg, along with sufficient epidural lidocaine to reach the T4 level, offers the advantages of both spinal and epidural anesthesia while avoiding their complications. Isobaric bupivacaine may be able to overcome the problem of unilateral spinal block, the result of the need to keep the patient in the lateral position.

▶ Combined spinal-epidural anesthesia is advantageous for selected patients undergoing cesarean section. Perhaps its greatest advantage is that it enables a rapid onset of reliable sacral blockade while it preserves the ability of the anesthesiologist to titrate the cephalad level of anesthesia and then use the epidural catheter to provide continuous postoperative analgesia. When using this technique, I typically give 6 mg of hyperbaric bupivacaine followed by incremental epidural doses of 2% lidocaine with 1:200,000 epinephrine.—D.H. Chestnut, M.D.

Anesthetic Management of Emergency Cesarean Delivery in a Patient With Noonan and Eisenmenger Syndromes: Case Report
Lawlor MC, Johnson C (Wayne State Univ, Detroit)
Reg Anesth 19:142–145, 1994   101-95-19-22

Introduction.—The rare genetic disorder, Noonan's syndrome, is characterized by facial, skeletal, and cardiovascular abnormalities. Eisenmenger's syndrome features pulmonary hypertension with a bidirectional or right-to-left shunt resulting from an intracardiac or aortopulmonary communication. Either of these syndromes can pose an anesthesiologic challenge. The combination of the 2 in a patient who required emergency cesarean section was described.

Case Report.—Woman, 29, was transferred for treatment of preterm labor at 25 weeks' gestation. She had both Eisenmenger's and Noonan's syndromes and had conceived and refused termination of the pregnancy contrary to medical advice. She was treated in the maternal special care unit with indomethacin for 1 week. She suddenly went into active labor, resulting a double footling breech presentation with feet in the vagina. Emergency cesarean delivery was chosen as the safest mode of delivery. Because there was no time for invasive monitoring or epidural anesthesia, the spinal route was selected as the best means of providing anesthesia, which was achieved with bupivacaine, 7.5 mg in 8.25% dextrose, plus fentanyl, 50 μg, administered at the L3–4 interspace with the patient in the left lateral position. This resulted in a T4 dermatomal level. The 750-g infant was delivered quickly; Apgar scores were 5 at 1 minute and 8 at 5 minutes. Maternal management also included the administration of oxygen, 10 L/min, by face mask and phenylephrine to stabilize blood pressure. The patient received intraoperative monitoring with ECG, pulse oximetry, and noninvasive blood pressure. After surgery, pain management was achieved with a continuous epidural infusion of fentanyl. The patient was discharged at 1 week and the infant at 24 weeks.

Discussion.—Eisenmenger's and Noonan's syndromes pose special challenges to the anesthesiologist. This is the first known case of a patient with the combination of these 2 syndromes who required an emergency cesarean delivery. Anesthesiologic management included spinal anesthesia with hyperbasic bupivacaine and fentanyl, oxygen, rapid correction of hypotension with phenylephrine, and postoperative pain management with continuous epidural fentanyl infusion. Important anesthesiologic considerations in Noonan's syndrome include thoracic deformities that leave the patient susceptible to hypoxia during induction of general anesthesia, orofacial abnormalities that complicate tracheal intubation, and kyphoscoliosis that complicates the performance of regional anesthesia. There is ongoing controversy about the use of Swan-Ganz catheter monitoring during delivery in patients with Eisenmenger's syndrome.

▶ I commend the authors for their skillful, successful management of this challenging case. Under controlled, elective circumstances, they probably would not have chosen single-shot spinal anesthesia for this patient. The successful outcome probably resulted in part from their understanding of the disease process and their experience with the management of high-risk parturients with cardiovascular disease.

One major question remains: Despite the good outcome, was it appropriate for the obstetrician and anesthesiologist to subject this mother to the risks of emergency cesarean section to deliver an infant at 25⁶/₇ weeks' gestation with a double footling breech presentation at 8 cm of cervical dilatation? The authors indicated that "the perinatologist considered emergency cesarean delivery to be the safest mode of delivery for this preterm infant." Was an emergency cesarean section the "safest mode of delivery" for this high-risk parturient?—D.H. Chestnut, M.D.

Is ST Segment Depression of the Electrocardiogram During Cesarean Section Merely Due to Cardiac Sympathetic Block?

Eisenach JC, Tuttle R, Stein A (Wake Forest Univ, Winston-Salem, NC)
Anesth Analg 78:287–292, 1994   101-95-19–23

Background.—Women undergoing cesarean delivery with regional anesthesia commonly have ST-segment depression, yet myocardial ischemia seems an unlikely cause of this finding in a healthy population. The possibility that ST-segment depression in this setting results from reduced sympathetic outflow to the heart was investigated.

Methods.—Electrocardiographic leads II and V_5 were monitored in 15 healthy women undergoing cesarean delivery with spinal anesthesia. Cardiac sympathetic tone was estimated by spectral analysis of heart rate variability, measuring the area under the power-frequency curve of the fast Fourier transform of heartbeat intervals.

Findings.—Five women (33%) had greater than 1-mm horizontal or downsloping depression of the ST segment, starting 5–30 minutes after spinal bupivacaine injection. Women with ST-segment depression had an elevated heart rate compared with women without ST-segment depression; the former group had received more ephedrine. All had similar areas in the low-frequency range of the heart rate power spectrum before spinal bupivacaine injection and after block resolution. During spinal anesthesia, women with ST-segment depression had less power in the low-frequency range than those without ST depression.

Conclusion.—The density of cardiac sympathetic block appears to vary considerably during high spinal anesthesia. The cause of ST-segment depression during cesarean delivery with regional anesthesia is usually reduced cardiac sympathetic tone, probably with different densities of right and left cardiac sympathetic neural block. Because myocardial ischemia causes an increase rather than a reduction in cardiac sympathetic tone, ST-segment depression during cesarean section is not the result of myocardial ischemia.

▶ Nonspecific ECG changes commonly occur among healthy women who receive regional anesthesia for cesarean section. Many years of clinical experience (i.e., millions of uneventful regional anesthetics administered by thousands of anesthesiologists) suggest that these ECG changes are usually benign and clinically insignificant in healthy pregnant women.

This study supports other studies that suggest that ST-segment depression during cesarean section is not the result of myocardial ischemia. It suggests, but does not prove, a possible mechanism for the etiology of these changes, and it should stimulate these and other investigators to perform additional studies of the cardiovascular effects of regional anesthesia in patients who are at high risk for morbidity from cardiovascular disease.—D.H. Chestnut, M.D.

Intrathecal Meperidine for Elective Caesarean Section: A Comparison With Lidocaine

Kafle SK (Tribhuvan Univ, Kathmandu, Nepal)
Can J Anaesth 40:718–721, 1993   101-95-19–24

Background.—Both epidural and intrathecal opioids are commonly used for postoperative pain control; however, meperidine is the only opioid used to provide analgesia for surgery. Its use as the sole agent in patients who are having a cesarean section has been reported. The safety and efficacy of spinal meperidine and 5% heavy spinal lidocaine in mothers and newborns were compared.

Methods.—Fifty full-term pregnant women with American Society of Anesthesiologists physical status I or II who were having elective cesarean section under spinal anesthesia were enrolled. By random assignment, 25 women received intrathecal meperidine, and 25 received lidocaine. All patients received premedication with oral ranitidine, 150 mg, the night before and 2 hours before surgery. Women in the meperidine group also received IV metoclopramide, 10 mg, 1 hour before surgery. After IV Ringer's lactate was administered, patients received 5% meperidine, 1 mg/kg^{-1}, or 5% heavy lidocaine, 1.2–1.4 mL, intrathecally.

Findings.—In all but 2 patients in each group, the sensory and motor blockades were adequate for surgery. Patients in whom blockades were inadequate needed sedation at the time of skin incision. The women experienced no major side effects. The lidocaine group had a higher incidence of hypotension than the meperidine group. Pruritus and drowsiness occurred more often in the meperidine group than in the lidocaine group. In both groups, all the newborns cried immediately after birth. All Apgar scores exceeded 7. The mean duration of postoperative analgesia in the meperidine and lidocaine groups was 6 hours and 1 hour, respectively. The postoperative analgesia requirement was lower in the meperidine group.

Conclusion.—Intrathecal 5% meperidine, 1 mg/kg^{-1}, is better than 5% heavy lidocaine in women who are having elective cesarean sections. The former provides a longer duration of analgesia after surgery. The 5% commercial solution of meperidine can be used for this purpose without additions.

▶ Meperidine differs from other opioids because it has local anesthetic qualities. This study represents the largest series in which intrathecal meperidine was administered as the sole anesthetic agent for cesarean section.

The major advantage of intrathecal meperidine is that it provides longer (i.e., approximately 5–6 hours) postoperative analgesia than intrathecal lidocaine. Of course, this limitation can be overcome by adding .2 mg of morphine to the lidocaine solution.

I have no experience with this technique. Because I work in a teaching hospital, I must use an agent that reliably provides anesthesia for longer than

50–60 minutes. On balance, there seems to be no compelling reason to sub-stitute meperidine for hyperbaric lidocaine or bupivacaine; perhaps that is why no American anesthesiologist has published a large series of cases using this technique.—D.H. Chestnut, M.D.

The Premature Infant: Anesthesia for Cesarean Delivery

Rolbin SH, Cohen MM, Levinton CM, Kelly EN, Farine D (Univ of Toronto; Sunnybrook Health Science Centre, Toronto)
Anesth Analg 78:912–917, 1994   101-95-19–25

Background.—There are few data to guide the choice of anesthetic technique during cesarean delivery of a premature infant. The existing evidence suggests that regional anesthesia may be associated with less perinatal morbidity in premature infants. The effects on outcome of epidural vs. general anesthesia were compared in singleton premature neonates delivered by cesarean section.

Methods.—Five hundred nine infants delivered by cesarean section at a gestational age of 32 weeks or fewer were identified from 2 prospective clinical data bases. Epidural anesthesia was used in 341 cases and general anesthesia in 168. Ordinal logistic regression was used to assess

	1-min		5-min	
Apgar score	*n*	%	*n*	%
All infants				
0–3	153	30.0	30	5.9
4–6	156	30.7	85	16.7
7–10	200	39.3	394	77.4
Total	509		509	
Infants delivered with GA				
0–3	78	46.4	17	10.1
4–6	48	28.6	43	25.6
7–10	42	25.0	108	64.3
Total	168		168	
Infants delivered with EPI				
0–3	75	22.0	13	3.8
4–6	108	31.7	42	12.3
7–10	158	46.3	286	83.9
Total	341		341	

Distribution of Apgar Scores at 1 and 5 Minutes for Neonates Younger Than 32 Weeks of Gestation (Cesarean Delivery)

Abbreviations: GA, general anesthesia; *EPI,* epidural anesthesia.
(Courtesy of Rolbin SH, Cohen MM, Levinton CM, et al: *Anesth Analg* 78:912–917, 1994.)

the independent effects of anesthetic technique on low Apgar scores at 1 minute, after controlling for other neonatal, maternal, or associated neonatal risk factors.

Results.—Apgar scores were 3 or less at 1 minute in 30% of infants and at 5 minutes in 6%. In the general anesthesia group, 46% had low Apgar scores at 1 minute and 10% at 5 minutes; corresponding figures in the epidural group were 22% and 4% (table). After controlling for confounding factors, the relative odds of low 1-minute Apgar scores in the general anesthesia group compared with the epidural group were 2.92. A number of other factors showed a significant association with low 1-minute Apgar scores, including malpresentation, maternal diabetes, primiparity, low gestational age, and associated neonatal outcomes such as respiratory distress syndrome and intraventricular hemorrhage. Nonsignificant factors included birth weight, labor status, maternal infection, and patent ductus arteriosus.

Conclusion.—In premature infants that were delivered by cesarean section, epidural anesthesia was associated with better Apgar scores than general anesthesia at 1 and 5 minutes, a difference that persisted after controlling for the effects of confounding factors. When there is a choice to be made, epidural anesthesia is the preferred technique in this situation.

▶ Preterm delivery represents a major public health problem in the United States. Approximately 7% to 9% of all newborn infants in the United States are delivered preterm. In this study, the administration of general anesthesia was an independent risk factor for low 1-minute Apgar scores in singleton infants that were delivered before 32 weeks' gestation. It is unclear that the administration of general anesthesia was an independent risk factor for low 5-minute Apgar scores. Unfortunately, in the Discussion section, the authors implied that their study confirmed that general anesthesia was an independent risk factor for low 5-minute Apgar scores. They reported no other evidence of adverse neonatal outcome among infants whose mothers received general anesthesia.

I agree that epidural or spinal anesthesia is the preferred anesthetic technique for most women who require cesarean section before term. However, this study does not make a compelling argument that administration of epidural anesthesia results in improved *neonatal* outcome. Low Apgar scores are neither sensitive nor specific for neonatal hypoxemia, acidosis, or adverse long-term outcome, especially in preterm infants.—D.H. Chestnut, M.D.

Epidural Sufentanil Does Not Attenuate the Central Haemodynamic Effects of Caesarean Section Performed Under Epidural Anaesthesia

Crosby ET, Bryson GL, Elliott RD, Gverzdys C (Univ of Ottawa, Ont, Canada)
Can J Anaesth 41:192–197, 1994   101-95-19–26

Purpose.—During cesarean section under major regional anesthesia, some patients have visceral pain referred to the chest, which may lead to nausea and vomiting. This complication can be decreased by the addition of fentanyl to the local anesthetic solution used to establish epidural blockade. No previous studies have compared cardiac performance during cesarean section in parturients who received epidural anesthesia with and without added opioids. A randomized, double-blind study in which maternal hemodynamics were measured by thoracic electrical bioimpedance (TEB) cardiography was conducted.

Methods.—The patients were 21 healthy women undergoing cesarean section with epidural anesthesia. The patients were randomized to receive sufentanil (group S) or no sufentanil (group C). Both groups underwent IV prehydration and placement of an epidural catheter at the L2–3 or L3–4 interspace. After a negative test dose, patients in group S received sufentanil, 30 μg, in 4.4 mL of 2% lidocaine carbonate with 5 μg of epinephrine per mL^{-1}. Patients in group C received only 5 mL of 2% lidocaine carbonate with epinephrine. Lidocaine carbonate 2% with epinephrine was then introduced into the epidural space in increments to achieve a T4 anesthetic level. All patients underwent continuous, noninvasive measurement of hemodynamic variables throughout the perioperative period, including heart rate, mean arterial blood pressure, cardiac index, ejection fraction, and end-diastolic index.

Results.—None of these hemodynamic measures differed between the 2 groups at any time, although there were significant differences within groups when compared with baseline values. Those in both groups showed an intraoperative increase in heart rate. Patients in group S had an increased cardiac index throughout the intraoperative period; this measure was less often elevated in group C. Those in group S also showed an increased ejection fraction throughout the perioperative period, whereas those in group C did not. In both groups, the end-diastolic index increased after IV preloading, but it returned to baseline when an epidural block was induced. There were no significant differences between groups in intraoperative pain or in nausea and vomiting.

Conclusion.—The addition of sufentanil, 30 μg, to epidural anesthesia in women undergoing cesarean section does not appear to alter maternal hemodynamic variables, as measured by TEB. However, differences occur within groups during the perioperative period, but they are unlikely to be of any clinical importance. The addition of fentanyl or other opioids to the epidural solution improves intraoperative analgesia while it reduces the incidence of breakthrough pain, nausea, and vomiting.

▶ The results of this study, although interesting, are not surprising. However, I am surprised that the authors chose to give 30 μg of sufentanil during the administration of epidural lidocaine anesthesia for cesarean section. Why did they give such a large dose of sufentanil? I suspect that a smaller dose of sufentanil would have provided adequate enhancement of the epidural lidocaine anesthesia with less risk of maternal or neonatal respiratory depression.

The authors acknowledged that "epidural sufentanil probably offers little advantage over fentanyl as an adjunct to epidural anaesthesia for Caesarean section." Furthermore, they noted that "a misplaced, intravenous injection of 30 μg sufentanil presents a greater risk of respiratory compromise to the parturient than does 50–75 μg of fentanyl."—D.H. Chestnut, M.D.

The Use of Fentanyl Added to Morphine-Lidocaine-Epinephrine Spinal Solution in Patients Undergoing Cesarean Section
Connelly NR, Dunn SM, Ingold V, Villa EA (Tufts Univ, Springfield, Mass)
Anesth Analg 78:918–920, 1994   101-95-19–27

Objective.—Intrathecal morphine has a slow onset of action and therefore may not be the best choice for intraoperative analgesia during cesarean section and other short cases. The potential benefits of adding fentanyl to a morphine-lidocaine spinal solution in patients having cesarean section were investigated in a randomized, placebo-controlled study.

Methods.—Sixty-two women having elective cesarean section received intrathecal 5% lidocaine with dextrose, 50–70 mg; epinephrine, 200 μg; and preservative-free morphine, .2 mg. In addition, those in the study group received 10 μg of fentanyl, and those in the control group received .2 mL of preservative-free normal saline. The severity of pain was assessed on a 10-cm visual analogue scale during surgery as the uterus was exteriorized and again when the dermatomal level receded to L1. Patients who reported intraoperative discomfort were given IV fentanyl.

Results.—The mean pain scores at the time of uterine extrusion were .8 in the placebo group and .4 in the fentanyl group, a significant difference. Scores in the postanesthesia care unit were 2.3 and 2.7, respectively, a nonsignificant difference. Six patients in the placebo group and none in the fentanyl group received IV fentanyl.

Conclusion.—In women having elective cesarean section, the addition of fentanyl to a morphine-lidocaine-epinephrine spinal anesthetic solution significantly improved intraoperative anesthesia. No differences were noted in the sensory level, the incidence of pruritus, or hypotension with or without fentanyl. In addition, intrathecal fentanyl had no apparent adverse effects on the fetus.

▶ Perhaps I am old fashioned, but I think this represents polypharmacy. Why did the authors add epinephrine to the solution of lidocaine, morphine, and fentanyl? Surely we can provide effective spinal anesthesia for cesarean section without adding 3 more drugs to the solution of local anesthetic. My preferred technique for spinal anesthesia for cesarean section is to administer 12 mg of hyperbaric bupivacaine with .2 mg of preservative-free morphine.—D.H. Chestnut, M.D.

Prediction of Hemorrhage at Cesarean Delivery
Naef RW III, Chauhan SP, Chevalier SP, Roberts WE, Meydrech EF, Morrison JC (Univ of Mississippi, Jackson)
Obstet Gynecol 83:923–926, 1994   101-95-19–28

Background.—As many as 6.8% of women having cesarean delivery require blood transfusion for hemorrhage. Although surgical trauma undoubtedly explains why the mean blood loss with abdominal delivery is greater than that with vaginal delivery, little is known about specific risk factors for excessive bleeding during cesarean section.

Methods.—This retrospective, matched-control study included 1,610 women having cesarean delivery during a 2-year period. One hundred twenty-seven patients (7.9%) had hemorrhage. A comparison group included women without bleeding who were matched for age, parity, indication for cesarean delivery, type of anesthesia, type of skin incision, and antepartum hematocrit.

Findings.—Significant bleeding during abdominal delivery was associated with preeclampsia, disorders of active labor, Native American ethnicity, previous postpartum bleeding, and body weight of more than 250 lb. The presence of 2 or more of these factors was associated with a greatly increased risk for bleeding, with odds ratios of 18.4 or more.

Conclusion.—Patients at increased risk for hemorrhage during cesarean section can be identified before surgery. Such women would benefit from extended preoperative counseling, effective use of blood bank technology, and preventive measures to minimize blood loss during delivery.

▶ Curiously, the authors of this study did not describe the relationship between placenta previa/accreta and intrapartum hemorrhage. Placenta previa/accreta is the most common etiology for *massive* obstetric hemorrhage in the United States. Placenta previa/accreta now represents the most common reason for emergency obstetric hysterectomy in most hospitals in the United States. Other potential causes of major obstetric hemorrhage include uterine atony, uterine rupture, placental abruption, coagulopathy, and retained products of conception.—D.H. Chestnut, M.D.

Sequential Combined Spinal Epidural Block Versus Spinal Block for Cesarean Section: Effects on Maternal Hypotension and Neurobehavioral Function of the Newborn
Thorén T, Holmström B, Rawal N, Schollin J, Lindeberg S, Skeppner G (Örebro Med Ctr Hosp, Sweden)
Anesth Analg 78:1087–1092, 1994   101-95-19–29

Background.—No controlled studies have compared a spinal block with a sequential combined spinal-epidural (CSE) block for cesarean section. These 2 techniques were compared, with a focus on the quality of surgical anesthesia and the effect on maternal blood pressure and neonatal neurobehavioral function.

Methods.—Forty-two healthy parturients were divided into equal groups and given a spinal or sequential block. The spinal block included .5% hyperbaric bupivacaine, 2.5 mL, injected into the subarachnoid space through a 26-gauge Quincke needle. The sequential CSE block, consisting of 1.5 mL of .5% hyperbaric bupivacaine, was injected into the subarachnoid space through a long 26-gauge Quincke needle, which was introduced through an 8-gauge Tuohy needle. If the sequential CSE block did not reach the T4 level in 15 minutes, it was extended by fractionated doses through the epidural catheter. Ephedrine was administered intravenously to treat hypotension.

Findings.—The interval from block induction to the start of surgery and delivery was shorter in patients who were given the spinal block. Fifteen minutes after induction, cephalad spread occurred to T4 in the spinal group and to T7 in the sequential CSE group. All women who were given the sequential CSE block required a mean epidural bupivacaine dose of 53.8 mg. Surgical analgesia was good or excellent in all patients before delivery. After delivery, a similar amount of supplementary fentanyl and/or IV dixyranzine was needed in both groups. Sixty-two percent of the patients in both groups had hypotension, although it developed earlier in the spinal group. The effects on the neonates were similar in the 2 groups. None of the patients had a postdural puncture headache.

Conclusion.—Spinal and sequential CSE block both provide good surgical analgesia for cesarean delivery. Both techniques are associated with a risk of maternal hypotension. No differences in neonatal outcomes were observed as long as the maternal blood pressure was carefully monitored and hypotension was treated promptly.

▶ In this study, hypotension occurred with equal frequency in the group of patients that received CSE anesthesia and the group that received spinal anesthesia alone. This confirms my experience. Administration of 6 mg of hyperbaric buivacaine (or 7.5 mg of bupivacaine, as was administered in this study) results in an extensive sympathectomy of the sacral, lumbar, and lower thoracic dermatomes.

Sympathectomy of the lower extremities is the major reason for decreased venous return and hypotension after administration of spinal anesthesia. Extension of the level of sympathetic blockade from the lower to the upper thoracic spinal segments results in little additional venous pooling. As a result, it is not surprising that the authors found no difference in the incidence of hypotension between the 2 groups. However, I was surprised that the authors observed no cases of early-onset hypotension in the CSE group.—D.H. Chestnut, M.D.

Emergency Caesarean Section During Labour: Response Times and Type of Anaesthesia

Quinn AJ, Kilpatrick A (Glasgow Royal Maternity Hosp, Scotland)
Eur J Obstet Gynecol Reprod Biol 54:25–29, 1994   101-95-19–30

Background.—The delay between the decision to perform a cesarean section and delivery is generally perceived to be caused by the time spent administering the chosen anesthetic and the time spent delivering the infant. However, communication among staff members and patient preparation and transit to the operating area may also be significant factors. The contribution of each of these factors to the decision-delivery interval was investigated.

Methods and Findings.—Of 212 consecutive emergency cesarean deliveries performed in women whose pregnancies were carried to term, 18% were considered truly urgent and required delivery within 20 minutes. Intrapartum cardiotocographic interpretation was generally accurate, although 6 cases originally classified as urgent were later found to have Krebs scores of greater than 4. Among the urgent cases, the median total time from decision to delivery was 25 minutes. The delay in one third of the urgent deliveries exceeded 30 minutes; the longest delay was 56 minutes. Responses were most rapid when fetal blood sample results were acidotic and an antepartum hemorrhage occurred. Nine percent of the infants were admitted to the special care infant unit. Seven percent of the women received general anesthesia for surgery. Although a decision-delivery interval of 20–30 minutes could be achieved when regional anesthetic techniques were used, a general anesthetic was needed to reduce this interval to fewer than 20 minutes.

Conclusion.—With good communication and prompt action, the interval between the decision to do a cesarean section and delivery can be shortened. With regional anesthetic methods, acceptable response times can be achieved for most urgent cesarean sections. The use of a general anesthetic may sometimes be warranted to ensure fetal safety.

▶ Most cases with a fetal heart rate tracing that is not reassuring do not preclude the use of regional anesthesia for an emergency cesarean section. Cases of dire fetal distress (e.g., uterine rupture, placental abruption, and cord prolapse with unremitting fetal bradycardia) mandate the rapid administration of anesthesia. In many cases, this is best accomplished by rapid-sequence induction of general anesthesia. Of course, the mother should not be unnecessarily endangered to deliver a distressed fetus. A high index of suspicion of a difficult airway contraindicates the rapid-sequence induction of general anesthesia, regardless of the severity of fetal distress. In such cases, either regional anesthesia should be administered or an awake endotracheal intubation should be performed before the administration of general anesthesia.

At the University of Alabama at Birmingham, we encourage the early administration of epidural analgesia in patients who are at high risk for operative delivery. This facilitates the extension of epidural anesthesia for an emergency cesarean section.—D.H. Chestnut, M.D.

Patient-Controlled Epidural Analgesia With Sufentanil Following Caesarean Section: The Effect of Adrenaline and Clonidine Admixture

Vercauteren MP, Vandeput DM, Meert TF, Adriaensen HA (Univ Hosp Antwerp, Belgium)
Anaesthesia 49:767–771, 1994   101-95-19–31

Background.—Increasing experience is being gained in the use of patient-controlled analgesia using the epidural route. However, several studies have indicated that, when administered epidurally, lipophilic opioids exert their effect by a systemic rather than a spinal action. To reduce the side effects of opioids when used alone, especially when a high degree of systemic resorption is assumed, their efficacy in combination with other substances was investigated.

Method.—Sixty patients who were scheduled for cesarean section were randomly allocated to receive by the epidural route in a double-blinded fashion one of the following patient-controlled analgesia mixtures for relief of postoperative pain: sufentanil, 2 μg/mL^{-1} in .9% sodium chloride; sufentanil, 2 μg/mL^{-1}, with epinephrine, 2.5 μg/mL $^{-1}$; or sufentanil, 2 μg/mL^{-1} with clonidine, 3 μg/mL^{-1}. Visual analogue scale scores were recorded retrospectively at 10 and 24 hours, and assessments were made of the quality of night rest, sedation, and incidence of pruritus.

Results.—Patients who were treated with plain sufentanil used a mean of 208.2 μg of sufentanil during the first 24 hours. This dose was significantly reduced in the groups that received combination therapy with epinephrine and clonidine (a mean of 167.5 μg and 139.1 μg, respectively), with the difference between the epinephrine group and the clonidine group reaching statistical significance ($P < .05$). The patient-controlled analgesia settings were decreased in 8 patients in the clonidine group compared with only 1 patient in the plain sufentanil group ($P < .05$). Although the sufentanil requirements were lower in the groups treated with mixtures, this was not apparent in the improved quality of sleep. The group that received epinephrine experienced more pruritus than the plain sufentanil group and less sedation than the clonidine-treated patients; however, it scored significantly higher with regard to the quality of night rest. Two patients in the epinephrine mixture group requested naloxone treatment for pruritus, which did not appear to influence the quality of analgesia.

Conclusion.—The addition of epinephrine and clonidine to sufentanil in patient-controlled analgesia using the epidural route is beneficial in terms of reduced sufentanil consumption. The epinephrine mixture appears to have some advantages and causes a lower incidence of sedation and a better quality of sleep, despite greater pruritus.

▶ The limitation of this study is that it compared 2 recipes for administration of postcesarean patient-controlled epidural analgesia. It remains unclear whether patient-controlled epidural analgesia represents a more cost-effective means of providing postcesarean analgesia when compared with single-shot intraspinal opioid analgesia or patient-controlled IV analgesia.—D.H. Chestnut, M.D.

Improving Epidural Anesthesia During Cesarean Section: Causes of Maternal Discomfort or Pain During Surgery
Capogna G, Celleno D (Fatebenefratelli Gen Hosp, Rome)
Int J Obstet Anesth 3:149–152, 1994   101-95-19–32

Introduction.—Although epidural anesthesia has several advantages over general or spinal anesthesia for cesarean section, patients frequently experience intraoperative discomfort or pain. The most common causes of intraoperative discomfort and pain were reviewed and solutions were explored in an effort to improve the efficacy of epidural anesthesia for cesarean section.

Discomfort.—A sensation of pressure on the chest may result from a high level of block, usually greater than T2. Careful titration of the dose with frequent checks of the level of the block can prevent this sensation. If the patient's pain requires a high-level block, she should be prepared for this sensation. A sensation of pressure on the abdomen results from the manual pressure exerted by the obstetrician when extracting the infant; patients should be warned that this may occur. Shivering may compensate for the heat loss that attends increased cutaneous blood flow, or it may be a consequence of central hypothermia. Using epidural fentanyl, warmed local anesthetic solution, low-dose diazepam, and radiant heat treatment, or clonidine could prevent or resolve shivering. Nausea and vomiting may be the result of maternal hypotension or may occur with the administration of opioids. It can be controlled or prevented with metoclopramide and droperidol, transdermal scopolamine, ondansetron, or prevention of hypotension.

Pain.—Pain occurs with inadequate block. The extension of a sensory nerve block must be determined individually. Inadequate block or unblocked segments can be caused either by a misplaced catheter or too little local anesthetic. Most inadequate block problems can be prevented by inserting only 2–3 cm of catheter. The catheter should be withdrawn or replaced when the patient experiences unilateral analgesia. When short-acting local anesthetics are used, an additional dose may be required if intraoperative sensory block regression occurs. The use of epidural opioids may prevent visceral pain, while not compromising maternal alertness.

Discussion.—Understanding the factors that can contribute to intraoperative discomfort and pain may improve the reliability of epidural anesthesia for cesarean section. In addition to technical concerns, an important component in the success of regional anesthesia is the proper psychological preparation and gentle treatment of the patient.

▶ This is a useful review for all anesthesia care providers who administer epidural anesthesia for cesarean section. In my experience, the most common reasons for inadequate epidural anesthesia during cesarean section include malposition of the epidural catheter; administration of an inadequate dose of local anesthetic; failure to wait long enough between administration of local anesthetic and the skin incision; failure to ensure an adequate sacral blockade; and administration of bupivacaine rather than 2-chloroprocaine or lidocaine with epinephrine.

Lidocaine with epinephrine is my preferred local anesthetic for most cases involving epidural anesthesia for cesarean section. I cannot remember the last time that I gave .5% bupivacaine during administration of epidural anesthesia for cesarean section. Its onset is intolerably slow, and the density of anesthesia is not always adequate. In addition, administration of large doses of .5% bupivacaine results in an increased risk of maternal cardiovascular toxicity.—D.H. Chestnut, M.D.

An Isobolographic Study of Epidural Clonidine and Fentanyl After Cesarean Section
Eisenach JC, D'Angelo R, Taylor C, Hood DD (Wake Forest Univ, Winston-Salem, NC)
Anesth Analg 79:285–290, 1994   101-95-19–33

Objective.—Epidural administration of clonidine and fentanyl has been used for postoperative pain relief; however, the nature of their interaction in humans has still to be defined. An isobolographic study design was used to determine whether epidurally administered fentanyl and clonidine interact additively or synergistically for the postoperative relief of pain.

Treatment.—The study included 90 healthy women with moderate-to-severe pain after elective cesarean section. Epidural anesthesia with lidocaine was used, with IV alfentanil as needed. In a randomized, double-blind protocol, each patient received a single epidural injection of 1 of 3 doses of fentanyl (15, 45, or 135 μg), clonidine (50, 150, or 400 μg), or a combination of fenantyl (F) and clonidine (C) (7.5 μg F + 25 μg C; 22.5 μg F + 75 μg C; or 67.5 μg F + 200 μg C). Pain and sedation were assessed using a 10-cm visual analogue scale.

Outcome.—Each drug alone and in combination produced analgesia and reduced the need for IV morphine. Contrary to expectations, the largest doses of fentanyl and clonidine alone failed to produce near-

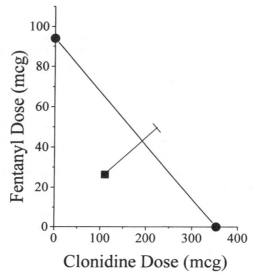

Clonidine Dose (mcg)

Fig 19–7.—Isobologram of epidural clonidine and fentanyl at the effective dose that produced analgesia in 50% of patients (ED$_{50}$). The *points* on each axis represent the ED$_{50}$ of each drug alone, and the *interconnecting line* is that of additivity. The confidence intervals of the observed point include the *line*, signifying that the combination does not differ from an additive one. (Courtesy of Eisenach JC, D'Angelo R, Taylor C, et al: *Anesth Analg* 79:285-290, 1994.)

complete pain relief, thereby decreasing the range of effect observed. Furthermore, there was a wide variability in pain relief scores. The effective dose that produced analgesia in 50% of patients (ED$_{50}$) for fentanyl was 94 µg and the ED$_{50}$ for clonidine was 353 µg. The ED$_{50}$ for the combination was 130 µg, which was only 52% of that predicted by an additive interaction (250 µg). However, the observed ED$_{50}$ did not differ significantly from the calculated ED$_{50}$ of an additive interaction (Fig 19-7). Clonidine, alone or in combination with fentanyl, reduced blood pressure, but it did not affect heart rate or cause more sedation than fentanyl.

Conclusion.—Epidurally administered clonidine and fentanyl have an apparent potency ratio of 3.8:1 for the treatment of acute postoperative pain in women after elective cesarean section. Contrary to studies in animals, this study in humans fails to demonstrate a synergy between fentanyl and clonidine. Instead, these drugs interact in an additive manner in humans. Whether this difference reflects a true species difference or is attributable to methodologic effects is not clear. Nevertheless, a reduced dose of fentanyl and clonidine can be combined to provide excellent analgesia with few side effects.

▶ In this study, the most surprising result was the authors' inability to demonstrate a synergistic interaction between epidurally administered clonidine and fentanyl. It represents one of a long series of systematic, well-designed studies that evaluated the mechanism, efficacy, and role of intraspinal clonidine for the treatment of either acute or chronic pain. I commend Dr. Eisenach for his systematic, painstaking approach and for his extensive contributions to our understanding of this subject. Unfortunately, epidural and intrathecal clonidine administration remains primarily an investigational tool that is not yet ready for routine clinical use.—D.H. Chestnut, M.D.

Epidural Butorphanol Does Not Reduce Side Effects From Epidural Morphine After Cesarean Birth

Gambling DR, Howell P, Huber C, Kozak S (Univ of British Columbia, Vancouver, Canada; Grace Hosp, Vancouver, BC, Canada)
Anesth Analg 78:1099–1104, 1994   101-95-19–34

Background.—Epidural morphine (EM) can result in pruritus, nausea, and respiratory depression. The addition of butorphanol to EM during cesarean delivery may reduce these common adverse effects of opioids.

Methods.—Seventy-one patients having elective cesarean deliveries were enrolled in a double-blind, randomized trial. All patients received a standard epidural anesthetic. Twenty minutes after delivery, patients received 3 mg of EM with either 1, 2, or 3 mg of butorphanol or 3 mL of normal saline. Patient assessments, which consisted of visual analogue scores for pain, satisfaction, nausea, itch, and somnolence, were made before surgery and at 2, 8, and 24 hours after surgery. A carbon dioxide (CO_2) challenge test was also done at each evaluation.

Findings.—The 4 groups did not differ significantly in terms of pain, satisfaction, nausea, or pruritus. The 3 groups that were given butorphanol had significantly greater somnolence scores at 8 hours than did the control group. Results of the CO_2 challenge test did not differ among groups at any time, but patients experienced an overall decreased sensitivity to CO_2 after opioid administration. No clinically significant incidence of respiratory depression occurred.

Conclusion.—The addition of epidural butorphanol in doses of 1, 2, or 3 mg to EM did not reduce adverse effects after cesarean delivery. Patients who received butorphanol had significantly greater levels of somnolence.

▶ The results of this study do not confirm those of an earlier study by Lawhorn and co-workers (1), who found that epidural butorphanol (i.e., 1–3 mg) did not reduce the side effects that resulted from epidural administration of 3 mg of morphine for postcesarean analgesia. Furthermore, patients who received epidural butorphanol had significantly greater somnolence than those who did not receive it. This negates one of the advantages of epidural opioid analgesia, which is that it allows patients to remain awake and alert during the postoperative period, facilitating maternal-infant bonding as well as early ambulation.—D.H. Chestnut, M.D.

Reference

1. Lawhorn CD, et al: *Anesth Analg* 72:53, 1991.

Extension of Epidural Blockade for Emergency Caesarean Section: Assessment of a Bolus Dose of Bupivacaine 0.5% 10 ml Following an Infusion of 0.1% for Analgesia in Labour
Dickson MAS, Jenkins J (Eastern Gen Hosp, Edinburgh, Scotland)
Anaesthesia 94:636–638, 1994   101-95-19–35

Background.—The routine method of maintained epidural analgesia for labor is by continuous infusion of bupivacaine, .1% at 20 mL/hr^{-1}, with additional top-up doses of .25% or .5% bupivacaine as needed. For emergency cesarean deliveries, the top-up dose routinely used is 10 mL of bupivacaine .5%. This dose of bupivacaine seems to result in a safe, reliable conversion from a block that is adequate for labor to an anesthetic block that is suitable for surgery.

Methods.—Eighteen patients (median age, 27 years) were enrolled in an observational, prospective study to test the efficacy of the routine clinical practice. The standard epidural analgesic regimen consisted of a 4-mL lidocaine 2% test dose followed by 8 mL of bupivacaine .5% to establish an analgesia block. Analgesia was maintained with an infusion of .1% bupivacaine at 20 mL/hr^{-1} and supplementary top-ups as needed.

Findings.—The 11 patients in group 1 had a block develop that was adequate for cesarean section. In group 2, 5 of the 7 patients with inadequate block needed a further top-up dose before surgery began; another 2 patients needed a general anesthetic after surgery was started, despite clinical evidence that the block was of sufficient density and height. The groups did not differ significantly in the duration or dosage of bupivacaine administered by infusion or in the number of top-up doses given during labor. The median additional top-up dose needed in group 2 was 35 mg of bupivacaine; the time required to produce a sufficient block was significantly longer in that group.

Conclusion.—In these patients, a 10-mL top-up dose of bupivacaine .5% did not reliably result in the conversion of an analgesic block maintained by a diluted infusion of local anesthetic to a block that was adequate for cesarean delivery. Five of the 18 patients needed an additional top-up dose, which delayed surgery and potentially increased the risk to mother and infant.

▶ It is difficult for me to imagine a circumstance in which one would want to use .5% bupivacaine to extend preexisting epidural anesthesia for an emergency cesarean section. Bupivacaine has a slower onset than either 2-chloro-procaine or lidocaine with epinephrine. Bolus administration of .5% bupivacaine is associated with an increased risk of maternal cardiac toxicity. This study was ill-conceived, and the results are not surprising. When time is of the essence, I extend preexisting epidural analgesia with 3% 2-chloroprocaine. Alternatively, a relatively rapid extension of epidural anesthesia can be achieved by giving alkalinized 2% lidocaine with epinephrine.—D.H. Chestnut, M.D.

A Two-Dose Epidural Morphine Regimen in Cesarean Section Patients: Pharmacokinetic Profile
Zakowski MI, Ramanathan S, Turndorf H (New York Univ)
Acta Anaesthesiol Scand 37:584–589, 1993   101-95-19–36

Objective.—It has been shown that 2 doses of 5 mg of epidural morphine administered 24 hours apart offer effective postoperative pain relief after cesarean section. The pharmacokinetics, maternal urinary excretion, breast milk concentration, and noenatal urinary excretion of epidural morphine in cesarean section patients were investigated.

Methods.—The first 5-mg epidural dose of morphine was administered after delivery, and the second dose was given 24 hours later. Maternal plasma, breast milk, and maternal and neonatal urine concentrations of unconjugated and conjugated (UM and CM) morphine were measured using radioimmunoassay, and pharmacokinetic values were calculated using noncompartmental analysis.

Results.—The mean serum concentrations of UM were 40% to 50% higher and concentrations of CM were 50% to 100% higher in the first hour after dose 2 compared with the corresponding values after dose 1. Compared with dose 1, values for dose 2 for the area under the curve increased by 28%, values for the area under the moment curve increased by 83%, the elimination half-time increased by 35%, and the mean residence time increased by 36%, but clearance decreased by 19%. The volume of distribution did not change significantly. The total urinary excretion of morphine progressively decreased on days 2 and 3, compared with day 1. Breast milk and neonatal urine contained negligible amounts of morphine, indicating minimal neonatal transfer.

Conclusion.—After epidural administration, morphine is rapidly absorbed into the systemic circulation and conjugated. Both UM and CM undergo renal elimination, but only negligible amounts of morphine enter the maternal breast milk.

▶ The authors defined the rationale for their study as follows: "It has been shown that two 5-mg doses of epidural morphine administered 24 h apart offers therapeutic advantages over a single-dose regimen." They cited their own study (1) to support this declarative statement. I know of no compelling reason to give such a large dose (i.e., 5 mg) of epidural morphine immediately after cesarean section, nor do I know of a compelling reason to give a second 5-mg dose of epidural morphine 24 hours after the first.—D.H. Chestnut, M.D.

Reference

1. Zakowski MI, et al: *Acta Anaesthesiol Scand* 36:698, 1992.

Epidural Anesthesia for Cesarean Delivery and Vaginal Birth After Maternal Fontan Repair: Report of Two Cases
Carp H, Jayaram A, Vadhera R, Nichols M, Morton M (Oregon Health Sciences Univ, Portland; Baylor College of Medicine, Houston)
Anesth Analg 78:1190–1192, 1994   101-95-19–37

Background.—More women who have undergone a Fontan procedure to repair a congenital heart defect are now reaching childbearing age. Epidural block has been used successfully to provide anesthesia for cesarean delivery and analgesia for vaginal birth in these women. Two patients who underwent Fontan repair were described.

Case 1.—Woman, 26, was a gravida 2, para 0-0-1-0 parturient. At 11 years of age, she had had a Fontan procedure to correct type III tricuspid atresia with associated single ventricle and levotransposition of the great vessels. Her activity level had been normal, but she had experienced recurrent episodes of symptomatic supraventricular tachycardia that were believed to be atrial flutter with variable conduction. Antepartum fetal contraction stress testing at 31 weeks of gestation showed late decelerations and persistent variable and late decelerations with subsequent contractions. Findings on ultrasonography indicated severe fetal growth retardation, so a cesarean delivery was planned. Radial artery, central venous pressure (CVP), and lumbar epidural catheters were placed using local anesthesia, and remote leads were applied to enable cardioversion if needed. To avoid aortocaval compression, an exaggerated left lateral tilt was used. The initial CVP reading of 18 mm Hg increased to 20 mm Hg after IV administration of 1,500 mL of lactated Ringer's solution. Two percent lidocaine, 25 mL, was administered over 30 minutes through the epidural catheter in 5-mL increments to achieve a sensory dermatome level of T4. The mean blood pressure declined by about 15% when the block reached a T4 level, and the CVP declined to 12 mm Hg. After another 500 mL of lactated Ringer's solution, the blood pressure and CVP promptly normalized. The fetal heart tracing was unchanged during this time. A boy weighing 1,030 g was delivered, with 1- and 5-minute Apgar scores of 2 and 7, respectively. The remainder of the surgery was uneventful.

Case 2.—Woman, 24, nulliparous, had undergone a palliative Blalock-Hanlon procedure at 3 months of age and a modified Fontan procedure at 11 years of age to correct a type III tricuspid atresia with associated single ventricle and levotransposition of the great vessels. Her activity had been somewhat limited since the Fontan repair and throughout her pregnancy, and she had experienced occasional palpitations. Premature rupture of the membranes occurred at 31 weeks' gestation and was treated with IV ampicillin. After 4 days, chorioamnionitis was diagnosed presumptively. The condition of the fetus worsened, and labor induction with oxytocin was planned. The patient's preoperative examination was unremarkable. A radial artery catheter and lumbar epidural catheter were inserted using local anesthesia. Over a 20-minute period, 10 mL of .25% bupivacaine was given through the epidural catheter in 5-mL increments to achieve a sensory dermatome level of T10. An epidural infusion of .10% bupivacaine containing 25 μg of alfentanil per mL was begun at 10 mL/hr. Maternal blood pressure was unaffected by the epidural block, and oxytocin infusion was begun. After about 1 hour, a male infant (weight, 1,500 g) was delivered over an intact perineum with minimal blood loss. One- and 5-minute Apgar scores were 5 and 8, respectively. The patient's recovery was uneventful.

Conclusion.—Pregnancy in patients who have had a congenital heart defect repaired by a Fontan procedure will probably become more common. This limited experience indicates that maternal cardiovascular status may not be adversely affected by pregnancy and that epidural anesthesia and analgesia can be used safely in such patients.

▶ An experienced anesthesiologist can probably give epidural analgesia/anesthesia safely to a pregnant patient with almost any kind of cardiovascular lesion, provided the block is established slowly enough. In the first case, the 25 mL of 2% lidocaine was administered in 5-mL increments over a period of 30 minutes. In the second case, the 10 mL of .25% bupivacaine was administered in 5-mL increments over a period of 20 minutes. The authors concluded that "the use of adequate prehydration, exaggerated uterine displacement, and the slow titration of the block may have compensated for the venodilatory effects of the epidural block and contributed to the hemodynamic stability observed in our patients." I agree. Slow induction of epidural analgesia/anesthesia is the key to successful management of these patients.—D.H. Chestnut, M.D.

Comparison of Prophylactic Angiotensin II Versus Ephedrine Infusion for Prevention of Maternal Hypotension During Spinal Anesthesia
Ramin SM, Ramin KD, Cox K, Magness RR, Shearer VE, Gant NF (Univ of Texas, Dallas)
Am J Obstet Gynecol 171:734–739, 1994   101-95-19–38

Background.—Regional anesthesia for cesarean delivery is associated with a high incidence of maternal hypotension. Ephedrine prophylaxis, although it maintains maternal blood pressure, has been shown to result in a 21% incidence of fetal acidemia, possibly because of its vasoconstrictor effect on the uteroplacental vascular bed. An alternative therapy with angiotensin II has been reported to have fewer vasoconstricting effects. The incidence of maternal hypotension and the fetal-neonatal outome were compared when ephedrine infusion or angiotensin II infusion was used as a prophylactic measure against maternal hypotension during regional anesthesia for cesarean delivery.

Methods.—Thirty healthy pregnant women who were admitted for elective repeat cesarean delivery were assigned to 1 of 3 groups of 10 each: control, prophylactic infusion of angiotensin II, and prophylactic infusion of ephedrine. Prophylactic infusions were titrated to a maternal diastolic blood pressure of 0–10 mm Hg above baseline, and cesarean delivery was performed. Maternal hypotension was defined as a decrease of more than 30% from baseline reading. The neonatal and fetal outcomes were assessed by Apgar scores, and the umbilical artery and umbilical venous blood samples for angiotensin II values were checked to determine whether maternal-to-fetal transport occurred.

Results.—Final results were obtained for all 30 women. Hypotension developed in 50% of the control group after injection of the spinal anesthetic, and bolus injections of ephedrine were required. The maternal baseline mean arterial blood pressure was increased after spinal anesthesia in the angiotensin II group (a mean of 79 compared with a mean of 89 mm Hg) and was maintained in the ephedrine group. The maternal and fetal angiotensin II levels were unchanged in the control and ephedrine groups, but they increased significantly with angiotensin II infusion from a mean of 159 to a mean of 647 pg/mL. The umbilical artery and vein angiotensin II levels were unaltered by angiotensin II infusions. However, the mean pH of the umbilical artery blood was lower in the ephedrine group than in the angiotensin II and control groups. No significant difference in Apgar scores was seen at 1 and 5 minutes among the 3 groups.

Conclusion.—In the healthy term fetus, the use of angiotensin II appears to be advantageous as an alternative to ephedrine in maintaining maternal blood pressure during regional anesthesia. Although the use of an angiotensin II infusion is not a familiar practice and can be time-consuming, its use in the preterm or compromised fetus, which is more susceptible to decreases in maternal systemic blood pressure, is likely to be more beneficial than ephedrine.

▶ The authors indicated that they had observed a 21% increase of fetal acidemia after the use of ephedrine prophylaxis during adminstration of spinal anesthesia for cesarean section. They cited an abstract that was presented in 1990, which has not yet been published as a full-length manuscript in a peer-reviewed journal. Others have not confirmed a problem with the use of ephedrine for the prophylaxis or treatment of hypotension during administration of spinal anesthesia for cesarean section.

The authors acknowledged that "the clinical application of an angiotensin II infusion is not a familiar practice and is more time-consuming. . . ." They go on to *speculate* that "the preterm or compromised fetus . . . likely would benefit from the use of angiotensin II rather than ephedrine." Where are the data? I think that ephedrine remains the vasopressor of choice for prophylaxis or treatment of hypotension for most obstetric patients who receive spinal anesthesia for cesarean section.—D.H. Chestnut, M.D.

A Survey of Airway Management During Induction of General Anaesthesia in Obstetrics: Are the Recommendations in the Confidential Enquiries Into Maternal Deaths Being Implemented?
Cook TM, McCrirrick A (Bristol Royal Infirmary, England)
Int J Obstet Anesth 3:143–145, 1994   101-95-19–39

Background.—Two recent reports on maternal deaths in England and Wales and in the United Kingdom have revealed 18 and 8 anesthetic-related deaths, respectively. Most resulted from difficulty in establishing and securing an airway. Recommendations were made in each report for improving patient care. These included the use of 2-handed cricoid pressure and its application by a trained anesthesiology assistant or a trained midwife with an additional anesthesiology assistant to help with intubation. Departmental protocols relating to airway management in obstetric anesthesia were investigated to determine whether such recommendations had been implemented.

Methods.—Forty-four British hospitals were randomly selected and contacted by telephone. Using a standard questionnaire, the obstetric anesthesiologist was interviewed about departmental codes of practice.

Results.—There was a 100% response to all questions. In all departments, an assistant was available to help the anesthesiologist at induction of anesthesia. In 88.6% of departments, the assistant was trained in anesthesiology. Cricoid pressure was always performed at intubation; single-handed cricoid pressure was used in 70.4% of cases. Two-handed cricoid pressure was always used in 13.6% of departments. In hospitals using 2-handed cricoid pressure for some or all cases (79.5%), a second assistant was not usually available. If one was present, the second assistant was a midwife in 3 departments and an operating department assistant in 1. Four anesthesiologists were unfamiliar with the term 2-handed cricoid pressure. Most anesthesiologists were aware of a departmental failed intubation protocol, but rehearsal was uncommon.

Conclusion.—The wide variation in airway management seen in 44 hospitals was demonstrated. Recommendations from the reports of 1982–1987 have not been fully implemented. Guidelines regarding the use of assistants and the existence of a failed intubation protocol have been largely implemented, but because they form a part of an accepted good practice in other areas of anesthesiology, it is not clear whether the reports have made an impact. More specific recommendations regarding 2-handed cricoid pressure, the number of and the roles of assistants involved in induction, and the practice of failed intubation drills do not appear to have been widely adopted.

▶ There is an old saying: "A low blood pressure is better than no pressure." I would like to offer a twisted version of that saying: "Incorrect application of cricoid pressure is *worse* than no cricoid pressure." I suspect that cricoid pressure is often applied incorrectly in hospitals throughout the United States. Such incorrect application of cricoid pressure may increase the likelihood of failed intubation and, in some cases, may prevent effective mask ventilation. We give lip service to the importance of cricoid pressure during rapid-sequence induction of general anesthesia in patients who are at risk for aspiration of gastric contents, but I fear that some of us spend little time ensuring that our assistants know how to apply cricoid pressure correctly.—D.H. Chestnut, M.D.

Intravenous Administration of the Proton Pump Inhibitor Omeprazole Reduces the Risk of Acid Aspiration at Emergency Cesarean Section
Rocke DA, Rout CC, Gouws E (Univ of Natal, Durban, South Africa; Inst for Biostatistics, Durban, South Africa)
Anesth Analg 78:1093–1098, 1994   101-95-19–40

Background.—Because of the potential for aspiration, a nonparticulate antacid is given to patients who are scheduled for cesarean section. However, antacids alone are not always effective. Many anesthesiologists use a combination of an antacid and a histamine H_2-receptor antagonist in patients who are having an urgent cesarean section to decrease the risk of acid aspiration. The proton pump inhibitors, a new class of agents, have recently been introduced into clinical practice. The efficacy of the proton pump inhibitor omeprazole, when given as part of a prophylactic regimen that includes IV metoclopramide and oral sodium citrate, was investigated.

Methods.—Patients were randomly assigned to receive IV omeprazole, 40 mg, or placebo when the decision was made to perform a cesarean section. All patients were given 10 mg of IV metoclopramide and 30 mL of .3 M sodium citrate. Gastric contents were aspirated just after endotracheal intubation (PI) and before tracheal extubation (PE). Women with pH levels lower than 3.5 and gastric volumes greater than 25 mL were considered to be at risk for acid aspiration if regurgitation occurred. Only patients with intervals from study drug to PI aspiration of greater than 30 minutes were assessed.

Findings.—Two hundred eighty-two patients in the study group and 259 in the control group could be evaluated. Immediately after PI, 11 patients in the control group and 4 in the study group were at risk. In these 4 patients, the interval from omeprazole to PI aspiration was 40 minutes or less. Before PE, 19 patients in the control group and 2 in the study group were at risk. The mean pH in patients who were given omeprazole was significantly greater than that in the control group. Gastric volumes in the omeprazole group were significantly lower after both PI and PE.

Conclusion.—Intravenous omeprazole, 40 mg, that is administered when a cesarean section has been decided on, significantly reduces the risk of acid aspiration when the time from injection to induction of anesthesia is greater than 30 minutes. If this interval can be extended to 40 minutes, patients' risk of aspiration is reduced even more. Omeprazole apparently also decreases the residual gastric volume.

▶ In this study, all patients also received 10 mg of IV metoclopramide and 30 mL of .3 M sodium citrate. The study is similar to the authors' earlier investigation of IV ranitidine (1).

It is unclear that omeprazole offers any advantage over an H_2-receptor antagonist. It is also unclear that omeprazole was as effective as ranitidine in the authors' earlier study. However, this is a fine point that does not have to be addressed in a future study. It would be a waste of time and money to perform a similar study that compares a sodium citrate–metoclopramide–ranitidine regimen with a sodium citrate–metoclopramide-omeprazole regimen.—D.H. Chestnut, M.D.

Reference

1. Rout CC, et al: *Anesth Analg* 76:156, 1993.

Gastric Emptying Is Delayed at 8–12 Weeks' Gestation
Levy DM, Williams OA, Magides AD, Reilly CS (Univ of Sheffield, England)
Br J Anaesth 73:237–238, 1994   101-95-19–41

Background.—Regurgitation of gastric contents and their aspiration into the lungs are major anesthetic hazards, and delayed emptying of the stomach is considered to be a significant risk factor. A previous study using the acetaminophen absorption method, which has been validated against scintigraphy, indicated delayed gastric emptying in the first trimester of pregnancy. The study has now been repeated using a larger population.

Method.—Gastric emptying was estimated by the acetaminophen absorption technique in 20 women with pregnancies at 8–12 weeks' gestation and in 20 nonpregnant controls. They received 1.5 g of acetaminophen in tablet form with 50 mL of water and remained semirecumbent for 2 hours as venous blood was sampled every 15 minutes.

Results.—The peak plasma acetaminophen concentration was significantly lower in pregnant women than in the controls, and the time to the peak was significantly longer. Areas under the time-concentration curve at 1 and 2 hours were significantly smaller in pregnant women.

Implications.—Gastric emptying is delayed at 8–12 weeks' gestation, and the duration of fasting before inducing anesthesia should probably not be compromised. In addition, the absorption of orally administered drugs may be delayed.

▶ This study contradicts at least one other that observed no difference in gastric emptying between nonpregnant controls and pregnant women at 8–10 weeks' gestation (1). I remain unconvinced that pregnancy per se substantially delays gastric emptying. By contrast, labor, and the administration of opioid analgesics during labor, clearly result in delayed gastric emptying. Before the onset of labor, I am more concerned with the decreased competence of the lower esophageal sphincter in pregnant women.—D.H. Chestnut, M.D.

Reference

1. Whitehead EM, et al: *Anaesthesia* 48:53, 1993.

Pulmonary Hypertension and Pregnancy: A Series of Eight Cases
Smedstad KG, Cramb R, Morison DH (McMaster Univ, Hamilton, Ont, Canada)
Can J Anaesth 41:502–512, 1994   101-95-19–42

Introduction.—Pulmonary hypertension (PH) during pregnancy, labor, and delivery presents a special challenge for health care providers. The cardiovascular changes that typically accompany pregnancy and childbirth represent an excessive burden for an already marginal cardiovascular system. Eight case studies of pregnancies complicated by PH were reported with emphasis placed on the benefits of a team approach to management of such cases.

Patients.—Five patients had Eisenmenger's syndrome. Primary PH and PH secondary to mitral valve disease had both been diagnosed in 1 patient. Pulmonary hypotension had been diagnosed before pregnancy in 6 patients and before delivery in all 7. The final patient required emergency treatment on the day of delivery and died of cyanosis and severe hypotension after cesarean section; a patent foramen ovale was found on postmortem. All of the infants survived.

Case Management.—The 7 survivors went to a high-risk obstetric unit early in pregnancy. They were hospitalized 4–8 weeks before delivery and received oxygen therapy for several hours daily while sleeping. Heparin (5,000–10,000 IU twice daily) was administered subcutaneously to prevent pulmonary embolism. Patients labored in left lateral recumbency. Instrumental delivery was performed and pushing did not occur. An interdisciplinary team was involved in case management, providing early, frequent consultation and patient contact.

Anesthetic Management.—When labor began, heparin therapy was stopped and protamine was administered to reestablish a normal coagultation profile. Oxygen was administered and oxygen saturation was monitored by ear oximetry. Electrocardiogram, intra-arterial, and central venous pressure were monitored. Bupivacaine (.125% to .375%) epidural anesthesia was administered before contractions became uncomfortable. Anticoagulation therapy resumed, antibiotic therapy began, and oxygen therapy continued post partum.

Conclusion.—This is the first report of 7 successful vaginal births in women with PH from 1 center. The multidisciplinary team approach is considered critical to the successful outcome of such complicated pregnancies. With this type of care, safe vaginal delivery can be conducted in women with PH.

Maternal Primary Pulmonary Hypertension Associated With Pregnancy
Martínez JM, Comas C, Sala X, Gratacós E, Torres PJ, Fortuny A (Hosp Clinic i Provincial de Barcelona)
Eur J Obstet Gynecol Reprod Biol 54:143–147, 1994   101-95-19-43

Background.—Primary pulmonary hypertension (PPH) is a rare clinical observation, but it has a high mortality when it is associated with pregnancy. The outcomes of 3 cases of PPH associated with gestation were reported, and the appropriate management of this association was assessed.

Case 1.—Woman, 33, in her fifth pregnancy with 4 previous uncomplicated gestations, was seen at 38 weeks' gestation with fatigue, increasing dyspnea, nonproductive coughing, and unspecific chest pain. Her blood pressure was 90/50 mm Hg and her pulse rate was 120 beats per minute. A systolic murmur was present at the pulmonic area. Elevated jugular pressure, an enlarged liver, generalized edema, distal cyanosis, and tachypnea were also evident. A chest x-ray showed a moderate cardiac enlargement, with pulmonary artery prominence and reduced vascularity in the distal half of the lung fields. Echocardiograpy showed thickening and dilatation of the right ventricular wall and severe incompetence of the tricuspid valve. Her mean pulmonary artery pressure was 45 mm Hg. A cesarean section was performed, during which her pulmonary arterial pressure continued to increase to 90/50 mm Hg, and her systemic pressure was 80/40 mm Hg. A healthy female infant was delivered; however, 6 hours later, the mother died of severe cardiovascular collapse.

Case 2.—Woman, 18, gravida 1, para 0, at 34 weeks' gestation was admitted with fatigue, increasing dyspnea at rest, chest pain, and syncopal episodes. Her blood pressure was 110/70 mm Hg and her pulse rate was 125 beats per minute. Distal cyanosis, tachypnea, hepatomegaly, high jugular pressure, and edema were all present. A radiographic scan showed slight cardiac enlargement, a prominent pulmonary artery, and tapered peripheral pulmonary arteries. Right axis deviation and right ventricular strain were also evident. A cesarean section was performed, and a healthy male infant was delivered. The mother continued to experience severe dyspnea and cyanosis for 24 hours. Hemodynamic monitoring showed dilatation of the right ventricle, with incompetence of the tricuspid valve and severe pulmonary hypertension. The patient died 48 hours later of irreversible cardiac failure.

Case 3.—Woman, 28, 13 weeks' gestation, had a medical history suggestive of PPH. Despite warnings of the risk of pregnancy, she rejected elective abortion. At 27 weeks' gestation, she experienced an increase in blood pressure to 150/95 mm Hg. Bed rest and hypotensive drugs were administered, bringing about a decrease of blood pressure. Ambroxol was given to induce lung maturity from the 30th week of gestation. Four weeks later, the lecitin-sphingomielin ratio was 3.1. At 35 weeks' gestation, her blood pressure increased to 160/110 mm Hg, her plasma uric acid level was 7.1 mg/dL, and proteinuria was .4 g/L. The patient was taken to the ICU and hemodynamic monitoring was set. Cesarean section was performed, and a healthy female infant was delivered. The mother remained in the ICU without any remarkable hemodynamic change. She was discharged 15 days later and remains healthy 6 months later.

Conclusion.—Primary pulmonary hypertension during pregnancy has a high mortality rate. Patients with this disease should be warned of the risk of pregnancy, and an early interruption must be considered if they become pregnant. If they choose to carry the pregnancy to term, a well-coordinated program of obstetric, cardiac, and anesthesiology care is essential to improve the course and outcome of this association.

▶ To my knowledge, the first of these 2 reports (Abstract 101-95-19–42) represents the largest single series of published cases that describes obstetric and anesthetic management of pregnant women with PH. Four points deserve emphasis. First, 7 of the 8 women labored and delivered vaginally without complication, underscoring that cesarean section should be reserved for obstetric indications. Second, the 7 women who labored all received epidural analgesia with a dilute solution of bupivacaine with fentanyl, emphasizing that carefully administered segmental epidural analgesia can be safely given to parturients with PH. Third, the authors successfully managed these patients without placing a pulmonary artery catheter. I think that use of a pulmonary artery catheter provides little benefit and may cause significant risk to the patient with PH. Fourth, the successful outcome for 7 of these 8 patients illustrates the utility of a multidisciplinary approach to the care of parturients with PH.

The second report (Abstract 101-95-19–43) contrasts with the first. All 3 women underwent cesarean section; 2 of the 3 received general anesthesia, and a pulmonary artery catheter was placed in all 3. Despite careful management, 2 of the 3 women died. It is difficult to compare results between these 2 series. Perhaps the patients in the second series were sicker. In the first series, 2 of the 8 women had PPH, whereas the remaining 6 had secondary PH. In the second series, all 3 women had PPH. Clearly, PH remains a disease that is associated with a high rate of maternal morbidity and mortality.—D.H. Chestnut, M.D.

The Risk of Pulmonary Edema and Colloid Osmotic Pressure Changes During Magnesium Sulfate Infusion
Yeast JD, Halberstadt C, Meyer BA, Cohen GR, Thorp JA (St Luke's Hosp, Kansas City, Mo)
Am J Obstet Gynecol 169:1566–1571, 1993   101-95-19–44

Introduction.—Magnesium sulfate is the primary therapy for the management of preterm labor at many perinatal centers, even though some reports suggest that its use as a tocolytic agent may increase the risk of pulmonary edema. Colloid osmotic pressure was measured in women who had received parenteral magnesium for preterm labor or preeclampsia to determine whether this therapy increases the likelihood of pulmonary edema. A decline in colloid osmotic pressure values may lead to pulmonary edema.

Patients and Methods.—Within a 1-year period, 294 patients—120 with preeclampsia and 174 with preterm labor—received magneisum sulfate. In the first group, the infusion rate was adjusted to maintain serum magnesium levels between 5 and 7 mg/dL. Treatment was continued for at least 24 hours after delivery. In cases of preterm labor, the infusion rate was adjusted to the minimum level needed to inhibit contractions but not to exceed 7 mg/dL. Magnesium levels and colloid osmotic pressure values were determined at 2 hours after the initial bolus and every 6 hours thereafter during therapy.

Results.—Those in the preeclampsia and preterm labor groups did not differ statistically in median age, gestational age, maternal weight, or initial hematocrit. Risk factors for pulmonary edema, including corticosteriod use, multiple gestation, and β-sympathomimetic therapy, were significantly more common in the preterm labor group. Serum magnesium levels were similar for both groups of patients, but colloid osmotic pressure values were consistently higher in the preterm labor group and in the 107 patients who were simultaneously treated with magnesium sulfate and corticosteriods. Pulmonary edema developed in 4 of the 294 patients, all of whom had preeclampsia and low colloid osmotic pressure values; 3 of the 4 had extremely low values.

Conclusion.—Pulmonary edema did not develop in any patient who received magnesium sulfate therapy with normal colloid osmotic pressure values. Measurement of colloid osmotic pressure is an inexpensive method of monitoring patients who are treated with magnesium sulfate. The risk of pulmonary edema can be reduced by vigorous fluid restriction.

▶ In the past, we thought that pulmonary edema was a specific complication of β-adrenergic tocolytic therapy. Subsequently, obstetricians and anesthesiologists have published case reports of pulmonary edema as a complication of other forms of tocolytic therapy, including that using magnesium sulfate. The current thought is that unrecognized infection (e.g., chorioam-

Moving?

I'd like to receive my *Year Book of Anesthesiology & Pain Management* without interruption. Please note the following change of address, effective:

Name: _____

New Address: _____

_____

City: _____ State: _____ Zip: _____

Old Address: _____

_____

City: _____ State: _____ Zip: _____

Reservation Card

Yes, I would like my own copy of *Year Book of Anesthesiology & Pain Management*. Please begin my subscription with the current edition according to the terms described below.* I understand that I will have 30 days to examine each annual edition. If satisfied, I will pay just $72.95 plus sales tax, postage and handling (price subject to change without notice).

Name: _____

Address: _____

City: _____ State: _____ Zip: _____

Method of Payment
O Visa   O Mastercard   O AmEx   O Bill me   O Check (in US dollars, payable to Mosby, Inc.)

Card number: _____ Exp date: _____

Signature: _____

LS-0909

---

*Your *Year Book* Service Guarantee:

When you subscribe to the *Year Book*, we'll send you an advance notice of future volumes about two months before they publish. This automatic notice system is designed to take up as little of your time as possible. If you do not want the *Year Book*, the advance notice makes it quick and easy for you to let us know your decision, and you will always have at least 20 days to decide. If we don't hear from you, we'll send you the new volume as soon as it's available. And, of course, the *Year Book* is yours to examine free of charge for 30 days (postage, handling and applicable sales tax are added to each shipment.).

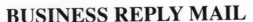

BUSINESS REPLY MAIL

FIRST CLASS MAIL   PERMIT No. 762   CHICAGO, IL

POSTAGE WILL BE PAID BY ADDRESSEE

Chris Hughes
Mosby-Year Book, Inc.
200 N. LaSalle Street
Suite 2600
Chicago, IL 60601-9981

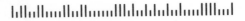

NO POSTAGE
NECESSARY
IF MAILED
IN THE
UNITED STATES

BUSINESS REPLY MAIL

FIRST CLASS MAIL   PERMIT No. 762   CHICAGO, IL

POSTAGE WILL BE PAID BY ADDRESSEE

Chris Hughes
Mosby-Year Book, Inc.
200 N. LaSalle Street
Suite 2600
Chicago, IL 60601-9981

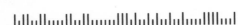

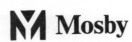 **Mosby**

Dedicated to publishing excellence

nionitis, urinary tract infection) may represent the proximate cause of pulmonary edema in patients who receive tocolytic therapy for treatment of preterm labor. Nontheless, β-adrenergic tocolytic therapy appears to be more likely to result in pulmonary edema than does tocolytic therapy with agents such as magnesium sulfate or indomethacin. This study is consistent with other studies that suggest that magnesium sulfate is associated with less maternal risk than β-adrenergic tocolytic therapy.—D.H. Chestnut, M.D.

Previous Wet Tap Does Not Reduce Success Rate of Labor Epidural Analgesia

Blanche R, Eisenach JC, Tuttle R, Dewan DM (Wake Forest Univ, Winston-Salem, NC)
Anesth Analg 79:291–294, 1994   101-95-19–45

Background.—It is still unclear whether an accidental dural puncture or "wet tap" during attempted epidural catheter insertion for labor analgesia increases the failure rate of epidural analgesia for subsequent deliveries. The records of women with a previous wet tap were reviewed to determine the success rate of epidural anesthesia for subsequent labor.

Methods.—The records of women who experienced a wet tap during attempted labor epidural analgesia were prospectively collected from 1981 to 1993. Three hundred women with wet taps were identified, 47 of whom received epidural anesthesia for a subsequent delivery. Two control groups were also examined. The first included 500 consecutive women who received epidural anesthesia during a 4-month period in 1991. Their charts were reviewed only for the incidence of catheter manipulation for inadequate block and removal for failed block and for the incidence of dural puncture. The second control group comprised women who were matched for the following factors: epidural analgesia for a previous delivery without a wet tap, epidural insertion by an anesthesiologist, and month and year. The records of these matched controls were compared with those of previous patients with a wet tap.

Results.—In comparison to the 500 women who received labor analgesia, women who had experienced a previous wet tap had a decreased incidence of epidural catheter manipulation, a similar incidence of epidural catheter replacement, and an increased incidence of wet tap. Among the 47 women with a previous wet tap, 44 were successfully matched to controls. The women with a previous wet tap did not differ from controls in demographic and epidural anesthetic characteristics or in the incidence of catheter manipulation or replacement, nor did they differ from controls in global assessment by the chart review of the success of epidural analgesia. Eight of the 47 women with a previous wet tap received a third epidural anesthetic for a further delivery, and 3 received a fourth. In 1 of these 11 anesthetics, the catheter was replaced, and all 11 procedures yielded successful analgesia.

Conclusion.—Parturients who have had a previous dural puncture and request epidural analgesia in a subsequent delivery have a 90% chance of good analgesia, but they may have a slightly increased risk of a repeat wet tap.

▶ These authors did not confirm the observations of Ong and associates (1), who noted a high incidence of failed epidural analgesia in patients with a history of unintentional dural puncture. The 2 most important findings of this study are the high likelihood of effective analgesia and the increased risk of an unintentional dural puncture in women with a history of unintentional dural puncture during administration of epidural analgesia.—D.H. Chestnut, M.D.

Reference

1. Ong BY, et al: *Anesth Analg* 70:76, 1990.

The Effects of Epidural Anesthesia on Uterine Vascular Resistance, Plasma Arginine Vasopressin Concentrations, and Plasma Renin Activity During Hemorrhage in Gravid Ewes
Vincent RD Jr, Chestnut DH, McGrath JM, Chatterjee P, Poduska DJ, Atkins BL (Univ of Iowa, Iowa City)
Anesth Analg 78:293–300, 1994   101-95-19-46

Background.—Epidural anesthesia has been found to increase uterine vascular resistance and fetal acidosis during bleeding in gravid ewes. It is not clear, however, whether epidural anesthesia modifies the uterine vascular resistance response during bleeding independent of arterial blood pressure changes. The effects of epidural anesthesia on the mean arterial pressure–uterine vascular resistance relationship and arginine vasopressin levels and plasma renin activity during hemorrhage in gravid ewes were investigated.

Methods.—Twenty-four experiments using 12 chronically instrumented ewes between .8 and .9 of timed gestation were performed. At baseline, .5% bupivacaine or normal saline was administered epidurally. Thirty minutes later, at time H, maternal bleeding of .5 mL/kg^{-1}/min^{-1} was started until a maternal mean arterial pressure of 60% of baseline measurements was obtained. At time H to H+60 minutes, hemorrhage was adjusted to maintain the maternal mean arterial pressure at 60% of baseline.

Findings.—In the epidural group, bupivacaine resulted in a median sensory level of T8 at 30 minutes. Uterine vascular resistance was comparable in both groups at that time, despite a lower mean arterial pressure in the epidural group. Uterine vascular resistance was lower between H and H+60 minutes in the epidural than in the control group. Fetal partial pressure of oxygen (PO_2) was also lower in the former group. However, fetal pH and PO_2 were not significantly different between groups. Compared with the control group, the epidural group did not have significantly lower levels of plasma arginine vasopressin and plasma renin activity during hemorrhage.

Conclusion.—Epidural anesthesia attenuates the increase in uterine vascular resistance during bleeding. However, no significant differences were observed in fetal PO_2 or pH between the control and epidural groups, suggesting that the clinical benefit of epidural anesthesia before hemorrhage is minimal.

▶ During maternal hemorrhage, fetal hypoxemia and acidosis are closely related to the reduction in maternal mean arterial pressure. The etiology of the maternal hypotension (i.e., sympathectomy and hemorrhage vs. hemorrhage alone) is of secondary importance. Vincent et al. noted that "anesthesiologists and obstetricians should take little comfort in the fact that hypotension in a bleeding parturient may be due in part to epidural anesthesia." Epidural anesthesia may attenuate the increase in uterine vascular resistance during hemorrhage. However, this may not be clinically relevant because the magnitude of maternal hemorrhage will probably not be diminished in obstetric patients who experience hemorrhage during epidural anesthesia.—D.H. Chestnut, M.D.

Ephedrine Remains the Vasopressor of Choice for Treatment of Hypotension During Ritodrine Infusion and Epidural Anesthesia

McGrath JM, Chestnut DH, Vincent RD, DeBruyn CS, Atkins BL, Poduska DJ, Chatterjee P (Univ of Iowa, Iowa City)
Anesthesiology 80:1073–1081, 1994   101-95-19–47

Introduction.—Most hypotensive obstetric patients who require a vasopressor have received ephedrine, but the best vasopressor to use in parturients who are given a β-adrenergic drug for tocolysis is uncertain. Ephedrine and phenylephrine were compared in chronically instrumented gravid ewes that had completed 80% to 90% of their gestations.

Methods.—The effects of ephedrine and phenylephrine on uterine blood flow and fetal oxygen were examined during ritodrine infusion and in the hypotensive state induced by epidural anesthesia. Ritodrine initially was infused intravenously, and, after 2 hours, the animals received 2% lidocaine epidurally to produce a sensory level of T6 or greater. An IV bolus of ephedrine, phenylephrine, or normal saline was given 15 minutes later, followed by a 30-minute infusion. The infusion rate was adjusted to maintain a stable maternal mean arterial blood pressure.

Results.—Infusion of ritodrine significantly increased the maternal heart rate and cardiac output and significantly reduced maternal systemic vascular resistance in all groups (Fig 19-8). Epidural anesthesia signifi-

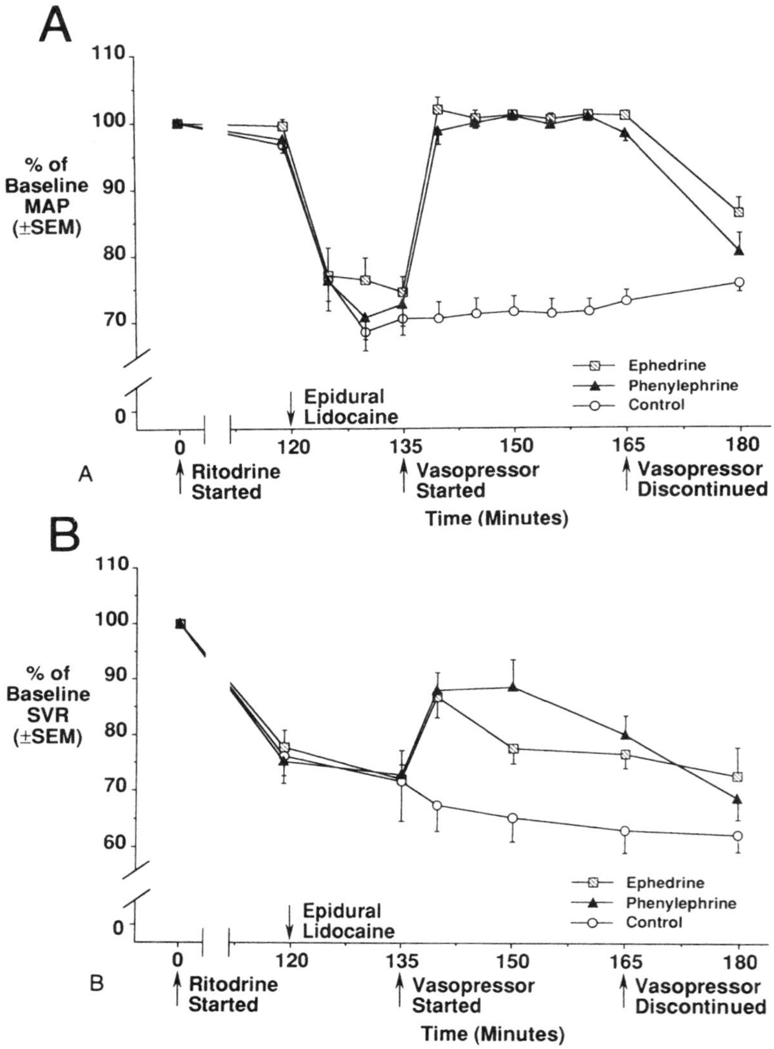

Fig 19–8.—A, maternal mean arterial pressure (MAP) over time for the ephedrine, phenylephrine, and normal saline (NS)–control groups. **B,** maternal systemic vascular resistance (SVR) over time for the ephedrine, phenylephrine, and NS–control groups. Each response is expressed as mean (± standard error of the mean [SEM]) percentage of baseline. *Standard error bars,* if not shown, are included within the height of the symbols for each data point. Both ephedrine and phenylephrine significantly increased maternal MAP when compared with NS-control. Both ephedrine and phenylephrine significantly increased maternal SVR when compared with NS-control. (Courtesy of McGrath JM, Chestnut DH, Vincent RD, et al: *Anesthesiology* 80:1073–1081, 1994.)

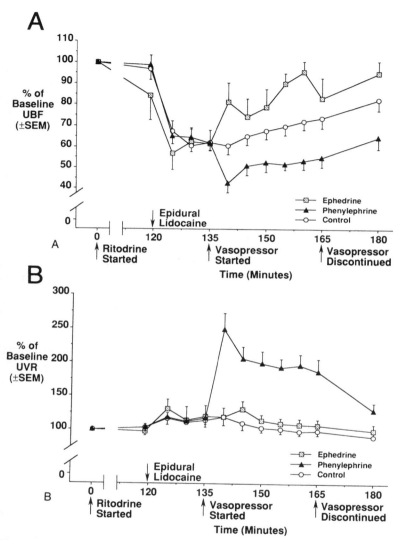

Fig 19–9.—A, uterine blood flow (*UBF*) over time for the ephedrine, phenylephrine, and normal saline (NS)–control groups. **B,** uterine vascular resistance (*UVR*) over time for the ephedrine, phenylephrine, and NS–control groups. Each response is expressed as mean (± standard error of the mean [SEM]) percentage of baseline. *Standard error bars,* if not shown, are included within the height of the symbols for each data point. Ephedrine significantly increased UBF when compared with NS–control, but phenylephrine did not. In addition, ephedrine significantly increased UBF when compared with phenylephrine. Phenylephrine increased UVR when compared with NS–control, but ephedrine did not. (Courtesy of McGrath JM, Chestnut DH, Vincent RD, et al: *Anesthesiology* 80:1073–1081, 1994.)

cantly reduced the maternal arterial pressure, uterine blood flow (UBF), and fetal partial pressure of oxygen in arterial blood (PaO_2) in all groups (Fig 19-9). Both ephedrine and phenylephrine returned the maternal mean arterial pressure to baseline without significantly altering the heart rate. Neither drug increased the maternal cardiac output significantly. Only ephedrine increased UBF significantly, and only phenylephrine increased uterine vascular resistance. Neither drug significantly altered the fetal pH or the partial pressure of arterial carbon dioxide; however, ephedrine was associated with a significantly higher fetal PaO_2.

Conclusion.—Ephedrine protects UBF during ritodrine infusion better than phenylephrine in hypotensive gravid ewes and promotes fetal oxygenation. Therefore, it may be the preferred vasopressor for hypotensive women who are receiving a β-adrenergic drug for tocolysis.

▶ There are at least 2 circumstances when anesthesiologists encounter patients who have recently received a β-adrenergic agent for tocolysis (i.e., the pharmacologic inhibition of uterine muscle contractions). First, the treatment of preterm labor is often unsuccessful, and patients who have received β-adrenergic tocolytic therapy often require administration of analgesia or anesthesia on an emergency basis. Second, obstetricians often given a β-adrenergic agonist to facilitate resuscitation of a distressed fetus in utero. The β-adrenergic agonists do not directly increase uteroplacental blood flow; rather, they improve uteroplacental perfusion by relaxing the uterus.

In this study, although ephedrine and phenylephrine provided similar restoration of the maternal mean arterial pressure, ephedrine was superior to phenylephrine in protecting uterine blood flow during ritodrine infusion and epidural anesthesia–induced hypotension in pregnant sheep. The study suggests that ephedrine remains the vasopressor of choice for the treatment of maternal hypotension in women who have recently received β-adrenergic tocolytic therapy.—D.H. Chestnut, M.D.

Sleeping Positions Adopted by Pregnant Women of More than 30 Weeks Gestation
Mills GH, Chaffe AG (Royal Hallamshire Hosp, Sheffield, England; Doncaster Royal Infirmary, England)
Anaesthesia 49:249–250, 1994   101-95-19–48

Background.—Late pregnancy brings the risk of compression of the aorta and inferior vena cava by the uterus and the subsequent reduction of venous return and cardiac output. The risk is heightened if the woman adopts a supine sleeping position. The sleeping position adopted by women of more than 30 weeks' gestation was investigated.

Methods.—The sleeping position of 52 pregnant women who were admitted to an antenatal unit was studied. An age-matched control population of 31 preoperative gynecologic patients sleeping in similar beds was observed in the same way. Sleeping positions were recorded as left tilt, right tilt, supine, or prone. In the pregnant group, the degree of any tilt was also noted. The statistical significance of the differences in sleeping positions between the 2 groups was analyzed with a chi-squared test.

Results.—Most of the pregnant women (76.9%) adopted a left-tilt position while sleeping. A smaller number adopted a right-tilt position (21.2%), whereas only 1.9% were supine. Among the nonpregnant controls, there was a more even distribution of supine, left-, and right-tilt sleepers (38.7%, 25.8%, and 32.3%, respectively), as well as a small number of women who slept in the prone position.

Conclusion.—These results show a significant difference in the sleeping positions adopted by pregnant and nonpregnant women. It appears that women with a pregnancy of more than 30 weeks' gestation adopt sleeping positions that are unlikely to produce aortocaval compression. However, some of these women were found to sleep in the supine position, and it would be useful to advise them to place a pillow under the right buttock to reduce the risk of caval compression.

▶ These results are not surprising; most pregnant women adopt a sleeping position that maximizes venous return, cardiac output, and cerebral and uteroplacental perfusion. Most anesthesia care providers recognize the importance of left uterine displacement during administration of regional anesthesia in pregnant women. I am concerned that some anesthesia care providers fail to ensure adequate left uterine displacement during administration of *general* anesthesia for cesarean section and other surgical procedures in pregnant women. It is important to avoid compression in pregnant women who undergo surgery, beginning at approximately 20 weeks' gestation.—D.H. Chestnut, M.D.

Factors Associated With Back Pain After Childbirth

Breen TW, Ransil BJ, Groves PA, Oriol NE (Charles A Dana Research Inst, Boston; Beth Israel Hosp, Boston; Harvard Med School, Boston)
Anesthesiology 81:29–34, 1994   101-95-19–49

Background.—Back pain after childbirth has been reported in 30% to 45% of women who receive epidural anesthesia. The incidence of such pain 1–2 months post partum was determined, and the relationship between postpartum back pain and epidural anesthesia was explored.

Methods.—Twelve to 48 hours post partum, 1,185 women who delivered a viable single infant were interviewed to document their history of back pain before or during the recent pregnancy, or both. The details of their delivery experience were also recorded. Two months later, these women were sent a follow-up questionnaire regarding the occurrence of back pain since giving birth. The response rate was 88%.

Findings.—The incidence of postpartum back pain in women who received epidural anesthesia and those who did not was 44% and 45%, respectively. In a multiple logistic regression model, postpartum back pain was associated with a history of back pain, younger age, and greater weight. New-onset postpartum back pain was associated with greater weight and shorter height. Postpartum back pain was unrelated to epidural anesthesia, number of attempts at epidural placement, duration of the second stage of labor, delivery mode, and birth weight.

Conclusion.—One to 2 months after delivery, the overall incidence of back pain was 44% in this population. Although predisposing factors were identified, epidural anesthesia did not appear to be associated with back pain 1–2 months post partum.

▶ In this, one of the most important obstetric anesthesia studies published during the past year, epidural analgesia during labor and delivery was found not to be a predisposing factor for postpartum back pain. Earlier studies of this subject were retrospective and subject to selective recall and selection bias. This study, although nonrandomized, was prospective. The authors observered that postpartum back pain occurs in 44% of the obstetric population and that it occurs with equal frequency in women who did and did not receive epidural analgesia during labor.—D.H. Chestnut, M.D.

Obstetric Hemorrhage and Blood Utilization
Sherman SJ, Greenspoon JS, Nelson JM, Paul RH (Univ of Southern California, Los Angeles)
J Reprod Med 38:929–934, 1993   101-95-19-50

Background.—A major cause of maternal death in the United States is obstetric bleeding. Such hemorrhage may occur unexpectedly, and it often requires homologous blood tranfusion. The frequency and type of obstetric conditions and interventions associated with blood product transfusion on a busy obstetric service were investigated.

Methods and Findings.—Data were obtained on 5,528 deliveries that occurred in the first 4 months of 1990. Fifty-five patients (1%) required blood transfusion during their pregnancy and puerperium. The conditions most often associated with transfusion were trauma from instrumental delivery in 16 patients, uterine atony in 15, placenta previa in 12, retained products of conception in 4, abruptio placentae in 4, and coagulopathy resulting from the hemolysis, elevated liver enzymes, and low platelet count syndrome in 1. Seven patients received platelets; 6, fresh frozen plasma; 1, whole blood; and 1, cryoprecipitate. The transfusion rates were 100% among those who had an emergency cesarean hysterectomy for bleeding placenta previa or atony, 6.1% among those who had a vacuum extraction, 4.2% among those who had a forceps delivery, 1.4% among those with an uncomplicated cesarean delivery, and .4% among those with spontaneous vaginal births. Bleeding and the subsequent need for blood transfusion were not necessarily caused by the procedure, except in patients with trauma from instrumental vaginal delivery. Women who had a vaginal instrumental delivery had a significantly greater rate of transfusion than women who had a cesarean delivery.

Conclusion.—Physicians should consider the risk of blood transfusion when determining the safest route of delivery in obstetric patients. The ability to predict which patients will need blood transfusions on the basis of antepartum factors is limited. For certain patients, such as those with placenta previa, autologous donation should be considered.

▶ The authors concluded that "the risk of blood transfusion should be one factor considered when determining the safest route of delivery." With the exception of patients with placental pathology (e.g., placenta previa, placenta abruption), it is hard for me to understand how an obstretrician would apply this recommendation to clinical practice. Cesarean section entails risks other than blood loss. Should an experienced obstetrician choose a cesarean section rather than a forceps delivery because of a possibly increased risk of blood loss associated with a forceps delivery? In this study, the operative vaginal deliveries were performed by obstetric residents who had varying levels of experience. On the other hand, I agree with the authors' recommendation that obstetricians should consider autologous blood donation in patients with a diagnosis of placenta previa.—D.H. Chestnut, M.D.

Epidural Analgesia and Uterine Rupture During Labour

Rowbottom SJ, Tabrizian I (Chinese Univ of Hong Kong)
Anaesth Intensive Care 22:79–80, 1994   101-95-19–51

Background.—Uterine rupture during labor rarely occurs in primigravid women. A nulliparous patient was described in whom an incomplete uterine rupture with intraperitoneal hemorrhage occurred during labor.

Case Report.—Woman, 33, was seen at 39 weeks' gestation in early labor. Her cervical dilation was 2 cm, and her contractions were irregular. The membranes were ruptured artificially. Uterine contractions were augmented by synthetic oxytocin (Syntocinon) infusion, which was initially given at 8 mU/hour. The patient asked for epidural analgesia. An IV Ringer's lactate solution preload of 500 mL was followed by a continuous IV infusion of 500 mL over 8 hours. Analgesia through an epidural catheter at the L3–L4 interspace was provided with 10 mL of .2% bupivacaine containing meperidine, 20 mg, and an infusion of .125% bupivacaine with meperidine, .1%, at 10 mL/hr. After 3.5 hours, the cervix had dilated to 6 cm, and the patient was given an epidural top-up of 10 mL of .2% bupivacaine with meperidine, 20 mg, to alleviate breakthrough pain. Contractions were still irregular, and 3 hours later, another epidural top-up for breakthrough pain was delivered. The patient reported pain again 1.5 hours later, and a top-up of 10 mL of .2% bupivacaine with meperidine, 20 mg, was administered. The patient described her pain as a continuous tight feeling in the lower abdomen that was different from labor pain; a cesarean delivery was planned. The patient requested a general anesthetic for the procedure. At surgery, 500 mL of fresh blood was discovered in the peritoneal cavity. Active bleeding was noted from a 3–4-cm incomplete tear in the posterior uterine wall above the uterosacral ligament. The infant was born with 1- and 5-minute Apgar scores of 9 and 10, respectively, and the uterine tear was repaired. The patient lost another 1.5 L of blood. The mother and infant had an uneventful postoperative course.

Conclusion.—Continuous epidural analgesia with low concentrations of epidural bupivacaine and meperidine does not mask abnormal pain associated with intraperitoneal bleeding during labor. However, medical personnel must be aware of the significance of a change in the nature of a patient's pain before administering additional epidural analgesia. Alternative diagnoses of abdominal pain during labor should be considered.

▶ The most important observation in this case report was that epidural analgesia did not mask the pathologic pain associated with intraperitoneal hemorrhage secondary to uterine rupture during labor. The presence of "breakthrough pain" should prompt anesthesiologists and obstetricians to consider alternative causes of abdominal pain during labor (e.g., placental abruption, uterine rupture).—D.H. Chestnut, M.D.

The Incidence of Herpes Simplex Virus Labialis After Cesarean Delivery
Norris MC, Weiss J, Carney M, Leighton BL (Thomas Jefferson Univ, Philadelphia)
Int J Obstet Anesth 3:127–131, 1994   101-95-19–52

Background.—Three recent studies have reported an increased incidence of recurrent oral herpes simplex viral lesions in patients who received epidural morphine for analgesia after cesarean section. Some anesthesiologists have subsequently avoided the use of neuraxial morphine in parturients with a history of herpes simplex virus labialis. The risk of oral herpes lesions was investigated in a large group of parturients after cesarean delivery.

Method.—Of 357 consecutive parturients who underwent cesarean delivery, 201 women received either spinal or epidural morphine, and the remaining 156 parturients received only systemic opioids for postoperative analgesia. All the women were all seen daily by an investigator until discharge.

Results.—Eleven patients had cold sores during their hospital stay. Eight of the 11 reported a history of facial lesions, but 3 denied having had previous cold sores. None of the women had severe lesions. The women who received neuraxial morphine had a 3.5% incidence of oral lesions compared with 2.6% among those who did not. Among the women who did not receive neuraxial morphine, only those with a history of cold sores had them after cesarean delivery.

Conclusion.—The use of epidural or intrathecal morphine did not significantly increase the incidence of cold sores. Among women who received neuraxial morphine, only 3.5% had cold sores compared with 2.6% of those who did not receive neuraxial morphine. Although this study does not prove that neuraxial opioids have no influence on the risk of recurrent oral herpes lesions, it indicates that, in this patient population, neuraxial opioids were not associated with a significant increase in the risk of facial cold sores.

▶ Neither epidural nor intrathecal morphine administration resulted in an increased incidence of herpes simplex virus labialis in these women after cesarean delivery. These results are in contrast with at least 3 earlier studies that noted an increased incidence of recurrent oral herpes simplex viral lesions in patients who had received epidural morphine for postcesarean analgesia. Thus, this study suggests that the increased risk of recurrent herpes simplex virus labialis in patients who received intraspinal morphine may be population-specific. This study should encourage other anesthesiologists to evaluate the incidence of this complication in their patient populations.—D.H. Chestnut, M.D.

Intravenous Nitroglycerin for Intrapartum External Version of the Second Twin

Abouleish AE, Corn SB (Harvard Med School, Boston)
Anesth Analg 78:808–809, 1994   101-95-19–53

Background.—Intrapartum external version is possible only when the uterus is not contracting. β-Agonists, such as ritodrine or terbutaline, have been used for external version of the singleton fetus or second twin; these agents are given by infusion over 15 minutes or more to reduce the risk of side effects. The use of IV nitroglycerin to achieve uterine relaxation for intrapartum external version of a second twin was described in a case report.

Case Report.—Woman, 34, with vertex-transverse diamniotic-dichorionic twins, was admitted at term in active labor with complete cervical dilatation. Lactated Ringer's solution, 1 L, was infused before epidural needle placement and again before delivery of the first twin. The patient was given epidural analgesia with 9 mL of 1.5% alkalinized lidocaine, which was reinforced at 50 and 100 minutes with 4 mL of 2% lidocaine. At the time of the first reinforcement, 50 μg of fentanyl was given as well. About 30 minutes after the start of epidural analgesia, the first twin was delivered in a healthy condition. After the transverse position of the second twin was confirmed by ultrasound, 50 μg of IV nitroglycerin was given to relax the uterus. External version was successfully performed, with no significant changes in the patient's blood pressure and heart rate and no headache or dizziness. The second twin, who was also healthy, was delivered 45 minutes later. Blood loss was normal for the vaginal delivery of twins.

Discussion.—The use of IV nitroglycerin to achieve uterine relaxation for intrapartum external version was reported. The advantages of nitroglycerin include its rapid onset, short half-life, and lack of undersirable maternal or fetal effects.

▶ A skilled obstetrician can often successfully perform either internal or external version of the second twin without pharmacologic uterine relaxation, provided it is performed immediately after delivery of the first twin. This case does not prove that nitroglycerin is either effective or necessary to accomplish intrapartum external version of the second twin. However, after an initial period of personal skepticism, I now acknowledge that the weight of anecdotal evidence supports the efficacy of nitroglycerin as a uterine relaxant. Both anesthesiologists and obstetricians should understand that the uterine-relaxing effect of nitroglycerin is very transient. This is both good news and bad news. The good news is that small bolus doses of nitroglycerin are unlikely to result in postpartum uterine atony. The bad news is that the obstetrician must be quick or the anesthesiologist must give repeated doses of 50–100 µg of nitroglycerin during difficult procedures.—D.H. Chestnut, M.D.

The Effect of Epidural Anesthesia on Safety and Success of External Cephalic Version at Term
Carlan SJ, Dent JM, Huckaby T, Whittington EC, Shaefer D (Arnold Palmer Hosp for Children and Women, Orlando, Fla; Orlando Regional Healthcare System, Fla)
Anesth Analg 79:525–528, 1994   101-95-19-54

Background.—Performing external cephalic version (ECV) late in pregnancy may decrease the incidence of intrapartum breech presentation and cesarean delivery. To limit the use of excessive force, which has been associated with severe pain and injury during this procedure, analgesia is usually not given. The effect of epidural anesthesia on the success and safety of ECV at term was investigated.

Methods.—The records of all pregnant women who were at greater than 36 weeks of gestation and giving birth at 1 center between April 1992 and April 1993 were reviewed retrospectively. The standard contraindications to ECV were observed. The use of tocolytics and lumbar epidural anesthesia was based on physician preference.

Findings.—Sixty-nine ECVs were attempted in 61 patients. Thirty-seven attempts were made without epidural anesthesia and 32 were made with it. Ten percent of those without epidural anesthesia and 34% with it were either in labor or had a cervical dilatation of greater than 3 cm when the attempt was made. Other major patient variables that were likely to affect ECV success did not differ between the groups. The success rates for the epidural and nonepidural groups were 59% and 24%, respectively. The groups had similar incidences of abruptio placenta, fetal bradycardia, low Apgar scores, and low umbilical artery pH.

Conclusion.—Epidural anesthesia may increase the success rate of ECV and reduce the cesarean delivery rate without increasing morbidity or mortality among mothers or neonates. Another advantage of regional anesthesia is that it can be extended rapidly if intervention is needed.

▶ External cephalic version does hurts. I agree with the authors' observation "that many attempts at ECV are terminated at the patient's request because of pain." Undoubtedly, the use of epidural analgesia makes the procedure more tolerable for the mother. On the other hand, some obstetricians worry that the use of epidural analgesia will encourage the use of excessive force and increase the risk of a placental abruption or cord accident. Clearly, ECV should be performed with ultrasonography guidance, which includes continuous monitoring of fetal heart rate activity, and should be followed by approximately 1 hour of continuous electronic fetal heart rate monitoring after completion of the procedure.—D.H. Chestnut, M.D.

Amnioinfusion During Labor Complicated by Particulate Meconium-Stained Amniotic Fluid Decreases Neonatal Morbidity

Cialone PR, Sherer DM, Ryan RM, Sinkin RA, Abramowicz JS (Univ of Rochester, NY)

Am J Obstet Gynecol 170:842–849, 1994   101-95-19–55

Introduction.—Studies suggest that meconium passage occurs in utero in 8% to 17% of deliveries. Of these deliveries, 54% are complicated by light meconium and 46% by moderate or thick meconium. Transcervical amnioinfusion has shown promising results in the management of labor that is complicated by meconium-stained amniotic fluid. The safety and efficacy of prophylactic amnioinfusion in decreasing neonatal morbidity associated with particulate meconium-stained amniotic fluid were evaluated in a randomized, controlled study.

Methods.—The study sample comprised 105 women in labor with particulate (moderate or thick) meconium staining. The presence of meconium was assessed by subjective clinical analysis and represented the patients' only obstetric risk factor; patients with any other antepartum complications were excluded. Forty-seven patients who were assigned to the study group received transcervical amnioinfusion with warmed normal saline solution, which was administered through an intrauterine pressure catheter at a rate of 600 mL for the first hour, followed by continuous infusion of 150 mL/hr thereafter until the cervix was fully dilated. The other 58 patients served as controls. Neonatal outcomes and other variables were compared in the 2 groups.

Results.—All patients in the study group had decreased meconium concentrations between rupture of membranes and delivery compared with 26% of the control group. By objective analysis, the relative dilution of meconium consistency decreased 77% in the study group, whereas it increased by 9% in the control group. Only 4% of infants in the study group had meconium below the vocal cords compared with 62% in the control group. The study group also had a higher umbilical artery pH (7.29 compared with 7.25) and a reduced rate of neonatal acidemia (9% compared with 24%). The meconium aspiration syndrome developed in only 1 patient in the study group and in 14% of patients in the control group. However, maternal and neonatal morbidity rates did not significantly differ.

Conclusion.—For patients with particulate meconium-stained amniotic fluid, prophylactic amnioinfusion may be a useful addition to intrapartum management. This treatment decreases the incidence of meconium below the vocal cords, lessens the incidence of neonatal acidemia, increases unbilical artery cord pH, relieves repetitive moderate- or severe-variable decelerations during labor, and reduces the incidence of fetal distress. Further study is needed to determine whether it significantly reduces the rate of the meconium aspiration syndrome.

▶ I am a strong advocate of saline amnioinfusion in patients with severe-variable decelerations secondary to cord compression. I am convinced that this technique spared my wife an emegency cesarean section before the delivery of our fourth child. This study supports the growing body of literature that suggests that prophylactic amnioinfusion decreases neonatal morbidity associated with labor that is complicated by thick meconium-stained amniotic fluid. Intuitively, it seems logical that prophylactic amnioinfusion might result in a reduction of the incidence of meconium aspiration syndrome, although the authors correctly acknolwedged that this potential benefit remains unproven.—D.H. Chestnut, M.D.

Vulvar Application of Lidocaine for Pain Relief in Spontaneous Vaginal Delivery

Collins MK, Porter KB, Brook E, Johnson L, Williams M, Jevitt CM (Univ of South Florida, Tampa; Tampa Gen Hosp, Fla)
Obstet Gynecol 84:335–337, 1994   101-95-19–56

Introduction.—Much of the pain that is experienced in the second stage of labor arises from the lower genital tract by way of pudendal nerve branches. The methods commonly used to control pain in the first stage of labor or to facilitate assisted vaginal delivery are not often used to lessen pain associated with the actual delivery of the infant. Topical analgesia is a potential means of avoiding inadvertent IV injection and the adverse maternal outcomes that are sometimes associated with injected anesthesia.

Study Plan.—Peripartum analgesia with topical 2% lidocaine was evaluated in 203 women who had uncomplicated vaginal deliveries. In a double-blind design, either lidocaine jelly or a placebo formulation of chlorhexidine gluconate was massaged into the perineum, labia minora, and the base of the clitoris, and the treatment was repeated if it was considered necessary. Application began at the start of the second stage of labor in multiparas and in primagravidas when delivery was expected within 15–20 minutes. Perineal pain was rated 30 minutes after delivery using a 4-point analogue scale.

Results.—When topical lidocaine was used, patients had less pain than placebo recipients and were less likely to have moderate or severe perineal pain. Moderate-to-severe pain was more frequent in women of lesser parity and when a vaginal laceration was present.

Conclusion.—Topical application of a 2% lidocaine gel effectively lessens perineal pain in the immediate postpartum period.

▶ In this study, 52% of the women who received topical lidocaine experienced either moderate or severe pain, compared with 67% of the patients who received placebo. These underwhelming results hardly represent a compelling argument to use topical lidocaine to provide intrapartum analgesia.—D.H. Chestnut, M.D.

20 Pediatric Anesthesia

The Pharmacology of Sevoflurane in Infants and Children
Lerman J, Sikich N, Kleinman S, Yentis S (Univ of Toronto)
Anesthesiology 80:814–824, 1994

101-95-20–1

Introduction.—Previous studies have shown that the minimum alveolar concentration (MAC) for halothane, isoflurane, and desflurane increases as age decreases. However, the MAC for sevoflurane has not been determined for pediatric patients except for those who are 3–5 years of age. The MAC of sevoflurane was examined in neonates, infants, and children younger than 12 years of age.

Methods.—Ninety neonates, infants, and children with American Society of Anesthesiologists physical status I or II who were scheduled for surgery of no longer than 1 hour's duration were studied. The patients were age-stratified: full-term neonates 30 days of age or younger; infants older than 1 month of age but younger than 6 months; infants older than 6 months of age but younger than 1 year; children older than 1 year of age but younger than 3 years; children older than 3 years of age but younger than 5 years; and children older than 5 years of age but younger than 12 years. The MAC of sevoflurane in oxygen was determined for each age group. The MAC of sevoflurane in nitrous oxide was deter-

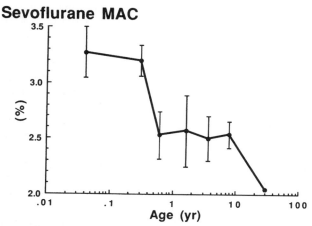

Sevoflurane MAC

Fig 20–1.—Mean (± standard deviation) end-tidal concentration of sevoflurane in oxygen for each of 6 age groups from neonates to children as old as age 12 years. (Courtesy of Lerman J, Sikich N, Kleinman S, et al: *Anesthesiology* 80:814–824, 1994.)

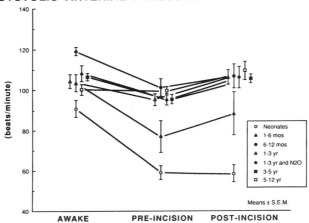

SYSTOLIC ARTERIAL PRESSURE

Fig 20–2.—Systolic arterial pressure (mean ± standard error of mean) for each of the 6 age groups while awake and at approximately 1 minimum alveolar concentration (MAC) of sevoflurane before and after a skin incision. The systolic pressure decreased significantly at approximately 1 MAC, compared with the awake values in all infants and children except children aged 1–3 years with nitrous oxide and children aged 5–12 years ($P < 1.05$). Systolic pressure returned toward awake values after the skin incision but remained significantly less than awake values in the neonate and the groups aged 6–12 months. (Courtesy of Lerman J, Sikich N, Kleinman S, et al: *Anesthesiology* 80:814–824, 1994.)

mined in a separate group of children aged 1–3 years. Dixon's up-and-down technique was used to determine the MAC. Hemostatic parameters were monitored. The renal-concentrating capability was assessed by measuring plasma concentrations of inorganic fluoride.

Results.—Neonates and infants aged 1–6 months required the highest mean MAC of sevoflurane in oxygen, which was reduced by about 25% in children older than 6 months of age but younger than 12 years (Fig 20–1). The MAC of sevoflurane in 60% nitrous oxide required by children older than 1 year of age but younger than 3 years was approximately 24% lower than the MAC of sevoflurane in oxygen for the same age group. The induction of anesthesia with sevoflurane could be accomplished without complications in all age groups. All infants and children younger than 5 years of age experienced a decreased systolic arterial pressure at 1 MAC before skin incision; the decrease was most pronounced in neonates. The systolic pressure recovered after the skin incision, but it remained lower than awake values in neonates and infants 6–12 months of age (Fig 20–2). The heart rate was unaffected before skin incision at 1 MAC in infants and children younger than 3 years of age, but it increased before skin incision in children older than 3 years of age. The patients experienced rapid emergence from anesthesia without airway reflex responses. Plasma concentrations of inorganic fluoride were highest 30 minutes after sevoflurane was discontinued, and they returned to baseline by 3.5 hours after surgery.

Discussion.—The MAC of sevoflurane was 3.3% for neonates, 3.2% for infants 1–6 months of age, and 2.5% for infants 6 months of age up to children 12 years of age. The smooth and uncomplicated induction and emergence from anesthesia recommend sevoflurane as an appropriate induction agent for pediatric patients as does the circulatory and renal stability exhibited by this study population.

▶ This well-done study again points out the very real possibility that sevoflurane may completely replace halothane, at least in the United States, because halothane's residual usage is almost entirely in this age group. This article also points out that, at least in infants and children, the MAC of sevoflurane may be somewhat higher than previously thought.—J.H. Tinker, M.D.

End-Tidal Sevoflurane Concentration for Tracheal Intubation and Minimum Alveolar Concentration in Pediatric Patients
Inomata S, Watanabe S, Taguchi M, Okada M (Mito Saiseikai Gen Hosp, Mito City, Ibaraki, Japan)
Anesthesiology 80:93–96, 1994   101-95-20–2

Introduction.—Inhalation agents alone are often used for induction of anesthesia and tracheal intubation in pediatric patients. A new inhalation

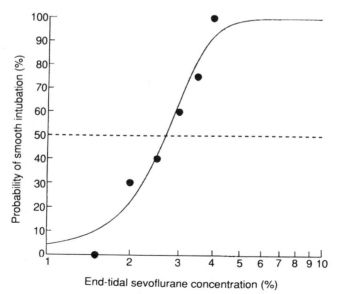

Fig 20–3.—Dose-response curve for sevoflurane plotted from logit analyses of individual end-tidal concentrations and the respective reactions to tracheal intubation. The sigmoid curve revealed that the minimum alveolar concentration is 2.69%. (Courtesy of Inomata S, Watanabe S, Taguchi M, et al: *Anesthesiology* 80:93–96, 1994.)

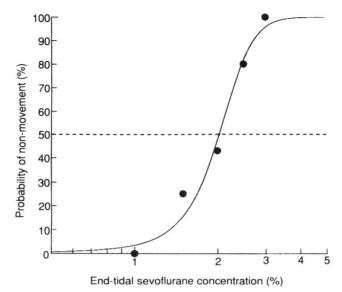

Fig 20–4.—Dose-response curve for sevoflurane plotted from logit analyses of individual end-tidal sevoflurane concentrations and their respective reactions to the skin incision. The maximum likelihood solution for minimum alveolar concentration (MAC) is presented by sigmoid curve; the MAC is 2.03% (95% fiducial limits: 1.51% and 2.53%). (Courtesy of Inomata S, Watanabe S, Taguchi M, et al: *Anesthesiology* 80:93–96, 1994.)

agent, sevoflurane, has a lower blood-gas partition coefficient, which may make it a more efficient induction agent. Pediatric patients were studied to determine the minimum alveolar concentration (MAC) of sevoflurane required for tracheal intubation and skin incision.

Methods.—A group of 36 pediatric patients, aged 1–9 years, with American Society of Anethesiologists physical status I who were undergoing elective surgery that required a skin incision were studied. Breath measurements of anesthetic and end-tidal carbon dioxide concentrations were continually monitored. Alveolar concentrations of sevoflurane were moved up and down by .5%, and the concentration at which tracheal intubation was attempted or accomplished smoothly without neuromuscular relaxants or other adjuvants was recorded. The process was repeated to record responses to skin incision. An absence of gross purposeful movements indicated adequate alveolar concentrations.

Results.—The logit analysis of patient responses indicated that the MAC of sevoflurane required for tracheal intubation was 2.69% (Fig 20–3). The skin incision required a MAC of sevoflurane of 2.03% (Fig 20–4).

Discussion.—The finding that the MAC of sevoflurane required for a tracheal intubation is about 30% higher than that required for a skin incision is consistent with the data for enflurane and halothane in pediatric patients. Sevoflurane seems to be an appropriate induction agent for the pediatric population, because it enables tracheal intubation without the use of muscle relaxants.

▶ On the surface, this article points out that the concentrations needed to do routine anesthesia maneuvers using sevoflurane will be somewhat higher than those required for isoflurane. I included this article because sevoflurane will be used for pediatric patients. It may indeed replace halothane for mask inductions in pediatric patients because its blood-gas solubility coefficient of .6 is so much lower than that of halothane, which is 2.24. Sevoflurane doesn't seem to be more pungent than halothane, so it could cause halothane to become almost an orphan drug, at least in the United States. I don't see anything wrong with that, because I am not one of those senior anesthesiologists who hangs onto old techniques and old drugs when it is obvious that there are better ways.—J.H. Tinker, M.D.

Recovery Characteristics of Desflurane Versus Halothane for Maintenance of Anesthesia in Pediatric Ambulatory Patients
Davis PJ, Cohen IT, McGowan FX Jr, Latta K (Univ of Pittsburgh, Pa; Children's Hosp, Pittsburgh, Pa)
Anesthesiology 80:298–302, 1994   101-95-20–3

Introduction.—Desflurane is a potent inhalational anesthetic that has low solubility in blood gases, which allows the rapid induction of and emergence from anesthesia. However, its pungency limits its acceptability for use as an induction agent in children. The practice of inducing anesthesia with halothane and nitrous oxide and subsequently giving desflurane by mask was evaluated in 45 children who had inguinal hernia repair, orchiopexy, or circumcision on an outpatient basis.

Methods.—In all patients, anesthesia was induced by halothane and nitrous oxide in oxygen. A caudal block was done with bupivacaine, after which 22 patients were switched to desflurane in a 60:40 mixture of nitrous oxide and oxygen. The remaining 23 patients continued to receive halothane in nitrous oxide/oxygen. Patient and surgical characteristics were similar in the 2 groups.

Results.—Anesthesia lasted longer in the desflurane group, and the time to first response and the time in the recovery room were both shorter than in patients who were given only halothane. Patients who were given desflurane anesthesia were somewhat more likely to be delirious at the time of emergence from anesthesia. There were no significant differences in the frequency of airway complications, nausea or vomiting, or the need for fentanyl in the recovery room. The time to discharge from the hospital was also similar in the 2 groups.

Conclusion.—Desflurane may be used in pediatric patients having day surgery if it is used for maintenance after anesthesia with halothane is induced.

▶ The pungency of desflurane causes upper-airway irritation and a high incidence of laryngospasm, cough, and hypoxemia when it is induced in children. These clinical investigators used a halothane induction and then switched to desflurane for maintenance of anesthesia. It is salutatory to note the rapid recovery that is associated with desflurane, even when anesthesia has been induced by halothane. Sevoflurane, another potent new inhaled anesthetic that is currently undergoing investigation in the United States, has a nonirritating and more pleasant odor, and therefore it may be well tolerated by children for inhalational induction (1). Its speed of induction is also likely to be rapid.—M. Wood, M.D.

Reference

1. Sury MRJ, Hatch DJ: *Anaesth Pharmacol Rev* 2:68, 1994.

Minimum Alveolar Concentration of Isoflurane for Tracheal Extubation in Deeply Anesthetized Children

Neelakanta G, Miller J (Univ of California, Los Angeles)
Anesthesiology 80:811–813, 1994   101-95-20–4

Objective.—There has been no documentation of precisely what end-tidal concentrations of inhalational anesthetics are required to prevent patients from coughing and moving during or immediately after tracheal extubation. Nineteen children 4–9 years of age in American Society of Anesthesiologists physical status I or II who were scheduled for strabismus surgery were studied.

Methods.—No premedication was given. Anesthesia was induced by halothane, nitrous oxide, and oxygen, and the patient was intubated. Twelve patients were maintained with isoflurane, nitrous oxide, and oxygen and 7 with isoflurane, air, and oxygen. Nitrous oxide was withdrawn before the end of surgery. After a predetermined end-tidal isoflurane concentration was achieved and maintained for at least 10 minutes, the trachea was extubated.

Results.—Extubation was considered to be satisfactory if the patient did not cough or buck on the tube when the pharynx or stomach was suctioned, did not move or cough within 1 minute of extubation, and did not stop breathing or have laryngospasm. Two patients had laryngospasm after extubation, but there were no other study-related complications. The estimated minimal alveolar concentration of isoflurane at which half the patients were satisfactorily extubated was 1.27%, and the corresponding value for 95% of patients was 1.46%.

Conclusion.—It can be expected that half the children 4–9 years of age can be satisfactorily extubated at an end-tidal isoflurane concentration of 1.27%.

▶ This article bothers me very much. I do not understand what the authors mean by "successful" extubation in a deeply anesthetized child. If I get a deeply anesthetized child (or anyone else) who is spontaneously breathing in an adequate manner, I suppose I can extubate darn near anybody. Why would I want to? Is avoidance of coughing really all that important? After delicate eye muscle surgery or any other kind of surgery, sooner or later these children will have to cough. Why is "bucking" on the endotracheal tube with an open airway any worse than coughing on the first or second postoperative day? Isn't it true that the sutures are strongest during the earliest postoperative days and progressively weaken as time goes by? I simply do not understand risking massive vomiting and aspiration in these children. I would not permit this to be done in my child.—J.H. Tinker, M.D.

Bradycardia During Anesthesia in Infants: An Epidemiologic Study

Keenan RL, Shapiro JH, Kane FR, Simpson PM (Virginia Commonwealth Univ, Richmond)
Anesthesiology 80:976–982, 1994

101-95-20–5

Introduction.—That heart rate is the chief determinant of cardiac output in the first year of life suggests that bradycardia occurring during anesthesia might have adverse effects.

Objective.—The prevalence of bradycardia and asystole during anesthesia was examined in a computerized data base of 7,979 patients aged 45 years and younger who underwent noncardiac operations. Bradycardia, which is defined as a heart rate of less than 100 beats per minute, was analyzed in 4,645 anesthetics given to infants in the first year of life. Causes and co-morbid conditions were studied in the 59 infants who had bradycardia during anesthesia.

Table 1.—Frequency of Bradycardia During Anesthesia in Children, by Age

	0–1 yr	1–2 yr	2–3 yr	3–4 yr
Total anesthetics	4,645	1,932	774	628
With bradycardia	59	19	5	1
% Bradycardia	1.27	0.98	0.65	0.16

Note: The observed decrease in frequency with age is significant ($P = .041$, chi-square).
(Courtesy of Keenan RL, Shapiro JH, Kane FR, et al: *Anesthesiology* 80:976–982, 1994.)

TABLE 2.—Causes, Co-Morbidity, and Treatment of Bradycardia (Heart Rate < 100 Beats/Min) Occurring in Infants (Newborn to 1 Year) During Anesthesia

	Total (n = 59)	Hypoxemia (n = 13)	Excessive Dose of Inhalation Agent (n = 21)	Disease or Surgery (n = 21)	Other Anesthesia Cause (n = 4)
Comorbidity					
Hypotension	19	2	6	11	0
Asystole/ventricular fibrillation	8	0	2	6	0
Operating room death	5	0	0	5	0
Therapy					
Atropine	46	9	19	15	3
Epinephrine	18	2	5	11	0
Chest compression	15	1	5	9	0

(Courtesy of Keenan RL, Shapiro JH, Kane FR, et al: *Anesthesiology* 80:976–982, 1994.)

Findings.—Bradycardia occurred in 1.3% of infants in the first year of life and at declining rates subsequently (Table 1). Hypoxemia caused bradycardia in 22% of episodes (Table 2). Anesthesia-related problems accounted for 8 episodes. The dose of inhalational anesthetic was considered to be a factor in 35% of episodes, and the same percentage was related to severe disease or surgical factors. The morbidity associated with bradycardia included hypotension in 30% of infants and asystole or ventricular fibrillation in 30%; 8% of infants died. One fourth of infants with bradycardia had received atropine before the episode took place. On logistic regression analysis, bradycardia correlated with American Society of Anesthesiologists physical status III–V, longer surgery, and whether surgery was done electively or on an emergency basis. Bradycardia was less likely to occur when the supervising anesthesiologist was a member of the Pediatric Anesthesia Service.

Conclusion.—Bradycardia, which produces substantial morbidity during anesthesia, is more likely to occur in the first year of life than in older children.

▶ So bradycardia is less likely to occur when a supervising pediatric anesthesiologist is present. Bradycardia that is related to the dose of inhalational agent was less likely to occur in the presence of a pediatric anesthesiologist, because experienced pediatric anesthesiologists appear to more readily recognize the dangers of high doses of inhalational anesthetic agents (especially halothane) on the heart. I have observed that occasional pediatric anesthesiologists tend to feel more comfortable using inhalational anesthesia alone (with the resultant higher dosage) to avoid the use of muscle relaxants. This epidemiologic study has obvious implications for subspecialty pediatric practice, and it highlights serious quality assurance issues for departments of anesthesia.—M. Wood, M.D.

Enlarging Pediatric IV Catheters

Mapes A, Jones BR (Univ of California at Davis)
Pediatr Emerg Care 10:18–19, 1994   101-95-20–6

Background.—The flow through an IV catheter is a function of its length and internal diameter. The Streamline IV catheter is made of an elastomer hydrogel that softens and increases in diameter when it is exposed to aqueous solutions.

Methods.—The flow rates of Streamline IV catheters of 3 sizes, 22-gauge × 1 in., 24-gauge × .7 in., and 26-gauge × .625 in., were studied during 90 minutes of hydration in 37°C normal saline. Ten tests of each size catheter were performed every 15 minutes starting at 0 minutes and ending at 90 minutes, with each test measuring the time for 10 mL of saline to flow through the catheter.

Results.—All 3 gauges showed significant increases in flow rates, which reached a maximum in the 75-minute test. The percentage increase in flow and the flow rate variability increased with larger gauge sizes. The maximum flow increase was 43%, 39%, and 32% for the 22-, 24-, and 26-gauge catheters, respectively, but none of the catheters equaled or exceeded the initial flow rate of the next larger gauge catheter.

Implications.—Patients who have difficult IV access, such as an infant or small child, may preclude the placement of a large catheter for rapid fluid administration. The Streamline IV catheter should facilitate fluid administration. In addition to enlarging, these catheters also appear to soften and not kink, and they have been shown to be useful in neonatal ICUs and home health care settings.

▶ Insertion of large-bore, peripheral IV catheters for volume infusion in the neonate or small infant is at best a difficult task. Small-bore catheters that are easier to place slow resuscitative efforts by limiting the speed by which volume can be administered. This problem can be minimized to a certain extent by use of these Streamline catheters. (It is unclear from the authors' statistical analysis, but I assume the flow rate increases were significant.) Although none of the catheters tested lived up to the manufacturer's claim of expanding a full gauge within 30 minutes of hydration, I believe that they may play a role in the operating room when IV access is limited and volume expansion is critical. Future clinical trials and cost analyses are warranted.—D.M. Rothenberg, M.D.

21 Transfusion, Fluids, and Electrolytes

Efficacy and Cost-Effectiveness of Autologous Blood Predeposit in Patients Undergoing Radical Prostatectomy Procedures
Goodnough LT, Grishaber JE, Birkmeyer JD, Monk TG, Catalona WJ (Washington Univ, St. Louis, Mo; Dartmouth Hitchcock Med Ctr, Lebanon, NH)
Urology 44:226–231, 1994   101-95-21–1

Introduction.—Preoperative autologous blood donation (PAD) to reduce allogeneic blood exposure in patients undergoing major elective surgery is routine practice. The efficacy and cost-effectiveness of PAD for radical prostatectomy were examined.

Methods.—During a 3-year period, 394 patients with clinical stage A or B prostate cancer underwent radical prostatectomy and 384 (97%) of them predonated autologous blood. A Markov decision-analysis model was used to calculate the costs, benefits, and cost-effectiveness of PAD.

Results.—Patients predonated a mean of 3.5 autologous blood units, 2.1 (60%) of which were retransfused. Thirty-five (9%) patients who predonated blood and 7 (70%) nondonors also received allogeneic blood units. The net costs of PAD ranged from $83 to $303. The quality-adjusted life expectancy benefit of PAD ranged from .05 to .07 days per patient. The estimated overall cost-effectiveness of PAD was $1,813,000 per quality-adjusted year of life saved. However, PAD was considerably more cost-effective for 2-unit donations than for 3- or 4-unit donations.

Conclusion.—The cost-effectiveness of PAD does not compare favorably with the cost-effectiveness that has been estimated for other commonly used medical interventions.

▶ Ninety-seven percent of patients predonated autologous blood (3.5 units per patient), and only 9% of autologous blood donors required and received allogeneic blood. However, it appears that the most cost-effective policy is to collect 2 blood units per patient, even though 18% of these patients would then receive allogeneic blood.

This study poses the question of safety vs. cost. I don't know the answer, but just as there is no doubt that donation of autologous blood is beneficial to the individual, I think that in the not too distant future we will see national policies defined for such issues.—M. Wood, M.D.

Reduction in the Homologous Blood Requirement for Abdominal Aortic Aneurysm Repair by the Use of Preadmission Autologous Blood Donation

O'Hara PJ, Hertzer NR, Krajewski LP, Cox GS, Beven EG (Cleveland Clinic Found, Ohio)
Surgery 115:69–76, 1994   101-95-21–2

Objective.—Conserving blood has become increasingly important in vascular surgery, partly because of unwarranted fears by some potential blood donors that they may acquire HIV. The value of preadmission autologous blood donation (PABD) for lessening homologous transfusion needs was examined in 145 patients who were having resection of an abdominal aortic aneurysm.

Methods.—Seventy-three patients had surgery after PABD. Intraoperative autotransfusion (IAT) was routinely done. The need for homologous blood was compared with that for 72 patients who had similar surgery with IAT alone. The groups were similar with respect to age, cardiovascular risk factors, complexity of surgery, and intraoperative blood loss. The IAT volumes were also comparable. The study patients received a mean of 1.9 units of predeposited autologous blood.

Results.—Patients in the PABD group had a mean hematocrit of 33.4% at discharge and a mean hemoglobin of 11 g/dL. The respective figures for the comparison group were nearly identical at 33.3% and 11.1 g/dL. The study patients required a mean of 1.3 units of homologous blood compared with 1.9 units for comparison patients. Two thirds of the study patients and 36% of those in the comparison group required no homologous blood. There were no significant group differences in the need for platelets, fresh frozen plasma, or cryoprecipitate.

Conclusion.—The PABD significantly reduces the need for homologous blood in patients who are having elective aortic aneurysm surgery. When combined with IAT, it eliminated the need for homologous blood in two thirds of these patients.

▶ Why was a variable technique used for PABD of 1–4 units? Even with this methodologic flaw, it is both significant and important that 67% of the patients in the study group (i.e., the predeposit group) required no homologous blood transfusion vs. 36% of the comparison patients in whom only intraoperative blood salvage was used. Furthermore, it is interesting that the discharge hematocrit in both groups was approximately 33%, a number that was seen in both the Yale and Hopkins series to be associated with optimal or close-to-optimal myocardial function in patients with ischemic cardiovascular disease.—M.F. Roizen, M.D.

Efficacy of Autotransfusion in Hepatectomy for Hepatocellular Carcinoma

Fujimoto J, Okamoto E, Yamanaka N, Oriyama T, Furukawa K, Kawamura E, Tanaka T, Tomoda F (Hyogo College of Medicine, Nishinomiya, Japan)

Arch Surg 128:1065–1069, 1993   101-95-21–3

Background.—Autologous blood transfusion reduces the need for banked blood in many surgical procedures and eliminates infectious risk. Although concerns of metastasis have contraindicated intraoperative blood salvage in patients with cancer, the procedure has been safely used in this patient group. The safety and clinical usefulness of autoinfusion in hepatectomy for hepatocellular carcinoma were evaluated.

Methods.—Among 104 patients who were undergoing hepatectomy for hepatocellular carcinoma, 54 received autologous blood transfusion and 50 received homologous blood. Physical examination, chest radiography, hematology, and ultrasonography were performed quarterly until patient death or December 1991.

Results.—Of the mean 831 mL of autotransfused blood used, 394 mL was obtained by preoperative donation and 439 mL by intraoperative salvage. Fifteen patients who received autologous blood transfusion required no homologous blood components during the operation, and 11 avoided homologous blood products during the entire hospitalization. Despite comparable intraoperative blood losses, patients undergoing autotransfusion required significantly less homologous blood, 814 mL, compared with patients undergoing homologous transfusion, 3,466 mL. The groups had similar mean postoperative hemoglobin levels, platelet counts, prothrombin times, and partial thromboplastin times. A cytology study that was performed using 5 samples from 20 patients undergoing autotransfusion revealed all class 1 specimens. Seventeen autotransfusion patients remained disease-free 32 months after follow-up. Intrahepatic or extrahepatic recurrence rates and 3-year cumulative survival rates were comparable for the 2 groups. Extrahepatic metastasis did not occur in the absence of intrahepatic metastasis in patients undergoing autotransfusion.

Conclusion.—Autotransfusion is safe, effective, and practical when it is used in liver surgery for hepatocellular carcinoma. Additional study is required to determine the long-term safety and potential benefits.

▶ Intraoperative blood salvage for oncologic surgery is rarely used because of the fear of seeding tumors. This study is one of the early examinations of this assumption, in which oncologic tumor resection and intraoperative blood salvage were compared with nonintraoperative blood salvage for recurrence rate, metastases, and survival. Although the lack of difference doesn't mean one did not occur in this small series, the series is large enough—more than 100 patients—that it has some meaning at least for hepatectomy. The advantage of autologous transfusion in the prevention of immunosuppression may mean that autotransfusion leads to better survival if the volume of homologous transfusion can essentially be reduced to zero. I look forward to further studies on this topic.—M.F. Roizen, M.D.

Effect of Postoperative Reinfusion Systems on Hemoglobin Levels in Primary Total Hip and Total Knee Arthroplasties: A Prospective Randomized Study

Mauerhan DR, Nussman D, Mokris JG, Beaver WB (Miller Orthopaedic Clinic, Charlotte, NC; Carolinas Med Ctr, Charlotte, NC)
J Arthroplasty 8:523–527, 1993   101-95-21-4

Introduction.—Blood transfusion is often required because of perioperative blood loss in patients undergoing total hip arthroplasty (THA) and total knee arthroplasty (TKA). Because of the risk of viral disease transmission, a number of studies have examined the feasibility of postoperative collection and reinfusion of shed blood in these procedures. The effect of reinfusion of postoperative shed blood drainage on hemoglobin levels in patients undergoing elective primary THA and TKA was quantified.

Patients and Methods.—Controls were assigned to a standard postoperative collection-drainage system (ConstaVac) and patients to a blood collection-reinfusion system (CBC ConstaVac). The difference in the systems is that the latter has an umbrella valve that ensures the top 100 mL of fluid containing serum, fat, and bone debris does not leave the reservoir. All patients were encouraged to donate 2 units of autologous blood before surgery. Intraoperative blood transfusion was left to the discretion of the operating surgeon. Postoperative drainage volumes for both groups and the volume of reinfused blood for the patient group were recorded.

Results.—Fifty-seven patients (35 TKAs and 22 THAs) received the CBC ConstaVac reinfusion system and 54 (34 TKAs and 20 THAs) received a ConstaVac collection unit. Postoperative hemoglobin levels, which were recorded on postoperative days 1, 3, and 6, revealed no statistically significant difference between the control and patient groups. Hemoglobin levels and drainage volumes were similar in both THA and TKA patient groups compared with their respective control groups. The mean volume of blood available for reinfusion in the first 6 hours was 360 mL in the patient group. Only 2 of 57 patients would have had a significant enough volume in the second 6-hour period to allow additional reinfusion. Ninety-three percent of the units transfused were autologous. Nine patients required homologous blood transfusion.

Conclusion.—Most transfusion requirements for elective primary THA and TKA can be met by a well-designed and administered autologous blood program. The risk of receiving homologous blood appeared to be a factor in whether autologous blood was available rather than whether a reinfusion unit was used. Thus, reinfusion units are not routinely needed in THAs and TKAs and should not be relied on to supply blood in the postoperative period.

▶ This article demonstrates that when a study of bleeding abnormalities and autotransfusion is attempted, the anesthesiologist should be involved so that the type of anesthesia is known, as well as whether intraoperative hypotension and intraoperative blood salvage were used. The failure of this study to find a benefit in postoperative reinfusion may well be the result of such good care having been taken intraoperatively or that there is no effect.

Another thought on this study comes from the authors' statement: "Homologous blood transfusion was required in nine patients. . . . Five patients who received homologous blood were in the reinfusion study group and six were in the control group." I don't understand how patients could be in both groups, but the reviewers and editors, if they exist for this journal, should be ashamed that they let this confusing statement, if not outright error, slip through.—M.F. Roizen, M.D.

Blood Transfusion in Total Hip Arthroplasty: Guidelines to Eliminate Overtransfusion
McSwiney MM, O'Farrell D, Joshi GP, McCarroll SM (Cappagh Hosp, Dublin)
Can J Anaesth 40:222–226, 1993   101-95-21–5

Introduction.—Blood transfusion is considered a "high volume, high risk, and error prone" procedure. Critical review is needed to identify areas in which blood transfusion may be overused in an effort to reduce patient risk and hospital costs. The use of routine blood transfusion during total hip arthroplasty has only recently been questioned. The transfusion guidelines for patients undergoing elective total hip arthroplasty were evaluated for their effects on both overtransfusion and perioperative morbidity.

Methods.—Eighty consecutive patients who were scheduled for total hip arthroplasty and had normal hemoglobin concentrations were studied. There were 44 women, with a mean age of 66 years, and 36 men, with a mean age of 69 years. For each patient, the investigators calculated the maximum allowable blood loss (MABL) according to the formula of Kallos and co-workers. Up to this volume, blood loss was replaced with polygeline colloid solution (Haemaccel). After the MABL was reached, replacement with Haemaccel continued unless the hematocrit declined to less than 30 in men and 27 in women. The results were assessed in terms of postoperative complications, length of hospital stay, and compliance with physiotherapy; overtransfusion was defined as a discharge hematocrit of greater than 36. The findings were compared with those of a group of patients undergoing hip replacement before the institution of the transplantation guidelines.

Results.—Thirty-two percent of the study sample received blood transfusion compared with 97% of the retrospective control group. The volume of blood transfused was 2.7 units for controls vs. 1.3 units for the study group. Overtransfusion occurred in 45% of the control group vs. only 5% of the study group. The 2 groups were no different in terms of complications, length of stay, or progress in physiotherapy.

Conclusion.—These blood transfusion guidelines can significantly reduce blood use by patients undergoing total hip arthroplasty. They have no adverse effects on patients and reduce costs considerably. The hospital nursing staff are now using hematocrit machines to assess not only hip arthroplasty, but also knee arthroplasty patients.

▶ In this article, the authors fell into what I consider to be a classic trap. They set up stringent guidelines for blood transfusion during total hip arthroplasty and followed them. They then compared their transfusion results with those for a group of patients in whom blood was administered previously without protocol for the same operation. I hope it is no surprise to anyone that they were able to significantly lower the amount of blood administered in the "treatment" group. This article is an example of what I call the "academic straw man" syndrome (perhaps it would be politically correct today to say "academic straw person"). It involves setting up a straw man (person) by creating a set of study conditions that cannot lose. The authors were well aware that if they instituted stringent transfusion criteria they could decrease the amount of transfusion. To use a previously performed group of surgeries, which were done without this protocol, as a "retrospective control" is neither important nor useful.

Total hip arthroplasty is among the many surgical operations during which blood is given in far smaller quantities today than only a few years ago. This particular article reflects my least favorite kind of "science," because the authors set out to teach us a lesson: that they could do this operation with less blood than they could have previously. I would rather see science designed to answer questions in as unbiased a manner as possible.—J.H. Tinker, M.D.

Blood Transfusions and Prognosis in Colorectal Cancer
Busch ORC, Hop WCJ, Hoynck van Papendrecht MAW, Marquet RL, Jeekel J (Univ Hosp Rotterdam-Dijkzigt, The Netherlands; Erasmus Univ, Rotterdam, The Netherlands)
N Engl J Med 328:1372–1376, 1993   101-95-21–6

Background.—Blood transfusion seems to adversely affect the prognosis of patients undergoing surgery for cancer, although it has not been proved. A randomized, multicenter trial was done in patients with colorectal cancer to determine whether autologous blood transfusion reduces the rate of cancer recurrence and improves survival compared with allogeneic transfusion.

Methods.—Of 475 patients, 236 received allogeneic transfusions and 239 received autologous transfusions. Patients in the autologous transfusion group each donated 2 units of blood before surgery.

Findings.—Four-year colorectal cancer–specific survival rates were 67% and 62% in the allogeneic and autologous transfusion groups, respectively. Of the 423 patients who had curative surgery, 66% in the allogeneic transfusion group had no colorectal cancer recurrence at 4 years compared with 63% in the autologous transfusion group. The recurrence risk was significantly higher in patients who received blood transfusions of either type compared with patients who did not. Relative recurrence rates were not significant at 2.1 and 1.8, respectively.

Conclusion.—The use of autologous blood rather than allogeneic blood for transfusion in patients undergoing surgery for colorectal cancer does not improve prognosis. Either type of transfusion is associated with a poor prognosis, probably because of the circumstances necessitating it.

▶ As an anesthesiologist, I have been constantly told by surgeons that blood transfusions may adversely affect the prognosis of cancer patients, but I never understood the reason. This study confirms my suspicions. I can now ask, "Have you read the article in the *New England Journal of Medicine?*" The use of autologous blood compared with allogeneic blood for transfusion did not improve survival rates. However, the risk of recurrence was significantly increased in patients who received blood transfusions of either type. The authors point out that transfusions of both types are associated with poor prognosis, probably because of the circumstances that necessitate them. Standard rules for transfusion were used for both groups. Packed red cells were given if blood loss exceeded 500 mL or if the hemoglobin concentration decreased to less than 10.5 g/dL. Thus, there was a strong relationship between blood loss and transfusion.—M. Wood, M.D.

Successful Hemostasis During a Major Orthopedic Operation by Using Recombinant Activated Factor VII in a Patient With Severe Hemophilia A and a Potent Inhibitor
O'Marcaigh AS, Schmalz BJ, Shaughnessy WJ, Gilchrist GS (Comprehensive Hemophilia Ctr, Rochester, Minn; Mayo Clinic, Rochester, Minn)
Mayo Clin Proc 69:641–644, 1994   101-95-21–7

Introduction.—Management of intraoperative bleeding and providing perioperative hemostasis in hemophilic patients in whom coagulation factor inhibitors have developed is a major challenge. The case of a patient with severe hemophilia A who required major orthopedic surgery and was effectively managed with recombinant activated factor VII (rFVIIa) was reported.

Case Report.—Boy, 16 years, with a fixed-flexion contracture of his right knee that developed as a result of hemophilic arthropathy was confined to a wheelchair. Severe hemophilia A had been diagnosed at age 14 months, and an FVIII inhibitor was detected at age 2 years. Attempts at replacement with prothrombin complex concentrate had proved ineffective, and an attempt to induce immune tolerance to FVIII by low-dose infusion also failed. A porcine FVIII concentrate did not provide adequate perioperative coverage. Purified rFVIIa was then given in IV bolus doses of 102 µg/kg at 2-hour intervals for 24 hours and then every 3 hours for a total of 9 days. Tranexamic acid was also given. The operation lasted 3 hours and resulted in full knee extension. The estimated operative blood loss was 400 mL, and the patient did not bleed excessively after surgery. There were no adverse effects of rFVIIa. Fibrin split products increased transiently in the first week after surgery.

Conclusion.—This case provides further evidence that rFVIIa is an effective means of controlling bleeding in severely hemophilic patients who have inhibitors and must undergo surgery.

▶ Plasma products that are rich in factor VIII are used as therapy for hemophilia patients. Patients are screened for the presence of an inhibitor to factor VIII before surgery. The patient described in this case report had an inhibitor to factor VIII that prevented effective transfusion therapy. Use of recombinant factor VII represents a new and interesting mode of treatment for this group of patients.—M. Wood, M.D.

Hemoglobin Blood Substitutes in Extended Preoperative Autologous Blood Donation: An Experimental Study
Slanetz PJ, Lee R, Page R, Jacobs EE Jr, LaRaia PJ, Vlahakes GJ (Harvard Med School, Boston)
Surgery 115:246–254, 1994   101-95-21–8

Background.—Polymerized bovine hemoglobin solution (PBHg) is a stroma-free blood substitute material that appears to lack the renal and coagulation system toxicities of hemoglobin. Because of known risks of infectious disease transmission by homologous transfusion, optimization of autologous donation and transfusion techniques has been attempted. The feasibility of extensive autologous blood donation and transfusion was explored using PBHg as a hemoglobin substitute.

Methods.—Twenty-four sheep that were splenectomized were divided into 4 groups of 6 animals each. All animals underwent a standardized exploratory laparotomy with a planned loss of 3 units of blood. In group 1, surgical blood loss was replaced with 6% hetastarch (Hespan) solution. Group 2 animals donated 45% of calculated blood volume, which was replaced with 6% hetastarch. Surgical blood loss was replaced by autologous blood. Group 3 sheep were similarly treated, except that preoperative blood donation was replaced by PBHg. Group 4 sheep donated 80% or more of blood volume, which was replaced by PBHg. Surgical blood loss was replaced by 6% hetastarch and autologous packed red blood cells. Blood samples and hemodynamic data were recorded periodically until 24 hours after surgery. The animals were killed and necropsied.

Results.—Blood donation and surgery were well tolerated by all sheep. No unplanned intraoperative or postoperative bleeding was noted. Oxygen consumption and cardiac output remained relatively stable in groups 3 and 4 sheep, despite initial reductions in hematocrit to 13.3% and 5.6%, respectively. There was no significant difference in oxygen delivery between any groups. The contribution of PBHg to arterial oxygen content was calculated to be 44.8% in group 3 and 65.5% in group 4. Hematocrits 2 days after surgery were 20.8%, 21.5%, 19.5%, and 25.7% for groups 1–4, respectively. Serum creatinine and blood urea nitrogen concentrations were not increased in PBHg-treated animals.

Conclusions.—Polymerized bovine hemoglobin solution was effective in transporting oxygen after extensive (80%) blood donation. Use of this product can safely increase preoperative blood donation for autologous transfusion, thereby decreasing the need for homologous transfusion and the associated risk of infectious disease transmission.

▶ This well-done study shows that if we have an efficacious, nontoxic blood substitute, we can increase preoperative autologous blood transfusion programs to the point that even in surgery where huge volumes of blood are lost, patients do not have to be exposed to the immune and infectious risks of homologous transfusion. The authors argue (remember this study is supported by a company that uses bovine blood) that bovine blood is better as a blood substitute, because of its large availability and reduced infectious transmission risk. Genetically engineered hemoglobin substitutes are probably even better.—M.F. Roizen, M.D.

A Review of Transfusion-Associated AIDS Litigation: 1984 Through 1993

Kern JM, Croy BB (Crosby, Heafey, Roach & May, San Francisco)
Transfusion 34:484–491, 1994   101-95-21–9

Background.—New cases of transfusion-associated AIDS (TA-AIDS) will continue to be diagnosed as patients who received transfusions before the availability of antibody testing become symptomatic. Information on TA-AIDS lawsuits was reviewed to identify trends in TA-AIDS litigation.

Methods.—One hundred sixty-three legal actions were analyzed. Legal defense or consultation was provided in 79; the remaining 84 were nationally reported cases.

Findings.—The defendants were blood centers in 74% of the cases, hospitals in 58%, and physicians in 53%. Surgeons were named in 78% of the lawsuits against physicians; 42% of these were cardiothoracic surgeons. Fourteen of the national cases resulted in total plaintiff awards of $75,420,798. Physicians were liable for 41% of that amount, blood banks for 31%, and hospitals for 26%. Ten liability theories were used in the lawsuits, the most common being claims of medical negligence, which were raised in 46% of the cases; failure to identify high-risk donors, which figured in 45%; lack of informed consent, which was a factor in 39%; and failure to conduct surrogate testing, which was claimed in 39%. In 26 of the national trials, the results were favorable to health care providers. Seventeen of these occurred in the San Francisco Bay area, where case filings peaked before 1990 and new case filings declined as verdicts favoring health care providers were reported.

Conclusion.—Transfusion-associated AIDS litigation initially began with verdicts against blood banks, but it has now expanded to suits against physicians and hospitals. Such suits are based on medical negligence and informed consent issues. Health care professionals have successfully defended these lawsuits, despite widely publicized verdicts favoring plaintiffs.

▶ This article is important in revealing how the prospect of a huge verdict can trigger more lawsuits, and the success in defending lawsuits can stop such a search for lottery-like winning. Does this stop the suits because lawyers realize that they will have to spend a lot of money and may not win much, or because the defense learns how to defend such lawsuits better?

I know from this article that if I needed a lawyer to defend me in a lawsuit in relation to AIDS, I would get Kern and Croy to help with my defense.—M.F. Roizen, M.D.

Immediate Versus Delayed Fluid Resuscitation for Hypotensive Patients With Penetrating Torso Injuries
Bickell WH, Wall MJ Jr, Pepe PE, Martin RR, Ginger VF, Allen MK, Mattox KL
(Saint Francis Hosp, Tulsa, Okla; Baylor College of Medicine, Houston; Ben Taub Gen Hosp, Houston; et al)
N Engl J Med 331:1105–1109, 1994   101-95-21–10

Introduction.—Hypotensive trauma victims routinely receive IV isotonic fluids before surgery, but there is concern that this practice may have adverse effects if it is applied before the bleeding is controlled.

Objective.—The effects of delaying fluid resuscitation until the time of surgery were studied in a prospective series of 598 patients 16 years of age and older who had penetrating torso injuries and a prehospital systolic blood pressure of 90 mm Hg or less. The patients underwent thoracotomy, laparotomy, or neck or groin exploration.

TABLE 1.—Total Volumes of Fluids Administered to Patients With Penetrating Torso Injuries, According to Treatment Group

Variable	Immediate Resuscitation (N = 309)	Delayed Resuscitation (N = 289)	P Value
Before arrival at the hospital			
Ringer's acetate (ml)	870±667	92±309	<0.001
Trauma center			
Ringer's acetate (ml)	1608±1201	283±722	<0.001
Packed red cells (ml)	133±339	11±88	<0.001
Operating room*			
Ringer's acetate (ml)	6772±4688	6529±4863	0.31
Packed red cells (ml)	1942±2322	1713±2313	0.07
Fresh-frozen plasma or platelet packs (ml)	357±1002	307±704	0.45
Autologous-transfusion volume (ml)	95±486	111±690	0.76
Hetastarch (ml)	499±717	542±696	0.41
Rate of intraoperative fluid administration (ml/min)	117±126	91±88	0.008

Note: Plus-minus values are means ± standard deviation.
*For these analyses, there were 268 patients in the immediate resuscitation group and 260 patients in the delayed resuscitation group.
(Courtesy of Bickell WH, Wall MJ Jr, Pepe PE, et al: *N Engl J Med* 331:1105–1109, 1994.)

Management.—Patients received either Ringer's acetate solution before admission to the hospital or no fluid other than what was needed to keep the line open before surgery. After induction of anesthesia, all patients received crystalloid and packed red cells as required to maintain a systolic arterial pressure of 100 mm Hg, a hematocrit of 25% or greater, and a urine output of at least 50 mL/hr.

Results.—In the prehospital phase, the 309 patients who were assigned to immediate fluid resuscitation received an average of 870 mL of isotonic solution, whereas the 289 in the delayed resuscitation group received 92 mL (Table 1). The 2 groups received comparable amounts of Ringer's acetate and hetastarch during surgery. Survival was 70% in the delayed-resuscitation group and 62% in patients who were immediately resuscitated, a significant difference (Table 2). Intraoperative blood losses were similar in the 2 groups, and complication rates did not differ substantially. The difference in survival persisted after adjustment for prehospital and trauma center intervals.

Implications.—The traditional practice of aggressive preoperative fluid resuscitation in hypotensive trauma victims is questionable. It is not the

TABLE 2.—Outcome of Patients With Penetrating Torso Injuries, According to Treatment Group

VARIABLE	IMMEDIATE RESUSCITATION	DELAYED RESUSCITATION	P VALUE
Survival to discharge — no. of patients/total patients (%)	193/309 (62)*	203/289 (70)†	0.04
Estimated intraoperative blood loss — ml‡	3127±4937	2555±3546	0.11
Length of hospital stay — days§	14±24	11±19	0.006
Length of ICU stay — days§	8±16	7±11	0.30

*95% confidence interval, 57% to 68%.
†95% confidence interval, 65% to 75%.
‡Estimated intraoperative blood loss was calculated for patients who survived the operation: 268 in the immediate resuscitation group and 260 in the delayed resuscitation group.
§The lengths of stays in the hospital and ICU were calculated for patients who survived the operation: 227 in the immediate resuscitation group and 238 in the delayed resuscitation group.
(Courtesy of Bickell WH, Wall MJ Jr, Pepe PE, et al: N Engl J Med 331:1105–1109, 1994.)

value of fluid resuscitation that is being questioned, but the appropriate timing and extent of this treatment.

▶ This study suggests that the preoperative use of isotonic crystalloid solutions (approximately 2.5 L over 1 hour and 15 minutes) in patients with penetrating torso trauma may promote fatal secondary hemorrhage by precipitating thrombus disruption and/or a coagulopathy before surgical control of bleeding. If this hypothesis is true, I would have expected a greater discrepancy in estimated intraoperative blood loss between the 2 groups, but that was not the case.

With regard to the conclusion that outcome was improved in the delayed resuscitation group, it would have been interesting to have broken down survival rates by site of injury, with the question being: Were there more groin injuries than thoracic or abdominal injuries in the delayed resuscitation group to explain its improved survival? Finally, I wonder, if the authors had excluded the 22 patients who violated their delayed resuscitation protocol, would their results still have achieved statistical significance?—D.M. Rothenberg, M.D.

Dilutional Hyponatremia During Endoscopic Curettage: The "Female TURP Syndrome"?
Marino J, Kelly D, Brull SJ (Yale Univ, New Haven, Conn)
Anesth Analg 78:1180–1181, 1994   101-95-21-11

Introduction.—A frequently cited complication of transurethral prostatectomy is hyponatremia because of absorption of the irrigation fluid in open venous sinuses. A woman undergoing endoscopic uterine surgery had a similar occurrence. The increasingly large number of laparoscopic procedures and the small number of cases presented warrant presentation of this case.

Case Report.—Woman, 32, was scheduled for endoscopic uterine myomata resection. Admission sodium of 138 mEq/L was normal. She was medicated with midazolam, metoclopramide, and droperidol. Anesthesia was induced and maintained with 66% nitrous oxide, 1% isoflurane, and oxygen. Lactated Ringer's solution was given at a rate of 200 mL/hr. The infusion bag of the hysteroscope contained 3% sorbitol Urological Irrigating Solution, which was infused into the uterine cavity at 150 mm Hg of pressure. After 80 minutes of surgery and a positive fluid balance of 1,100 mL of sorbitol, the serum sodium was 111 mEq/L, which changed to 112 with discontinuation of the sorbitol. Because of hyponatremia, the endoscopic resection was halted and continued through a vertical suprapubic incision. A solution of .9% sodium chloride was substituted for the Ringer's solution, and serum sodium increased to 114 mEq/L. Thus, a 3% sodium chloride infusion of 40 mL/hr was begun. Postoperatively, physical and mental functions were normal. On transfer to her room, serum sodium was 122 mEq/L, hypertonic infusion was discontinued, and fluids were restricted. The patient was discharged 2 days later with a serum sodium of 140 mEq/L.

Comment.—The likelihood of the irrigation fluid being absorbed is increased in hysteroscopic surgery because of the pressure needed for uterine distention, the prolonged resection time, and the exposure of raw tissue. In transurethral prostatectomy, the patient is usually given spinal anesthesia and the mental status is used as an indicator of dilutional hyponatremia. In this case, the patient preferred general anesthesia. Frequent monitoring of serum sodium and the determination of early fluid absorption by methods such as ethanol labeling may be useful when the mental status of the patient cannot be used as a monitor of dilutional hyponatremia.

▶ I continue to be amazed by the lack of understanding of how to manage the hyponatremia associated with transurethral prostatectomy (TURP), or for that matter "female TURP" surgery. In this case report, the authors empirically measured serum sodium, and when they obtained a lower value, a number of "therapeutic" decisions were made. The first was a drastic change in the surgical approach. Why the authors recommended this is unclear, because the patient was quite stable. The second was the change in IV fluids from lactated Ringer's to .9 sodium chloride and then eventually to hypertonic (3%) saline. Why this was done is just as unclear.

If it is systemically absorbed, 3% sorbitol solution is osmotically active and impermeable to the blood-brain barrier. Therefore, the dilutional hyponatremia that occurs does so in the face of isotonicity, thereby preventing the development of cerebral edema. This phenomenon could have been diagnosed easily by measuring a simultaneous serum osmolarity, which most certainly would have revealed a normal, if not high, level, even though the patient was hyponatremic (also known as an osmolar gap = [measured-calculated osmolarity]). This is the probable explanation why the patient's postoperative neurologic examination was normal despite the acute hyponatremia. Administering hypertonic saline to a patient with a normal or high serum osmolarity could have rendered the patient hyperosmolar and precipitated the syndrome of central pontine myelinolysis, which the authors themselves describe as an often-fatal complication of rapid correction of hypotonic hyponatremia. It is imperative that use of hypertonic saline be reserved only for patients who manifest neurologic symptoms of acute hyponatremia and who have documented low serum osmolarities. In patients with cardiopulmonary disease or renal insufficiency who manifest the changes of pulmonary edema, furosemide may be more effective in creating a free-water clearance. These otherwise-healthy patients should be treated solely with free-water restriction and a "tincture of time" to correct the laboratory abnormality of hyponatremia.—D.M. Rothenberg, M.D.

Call Mosby Document Express at **1 (800) 55-MOSBY** to obtain copies of the original source documents of articles featured or referenced in the YEAR BOOK series.

22 Critical Care Medicine

Pulse Oximetry Monitoring Can Change Routine Oxygen Supplementation Practices in the Postanesthesia Care Unit
DiBenedetto RJ, Graves SA, Gravenstein N, Konicek C (Univ of Florida, Gainesville)
Anesth Analg 78:365–368, 1994   101-95-22–1

Introduction.—The routine use of supplemental oxygen in the postanesthesia care unit (PACU) is costly and time-consuming. With the widespread use of pulse oximeters to determine oxygen saturation (SpO_2), the need for this practice was examined.

Methods.—During a 4½-week period, patients did not receive supplemental oxygen when the SpO_2 was 94% or greater. Supplemental oxygen was administered by face mask whenever the SpO_2 declined to less than 94%. When the preoperative SpO_2 was less than 94% and the postoperative SpO_2 was greater than the preoperative level, no supplemental oxygen was given.

Results.—Of the 491 patients included in the study, 307 (63%) did not receive supplemental oxygen because their SpO_2 remained at least 94% or their preoperative level was less than 94% during their stay in the PACU. A total of 184 patients (37%) required supplemental oxygen because their SpO_2 was less than 94% at some time in the PACU.

Discussion.—Some patients require supplemental oxygen after surgery, but most do not. Although an SpO_2 of 90% has historically been used to define hypoxia, an SpO_2 of 94% was chosen as a conservative cutoff point because of concern that even a single negative reaction would negate the benefits of the investigation. Additionally, patient safety was augmented by a standard ECG, blood pressure monitoring, and nurse observation. A savings of $31,928 in potential patient charges was realized for the 307 patients who did not require supplemental postoperative oxygen.

Conclusion.—If supplemental oxygen was not required for 63% of the 10,000 patients who are admitted to the PACU yearly, $623,272 could be saved in potential patient charges. The cost savings of administering supplemental postoperative oxygen only to patients who need it could yield considerable savings without compromising the quality of patient care.

▶ Despite the lack of additional demographic data in this study (e.g., duration and type of surgery, tobacco history, or preoperative weight assessment), I would agree that it would make medical *sense* to titrate oxygen therapy in the postoperative setting, based on the results of pulse oximetry. It is quite likely that most healthy patients undergoing general anesthesia would not require supplemental oxygen. However, the authors' contention that this practice could translate into a real hospital "savings" is questionable. Although the actual direct costs of oxygen therapy per patient in most centers is small, the indirect costs (i.e., that of PACU nurses, respiratory therapists, and personnel necessary to maintain oxygen pipelines) often lead to patient charges in excess of $100 to $200. The authors include these indirect costs in reaching their conclusion that an annual savings of $655,200 could be achieved. Unless these indirect costs are addressed by eliminating salaries, I remain unconvinced that this study makes "medical *cents*."—D.M. Rothenberg, M.D.

Name That Tone: The Proliferation of Alarms in the Intensive Care Unit
Cropp AJ, Woods LA, Raney D, Bredle DL (St Elizabeth Hosp, Youngstown, Ohio; Northwestern Ohio Univs, Rootstown)
Chest 105:1217–1220, 1994   101-95-22–2

Introduction.—Sophisticated critical care units are equipped with numerous monitoring devices that audibly warn the staff of changes in patient status or equipment malfunctions. In an 11-bed medical ICU, an average of 50 alarms from 33 sources was noted during an average day-shift hour. The ability to discern audible signals, particularly those that indicate life-threatening situations, was questioned.

Methods.—In a quiet room, 100 staff members, including physicians, registered nurses (RNs), registered respiratory therapists (RRTs), and nonregistered respiratory therapists (RTs), each listened alone to an audiotape with 33 different sounds from ICU equipment. Each person listened only once and did so without previous knowledge of the tape or study. Ten seconds were allowed for listening, and then 10 more were allowed for a written response before the next sound. Seven of the 10 sounds that were considered to be critical to patient safety involved ventilators.

Results.—Overall, 43% of sounds were identified correctly, with a mean correct response rate of 50% for critical alarms and a mean of 40% for noncritical alarms. By occupation, the RRTs scored highest in correctly identifying sounds, followed by the RNs, and then the RTs; physicians scored lowest. Staff members with less than 1 year of experience scored lower in all sounds than those with more experience, but there was no significant difference between groups in identifying critical alarms. Full- or part-time employment had no impact on the ability to identify the sounds.

Conclusion.—Most critical alarms tested were ventilator-related, so it is understandable that RRTs would recognize them best. The benefit of alarms is questioned, because a large number of signals are not identified by the typical caregiver. To increase recognition of audible alarms, the noise levels in the ICU should be reduced by eliminating unnecessary alarms and staff members should receive regular inservice training for critical alarms. The decrease in noise would be beneficial to staff and patients alike.

▶ As a resident in anesthesiology, I was subject to an audible quiz of sorts in which I was asked to identify from a tape a number of operating room alarms. I failed miserably; however, I fared no worse than my resident colleagues or, for that matter, my attendings. This study suggests that low-intensity flashing lights seem to be a more viable alternative to noncritical audible alarms that are consistently not recognized by trained health care professionals and that simply do no more than add to the already intolerable level of noise in the ICU.—D.M. Rothenberg, M.D.

Delivery and Monitoring of Inhaled Nitric Oxide in Patients With Pulmonary Hypertension

Wessel DL, Adatia I, Thompson JE, Hickey PR (Children's Hosp, Boston; Harvard Med School, Boston)
Crit Care Med 22:930–938, 1994   101-95-22-3

Introduction.—A portable and adaptable system has been designed for the delivery of nitric oxide at any concentration between 5 and 100 ppm with a forced expiratory oxygen (FIO_2) range of .21–.97 to patients with pulmonary hypertension. Nitric oxide has been shown to be useful in the perioperative care of children with congenital heart disease, neonates with persistent pulmonary hypertension, and adults with pulmonary hypertension or adult respiratory distress syndrome. The formation of nitrogen dioxide and methemoglobinemia are the major recognized potential toxicities of inhaled nitric oxide. These hazards can be reduced by a system that minimizes the duration of gas in the delivery circuit; allows precise control of the dose; permits online analysis of nitric oxide, nitrogen dioxide, and oxygen concentrations; and has stringent controls for treating exhaust gases and inhaled gas.

Methods.—A sample of 123 patients aged 1 day to 72 years with pulmonary hypertension (88 had congenital heart disease) was given nitric oxide at 10–80 ppm with an FIO_2 ranging from .21 to .97. The basic delivery system ensured that alterations in gas exchange, ventilatory variables, or hemodynamics during changes of inhaled concentrtions of ni-

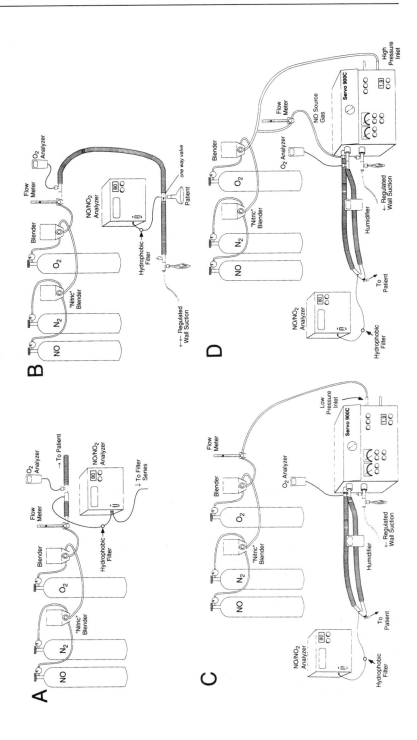

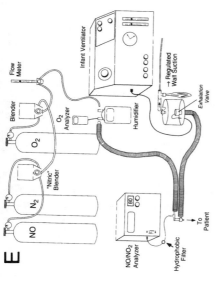

Fig 22-1.—A, basic nitric oxide (NO) delivery system, using a double-blender technique and chemiluminescence analysis. Modified systems for **B,** the patient who is breathing spontaneously and without assistance; **C,** the mechanically ventilated patient in the volume control mode when low tidal volumes are required; **D,** the mechanically ventilated patient in the volume control mode when large tidal volumes are required (Note that the additional flowmeter and continuous flow line are inserted if the positive end-expiratory pressure is to be maintained.); **E,** the patient requiring a time-cycled, pressure-limited infant ventilator. Currently, the use of a low flowmeter attached to the nitric oxide source tank permits elimination of the nitrogen tank and 1 blender, thus simplifying the delivery of nitric oxide with continuous flow infant ventilators. (Courtesy of Wessel DL, Adatia I, Thompson JE, et al: *Crit Care Med* 22:930-938, 1994).

tric oxide could be ascribed to the effect of nitric oxide alone. It was adapted to a variety of circumstances (Fig 22–1).

Results.—Thirty-two patients breathed spontaneously through a mask. Ninety-one were mechanically ventilated: 53 had a volume-controlled ventilator; 5 had a pressure-controlled ventilator; 25 had a pressure-limited, time-cycled continuous flow infant ventilator; 2 had high-frequency oscillator ventilation; 6 received the gas during surgery through an anesthesia machine; and 7 were hand-ventilated by bag through an endotracheal tube. Nitric oxide doses remained stable, independent of minute ventilation, and were changed quickly and easily. Nitrogen dioxide was continuously monitored, and in 83 patients, it was less than or equal to 1 ppm; in 19 patients, it was less than or equal to 2 ppm; in 10 patients, it was 3 ppm or less; and in 4 patients, it was 4 ppm or less. The concentrations of methemoglobin exceeded 5% in 4 patients.

Conclusion.—With such a system, nitric oxide can be delivered safely and effectively to patients of any size, whether they are breathing spontaneously or unassisted or during pressure- or volume-limited modes of mechanical ventilation.

▶ Despite the number of modalities available to administer and monitor nitric oxide, I know of no commercially available delivery systems. The chemiluminescence analyzer is designed for industrial use and is quite expensive (over $20,000). It will take some time (and Food and Drug Administration approval) before we can use nitric oxide routinely.—D.M. Rothenberg, M.D.

Inhaled Nitric Oxide Reverses the Increase in Pulmonary Vascular Resistance Induced by Permissive Hypercapnia in Patients With Acute Respiratory Distress Syndrome
Puybasset L, Stewart T, Rouby J-J, Cluzel P, Mourgeon E, Belin M-F, Arthaud M, Landault C, Viars P (Univ of Paris VI)
Anesthesiology 80:1254–1267, 1994   101-95-22–4

Introduction.—It has been hypothesized that ventilatory management of patients with acute respiratory distress syndrome (ARDS) that includes both permissive hypercapnia and inhaled nitric oxide (NO) may limit oxygen toxicity and barotrauma. Whether inhaled NO can reduce the increase in pulmonary arterial pressure and improve oxygenation in ARDS patients who are also managed with permissive hypercapnia was examined.

Methods.—Eleven patients with severe ARDS were studied under 4 conditions: normocapnia, normocapnia during mechanical ventilation with 2 ppm of inhaled NO, hypercapnia, and hypercapnia during mechanical ventilation with 2 ppm of inhaled NO. Arterial pressure, pulmonary artery pressure, and tidal volume were monitored continuously. When a steady state was reached in each condition, arterial and mixed

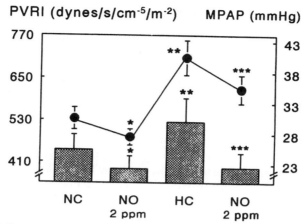

Fig 22–2.—Effects of inhaled nitric oxide (NO) at a concentration of 2 ppm on pulmonary vascular resistance index (PVRI) (*bars*) and mean pulmonary arterial pressure (MPAP) (*circles*) during the 4 phases of the study: normocapnia (NC), NC + NO 2 ppm, hypercapnia (HC), and HC + NO 2 ppm. *P < .05 NC + NO 2 ppm vs. NC; **P < .05 HC vs. NC; ***P < .05 HC + NO 2 ppm vs. HC. (Courtesy of Puybasset L, Stewart T, Rouby J-J, et al: *Anesthesiology* 80: 1254–1267, 1994.)

venous blood was drawn and hemodynamic and respiratory parameters were measured.

Results.—Patients in the normocapnic state demonstrated significant increases in the pulmonary vascular resistance index (PVRI) and the mean pulmonary arterial pressure (MPAP); the administration of 2 ppm

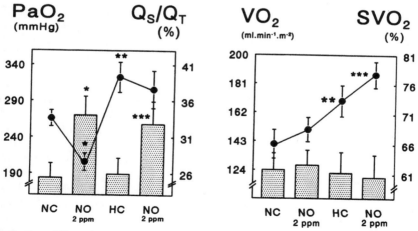

Fig 22–3.—Effects of inhaled nitric oxide (NO) at a concentration of 2 ppm (**left**) on arterial oxygen tension (PaO$_2$, *bars*) and pulmonary shunt (Q$_s$/Q$_T$, *circles*) and (**right**) on oxygen consumption (VO$_2$, *bars*) and mixed venous hemoglobin oxygen saturation (SvO$_2$, *circles*) during 4 phases of study: normocapnia (NC), NC + NO 2 ppm, hypercapnia (HC), and HC + NO 2 ppm. *P < .05 NO 2 ppm vs. NC; **P < .05 HC vs. NC; ***HC + NO 2 ppm vs. HC. (Courtesy of Puybasset L, Stewart T, Rouby J-J, et al: *Anesthesiology* 20:1254–1267, 1994.)

of inhaled NO induced significant reductions in both PVRI and MPAP in both normocapnic and hypercapnic patients (Fig 22–2). The reductions were more pronounced in the hypercapnic state. Although oxygen consumption remained relatively steady, arterial oxygen tension and-mixed venous hemoglobin oxygen saturation increased significantly, and the pulmonary shunt decreased with inhaled NO in both normocapnic and hypercapnic patients (Fig 22–3). Serum concentrations of methemoglobin and nitrogen dioxide in the trachea did not increase in any condition. Alveolar dead space was reduced with the administration of NO in the 5 patients who were studied for changes.

Conclusion.—Inhalation of NO mitigates some of the effects of permissive hypercapnia by reversing the increase in PVRI, lessening pulmonary hypertension, and improving arterial oxygenation. A concentration of 2 ppm is sufficient to produce these therapeutic effects, which reduce the risk of toxicity.

Prolonged Inhalation of Low Concentrations of Nitric Oxide in Patients With Severe Adult Respiratory Distress Syndrome: Effects on Pulmonary Hemodynamics and Oxygenation
Bigatello LM, Hurford WE, Kacmarek RM, Roberts JD Jr, Zapol WM (Harvard Med School, Boston)
Anesthesiology 80:761–770, 1994   101-95-22–5

Introduction.—Studies have shown that inhaled nitric oxide (NO) can induce selective pulmonary vasodilatation in patients with pulmonary artery hypertension, whereas it does not affect systemic arterial pressure. The effects of NO were examined by investigating the dose-response effect of inhaled NO on pulmonary hypertension and oxygen exchange, identifying the persistent effects with prolonged NO inhalation, and calculating the correlation between baseline and postinhalation physiologic characteristics.

Methods.—Thirteen patients with adult respiratory distress syndrome (ARDS) and pulmonary hypertension were monitored throughout the studies using radial and pulmonary artery catheters. Inhaled NO was administered in concentrations of 5, 10, 20, and 40 ppm, with each concentration being inhaled for 20 minutes. After the dose-response trial, 7 patients were given continuous NO inhalation therapy at concentrations of 2–20 ppm for 2–27 days.

Results.—The mean pulmonary artery pressure demonstrated a dose-related decrease (Fig 22–4). During inhalation of 5–40 ppm of NO, the ratio of arterial oxygen tension to inspired oxygen fraction increased and the venous admixture decreased, although not in a dose-dependent fashion. These effects persisted throughout prolonged administration and occurred with NO concentrations as low as 2 ppm. There were no significant changes at any dose in the heart rate, mean systemic arterial

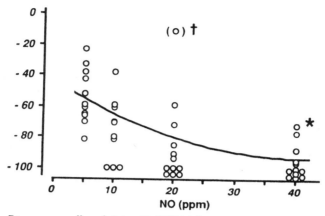

% MAXIMUM CHANGE MPAP

Fig 22–4.—Dose-response effect of nitric oxide (NO) inhalation on the mean pulmonary artery pressure (MPAP) in 11 patients with adult respiratory distress syndrome (12 observations). Values are expressed as the percentage of maximal response. Analysis of variance for repeated measures: $P < .0001$. *Mean value at 40 ppm of NO was significantly different from mean value at 5 ppm of NO. †Positive value (100%). (Courtesy of Bigatello LM, Hurford WE, Kacmarek RM, et al: *Anesthesiology* 80:761-770, 1994.)

pressure, cardiac output, central venous pressure, pulmonary artery occlusion pressure, oxygen delivery, inspiratory airway pressures, tidal volume, respiratory dynamic compliance, or methemoglobin concentration. Prolonged NO inhalation did not induce tachyphylaxis. The degree of physiologic response to inhaled NO was predicted by baseline levels.

Discussion.—Inhaling NO at concentrations of 2–40 ppm selectively decreased pulmonary artery pressure (in a dose-related fashion) and improved arterial oxygenation in patients with ARDS, but the effects were quickly reversed after the discontinuation of NO. Improved arterial oxygenation allowed reduction of the inspired oxygen fraction or the positive end-expiratory pressure, or both, which can make respiratory management easier. There was no evidence of NO toxicity; however, survival was not improved in these patients.

▶ Permissive hypercapnia, a technique designed to minimize lung damage in patients with ARDS, is gaining popularity, although hemodynamic alterations associated with low arterial pH and increased pulmonary vascular resistance are often cited as potentially deleterious systemic effects that may limit its application. In the first study (Abstract 101-95-22–4), low levels of inhaled NO were used to attenuate the effects of hypercapnia. Even at low levels (2 ppm) for a short duration (30 minutes), NO showed a pronounced effect in decreasing pulmonary vascular resistance. Although the partial pressure of oxygen in arterial blood improved, the mechanism was apparently unrelated to a decrease in the pathophysiologic shunt.

In the second study (Abstract 101-95-22–5), a similar improvement in pulmonary vascular tone and oxygenation was achieved, although in a dose-dependent fashion and with prolonged use of NO. Neither toxicity, as measured by methemoglobin levels, nor tachyphylaxis occurred with prolonged use.

Although neither study was designed to assess mortality, the ultimate goal of any type of therapy for ARDS is to improve outcome. Perhaps future controlled studies that use both permissive hypercapnia and NO for a prolonged period will prove successful in improving survival from ARDS.—D.M. Rothenberg, M.D.

High-Dose Intravenous Magnesium Sulfate in the Management of Life-Threatening Status Asthmaticus
Sydow M, Crozier TA, Zielmann S, Radke J, Burchardi H (Georg-August Univ of Göttingen, Germany)
Intensive Care Med 19:467–471, 1993   101-95-22–6

Introduction.—Life-threatening status asthmaticus is often unresponsive to conventional conservative medical treatment. The resultant tracheal intubation and mechanical ventilation are associated with severe complications and a mortality of 22%. The bronchodilatory effects of moderate doses of magnesium sulfate ($MgSO_4$) have been demonstrated, and the effects of larger doses in 5 patients for whom maximal conservative treatment had failed were investigated.

Case Report.—Man, 25, with a 10-year history of allergic asthma was asymptomatic and received no medication before a scheduled elective inguinal herniorrhaphy. The induction of anesthesia with fentanyl, .25 mg, and 100 mg of methohexital was followed by difficulty in ventilating with a face mask, chest flushing, severe bronchospasm, and hypoxia. The patient was intubated and put on mechanical ventilation with halothane. The bronchospasm was not relieved by theophylline and methylprednisolone, and a bilateral tension pneumothorax and skin emphysema developed within 15 minutes. Bilateral chest tubes were inserted and salbutamol was administered by nebulizer. Because of the poor response, $MgSO_4$ was started at 10 g/hr for 1 hour. In fewer than 30 minutes, the patient's peak airway pressure decreased from 45 to 32 cm H_2O and continued to decrease. Mild hypotension was corrected by reducing the infusion rate to .4 g/hr. Within 12 hours, the patient was extubated.

Discussion.—It is possible that $MgSO_4$ acts as a calcium antagonist to relax airway smooth muscles. The hypotensive response to high-dose administration indicates the need for continuous on-line blood pressure monitoring. After this favorable response by 5 patients, consideration should be given to high-dose administration of $MgSO_4$ as an adjunct to management of severe bronchospasm during mechanical ventilation. Larger controlled, randomized, blind studies are needed.

Rapid Infusion of Magnesium Sulfate Obviates Need for Intubation in Status Asthmaticus
Schiermeyer RP, Finkelstein JA (Brooke Army Med Ctr, San Antonio, Tex)
Am J Emerg Med 12:164–166, 1994   101-95-22–7

Background.—Magnesium sulfate ($MgSO_4$) causes bronchodilation. Recently, it has been administered with variable success as a slow infusion over 20 minutes for the treatment of acute asthmatic exacerbations. The first successful emergency room use of a rapid infusion of $MgSO_4$ to avoid endotracheal intubation in patients with status asthmaticus leading to impending respiratory failure was reported.

Case 1.—Girl, 16 years was brought to the emergency room in severe respiratory distress as a result of an asthmatic exacerbation. She was progressively given an albuterol nebulizer; 250 mg of IV methylprednisolone sodium succinate (Solu-Medrol); a nebulizer of albuterol and glycopyrrolate; subcutaneous terbutaline; and continuous albuterol nebulization. Because there was no significant improvement, the patient was electively intubated. She was given 2 g of IV $MgSO_4$ over a 2-minute period as a last treatment measure before intubation. After the infusion, the patient felt flushed and then immediately better. Intubation was avoided.

Case 2.—Man, 22, was brought to the emergency room in significant respiratory distress. The patient was given nebulized albuterol, 2 L of oxygen by nasal cannula, another nebulizer composed of albuterol and glycopyrrolate, 125 mg of IV methylprednisolone sodium succinate, and continuous β_2-agonist therapy. The clinical impression was that of impending respiratory failure. As a last treatment measure before elective intubation, the patient was given 2 g of IV $MgSO_4$ over a 2-minute period. After the infusion, the patient reported feeling flushed and experienced marked immediate improvement. Intubation was no longer required.

Conclusion.—In the 2 young adults with status asthmaticus that resulted in impending respiratory failure, both were unresponsive to conventional therapy. After they were given 2 g of IV $MgSO_4$ over a 2-minute period, significant improvement occurred in both and intubation was averted.

▶ The clinical use of magnesium to treat ventricular arrhythmias as well as its experimental use in mitigating oxygen-induced lung toxicity were presented in last year's YEAR BOOK (Abstracts 101-94-5–44 and 101-94-12–4). These 2 additional studies (Abstracts 101-95-22–6 and 101-95-22–7) focus on magnesium's bronchodilatory properties. In the first study, extremely high doses of magnesium (10–20 g followed by .4 g/hr) were used to improve airway resistance in patients with severe status asthmaticus. Few side effects of this therapy were noted. (Monitoring for hypotension secondary to the intrinsic vasodilatory effect as well as from the relief of bronchospasm is in order. The need for close train-of-four monitoring to detect prolongation of neuromuscular blockade also seems warranted.)

The second study suggests that the rapidity of administration may add to the drug's beneficial effect. With magnesium being recommended as a first-line therapy for torsade-de pointes, it is now routinely provided in all our operating room carts. This readily available drug can now be used with minimal risk for the rapid treatment of intraoperative bronchospasm in a probable dose-dependent manner.—D.M. Rothenberg, M.D.

Elevation of Systemic Oxygen Delivery in the Treatment of Critically Ill Patients

Hayes MA, Timmins AC, Yau EHS, Palazzo M, Hinds CJ, Watson D (St Bartholomew's Hosp, London; Charing Cross Hosp, London)
N Engl J Med 330:1717–1722, 1994   101-95-22–8

Background.—To replete tissue oxygen and prevent loss of organ function in patients who are critically ill, it has been recommended that cardiac index, oxygen delivery, and oxygen consumption be increased to levels that are median maximal values in survivors (> 4.5 L/min/m² of body surface area, > 600 mL/min/m², and > 170 mL/min/m², respectively). The effectiveness of that strategy was evaluated.

Methods.—A prospective study was conducted of patients who were admitted to the ICU for a variety of critical illnesses. If, after fluid resuscitation, the cardiac index, oxygen delivery, and oxygen consumption did

	Outcome Data		
OUTCOME	CONTROL GROUP (N = 50)	TREATMENT GROUP (N = 50)	NOT RANDOMIZED (N = 9)
Days in unit — median (range)	10 (1–64)	10 (1–48)	10 (1–29)
Ventilation			
No. of days — median (range)	8 (0–54)	8 (0–41)	2 (0–26)
No. of patients	44	46	7
Days in hospital — median (range)	23.5 (1–244)	19 (1–187)	20 (11–102)
Mortality — %			
In intensive care unit	30	50*	—
In hospital	34	54*	—
Predicted risk of death — median % (range)	34 (3–91)	34 (3–85)	6 (3–32)
Cause of death — no. of patients			
Intractable hypotension	4	4	—
Cardiac event	2	4	—
Multiple organ failure	9	17	—

* $P = .04$ for comparison between control and treatment groups.
(Courtesy of Hayes MA, Timmins AC, Yau EHS, et al: N *Engl J Med* 330:1717–1722, 1994.)

not reach the levels cited, the patients were randomized to treatment with dobutamine, 5–200 µg/kg/min, or to the control group, which received dobutamine only if the cardiac index was less than 2.8 L/min/m².

Results.—One hundred nine patients were studied (table). Nine patients were not randomized because fluid resuscitation achieved the therapeutic goals. Fifty patients were randomized to the treatment group and 50 were randomized to the control group. For cardiac index and oxygen delivery, the 48-hour incremental area under the curve was significantly higher in the treatment group than in the control group. There was no significant difference between the 2 groups in oxygen consumption. All 9 patients who were not randomized survived their hospital stay. Fifty-four percent of the treatment group died in the hospital compared with 34% of the control group.

Conclusion.—When admitted to the ICU, critically ill patients who have had adequate volume replacement and have sufficient perfusion pressure do not benefit from the use of dobutamine to reach target values for cardiac index, oxygen delivery, and oxygen consumption.

A Randomized Clinical Trial of the Effect of Deliberate Perioperative Increase of Oxygen Delivery on Mortality in High-Risk Surgical Patients

Boyd O, Grounds RM, Bennett ED (St George's Hosp, London)
JAMA 270:2699–2707, 1993   101-95-22–9

Background.—Safety concerns persist about perioperative hemodynamic management to increase cardiac output and oxygen delivery. The effect of goal-directed therapy on mortality and morbidity in high-risk surgical patients was evaluated.

Methods.—Fifty-three patients underwent a perioperative protocol that included a deliberate increase of oxygen delivery index exceeding 600 mL/min/m² using dopexamine hydrochloride infusion; 54 patients

Treatment Goals	
Variable	**Goal**
For Both Study Groups	
Mean arterial pressure, mm Hg	80-110
Pulmonary arterial occlusion pressure, mm Hg	12-14
Arterial oxygen saturation, %	>94
Hemoglobin, g/L	>120
Urine output, mL/kg per h	>0.5
Additional for Protocol Patients	
Oxygen delivery index, mL/min per m²	>600

(Courtesy of Boyd O, Grounds RM, Bennett ED: *JAMA* 270:2699–2707, 1993.)

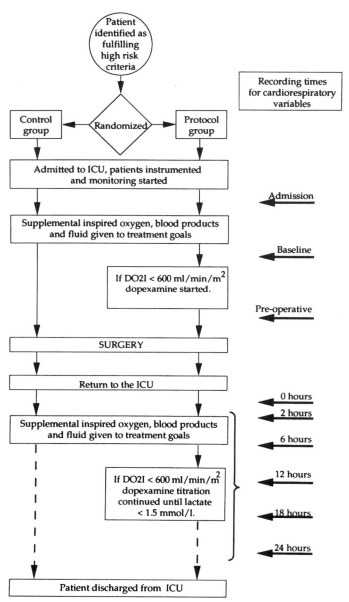

Fig 22–5.—Diagnostic representation of trial regimen and data recording times. *Abbreviation:* DO2I, oxygen delivery index. (Courtesy of Boyd O, Grounds RM, Bennett ED: *JAMA* 270:2699–2707, 1993.)

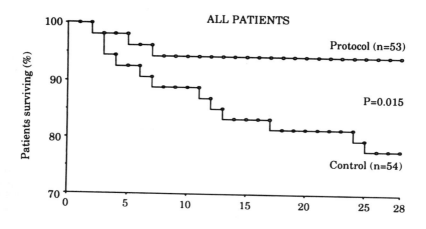

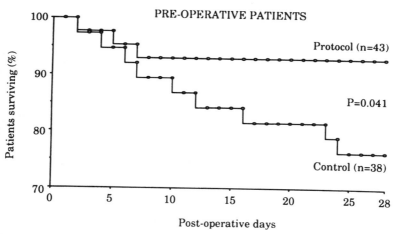

Post-operative days

Fig 22–6.—Survival curves for protocol and control groups for all patients and for patients preoperatively allocated to the study. (Courtesy of Boyd O, Grounds RM, Bennett ED: *JAMA* 270:2699–2707, 1993.)

served as controls. Mortality and complications were assessed during the subsequent 28 days.

Results.—Goal-directed therapy reduced mortality in the protocol group to 5.7%, a rate that was significantly lower than that of controls, 22.2%, and the 25% to 40% mortality rates demonstrated in similar groups of high-risk patients. Patients who had previous abdominal surgery demonstrated the greatest difference in mortality: no protocol patients vs. 25% of control patients. Ten percent of protocol patients and 21% of controls died after vascular surgery. Protocol patients had significantly fewer complications per patient. Among survivors, there was a trent toward a shorter median hospital and ICU stays in the protocol group (Figs 22–5 and 22–6, table).

Conclusion.—Increasing perioperative oxygen delivery with dopexamine hydrochloride significantly reduces mortality and morbidity in high-risk surgical patients.

▶ It has been suggested that in certain critical states, such as adult respiratory distress syndrome (ARDS) and sepsis syndrome, oxygen consumption ($\dot{V}O_2$) appears to be dependent on the rate of oxygen delivery ($\dot{D}O_2$). This pathologic supply dependency of oxygen consumption is thought to indicate an oxygen debt. The ability to increase $\dot{D}O_2$ to a point where $\dot{V}O_2$ plateaus may correspond to relief from this occult oxygen debt. However, previous studies measured $\dot{V}O_2$ indirectly using the Fick equation and thereby called into question whether supply dependency is a true clinical finding or simply an inherent coupling error that results from calculating both $\dot{V}O_2$ and $\dot{D}O_2$ from the same set of thermodilution-derived variables.

In the Hayes study (Abstract 101-95-22–8), increasing $\dot{D}O_2$ to 600 mL/min/m² with high-dose dobutamine (in association with norepinephrine and low-dose dopamine) failed to improve outcome. Indeed, the treatment group had a higher mortality, suggesting a dobutamine-induced maldistribution of blood flow within the microcirculation. As was seen in another study, predicting the individual response to dobutamine was difficult (1), although in general it appears that this type of therapy during the later stages of ARDS or sepsis is of little benefit and may be detrimental.

The results of the Boyd study (Abstract 101-95-22–9) tend to refute these data by showing an improved survival rate in patients who are treated preoperatively with dopexamine for high-risk surgery. The difference in outcomes may be related to the difference between dopexamine and dobutamine, the earlier institution of treatment, and the lower severity of illness in this presurgical group.

Both studies show that if supraphysiologic $\dot{D}O_2$ and $\dot{V}O_2$ can be achieved, either with IV fluids or pharmacologically, then survival rates can be improved.

Economically speaking, these concepts are similar to a variable-rate mortgage, because as interest rates rise ($\dot{V}O_2$), so too must the mortgage payment ($\dot{D}O_2$). However, by prepaying the mortgage (with IV fluids, dobutamine, or dopexamine), it may be possible to lower the oxygen debt.—D.M. Rothenberg, M.D.

Reference

1. Krachman SL, et al: *Intensive Care Med* 20:130, 1994.

Hemodynamic Effects of Manual Hyperinflation in Critically Ill Mechanically Ventilated Patients

Singer M, Vermaat J, Hall G, Latter G, Patel M (Bloomsbury Inst, London; Univ College London)
Chest 106:1182–1187, 1994

101-95-22–10

Background.—It has been suggested that manually inflating a patient's lungs to tidal volumes 50% greater than those delivered by ventilation will help mobilize secretions, prevent atelectasis, and promote oxygenation. Hyperinflation can potentially lead to hemodynamic instability, increase intracranial pressure, or produce barotrauma. Most physical therapists recommend a 3-phase process of slow inspiration, an inspiratory hold of 1–2 seconds, and then a rapid release of the bag.

Objective and Methods.—The effects of manual hyperinflation of the lungs were studied in 18 patients who were receiving mechanical ventilation and were normovolemic and hemodynamically stable. The patients were disconnected from the ventilator for 6 manual hyperinflations, increasing the tidal volume by 50%. Aortic blood flow was estimated by esophageal Doppler ultrasonography. Cardiorespiratory measurements were made at 5-minute intervals after reconnecting the patient to the ventilator.

Results.—In only 10 of 20 attempts did the tidal volume increase by more than 50% of the ventilator-set level. The highest tidal volumes exceeded 2 L, and the highest peak inspiratory pressure recorded was 60 mm Hg. Baseline hemodynamics did not predict the effects of hyperinflation, but during hyperinflation, the cardiac output decreased more, and for a longer time, in patients in whom the tidal volume increased more than 50% (Fig 22–7).

Conclusion.—Manual hyperinflation of the lungs can lead to significant hemodynamic changes in patients receiving mechanical ventilatory assistance.

▶ As a form of chest physiotherapy, manual hyperinflation fails to achieve its effects and may cause detrimental hemodynamic changes. I see no reason to encourage this practice.—D.M. Rothenberg, M.D.

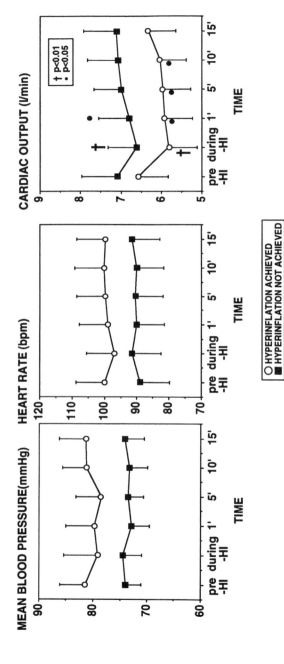

Fig 22-7.—Hemodynamic changes with hyperinflation. (Courtesy of Singer M, Vermaat J, Hall G, et al: *Chest* 106:1182–1187, 1994.)

Therapeutic Efficacy of Tirilazad in Experimental Multiple Cerebral Emboli: A Randomized, Controlled Trial

Clark WM, Hotan T, Lauten JD, Coull BM (Oregon Health Sciences Univ, Portland)

Crit Care Med 22:1161–1166, 1994

101-95-22-11

Background.—The effect of free oxygen radicals in augmenting lipid peroxidation appears to be a promotion of tissue injury during cerebral ischemia. Tirilazad mesylate is a 21-aminosteroid that strongly inhibits this effect of oxygen free radicals. Benefit has been confirmed in experimental models of transient focal and global cerebral ischemia. The drug seems to have few or no physiologic or behavioral side effects.

Study Plan.—The functional effects of tirilazad were examined in a rabbit model of microembolic cerebral ischemia. Multiple emboli were produced with microspheres. Pretreated animals received IV tirilazad mesylate, 3 mg/kg, 5 minutes before embolization, followed by 3 doses of tirilazad mesylate, 1.5 mg/kg, at 5-hour intervals. Other animals received tirilazad 30 minutes after embolization. The adherence of neutrophils to the basement membrane protein laminin was determined.

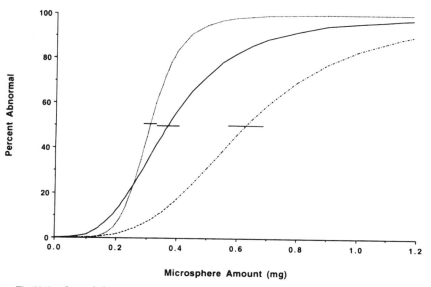

Fig 22–8.—Quantal dose-response curves for tirilazad pretreatment (*broken line*), post-treatment (*heavy line*), and control (*light line*) groups in the rabbit multiple cerebral embolism model: calculated percentage of animals expected to be abnormal vs. weight of injected microspheres in the brain. The effective stroke dose (*midpoint of curve*) is the calculated average quantity of microspheres that is expected to produce impairment in 50% of the animals in the group. The *error bar* shows the standard error of the effective stroke dose. (Courtesy of Clark WM, Hotan T, Lauten JD, et al: *Crit Care Med* 22:1161–1166, 1994.)

Results.—Pretreatment with tirilazad significantly reduced neurologic deficits, but treatment after embolization was ineffective (Fig 22–8). Tirilazad administration also decreased the postischemic increase in neutrophil adhesion observed in control animals.

Conclusion.—Pretreatment with tirilazad significantly improved the neurologic outcome in this rabbit model of multiple cerebral microembolism. This approach might prove helpful in clinical settings where there is a high risk of cerebral embolism.

The Effect of Tirilazad Mesylate (U74006F) on Cerebral Oxygen Consumption, and Reactivity of Cerebral Blood Flow to Carbon Dioxide in Healthy Volunteers

Skovgaard Olsen K, Videbaek C, Agerlin N, Krøll M, Bøge-Rasmussen T, Paulson OB, Gjerris F (Univ of Copenhagen)
Anesthesiology 79:666–671, 1993   101-95-22–12

Background.—The 21-aminosteroids are a family of compounds that inhibit lipid peroxidation in cells. The first in the series to be tested, tirilazad mesylate (U74006F), exerts this effect by scavenging lipid free radicals. It also stabilizes the injured cell membrane by blocking the release of free arachidonic acid. As a result, it may have value in treating cerebral ischemia and vasospasm.

Objective and Methods.—The effects of tirilazad mesylate on cerebral blood flow (CBF), oxygen metabolism, and the reactivity of CBF to changes in blood gas tension were studied in 16 healthy young men, half of whom received an infusion of tirilazad mesylate, 1.5 mg/kg, over a 10-minute period. The controls received the citrate vehicle. A double-blind design was used. Regional CBF was estimated by the radioxenon inhalation technique as the arterial carbon dioxide (CO_2) tension was reduced by hyperventilation and increased by inhaling a mixture of air and CO_2. The absolute regional CBF was determined by single-photon emission CT.

Results.—Neither CBF nor the cerebral metabolic rate of oxygen changed after tirilazad infusion, and there were no changes in the mean arterial blood pressure, pulse rate, or partial pressure of CO_2 in arterial blood. The tirilazad-treated patients and placebo recipients showed no significant differences in CO_2 reactivity before or after the infusion.

Conclusion.—Infusion of tirilazad mesylate did not alter CBF, cerebral oxygen consumption, or cerebrovascular reactivity to CO_2 in normal controls, but the results are not necessarily applicable to patients who have a CNS injury or ischemic cerebrovascular disease.

▶ Pretreatment with tirilazad may protect the brain from microemboli during carotid or open heart surgery. It can also be used to mitigate vasospasm without increasing intracranial pressure in the setting of an aneurysm-induced subarachnoid hemorrhage. The potential benefits of this lipid peroxidase inhibitor would be enormous if future studies show clinical efficacy without untoward side effects.—D.M. Rothenberg, M.D.

Effect of Postoperative Low-Dose Dopamine on Renal Function After Elective Major Vascular Surgery

Baldwin L, Henderson A, Hickman P (Princess Alexandra Hosp, Woolloongabba, Brisbane, Queensland, Australia)
Ann Intern Med 120:744–747, 1994   101-95-22–13

Introduction.—The effect on renal function of postoperative low-dose dopamine in patients who are volume-repleted after elective vascular abdominal surgery was determined. The adverse effects of dopamine have included arrhythmias, depression of respiratory drive, increased intrapulmonary shunt, myocardial ischemia in patients with obstructive coronary artery disease, and increased pulmonary wedge pressure.

Methods.—The 5-day analysis divided 37 patients who were having elective repair of an abdominal aortic aneurysm or having aortobifemoral grafting into 2 groups: 18 received a low-dose infusion of dopamine, 3 µg/kg/min, in saline and 19 received placebo. All patients were given crystalloid to maintain a urine flow of more than 1 mL/kg/hr during the first 24 hours after surgery. Plasma creatinine levels, urea levels, and creatinine clearance were measured before surgery and 24 hours and 5 days after surgery.

Results.—One patient from the placebo group and 3 from the dopamine group had myocardial infarctions; 2 from the dopamine group died. The mean fluid requirements were slightly less in the first 24 hours in those in the dopamine group, whereas the mean urine volumes were slightly higher. There was no statistical difference in plasma creatinine levels. Preoperative and 5-day plasma urea levels were not statistically different. At 24 hours, a small decrease in urea levels was noted in both groups. The preoperative creatinine clearance in the placebo group was 18% lower than in the dopamine group. By 24 hours, it increased in both groups. By the fifth day it had decreased to baseline level in the dopamine group, although the increase was sustained in the placebo group.

Conclusion.—Low-dose dopamine offers no advantage to euvolemic patients after elective abdominal aortic surgery, suggesting that generous fluid replacement alone is as effective as fluid combined with low-dose dopamine. Nevertheless, the trend indicates that the addition of dopamine might enable production of more urine per unit of fluid infused, supporting the view that dopamine has a mild diuretic effect, which could be deleterious to hypovolemic patients. Hypovolemia should be excluded before using dopamine in oliguric patients. Patients with acute oliguric renal failure were not included in this study, so results cannot be extrapolated for treating this condition.

▶ In this study, low-dose dopamine (LDD) was used postoperatively in patients who underwent abdominal aortic surgery to assess its effect on renal function in patients without evidence of preoperative renal insufficiency. These results are similar to those reported in a study involving patients who received LDD during cardiopulmonary bypass that was critiqued in the 1994 YEAR BOOK (Abstract 101-94-12-5). Once again I must conclude that the lack of efficacy of LDD was related to the lack of need. I seriously doubt that I can show an improvement in myocardial function in patients who are given nitroglycerin who have clinically insignificant coronary artery disease. Therefore, should I conclude that nitroglycerin would not protect the patient who *does* have significant coronary artery disease?

Finally, I must profess my ignorance as to why the authors set a goal of maintaining a urine output of 1–1.5 mL/kg/hr. Is this supposed to be a sign of adequate intravascular volume, or does this so-called good urine imply a lower risk of renal failure? To my knowledge, neither correlates. The suppositions that a low urine volume can cause renal failure, as opposed to it potentially being a manifestation of renal failure, and that merely making urine appear will prevent this occurrence have no basis in science.—D.M. Rothenberg, M.D.

The Contrasting Effects of Dopamine and Norepinephrine on Systemic and Splanchnic Oxygen Utilization in Hyperdynamic Sepsis
Marik PE, Mohedin M (Detroit Receiving Hosp; Wayne State Univ, Detroit)
JAMA 272:1354–1357, 1994   101-95-22–14

Background.—Many patients with sepsis continue to be hypotensive and exhibit poor tissue oxygen utilization, even after adequate fluid resuscitation. Many consider dopamine to be the best choice in this setting; however, it may augment splanchnic oxygen needs. Norepinephrine might exert more desirable action on splanchnic microcapillary flow and tissue oxygen utilization, but it has not been widely used because of fear of excessive vasoconstriction.

Patients.—The short-term hemodynamic and metabolic effects of infused dopamine and norepinephrine were compared in 20 patients with hyperdynamic sepsis. All had a cardiac index greater than 3.2 L/min^{-1}/m^{-2} and either a mean arterial pressure (MAP) less than 60 mm Hg or a systemic vascular resistance index less than 1,200 dynes/sec/cm^{-5}/m^{-2}.

Methods.—After fluids were given to achieve a pulmonary capillary wedge pessure greater than 12 mm Hg, each of the vasoactive agents was titrated over a period of 20 minutes to elevate the MAP to greater than 75 mm Hg. The dose of dopamine was also adjusted to keep the

Hemodynamic and Oxygenation Data

	Norepinephrine (n=10)			Dopamine (n=10)			Changes at 3 Hours, P*
	Baseline	3 Hours	P	Baseline	3 Hours	P	
Heart rate, beats/min	105±5	102±3	.20	121±4	139±3	.001	.002
Mean arterial pressure, mm Hg	65±4	87±4	<.001	63±2	87±3	<.001	.60
Mean pulmonary arterial pressure, mm Hg	27±3	31±2	.03	29±2	34±3	.005	.70
Pulmonary capillary wedge pressure, mm Hg	15±1	16±1	.20	15±1	16±1	.10	.70
Cardiac index, $L \cdot min^{-1} \cdot m^{-2}$	4.2±0.5	4.7±0.4	.01	4.2±0.4	5.3±0.7	.008	.05
Right ventricular ejection fraction	28.6±3.2	31.1±3.0	.008	28.4±3.4	33.3±3.71	.02	.50
Left ventricular stroke work index	29±4	44±7	.007	25±4	37±5	<.001	.50
Systemic vascular resistance index, $dyne \cdot s \cdot cm^{-5} \cdot m^{-2}$	1110±109	1405±107	.005	1035±77	1221±130	.10	.60
Oxygen delivery index, $mL \cdot min^{-1} \cdot m^{-2}$	498±77	569±68	.02	573±54	703±89	.02	.20
Oxygen consumption index, $mL \cdot min^{-1} \cdot m^{-2}$	145±21	162±22	.05	183±29	221±38	.001	.20
Intramucosal pH	7.16±0.07	7.23±0.07	.008	7.24±0.04	7.18±0.05	.001	<.001
Lactate, mmol/L	1.8±0.5	1.9±0.43	.60	2.2±0.4	2.1±0.4	.02	.60

Note: Values are mean ± standard error of the mean.
* Difference between the 3-hour values of dopamine and norepinephrine correcting for baseline values.
(Courtesy of Marik PE, Mohedin M: *JAMA* 272:1354–1357, 1994.)

pulse rate less than 150 beats per minute. The mean infusion rate was dopamine, 26 μg/kg/min, and norepinephrine, .18 μg/kg/min.

Results.—Dopamine infusion increased the MAP by 38%, mainly by an increase in the cardiac index (table). Norepinephrine increased the MAP by 33%, chiefly through an increase in systemic vascular resistance. Oxygen delivery and oxygen consumption increased in both groups. The gastric mucosal pH increased significantly in patients who were given norepinephrine, but it decreased significantly in those given dopamine.

Conclusion.—Infused dopamine may adversely affect the balance between splanchnic oxygen delivery and utilization in hyperdynamic patients with sepsis. By contrast, norepinephrine may improve splanchnic oxygen utilization.

▶ It is apparent from this well-designed clinical study that measurements of oxygen delivery and oxygen uptake must be interpreted in conjunction with indices of tissue oxygenation, for example, gastric intramucosal pH (pH_i). The decrease in pH_i in the high-dose dopamine group suggested an increase in splanchnic oxygen debt, possibly as a result of a redistribution of blood flow away from gut mucosa. (This theory may also apply to patients who had poor outcomes after high-dose dobutamine [Abstract 101-95-22–8].) Long-term outcome studies are now required to validate these preliminary data.—D.M. Rothenberg, M.D.

Continuous Intravenous Infusions of Lorazepam Versus Midazolam for Sedation During Mechanical Ventilatory Support: A Prospective, Randomized Study
Pohlman AS, Simpson KP, Hall JB (Univ of Chicago)
Crit Care Med 22:1241–1247, 1994   101-95-22–15

Introduction.—For most critically ill patients receiving life support measures, sedation is ultimately required to ensure comfort, optimal management, and safety. The use of continuous IV infusions of lorazepam was compared with use of midazolam for sedation in the ICU.

Treatment.—Twenty adult patients in the medical ICU who were receiving mechanical ventilatory support required benzodiazepines by continuous infusion for control of agitation syndromes. A standardized protocol was adopted for titrating the infusions. For lorazepam, an IV bolus load of 2 mg and an initial infusion of 1 mg/hr were required with assessment of the adequacy of sedation every 30 minutes, an administration of repeat boluses of 2 mg, and an increase in the infusion rate of 1 mg/hr until adequate sedation was achieved. For midazolam, a bolus load of 3 mg and infusion at 2 mg/hr were required, with assessment of adequacy sedation every 15 minutes, administration of repeat boluses of 3 mg, and increases in the infusion rate of 2 mg/hr until adequate seda-

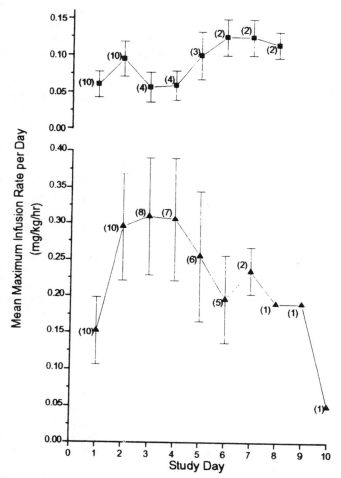

Fig 22–9.—Top, mean maximum infusion rate per day (mg/kg/hr) for lorazepam; **bottom,** mean maximum infusion rate per day (mg/kg/hr) for midazolam. *Error bars* indicate standard deviation. *Numbers* in *parentheses* represent the number of patients completing that day of study. Note the relatively high doses of both agents required for sedation in this patient group. (Courtesy of Pohlman AS, Simpson KP, Hall JB: *Crit Care Med* 22:1241–1247, 1994.)

tion was achieved. The infusion rate was adjusted to maintain sedation at Ramsay's sedation level 2 or 3.

Results.—Ten patients received lorazepam and 10 received midazolam; both groups had similar demographics, Acute Physiology and Chronic Health Evaluation II scores, ICU admission diagnoses, underlying disease processes, and supplemental analgesic administration. The mean time to achieve initial adequate sedation did not differ significantly for lorazepam (124 minutes) and midazolam (105 minutes), and the mean infusion rate at the point of initial sedation was lorazepam, .06

mg/kg/hr, and midazolam, .15 mg/kg/hr. The infusion rates were quite large for the entire study period, with maximum and mean infusion rates of .1 and .06 mg/kg/hr, respectively, for lorazepam, and .29 and .24 mg/kg/hr, respectively, for midazolam (Fig 22–9). The number of infusion rate adjustments per day was 1.9 mg/kg/hr for lorazepam and 3.6 mg/kg/hr for midazolam. Among survivors, the mean to return to baseline mental status after discontinuing the benzodiazepene infusion was 261 minutes for lorazepam and 1,815 minutes for midazolam. All 7 patients who received lorazepam and returned to baseline mental status did so in fewer than 12 hours, whereas half the patients who received midazolam who returned to baseline mental status did so only after more than 24 hours of discontinuing the infusions. Furthermore, a large volume of fluid was required to deliver the benzodiazepines by infusion: 1.2 L for lorazepam (maximum, 2.4 L) and 1.3 L for midazolam (maximum, 3.6 L).

Conclusion.—For both lorazepam and midazolam, the time required to achieve adequate sedation was longer than desired, and the dose necessary to maintain sedation was larger than expected. Furthermore, the time needed to awaken after discontinuation of the infusion occasionally may be delayed for more than 24 hours, and large volumes of fluid are required for continuous infusion of these benzodiazepines. These findings cast doubt on whether the routine use of continuous infusions of benzodiazepines to sedate patients in the ICU is optimal.

▶ This study highlights the difficulties encountered when attempting to sedate the critically ill patient. Altered volumes of distribution and clearances, and concomitant drug therapy all contribute to pronounced patient variations in response to sedative therapy. The more frequent use of shorter-acting benzodiazepines in the ICU appeared to be an ideal alternative to longer-acting agents such as diazepam. However, this study and another recent study that compared the duration of action of diazepam and midazolam in the ICU (1) would question this popular belief. Therefore, the quest continues for the ideal sedative agent or "cocktail" that will ensure patient comfort, lessen anxiety, lower oxygen consumption, prevent increases in intracranial pressure, decrease the work of breathing and the risk of barotrauma, as well as minimize the use of neuromuscular-blocking agents.—D.M. Rothenberg, M.D.

Reference

1. Ariano RE: *Crit Care Med* 22:1492, 1994.

A Double-Blind, Prospective, Randomized Trial of Ketoconazole, a Thromboxane Synthetase Inhibitor, in the Prophylaxis of the Adult

Respiratory Distress Syndrome
Yu M, Tomasa G (Univ of Hawaii, Honolulu)
Crit Care Med 21:1635-1642, 1993   101-95-22-16

Introduction.—A prospective, randomized, double-blind, placebo-controlled study was planned to determine whether the thromboxane-A_2 synthetase inhibitor ketoconazole could reduce the risk of adult respiratory distress syndrome (ARDS) developing in patients with sepsis if it was given within 24 hours after diagnosis.

Study Plan.—Fifty-four consecutive patients who were admitted to a surgical ICU with a diagnosis of sepsis received either 400 mg of ketoconazole or a placebo, either orally or by a nasogastric tube, within 24 hours.

Results.—The frequency of ARDS was reduced from 64% in the placebo recipients to 15% in the ketoconazole-treated patients. Active treatment was also associated with a decline in mortality from 39% to 15%. The time in the ICU and the need for ventilatory assistance were not significantly different in the treatment and placebo groups.

Conclusion.—Administration of a single dose of ketoconazole early in the course of sepsis may prevent the development of ARDS and lower the mortality rate in high-risk patients with sepsis. Problems with gastrointestinal absorption might be circumvented by using miconazole, an IV antifungal imidazole.

▶ Ketoconazole, by decreasing the thromboxane-A_2 concentration, may improve outcome in patients who have sepsis syndrome by preventing ARDS. Other studies have also shown that this drug inhibits the 5-lipoxygenase metabolites of arachidonic acid. These effects may also indirectly block the adverse effects of tumor necrosis factor and interleukin-1, cytokines that contribute to the inflammatory response of sepsis.

The risks of ketoconazole therapy appear to be minimal, with no cases of hepatotoxicity being reported here or in other similar studies. In this regard, oral ketoconazole therapy may offer select patients a simple, relatively nontoxic and inexpensive form of therapy to prevent the development of ARDS from sepsis.—D.M. Rothenberg, M.D.

Risk Factors for Gastrointestinal Bleeding in Critically Ill Patients
Cook DJ, for the Canadian Critical Care Trials Group (McMaster Univ, Hamilton, Ontario, Canada)
N Engl J Med 330:377-381, 1994   101-95-22-17

Introduction.—Measures that are used to prevent stress ulceration are expensive and may themselves have adverse effects. The frequency of significant gastrointestinal bleeding in patients who are critically ill was investigated in a prospective study.

Study Population.—Consecutive patients older than age 16 years who, in a 1-year period, were admitted to 4 university-affiliated medical-surgical ICUs were studied. Patients with evidence of upper gastrointestinal bleeding were excluded. Physicians were asked to withhold measures intended to prevent stress ulceration except in patients with a head or burn injury, organ transplant recipients, and those who had received a diagnosis of peptic ulcer or gastritis in the past 6 weeks.

Findings.—Of the 2,252 eligible patients, 674 received prophylaxis against stress ulceration. Their Acute Physiology and Chronic Health Evaluation (APACHE) scores were comparable to those of the other patients, although their mortality was higher (16.8% vs. 6.7%). The 100 overt bleeding episodes included 33 that were clinically significant, which was defined as overt bleeding with either hemodynamic compromise or a need for transfusion. On multiple regression analysis, the only independent risk factors for clinically important bleeding were prolonged respiratory failure necessitating mechanical ventilation and coagulopathy. Only 2 affected patients lacked both risk factors. Bleeding occurred in 3.4% of the patients who were given prophylaxis and in .6% of the others.

Conclusion.—Because relatively few patients who are critically ill have clinically important gastrointestinal bleeding, prophylaxis against stress ulceration may be withheld unless coagulopathy is present or the patient requires mechanical ventilation.

Prophylaxis for Stress-Related Gastric Hemorrhage in the Medical Intensive Care Unit

Ben-Menachem T, Fogel R, Patel RV, Touchette M, Zarowitz BJ, Hadzijahic N, Divine G, Verter J, Bresalier RS (Henry Ford Hosp and Health Sciences Ctr, Detroit)
Ann Intern Med 121:568–575, 1994   101-95-22–18

Introduction.—Measures designed to prevent stress-related gastrointestinal bleeding were evaluated in 300 patients who were admitted to the medical ICU of a university-affiliated teaching hospital during a 10-month period. Only adults who were expected to stay for at least 24 hours and who had no evidence of gastrointestinal bleeding at the outset were included.

Management.—Patients were randomly assigned to receive 1 g of sucralfate orally or by nasogastric tube at 6-hour intervals, or to receive 300 mg of IV cimetidine followed by infusion of a dose adjusted to the creatinine clearance or to a control group. The controls received no antacids, sucralfate, omeprazole, or H_2-receptor antagonists.

Results.—Risk factors were equally distributed except for a higher rate of sepsis syndrome in patients who were assigned to receive cimetidine (table). About one third of each group had 3 or more risk factors (Fig

Distribution of Risk Factors for Stress-Related Hemorrhage

Variable	Control (n = 100)	Sucralfate (n = 100)	Cimetidine (n = 100)
		n/n	
Respiratory failure	60/65	64/72	66/76
Shock	18/28	14/24	23/35
Sepsis syndrome	15/17	15/20	26/27
Cardiac arrest	0/6	1/6	1/6
Acute hepatocellular impairment	7/13	6/13	8/20
Acute renal failure	13/14	13/15	19/22
Coagulopathy	16/20	14/17	21/22
Pancreatitis	1/1	1/2	2/2
High-dose corticosteroids	17/41	19/40	15/37
Systemic anticoagulation	0/3	0/3	0/4

Note: Values represent the number of patients with a specific risk factor. Baseline denotes risk factors present at time of admission to the ICU. Total represents risk factors present at admission to the ICU or anytime during the ICU stay. There were no statistically significant differences among the 3 groups ($P > .05$), except sepsis syndrome at baseline ($P = .04$).
(Courtesy of Ben-Menachem T, Fogel R, Patel RV, et al: Ann Intern Med 121:568–575, 1994.)

22–10). Stress-related hemorrhage occurred in 5% of the actively treated patients and in 6% of the controls. Those in the groups did not differ significantly with respect to transfusion requirements, duration of stay in the medical ICU, or mortality. Nosocomial pneumonia was diagnosed in

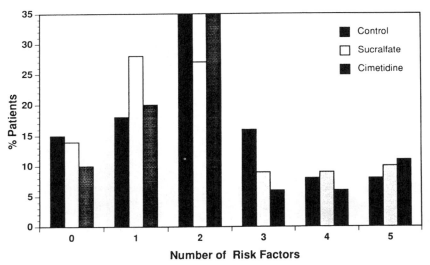

Fig 22–10.—Number of risk factors per patient in the 3 study groups. There were no statistically significant differences in the distributions among the 3 groups (P > .05). (Courtesy of Ben-Menachem T, Fogel R, Patel RV, et al: *Ann Intern Med* 121:568–575, 1994.)

6% of controls, 12% of those given sucralfate, and 13% of cimetidine recipients.

Conclusion.—Prophylactic administration of cimetidine or sucralfate failed to lessen the risk of stress-related gastrointestinal bleeding in medical ICU patients. Nosocomial pneumonia was more prevalent in patients who were given prophylaxis, although not significantly so. Routine prophylaxis is not warranted in this setting.

The Virtual Absence of Stress-Ulceration Related Bleeding in ICU Patients Receiving Prolonged Mechanical Ventilation Without any Prophylaxis: A Prospective Cohort Study
Zandstra DF, Stoutenbeek CP (Onze Lieve Vrouwe Gasthuis, Amsterdam)
Intensive Care Med 20:335–340, 1994   101-95-22–19

Background.—The incidence of stress ulceration–related bleeding (SURB) in ICU patients appears to have decreased in the past decade. Some studies find prophylactic therapy against SURB to be effective, whereas other investigators attribute the change to improvement in the general support of the ICU patient. To determine whether specific preventive medication is needed, the incidence of SURB was examined in a cohort of ICU patients receiving prolonged mechanical ventilation (MV) without any prophylaxis.

Methods.—All patients who were admitted within the course of 1 year to a medical surgical ICU who required MV for more than 48 hours were studied. Patients with SURB on admission were not eligible, but stress ulceration prophylactic medications were continued in patients who were already receiving these medications. A total risk score (TRS) was calculated for each patient based on the number of risk factors for SURB. All patients received clinical treatment, including maintenance of adequate tissue perfusion, infection prevention, and suppression of generalized inflammatory reactions by steroids.

Results.—The 167 study patients who were not receiving any prophylaxis accounted for a total of 1,753 days on MV and 2,182 treatment days in the ICU. The mean TRS for SURB (Tryba score) was 38. Common primary risk factors were severe bacterial infection, cardiogenic shock, and respiratory insufficiency. There were 100 patients older than 65 years of age and 15 patients who required more than 21 days on MV. Stress ulceration–related bleeding developed in only 1 patient who did not receive prophylaxis, or .6% of the cohort. This patient had a TRS of 66 with 4 primary risk factors. Of the 17 patients who were already receiving prophylaxis, 2 had SURB.

Conclusion.—Only 1 of 167 ICU patients who received prolonged MV and had a high risk for SURB had this complication, despite the lack of specific prophylaxis. Integral ICU therapies, including aggressive shock resuscitation, selective decontamination of the digestive tract, and suppression of inflammatory response, are factors that probably contributed to the low incidence of SURB.

▶ Much to the delight of the pharmaceutical industry, H_2-antagonists have for years been routinely employed for all critically ill patients who are presumed to be at risk for SURB. However, taken collectively, the results of these 3 large, prospective studies (Abstracts 101-95-22–17 to 101-95-22–19) should herald the end of this practice.

Cook and co-workers (Abstract 101-95-22–17) identify 2 independent risk factors for critically ill patients to have SURB develop (i.e., prolonged mechanical ventilation [longer than 48 hours] and coagulopathy), as they support the contention that patients with head trauma, extensive burns, organ transplants, or preexisting peptic ulcer disease/gastritis are also at risk for upper gastrointestinal bleeding. Another recent study (1) would also support the use of SURB prophylaxis in patients with respiratory failure.

Another interesting aspect of these 3 studies was their failure to show that endogenous corticosteroid use was a risk factor for SURB. Indeed, Zandstra and Stoutenbeek's study (Abstract 101-95-22–19) would support its use to limit SURB.

Finally, in addition to decreasing cost, limiting the use of stress ulcer prophylaxis could decrease the incidence of ventilation-associated pneumonia, a controversial, although important, concern.—D.M. Rothenberg, M.D.

Reference

1. Eddleston JM, et al: *Crit Care Med* 22:1949, 1994.

Safety and Efficacy of Intravenous Carbicarb® in Patients Undergoing Surgery: Comparison With Sodium Bicarbonate in the Treatment of Mild Metabolic Acidosis

Leung JM, for the SPI Research Group (Univ of California, San Francisco; Univ of Massachusetts, Worcester)
Crit Care Med 22:1540–1549, 1994   101-95-22-20

Introduction.—There is debate as to the use of sodium bicarbonate in the treatment of patients with metabolic acidosis. Sodium bicarbonate has potential deleterious effects on organ function that are related in part to carbon dioxide (CO_2) production resulting from sodium bicarbonate breakdown, which leads to the development of other buffers to optimize arterial pH without producing CO_2. One of these is Carbicarb, an equimolar solution of sodium bicarbonate and sodium carbonate. Because it does not increase blood CO_2 concentrations to the same extent as sodium bicarbonate, it may be a better treatment for metabolic acidosis. The safety and efficacy of IV Carbicarb and sodium bicarbonate were compared in patients who had metabolic acidosis develop during major surgery.

Methods.—The double-blind, randomized, prospective, multicenter study included 36 patients who had metabolic acidosis during cardiac or major noncardiac surgery. All had arterial and pulmonary artery catheters

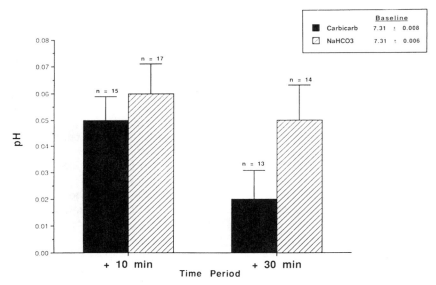

Fig 22–11.—Changes in arterial pH from baseline to 10 and 30 minutes after treatment with either Carbicarb (*black columns*, baseline pH 7.31 ± .008) or sodium bicarbonate (NaHCO3) (*slashed columns*, baseline pH 7.31 ± .006). The increases in pH from baseline to 10 minutes after treatment were statistically significant (P = .0001) for both groups. (Courtesy of Leung JM, for the SPI Research Group: *Crit Care Med* 22:1540–1549, 1994.)

in place for other indications. Metabolic acidosis was defined as a serum pH of less than 7.35 and a greater than 3-mmol decrease in serum bicarbonate concentration. Patients were assigned to receive either sodium bicarbonate or Carbicarb, 1 mEq of sodium per mL, with the dose calculated as base deficit (mEq/L) $\times$ .2 $\times$ kg of body weight = mEq sodium. Arterial blood gases and hemodynamic variables were measured before and as long as 60 minutes after drug administration. Drug administration was repeated if necessary at 10 and/or 20 minutes. The fractional inspiration of oxygen and the level of anesthesia were kept constant at all times. Anesthesia was with high-dose opioids in the cardiac surgical patients and with isoflurane in the noncardiac patients. None of the patients were taking any drugs that might affect hemodynamic status.

Results.—Both groups had significant increases in mean pH by 10 minutes after treatment, with no differences in the number of doses required to correct acidosis (Fig 22–11). The mean cardiac output increased in a subset of the Carbicarb group and decreased in a subset of the sodium bicarbonate group. The mean pulmonary artery occlusion pressure decreased to a greater extent and systemic lactate utilization increased to a greater extent with Carbicarb. None of the patients was withdrawn from the study because of adverse reactions.

Conclusion.—Carbicarb and sodium bicarbonate treatment yield similar increases in arterial pH for nonhypoxic patients with mild metabolic acidosis. More studies are needed to determine whether Carbicarb treatment of moderate-to-severe metabolic acidosis might yield better hemodynamic improvements for patients with cardiac dysfunction or hypoxia.

▶ In the 1994 YEAR BOOK (Abstract 101-94-21–6), a study described the use of Carbicarb in dogs. Carbicarb was shown to be beneficial in mitigating the hemodynamic and pH changes associated with hypoxic lactic acidosis. In the clinical study by Leung and associates, a statistical significance was achieved in a pH change after 10 minutes after a Carbicarb or sodium bicarbonate injection, although little if any clinical significance can be inferred from these findings. Also, the type of metabolic acidosis was never really elucidated, and the reader was left to assume that the acidosis being treated was a lactic acidosis. The increase in systemic utilization of lactate does not necessarily equate with clinically significant lactate levels (e.g., greater than 2.5 mmol/L). (Although the electrolye and lactate levels were measured, these data were not presented.)

Previous studies (1), including one from the SPI Research Group (2), suggest that most of these surgical patients have a hyperchloremic metabolic acidosis that is probably the result of the infusion of isotonic saline or Ringer's lactate during surgery. These solutions are unphysiologic relative to their chloride concentrations, and delivery of such solutions to the proximal tubule of the kidney can lead to a decrease in hydrogen ion secretion and therefore bicarbonate wasting. Limiting the amount of these high chloride–containing solutions by infusing 100 mL of sodium bicarbonate in 900 mL of

.45 saline should mitigate the degree of hyperchloremic metabolic acidosis.—D.M. Rothenberg, M.D.

References

1. Ernest D, et al: *Crit Care Med* 20:52, 1992.
2. Mark NH, et al: *Crit Care Med* 21:659, 1993.

Accuracy of Portable Chest Radiography in the Critical Care Setting: Diagnosis of Pneumonia Based on Quantitative Cultures Obtained From Protected Brush Catheter
Lefcoe MS, Fox GA, Leasa DJ, Sparrow RK, McCormack DG (Victoria Hosp Corp, London, Ont, Canada; Univ Hosp, London, Ont, Canada)
Chest 105:885–887, 1994   101-95-22–21

Introduction.—Accurate diagnosis of pneumonia in patients who are critically ill is difficult. The value of chest radiography in such instances has not been established because there is no gold standard. However, evidence suggests that the use of quantitative cultures obtained from protected brush catheter (PBC) specimens is a highly sensitive, specific test for diagnosing nosocomial pneumonia. The diagnostic accuracy of the portable chest radiograph was investigated using quantitative bacteriologic cultures as the gold standard.

Methods.—Sixty-six supine portable chest radiographs were obtained on the day of bronchoscopy from 62 patients in the critical care unit who were thought to have pneumonia. Two radiologists examined the radiographs in a blinded manner. Chest radiographic scores were then compared with quantitative culture results obtained from PBC specimens.

Findings.—For the 2 observers, the respective sensitivities of the chest radiograph for predicting the presence of positive culture findings were .6 and .64, specificities were .29 and .27, overall agreement was .41 and .41, positive predictive values were .34 and .35, and negative predictive values were .55 and .55. Interobserver reproducibility was marginal.

Conclusion.—When quantitative cultures obtained from PBC specimens were used as the gold standard, portable chest radiography in the critical care setting was not an accurate predictor of the presence of pneumonia. Because of the problems inherent in interpreting portable chest radiographs in the critical care setting, these findings were not surprising.

▶ The routine use of daily portable chest x-rays (CXRs) was reviewed in the 1994 YEAR BOOK (Abstract 101-94-23–6) and the lack of efficacy and major cost were noted. In this new article by Lefcoe et al., the simple finding of infiltrate on a portable CXR in association with a prevalent tracheal aspirate failed to correlate with the quantitative cultures obtained from a PBC during bronchoscopy. It is likely that by including the finding of an air bronchogram on CXR, a better correlation between the CXR and cultures might be achieved. Nonetheless, it is interesting to speculate just how often antibiotics are inappropriately prescribed for presumed pneumonia only to promote a more virulent and often resistant disease.—D.M. Rothenberg, M.D.

Effects of Insertion Depth and Use of the Sidearm of the Introducer Sheath of Pulmonary Artery Catheters in Cardiac Output Measurement

Boyd O, Mackay CJ, Newman P, Bennett ED, Grounds RM (St George's Hosp, London, England)
Crit Care Med 22:1132–1135, 1994   101-95-22–22

Introduction.—In a prospective, randomized, crossover study in a general ICU, the effects of various insertion depths and sidearm functions of the introducer sheath of pulmonary artery flotation catheters (Fig 22–12) on cardiac output measurements were investigated. A change in the sidearm function has been known to change the measurement of cardiac output, but the magnitude of the changes has never been measured. Error-induced variations in cardiac output measurements could lead to inappropriate treatment.

Methods.—In 10 patients with a pulmonary artery flotation catheter placed in the right internal jugular vein, cardiac output was measured at 3 insertion depths, 40-, 45-, and 50-cm of the pulmonary artery, each with a different rate of flow (open, 20 drops per minute, and closed) of .9% saline to the introducer sheath (Fig 23–13). The thermodilution technique was used to measure cardiac output. In the closed position, a maximum resistance to backflow of injectate fluid up the sidearm was evident. When fully open, with the saline running into the patient to equilibrate at the level of the central venous pressure, a minimum degree of resistance to injectate backflow was seen.

Results.—Significant differences occurred in cardiac output measured under the various conditions. Two new, potentially important errors in cardiac output measurement by thermodilution have been identified: position of the sidearm and the level of insertion depth. Cardiac output was higher with a 40-cm insertion depth than with the 45- or 50-cm level, and it also was higher with the sidearm open than with it closed or at the 20 drops per minute position. With the open sidearm position and a 40-cm insertion depth, measurements of cardiac output were 23% higher than those obtained with the closed sidearm position at a 50-cm level.

Conclusion.—In measurement of cardiac output with thermodilution, the errors highlighted here must be avoided. The cold saline injection port of the pulmonary artery catheter must be downstream of the introducer sheath, and the sidearm must be closed. Catheter placement can be achieved by using a vein that is more distal to the heart as the inser-

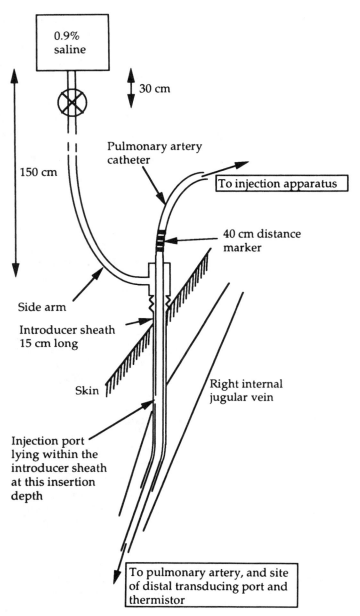

0.9% saline

30 cm

150 cm

Pulmonary artery catheter

To injection apparatus

40 cm distance marker

Side arm

Introducer sheath 15 cm long

Skin

Right internal jugular vein

Injection port lying within the introducer sheath at this insertion depth

To pulmonary artery, and site of distal transducing port and thermistor

Fig 22–12.—Schematic diagram of a pulmonary artery flotation catheter and introducer sheath. (Courtesy of Boyd O, Mackay CJ, Newman P, et al: *Crit Care Med* 22:1132–1135, 1994.)

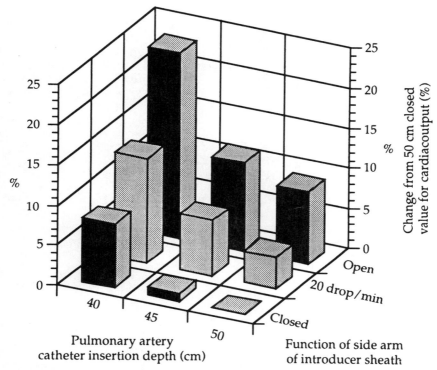

Fig 22–13.—Mean percentage difference in measured cardiac output for varying insertion depths and sidearm function of the pulmonary artery catheter, compared with cardiac output measured by thermodilution when the catheter is inserted to 50 cm and the introducer sidearm is closed. (Courtesy of Boyd O, Mackay CJ, Newman P, et al: *Crit Care Med* 22:1132–1135, 1994.)

tion site, allowing the catheter to be advanced further before wedging is obtained.

Effect of Injectate Temperature and Thermistor Position on Reproducibility of Thermodilution Cardiac Output Determinations
Williams JE Jr, Pfau SE, Deckelbaum LI (Yale Univ, West Haven, Conn; West Haven Veterans Affairs Med Ctr, Conn)
Chest 106:895–898, 1994   101-95-22–23

Background.—Serial estimates of cardiac output by the thermodilution technique often vary to a degree that limits their usefulness; the best measurement technique is uncertain. One potential error is a loss of the thermal indicator between the injection port and the thermistor. Warming the injectate as it passes through the catheter has been reported to cause a 3% to 12% overestimation of cardiac output.

Means for Cardiac Output (CO), Coefficient of Variation (CV), and Standard Error of the Mean Percentage (SEM%) for Each Experimental Condition of Thermodilution Cardiac Output Determination

Condition	CO ± SD, L/min	SEM%†	CV, %†	95% Confidence Interval for CV, %†
ICE EXT	6.29 ± 0.63*	5.86	10.16	8.8-16.8
ICE RA	5.15 ± 0.27	3.17	5.49	4.3-6.7
RM EXT	5.41 ± 0.72	7.42	12.85	6.4-14.0
RM RA	5.23 ± 0.42	4.53	7.85	6.1%-9.7

* P < .05 compared with all other conditions.
† P < .05 between thermistor locations.
Abbreviations: ICE, iced injectate; EXT, external; RA, right atrium; RM, room temperature.
(Courtesy of Williams JE Jr, Pfau SE, Deckelbaum LI: *Chest* 106:895–898, 1994.)

Objective and Methods.—Data from 20 consecutive, hemodynamically stable patients undergoing right and left heart catheterization were used to determine the effects of injectate temperature and thermistor position on the reproducibility of cardiac output estimates. Either an external thermistor in the injectate reservoir or an internal thermistor at the right atrial injectate port was used. Measurements were made with injectates of 5% aqueous dextrose that was either iced (0–5°C) or at room temperature (20–25°C).

Results.—Estimated cardiac output was significantly higher using an iced injectate and an external reservoir thermistor than with any other combination (table). More reproducible measurements were obtained when the injectate temperature was measured at the right atrial port than when it was measured in the reservoir.

Conclusion.—Thermodilution cardiac output is best measured using an iced injectate and an internal right atrial thermistor. The most reproducible measurements are obtained when the injectate temperature is measured at the right atrial port rather than externally at the injectate reservoir.

Assessment of Critical Care Nurses' Knowledge of the Pulmonary Artery Catheter

Iberti TJ, Daily EK, Leibowitz AB, Schecter CB, Fischer EP, Silverstein JH, Pulmonary Artery Catheter Study Group (Mount Sinai Med Ctr, New York; Univ of Arkansas, Little Rock; Bronx-VA Hosp, New York; et al)
Crit Care Med 22:1674–1678, 1994   101-95-22–24

Purpose.—Pulmonary artery catheters are widely used in patients who are seriously ill, despite the scarcity of data documenting their positive effects on morbidity and mortality. Some studies have described poor outcomes, but it is unclear whether this is the result of the device itself

	Subtest Scores		
Subtest Content	No. of Items	Score (mean ± SD)	%
Complications	3	1.9 ± 0.9	63.3
Waveforms	6	3.7 ± 1.5	52.2
Patient management	5	2.5 ± 1.3	50.5
Insertion technique	4	2.0 ± 1.1	49.9
Positioning	4	1.9 ± 1.2	47.2
Physiology	5	2.0 ± 1.2	40.9
Calculations	6	2.3 ± 1.4	38.6

(Courtesy of Iberti TJ, Daily EK, Leibowitz AB, et al: *Crit Care Med* 22:1674–1678, 1994.)

or of poor use. A previous survey of physicians found significant variations in their understanding of the safe and effective use of pulmonary artery catheters. In many centers, the critical care nurse is responsible for acquiring data from pulmonary artery catheters and for making subsequent management decisions. Critical care nurses were surveyed to determine how well they understood the use of the pulmonary artery catheter.

Methods.—A 37-question multiple-choice examination regarding the use of the pulmonary artery catheter was given to about 500 critical care nurses who were attending the National Teaching Institute Conference of the American Association of Critical Care Nurses. All attendees were preregistered for a workshop on hemodynamics. Responses were obtained from 216 nurses, for a response rate of 43%.

Results.—The mean test score was 16.5, or 48.5%. Univariate analyses showed that test scores were significantly associated with years of critical care experience, certification as a critical care registered nurse, responsibility for catheter repositioning and manipulation, frequency of catheter use, and self-assessed adequacy of knowledge. The nurses scored best on questions pertaining to the practical aspects of catheter use and lowest on those relating to physiologic interpretation and calculation of hemodynamic variables (table).

Conclusion.—Like physicians, critical care nurses vary widely in their understanding of the use of the pulmonary artery catheter. Nurses appear to have a lower overall understanding of this device, although they scored somewhat better on questions concerning the interpretation of pulmonary artery occlusion pressure. Nurses responsible for catheter positioning or repositioning had higher test scores; clinical nurse specialists had scores similar to those of physicians. The results suggest that critical care registered nurse certification might be considered as a requirement for using the pulmonary artery catheter. Until measures are taken to ensure the safe and effective use of this device, effective observational studies of its clinical value will be impossible to perform.

▶ The first 2 articles (Abstracts 101-95-22–22 and 101-95-22–23) highlight the tremendous potential for discrepancies in measuring thermodilution cardiac outputs using a pulmonary artery catheter (PAC). Taken together, the validity of previous studies that used this measurement to assess either efficacy of treatment or overall outcome must be questioned. Finally, when the third article (Abstract 101-95-22–24), as well as a similar study that documented the inability of physicians to interpret PAC data, are taken into consideration (1), there is reason to wonder whether anyone could interpret them even if the measurements were reliable!—D.M. Rothenberg, M.D.

Reference

1. Iberti TJ, et al: *JAMA* 264:2928, 1990.

Early, Routine Paralysis for Intracranial Pressure Control in Severe Head Injury: Is it Necessary?

Hsiang JK, Chestnut RM, Crisp CB, Klauber MR, Blunt BA, Marshall LF (Univ of Calif, San Diego and San Francisco)
Crit Care Med 22:1471–1476, 1994

101-95-22–25

Purpose.—Neuromuscular blocking agents are routinely used to manage intracranial pressure in patients with severe head injuries. Early pharmacologic paralysis facilitates transportation and allows mechanical hyperventilation of patients with head injuries who may be difficult to transport. This analysis was done because no clinical studies had examined the efficacy of this policy.

Methods.—Between 1984 and 1987, the Traumatic Coma Data Bank collected data on 1,030 patients with severe head injuries. Only patients with a Glasgow Coma Score of 8 or less were included in the analysis. Of 514 patients who met the inclusion criteria, 239 received early pharmacologic paralysis for the management of intracranial pressure. Early pharmacologic paralysis was defined as starting during the first ICU shift or 6 hours or fewer into the second shift and lasting at least 12 hours. The remaining 275 patients did not fulfill these criteria.

Results.—The mean ICU stay was 7.76 days for the paralyzed patients and 4.84 for the nonparalyzed patients, a statistically significant difference. In addition, pneumonia in paralyzed patients occurred significantly more often than in patients who were not paralyzed. The final Glasgow Outcome scores for survivors with good and moderate outcomes did not differ significantly between the 2 groups.

Conclusion.—Early, routine, long-term use of neuromuscular blocking agents in patients with severe head injuries prolongs the ICU stay, does not improve the overall outcome, and increases the frequency of extracranial complications associated with their use.

▶ This nonrandomized, retrospective study concluded that the use of neuromuscular blocking agents in the traumatic head-injured patient led to a prolonged ICU stay, a higher incidence of pneumonia, and a worse neurologic outcome. Regardless of whether these findings are valid, it is clear that many patients received neuromuscular blocking agents for inappropriate reasons. The use of muscle relaxants to lower intracranial pressure in head-injured patients is based on decreasing respiratory muscle activity and intrathoracic pressure, thereby allowing for improved cerebral venous outflow. However, in this study, 34% of group 1 patients and 15% of the subgroup of patients in group 2 who received such agents late but for longer than 12 hours did so without evidence of severe intracranial hypertension. This article once again calls into question the cavalier use of neuromuscular blocking agents in the critically ill patient.—D.M. Rothenberg, M.D.

Efficiency of Bronchodilator Aerosol Delivery to the Lungs From the Metered Dose Inhaler in Mechanically Ventilated Patients: A Study Comparing Four Different Actuator Devices

Fuller HD, Dolovich MB, Turpie FH, Newhouse MT (St Joseph's Hosp, Hamilton, Ont, Canada; McMaster Univ, Hamilton, Ont, Canada)

Chest 105:214–218, 1994   101-95-22-26

Introduction.—Therapeutic aerosol from a metered-dose inhaler (MDI) used in conjunction with an accessory chamber has been found to deliver the dose to the lung more efficiently than that from a jet nebulizer. However, the optimal size of the chamber for patients receiving assisted mechanical ventilation has not been determined. Several MDI actuator devices without chambers have recently been developed for use by patients who are ventilated. The effectiveness of 4 different actuator devices was compared in adult patients receiving ventilation.

Methods.—Forty-eight patients receiving assisted ventilation who required inhaled bronchodilators were randomly assigned to receive radioactively labeled fenoterol aerosol from an MDI by either a cylindrical

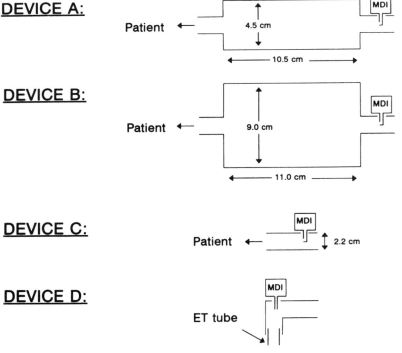

Fig 22–14.—Diagrams of the 4 devices for providing aerosol therapy to patients receiving ventilation. (Courtesy of Fuller HD, Dolovich MB, Turpie FH, et al: *Chest* 105:214–218, 1994.)

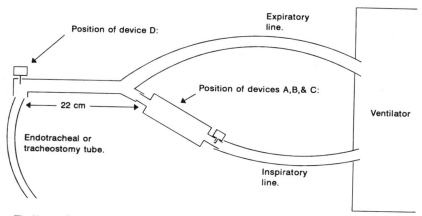

Fig 22–15.—Diagram of ventilator circuit with endotracheal tube, showing the position of the 4 MDI accessory devices. For each patient, only 1 device was present. (Courtesy of Fuller HD, Dolovich MB, Turpie FH, et al: *Chest* 105:214–218, 1994.)

chamber with a volume of 167 mL (device A), a cylindrical chamber with a volume of 700 mL (device B), a device without a chamber that affects MDI actuation from the inspiratory ventilator tubing (device C), or a device without a chamber that allows MDI actuation into the endotracheal or tracheostomy tube (device D) (Fig 22–14). Device D was positioned on the end of the tube (Fig 22–15). A mobile gamma camera measured lung deposition in 1-minute images, beginning 2 breaths after each aerosol puff.

Results.—There were significant differences in deposition with the nonchamber device attached to the ventilator tubing and each of the chamber devices. There were no other statistically significant differences between paired groups. The percentage of the dose delivered to the lungs was 5.53 with device A, 6.33 with device B, 1.67 with device C, and 3.89 with device D.

Discussion.—Among the devices positioned on the inspiratory ventilator line, those with a chamber delivered significantly higher doses of aerosol to the lung than did devices without a chamber. The inline connector for device C was relatively long and narrow, which may have reduced the available MDI dose by limiting the generation of particulate from the aerosol and allowing a loss of some aerosol through the outer envelope of the MDI flume. If 10% deposition, as occurs in spontaneously breathing patients, is considered optimal, then the optimal dose for patients who are ventilated would be 2 puffs with each of the chambered devices, 6 puffs with the nonchambered inline device, and 3 puffs for the nonchambered endotracheal device. Definitive determination of the optimal dose will require dose-response trials.

▶ Inhaled β_2-agonists are standard agents for patients who have broncho-spasm develop while being mechanically ventilated. This form of therapy has tended to replace the use of such IV bronchodilators as aminophylline, pri-marily because of concern over the drug's low therapeutic index. However, frequent dosing intervals or a continuous mode of inhalation therapy are of-ten required to treat the patient with persistent wheezing.

Often neglected in assessing the impact of inhalational treatment is the way in which the drug is deposited in the terminal bronchioles. All too often I have witnessed anesthetists administering 1–2 puffs of a β_2-agonist directly into the endotracheal tube via the handheld nebulizer for the spontaneously breathing patient. The resultant failure to reverse the bronchospasm is then often equated with lack of drug efficacy.

This study and other similar ones suggest that at least 50% more drug is needed to achieve a clinical benefit in a patient requiring mechanical ventila-tion compared with a spontaneously breathing patient. Metered-dose inhal-ers with actuator devices should be used in the ICU, and smaller inline de-vices should be avoided. In the operating room, the proximal end-tidal carbon dioxide port can be adapted to fit an MDI by luer-locking the cutoff end of a 5-cc syringe. By increasing the number of puffs administered (usually 3–6), a clinical effect is more likely to be achieved.—D.M. Rothenberg, M.D.

Closed Versus Open Endotracheal Suctioning: Costs and Physiologic Consequences
Johnson KL, Kearney PA, Johnson SB, Niblett JB, MacMillan NL, McClain RE (Univ of Kentucky, Lexington)
Crit Care Med 22:658–666, 1994   101-95-22–27

Introduction.—Endotracheal suctioning is routinely performed to clear secretions from the intubated patient's airway. However, there can be complications, such as decreased systemic venous oxygenation, al-tered mean arterial pressure, cardiac dysrhythmia, and nosocomial pneu-monia. Techniques such as open suctioning have been developed to pre-vent these complications. Open suctioning uses hyperinflation and hyperoxygenation breaths before and after suctioning, whereas closed suctioning uses a closed-circuit multiple-use ventilator catheter. The safety and costs of these 2 methods were evaluated in a prospective, ran-domized study.

Methods.—The patient's bedside nurse determined the type of suc-tioning to be performed. Data were collected on mean arterial pressure, heart rate and rhythm, arterial oxygen saturation, and systemic venous oxygen saturation in patients before suctioning, immediately after hyper-oxygenation and suctioning, and 30 seconds after suctioning (to detect hypoxia). The patients were monitored to detect nosocomial pneumo-

Comparison of Mean Arterial Pressure, Heart Rate, Arterial Oxygen Saturation, and Systemic Venous Oxygen (O_2) Saturation in Open and Closed Endotracheal Suctioning

Variable	After Hyperoxygenation		After Suctioning		30 Secs Postsuctioning	
	Open ET Suctioning*	Closed ET Suctioning†	Open ET Suctioning*	Closed ET Suctioning†	Open ET Suctioning*	Closed ET Suctioning†
Mean arterial pressure (mm Hg)‡	92 ± 1.7	89 ± 1.3	102 ± 1.7	97 ± 1.4	101 ± 1.6	96 ± 1.2
% Change from baseline	+4	+0.7	+17.3	+8.6	+15.2	+7.9
p value	.0019		.0001		.0001	
Heart rate (beats/min)‡	108 ± 1.8	98 ± 1.4	114 ± 1.7	102 ± 1.5	112 ± 1.8	100 ± 1.4
% Change from baseline	+2.2	+1.2	+8.1	5.7	+6.4	+3.6
p value	>.05		>.05		.0209	
Arterial O_2 saturation (%)‡	97 ± 0.3	98 ± 0.2	96 ± .04	99 ± 0.1	97 ± 0.1	99 ± 0.1
% Change from baseline	-0.4	+0.3	-1.1	+1.6	-0.4	+1.4
p value	.0005		.0001		.0001	
Systemic venous O_2 saturation (%)‡	72 ± 0.9	73 ± 0.9	67 ± 1.5	74 ± 0.9	67 ± 1.4	75 ± 1.0
% Change from baseline	-0.9	+0.3	-8.3	+2.1	-7.7	+3.4
p value	.0268		.0001		.0001	

* Based on 127 suctioning observations.
† Based on 149 suctioning observations.
‡ Values are means ± standard error of the mean.
Abbreviation: ET, endotracheal tube.
(Courtesy of Johnson KL, Kearney PA, Johnson SB, et al: *Crit Care Med* 22:658–666, 1994.)

nia. Patient costs and the nursing time required for each suctioning method were compared.

Results.—Open endotracheal suctioning was performed 127 times on 19 patients; closed endotracheal suctioning was performed 149 times on 16 patients. There were significant differences between the 2 groups in postprocedure physiologic complications (table). The mean arterial pressure increased less with closed suctioning than with open suctioning. Heart rate was comparable in the 2 groups until 30 seconds after suctioning, when the patients who underwent open suctioning demonstrated persistent tachycardia and had more evidence of dysrhythmia, particularly immediately after suctioning. The mean arterial and systemic venous oxygen saturation decreased after open suctioning and increased after closed suctioning. Ten of the patients who underwent open suctioning and 8 of the patients who underwent closed suctioning had pneumonia. Closed suctioning was performed at a lower patient cost and required less nursing time than open suctioning.

Conclusion.—Closed endotracheal suctioning resulted in less physiologic disturbances, did not increase the risk of nosocomial pneumonia, and was more cost-effective than open endotracheal suctioning.

▶ The experience of endotracheal suctioning was once described to me by a colleague who had required prolonged mechanical ventilation as if someone were passing a "red-hot branding iron into his trachea" (1). This intensivist was driven to forcibly restrain the nurse from performing what appeared to be a routine and innocuous task. Unfortunately, most caregivers who perform this procedure have little regard for the physiologic and psychological consequences that may ensue.

Whether closed-suction techniques are superior to open suctioning in terms of reducing morbidity from myocardial ischemia, increased intracranial pressure, or simply patient discomfort, cannot be answered by this study. A future study that assesses these outcome variables as well as the effects of both techniques in the *same* patients would be insightful.—D.M. Rothenberg, M.D.

Reference

1. Hayden WR: *Crit Care Clin* 10:651, 1994.

Noninvasive Nasal Mask Ventilation for Acute Respiratory Failure: Institution of a New Therapeutic Technology for Routine Use
Pennock BE, Crawshaw L, Kaplan PD (Allegheny Gen Hosp, Pittsburgh, Pa)
Chest 105:441–444, 1994   101-95-22–28

Introduction.—The successful use of a simplified pressure support ventilator (BiPAP) with a nasal mask for ventilatory assistance in patients with acute respiratory failure has been reported. In the hands of research personnel, this device avoided intubation and mechanical ventilation in 76% of patients. The successful transfer of this technology to the usual care providers has now been achieved.

Patients and Methods.—The study participants were 110 patients with acute respiratory failure who were being considered for intubation and mechanical ventilation; those with hemodynamic instability or multiple system failure were excluded. Ninety percent of the patients were in the medical or surgical ICU, and 80% were surgical patients, most of whom had hypercapnic failure. All patients received noninvasive ventilatory support with BiPAP applied by nasal mask. In the initial special-care phase, 31 patients received this intervention from members of the research team. In the next phase, the transition phase, BiPAP administration was transferred from the research team to the usual care providers. In the final, usual-care phase, the usual care providers administered the intervention almost exclusively.

Results.—Therapy was successful, that is, it allowed withdrawal of BiPAP for at least 48 hours, in 76% of patients in the special care and transition phases. In 110 recorded trials in all 3 phases, the success rate was 80%. In most cases, ventilator settings did not have to be readjusted from the initial choice of spontaneous ventilation, with an expiratory positive airway pressure of 5 cm H_2O and an inspiratory positive airway pressure of 10 cm H_2O. This mode of ventilation was not accepted by about 10% of patients. In the transition phase, the urgency of this type of support was stressed. Caregivers had to be made to understand that the mask seal did not have to be absolutely tight and that a looser mask was essential for patient comfort and support. Fifteen to 30 minutes of provider-patient interaction time was needed before the patient became comfortable with assisted ventilation.

Conclusion.—Administration of noninvasive mechanical ventilation for patients with acute respiratory failure has been transferred successfully from the research setting to the routine hospital setting. It is important for the caregivers to understand and accept the urgency of this type of support, the concept of leak tolerance, and the importance of a comfortable fit.

▶ The use of BiPAP ventilatory support is gaining popularity as a means to avoid endotracheal intubation for impending respiratory failure caused by atelectasis, pulmonary edema, or muscle fatigue. By delivering both inspiratory pressure support ventilation and positive end-expiratory pressure, the work of breathing and oxygenation is improved with this system. The ability of BiPAP to be easily applied without the need for a tight seal lends itself to patient tolerance and acceptance. Despite the need for careful monitoring during the initial application, this technique may offer the clinician an alternative for patients in whom respiratory failure is not immediately life-threatening.—D.M. Rothenberg, M.D.

Resuscitation of Multiple Trauma and Head Injury: Role of Crystalloid Fluids and Inotropes

Scalea TM, Maltz S, Yelon J, Trooskin SZ, Duncan AO, Sclafani SJA (State Univ of New York, Brooklyn)
Crit Care Med 22:1610–1615, 1994   101-95-22–29

Introduction.—Intracranial hypertension is a potentially devastating consequence of head injury. For head-injured patients with multiple injuries, the volume of fluid needed for resuscitation and its effects on intracranial pressure are important areas of concern. There are few data to guide therapy for these patients. The hemodynamic responses to multiple trauma with head injury were reviewed in 30 patients, including the effects of resuscitation on intracranial pressure and neurologic performance.

Methods.—The patients all had multisystem injuries, including a nonoperative closed-head injury requiring intracranial pressure monitoring (Table 1). Invasive hemodynamic monitoring was performed in all patients, serum lactate concentrations and oxygen transport variables were measured every 4 hours, and intracranial pressures and vital signs were recorded every hour (Table 2). Management was aimed at reaching a non–flow-dependent state of oxygen consumption and a normal serum lactate concentration.

Findings.—Eighty percent of patients had evidence of inadequate tissue perfusion, although they were normotensive and had neither tachycardia nor oliguria. Of the rest, only half had an adequate response to volume. The other half showed no increase in intracranial pressure, even with volume loading and inotropic agents and nowithstanding the presence of severe intracranial injuries and a potential alteration of the blood-brain barrier, as shown by CT. Six of the patients died; cardiac output and systemic oxygen delivery were significantly lower in nonsurvivors than in survivors. Oxygen consumption decreased despite therapy in the nonsurvivors, but it increased significantly in the survivors. On linear

TABLE 1.—Results of Initial Head CT Scan

Result	Number (n = 30)
Subarachnoid hemorrhage	11
Normal	9
Edema	6
Skull fracture	7
Contusion	3
Intraventricular bleeding	3

TABLE 2.—Hemodynamic Variables of All Patients

Variable	Initial	Stabilized	p Value
MAP (mm Hg)	99 ± 3.6	103 ± 2.1	NS
HR (beats/min)	109 ± 3.2	99 ± 3.4	.038
PAOP (mm Hg)	11 ± 0.9	13 ± 0.8	NS
CVP (mm Hg)	9 ± 0.9	10 ± 0.8	NS
SVR (dyne·sec/cm⁵)	1059 ± 80	861 ± 54	.021
Hgb (g/dL)	12.1 ± 0.4	11.1 ± 0.3	.028
Lactate (mmol/L)	5.2 ± 0.8	2.1 ± 0.3	.024
Cardiac output (L/min)	5.6 ± 0.5	7.6 ± 0.4	.020
$S\bar{v}_{O_2}$ (%)	70 ± 2.5	77 ± 1.2	.013
P_{O_2} (torr)	101 ± 8.6	111 ± 8.1	NS
(kPa)	13.4 ± 1.2	14.8 ± 1.1	NS
$\dot{V}_{O_2}$ (mL/min)	346 ± 35	426 ± 44	.015
ICP (mm Hg)	15 ± 2.7	13 ± 2.4	NS

Note: Initial/optimization; $n = 30$; mean ± standard error of the mean.
Abbreviations: MAP, mean arterial pressure; HR, heart rate; PAOP, pulmonary artery occlusion pressure; CVP, central venous pressure; SVR, systemic vascular resistance; Hgb, hemoglobin; $S\bar{v}_{O_2}$, mixed venous oxygen saturation; P_{O_2}, partial pressure of oxygen; $\dot{V}_{O_2}$, oxygen consumption; ICP, intracranial pressure.
(Courtesy of Scalea TM, Maltz S, Yelon J, et al: Crit Care Med 22:1610–1615, 1994.)

regression analysis, only the lactate concentration correlated significantly with intracranial pressure.

Conclusion.—For patients with multiple injuries, including head injury, volume infusion and vasodilating inotropic agents are safe treatments to support systemic oxygen delivery. Oxygen transport is best monitored invasively. Because the ability to achieve normal lactate values correlates with outcome, and the adequacy of resuscitation can affect neurologic performance, the correlation between intracranial pressure and lactate concentration is expected.

▶ This appears to be another study of pathologic oxygen supply dependency in which increases in oxygen delivery and utilization by IV volume expansion and inotropic support decrease serum lactate and improve survival in the head-injured patient. However, the retrospective, uncontrolled nature of this study does not allow for such conclusions to be substantiated. Whether large volumes of isotonic solutions can be safely used in these patients without the risk of elevating intracranial pressure (ICP) is still controversial. Indeed, the authors fail to cite previous experimental studies that reach the opposite conclusion. Many would suggest that the most ideal volume expander for patients with elevated ICP would be hypertonic saline, because it has been shown to actually decrease ICP as it restores circulating volume (1).—D.M. Rothenberg, M.D.

Reference

1. Freshman SP, et al: *J Trauma* 35:344, 1993.

Adult Respiratory Distress Syndrome Associated With Epidural Fentanyl Infusion

Goetz AM, Rogers PL, Schlichtig R, Muder RR, Diven WF, Prior RB (Univ of Pittsburgh, Pa; Veterans Affairs Med Ctr, Pittsburgh, Pa; Ohio State Univ, Columbus)
Crit Care Med 22:1579–1583, 1994   101-95-22-30

Background.—Six postoperative patients seen in a 6-week period had adult respiratory distress syndrome (ARDS) develop for reasons that were not clear. They were treated in the critical care center of a university-affiliated acute care facility. The patients had abruptly had hypoxemia and diffuse pulmonary infiltration develop 1–4 days after uneventful surgery; 2 of the 6 patients died.

Epidemiologic Investigation.—The study patients were compared with 17 patients who had vascular or thoracic operations in the same period and did not have ARDS develop. In no instance was the severity of hypoxemia explained by a purely cardiogenic cause (Table 1). Cultures were negative for fungi, *Mycobacteria*, and *Legionella*. The only significant association discovered in case-control comparisons was related to the use of analgesics, including parenteral morphine and oral oxycodone/acetaminophen, and of digoxin (Table 2). All 6 patients with ARDS but none of the controls had received fentanyl epidurally. No for-

---

TABLE 1.—Physiologic Variables of Patients With Unexplained Adult Respiratory Distress Syndrome

Pt.	Initial PAOP (mm Hg)	PAOP at 24 hrs (mm Hg)	CI (L/min)	Highest FIO₂	Highest PEEP (cm H₂O)	Highest P(A-a)O₂ (torr)
1	13	20	3.51	0.7	12.5	232 (30.9)
2	13	14	2.16	0.8	15	431 (57.5)
3	12	12	3.04	1.0	20	544 (72.5)
4	9	10	2.95	0.9	12	532 (70.9)
5	16	20	4.01	0.6	10	306 (40.8)
6	12	12	2.04	0.9	12.5	432 (57.6)

Note: Values in parentheses are kPa.
Abbreviations: Pt., patient; *PAOP*, pulmonary artery occlusion pressure; *CI*, cardiac index; *PEEP*, positive end-expiratory pressure; $P(A-a)O_2$, alveolar-arterial oxygen difference.
(Courtesy of Goetz AM, Rogers PL, Schlichtig R, et al: *Crit Care Med* 22:1579–1583, 1994.)

TABLE 2.—Results of Case-Control Study of Adult Respiratory
Distress Syndrome (ARDS)

Factor	ARDS Patients (n = 6)	Control Patients (n = 17)	p Value*
Epidural fentanyl	6	0	.0002
Morphine sulfate	0	10	.04
Oxycodone/acetaminophen	0	13	.007
Digoxin	0	11	.02

* Fisher's exact test, 2-tailed.
(Courtesy of Goetz AM, Rogers PL, Schlichtig R, et al: *Crit Care Med* 22:1579–1583, 1994.)

eign substances were detected in any materials, including urine and serum from the patients.

Control.—No similar outbreaks were known by the Food and Drug Administration or by the manufacturers of fentanyl. Fentanyl had, however, previously been stolen from the institution. After a tamperproof system for delivering parenteral fentanyl was instituted, 1 of 26 consecutive surgical patients had ARDS develop. Subsequently, 2 patients who were given fentanyl epidurally after uneventful vascular operations had ARDS develop for no apparent reason, and, at that time, fentanyl infusion was banned in the ICUs.

Conclusion.—It is possible that fentanyl infusate was removed from its infusion bottle and replaced with another substance. A health care provider was observed removing fentanyl from a bottle at a patient's bedside. If a patient who has been given fentanyl deteriorates unexpectedly, the infusion should be stopped and the possibility of tampering considered.

▶ This article not only highlights the degree to which drug abuse permeates our society, but it also shows the extremes to which people will go to get a "fix." Although the authors' exhaustive *medical* investigation was unable to conclusively prove cause and effect, it was clear that drug-tampering had occurred, despite attempts to secure and monitor access to the fentanyl infusions. What is most distressing about these cases is that the alleged tampering led to the eventual deaths of 2 patients; therefore, it appears that a *criminal* investigation was also in order. Random drug testing of all ICU personnel should have been performed, with anyone who tested positive being considered a potential suspect.—D.M. Rothenberg, M.D.

Diagnosis of Perioperative Myocardial Infarction With Measurement of Cardiac Troponin I

Adams JE III, Sicard GA, Allen BT, Bridwell KH, Lenke LG, Dávila-Román VG, Bodor GS, Ladenson JH, Jaffe AS (Washington Univ, St Louis, Mo; Vanderbilt Univ, Nashville, Tenn)

N Engl J Med 330:670–674, 1994   101-95-22-31

Introduction.—Among patients undergoing noncardiac surgical procedures, perioperative myocardial infarction is a common problem that can be difficult to diagnose. Detection of myocardial infarction in these patients would be facilitated by some serum marker for cardiac injury that was more specific than and just as sensitive as MB creatine kinase. Serum cardiac troponin I was evaluated for this purpose.

Methods.—Ninety-six patients undergoing vascular surgery and 12 undergoing spinal surgery were studied. Before surgery, each patient underwent measurement of MB creatine kinase, total creatine kinase, and cardiac troponin I. Electrocardiograms and 2-dimensional echocardiograms were also obtained. After surgery, blood samples were evaluated every 6 hours and ECGs were evaluated daily, with a second echocardiogram obtained 3 days postoperatively. An echocardiographic finding of a new abnormality in segmental wall motion was considered to indicate a perioperative infarction.

Results.—Based on this criterion, the diagnosis of perioperative myocardial infarction was made in 8 patients. Cardiac troponin I was elevated in all 8 and MB creatine kinase in 6 of 8. Of the remaining 100 patients, none of whom had evidence of perioperative myocardial infarction, 19 had elevated MB creatine kinase values and 1 had a slight elevation in cardiac troponin I (Figs 22–16 and 22–17). Specificities were 99% for cardiac troponin I vs. 81% for MB creatine kinase.

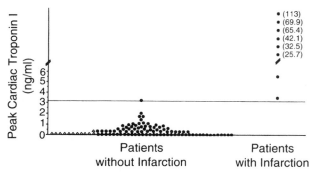

Fig 22–16.—Peak cardiac troponin I mass in patients with and without perioperative myocardial infarction. The upper reference limit for cardiac troponin I mass is 3.1 ng/mL. The *triangles* denote patients undergoing spinal surgery, and the *circles* those undergoing vascular surgery. (Courtesy of Adams JE III, Sicard GA, Allen BT, et al: *N Engl J Med* 330:670–674, 1994.)

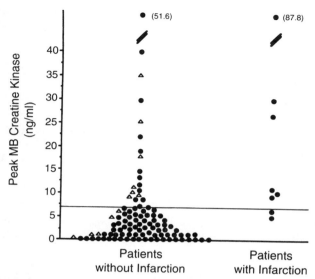

Fig 22–17.—Peak MB creatine kinase mass in patients with and without perioperative myocardial infarction. The upper reference limit for MB creatine kinase mass is 6.7 ng/mL. The *triangles* denote patients undergoing spinal surgery, and the *circles* those undergoing vascular surgery. (Courtesy of Adams JE III, Sicard GA, Allen BT, et al: *N Engl J Med* 330:670–674, 1994.)

Conclusion.—Cardiac troponin I is a sensitive and specific serum marker for perioperative myocardial infarction. Its greater specificity avoids the high false positive diagnostic rate that is observed with MB creatine kinase, and it should be simpler and more cost-effective to use than routine echocardiography.

▶ Defining inclusion criteria for the diagnosis of perioperative myocardial infarction (POMI) by assessing levels of creatine phosphokinase (CPK) MB has been a difficult if not an altogether arbitrary task. Most investigators have designated an absolute CPK-MB of greater than 80 mIU/mL in association with ECG changes as criterion for POMI after coronary artery bypass surgery. This is based primarily on studies in which CPK-MB levels correlate with myocardial infarct scintigraphy.

Unfortunately, CPK-MB can be elevated secondary to noncardiac injury and therefore occasionally be an unreliable indicator of POMI. Intramuscular injection, hypothyroidism, total hip arthroplasty, spinal surgery, and prostate surgery have all been known to lead to a false positive elevation in this isoenzyme. In this regard, cardiac troponin I appears to be a more specific (and still very sensitive) test for detecting cardiac injury in patients with POMI. (Troponin T, another cardiac contractile apparatus protein, is also released into the circulation in the event of myocardial cell injury, and elevated levels have been noted in patients with clinical diagnoses of unstable angina [1].) Although other assays, such as plasma myoglobin levels, have not been successful (because of poor predictability in patients with renal dysfunction), I think that cardiac troponin I, and perhaps troponin T, offer promise as early, accurate markers of POMI.—D.M. Rothenberg, M.D.

Reference

1. Mächler H, et al: *Anesthesiology* 81:1317, 1994.

Adverse Environmental Conditions in the Respiratory and Medical ICU Settings

Meyer TJ, Eveloff SE, Bauer MS, Schwartz WA, Hill NS, Millman RP (Rhode Island Hosp, Providence; VA Hosp, Providence, RI)
Chest 105:1211–1216, 1994   101-95-22–32

Introduction.—Recent studies have suggested that sleep deprivation may adversely affect respiratory muscle function and respiratory center sensitivity to carbon dioxide, which can impair weaning from mechanical ventilation. Normal sleep patterns are often disrupted in the hospital environment, possibly because the normal day/night environmental patterns are disrupted. To study the importance of environmental patterns, light, sound, and interruption rhythms were observed in the hospital.

Methods.—Environmental patterns were observed in a 3-bed medical ICU room, a 3-bed respiratory care unit (BRCU) room, a single RCU (SRCU) room, and a private room (PR). Patient interruptions by doctors, nurses, and respiratory therapists were recorded for a 24-hour period. Light and sound levels were monitored continuously for at least 7

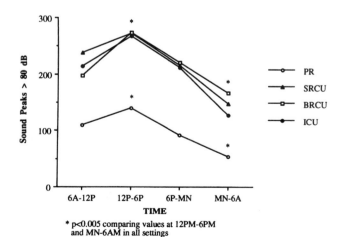

Fig 22–18.—Average number of sound peaks greater than 60 dB for each 6-hour period. *Abbreviations: BRCU,* 3-bed respiratory care unit; *SRCU,* single RCU; *PR,* private room. (Courtesy of Meyer TJ, Eveloff SE, Bauer MS, et al: *Chest* 105:1211–1216, 1994.)

days, and the values recorded at the same time each day were averaged to determine day/night patterns.

Results.—The light levels at night were significantly higher in the BRCU than in the ICU and the PR, and they were slightly higher than in the SRCU. Overall, the sound levels were very high in each of the hospital settings sampled, especially in the ICU, BRCU, and SRCU, although the levels decreased slightly at night. The lowest frequencies of sound bursts greater than 80 dB were recorded in the PR. Overall, the frequencies of sound bursts were highest in the afternoon and lowest at night (Fig 22–18). There were at least hourly interruptions in the ICU during both day and night. There were fewer interruptions in the PR, but no more than 4 hours passed without an interruption in any of the settings.

Discussion.—Although there was a day/night pattern for overall sound level and frequency of loud sound bursts, both were quite high; in the higher care areas, the sound levels were louder than the recommended Environmental Protection Agency values. Studies have shown that although younger patients may adjust their sleep patterns to hospital sound levels over time by increasing their arousal threshold, older patients may become more sensitive to sound levels. In addition, the interruptions were too frequent to allow enough time for condensed sleep. The hospital environment provides significant stimuli that induce sleep fragmentation, which can impair respiratory function.

▶ Am I the only one who still remembers that hospitals used to be considered quiet zones? That sounding one's car horn was strongly discouraged in the vicinity of a hospital? I have noticed over the years that the near-deafening sounds of multiple alarms, overhead pages, and routine everyday conversations during teaching rounds in the ICU have reached a point that often makes it impossible to hear even a bedside presentation. For those who claim that I am the problem and that I have simply become intolerant in my "old age," I offer this and other similar studies to support my contention that the noise level in the ICU is disruptive.

Sleep deprivation is a well-known phenomenon in the ICU (for the patient, not the house officer), and it may lead to muscle fatigue and the inability to wean the patient from mechanical ventilation. Frequent interruption of the patient's sleep cycle is the probable culprit in the development of so-called ICU psychosis. If efforts to ensure noise and light reduction fail, the use of earplugs, as the authors suggest, and perhaps blinders as well may have to become standard issue for all patients.—D.M. Rothenberg, M.D.

Complete Recovery After Prolonged Resuscitation and Cardiopulmonary Bypass for Hyperkalemic Cardiac Arrest

Lee G, Antognini JF, Gronert GA (Sacred Heart Med Ctr, Spokane, Wash; Univ of Calif, Davis)
Anesth Analg 79:172–174, 1994   101-95-22-33

Background.—Numerous episodes of cardiac arrest have been reported in apparently healthy young children after receiving succinylcholine. One girl had hyperkalemic cardiac arrest and underwent 2 hours of CPR and 2½ hours of cardiopulmonary bypass (CPB).

Case Report.—Girl, 11 years, in good health except for recurrent pharyngitis and tonsilitis, was seen for elective tonsillectomy. After induction of general anesthesia, IV succinylcholine, 40 mg, was administered to facilitate tracheal intubation. After intubation, the surgeon had difficulty opening the patient's mouth, her skin color was poor, and her ECG deteriorated, with progression to asystole over approximately 5 minutes. Cardiopulmonary resuscitation was initiated immediately, and she received atropine, bicarbonate, epinephrine, lidocaine, calcium chloride, multiple defibrillation attempts, and external pacing, all without response. Approximately 40 minutes after initiating CPR, her plasma concentration of potassium (K^+) was 10.2 mEq/L, and she was treated with insulin, dextrose, and cation-exchange resin. The repeat concentration of K^+ was 8.5 mEq/L, and the patient's asystole continued, alternating with ventricular fibrillation and runs of ventricular tachycardia that lasted approximately 5 seconds. Intravenous dantrolene, 50 mg, was administered and the patient was transported to a facility capable of performing CPB. Although during transport she had pulmonary edema and her pupils were dilated and minimally reactive, on arrival, successful bypass was instituted and continued for about 2½ hours until she maintained a sinus rhythm. On day 1 after her surgery, her rhabdomyolysis caused a compartment syndrome requiring fasciotomy. Renal failure developed and hemodialysis was required for approximately 6 weeks. The patient also had disseminated intravascular coagulation, requiring multiple units of blood platelets and fresh frozen plasma. A full recovery was eventually achieved without neurologic, pulmonary, muscular, or renal sequelae. An evaluation for malignant hyperthermia was conducted 20 months after this incident, using a muscle biopsy specimen from the right vastus lateralis. Histologic study did not reveal myopathy, although a thorough history revealed that the patient, her father, and 4 of her sisters had muscle cramping after exercise. Resting plasma creatine kinase levels were elevated in all 6, as well as in 2 cousins and 2 half-brothers.

Discussion.—When sudden cardiac arrest occurs in young children after receiving succinylcholine, hyperkalemia must be suspected, electrolytes measured, and treatment initiated. In addition to administering calcium, insulin, glucose, bicarbonate, and a cation-exchange resin, the use of dantrolene is recommended, because the connection between these cases and malignant hyperthermia is unclear. Subclinical myopathy is quite often subsequently demonstrated. Despite a complex postoperative course, this patient survived without sequelae. In similar cases, it is recommended that CPR be continued and CPB initiated when resuscitation is refractory to normal interventions.

▶ This case is extraordinary and worthy of review, if only for the heroic efforts made in resuscitating this child. Based on this case, the authors pose a number of recommendations, including persisting in resuscitation in otherwise young, healthy patients and strong consideration of CPB; treating hyperkalemia with insulin and glucose without concern for hyperglycemia-mediated neurologic injury; using dantrolene if there is a suspicion of malignant hypothermia (MH) as an etiology of the hyperkalemia; and administering inhaled anesthetics cautiously in patients with known non–MH-related myopathies.

In addressing these recommendations, there can be no question that an all-out, lengthy resuscitation, including CPB, is warranted for nonischemic etiologies of cardiac arrest, especially if there is evidence, as in this case, of neurologic function during resuscitation. However, I doubt that centers that do not have CPB capability (e.g., outpatient surgicenters or small community hospitals) will be as fortunate in transporting a patient who is 2 hours into CPR to a center that has such capability.

In treating hyperkalemia with glucose and insulin therapy, the goal is to drive potassium into the cell while buying time for more definitive therapy. However, hyperglycemia (and hyperosmolarity) should not be discounted as a potential risk for exacerbating neurologic injury. This viewpoint may be controversial, as the authors state, but I think that the avoidance of succinylcholine in children and the "cautious" use of inhalational anesthetics in patients with non–MH-related myopathies are more controversial but are nonetheless recommended by the authors.—D.M. Rothenberg, M.D.

23 Pain and Its Management

Pregnancy Enhances the Antinociceptive Effects of Extradural Lignocaine in the Rat
Kaneko M, Saito Y, Kirihara Y, Kosaka Y (Shimane Med Univ, Izumo, Japan)
Br J Anaesth 72:657–661, 1994   101-95-23–1

Introduction.—The dose of local anesthetic required for extradural anesthesia has been shown to be lower in pregnant than in nonpregnant animals. There is no experimental evidence to show that these drugs induce a higher level of analgesia during pregnancy, although most of the applicable research has involved somatic rather than visceral nociception. The influence of pregnancy on the antinociceptive effects of extradurally administered lidocaine was evaluated, using both somatic and visceral noxious stimuli.

Methods.—Tail-flick (TF) latency and colorectal distension (CD) threshold tests, indicators of somatic and visceral nociception, respectively, were measured before conception and at days 7, 14, and 19 of pregnancy in female rats. Lidocaine was administered on days 19, 20, and 21 of pregnancy, at 200, 400, or 800 μg, by a catheter implanted in the lumbar extradural space. Tail-flick and CD tests were performed 8 times over the course of 1 hour; a nonpregnant cohort was used as a control.

Results.—Both TF and CD increased over the course of pregnancy, indicative of a decreased response to somatic and visceral noxious stimuli. Lidocaine caused a dose- and time-dependent increase in TF and CD in both pregnant and nonpregnant animals. The increase in TF and CD produced by 800 μg was similar in the 2 groups, but it was of longer duration in pregnant rats. At 400 μg, TF and CD increases were greater in pregnant than in nonpregnant rats, whereas at 200 μg, only CD was significantly higher in pregnant rats.

Conclusion.—The response to noxious stimuli was decreased during pregnancy in the rat, and pregnant rats were more sensitive to the effects of extradural anesthesia than nonpregnant rats. This effect appears to be more marked for visceral than for somatic nociception.

▶ In the past, most studies of pain have evaluated the response to somatic nociception. This study evaluated both somatic and visceral nociception, using the model for colorectal distention in rats, which was originally described by Ness and Gebhart (1). In this new study, it appeared that epidural lidocaine had a greater effect on visceral nociception than somatic nociception in pregnant rats, which is consistent with the clinical observation that relatively small doses of epidurally administered local anesthetic relieve the pain of cervical dilation during the first stage of labor in pregnant women. However, this study did not provide new information regarding the mechanism for the enhanced efficacy of epidural local anesthetics during pregnancy.—D.H. Chestnut, M.D.

Reference

1. Ness TJ, Gebhart GF: *Brain Res* 450:153, 1988.

Spinal Nitric Oxide Synthesis Inhibition Blocks NMDA-Induced Thermal Hyperalgesia and Produces Antinociception in the Formalin Test in Rats

Malmberg AB, Yaksh TL (Univ of California, San Diego, La Jolla; Sahlgrenska Univ, Göteborg, Sweden)
Pain 54:291–300, 1993   101-95-23–2

Background.—In hyperalgesia, evidence suggests that peripheral afferent stimulation leads to increased excitability of spinal cord neurons and changes in peripheral afferent terminal sensitivity. The role of spinal nitric oxide synthesis was explored in modulating facilitatory states involved in behaviorally defined hyperalgesia generated by protracted afferent input and by spinal N-methyl-D-aspartate (NMDA) receptor activation in unanesthetized rats.

Methods.—Male rats received intrathecal injections of arginine analogues, which are alternate substrates for nitric oxide synthase and thereby inhibit the production of nitric oxide. Motor function, righting, ambulation, catalepsy, and allodynia were assessed. Rats were injected with formalin, and pain-related behavior was examined. Thermal sensitivity was also assessed.

Results.—A dose-dependent stereospecific inhibition of phase 2 of the formalin test (10–60 minutes; median effection dose [ED_{50}], 135 and 246 nmol) was produced by NG-nitro-L-arginine methyl ester (L-NAME) and NG-monomethyl-L-arginine, but with little effect on phase 1 (0–9 minutes; $ED_{50} > 1.1$ μmol). The inhibitory effect of L-NAME was dose-dependently reversed by a 5-minute pretreatment with high doses of L-arginine but not by D-arginine (Fig 23–1). Suppression of the second-phase formalin response by L-NAME was similar, regardless of administration before or after the injection of formalin. Spinal injection of L-NAME, but not NG-nitro-D-arginine methyl ester, blocked thermal hyperalgesia induced by NMDA. L-Arginine but not D-arginine reversed the effect of

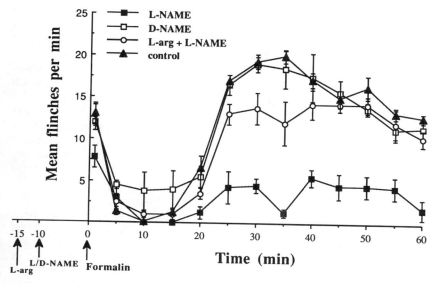

Fig 23–1.—Time-effect curve of intrathecal NG-nitro-L-arginine methyl ester (L-NAME) (370 nmol), D-NAME (3.7 μmol), and L-arginine (4.7 μmol) + L-NAME (370 nmol) on the formalin test. L- and NG-nitro-D-arginine methyl ester (D-NAME) were administered 10 minutes before formalin, and L-arginine was injected 5 minutes before L-NAME. The data are presented as the mean ± standard error of the mean (4–8 rats per line) of the number of flinches per minute vs. the time after the formalin infection. (Courtesy of Malmberg AB, Yaksh TL: *Pain* 54:291–300, 1993.)

L-NAME. When the compounds were injected alone, there was no effect on thermal response latencies.

Discussion.—The modulation of spinal nitric oxide synthesis can lessen facilitated processing of afferent activity induced by an acute afferent barrage. This component of hyperalgesia can be initiated by activation of a spinal NMDA receptor, which leads to augmented processing of afferent input and subsequent pain behavior.

▶ Although this study sheds some light on the mechanism by which noxious stimulation sensitizes dorsal horn neurons, it seems unlikely that such therapy will be clinically useful, because spinal cord injury can result from spinal administration of nitric oxide synthase inhibitors.—S.E. Abram, M.D.

Antinociceptive Effects of Spinal Cholinesterase Inhibition and Isobolographic Analysis of the Interaction With μ and α₂ Receptor Systems

Naguib M, Yaksh TL (King Saud Univ, Riyadh, Saudi Arabia; Univ of California, San Diego, La Jolla)
Anesthesiology 80:1338–1348, 1994

101-95-23–3

Background.—The spinal injection of cholinergic agonists leads to dose-related antinociceptive effects in animal studies, an effect that is mediated by spinal muscarinic receptors. It may be possible that spinal cholinergic systems inhibit transmitter release by sensory neurons.

Objective and Methods.—The antinociceptive properties of 2 cholinesterase inhibitors were examined in rats that were prepared with chronic intrathecal catheters. Nociceptive thresholds were estimated by the radiant heat-evoked hindpaw withdrawal technique. The agonists that were given intrathecally included neostigmine, edrophonium, carbachol, morphine, and clonidine. Animals were pretreated with the antagonists atropine, mecamylamine, naloxone, and yohimbine. Interactions between drug classes were defined by the method of equal dose-ratio isobolographic analysis.

Results.—All the antagonists led to a dose-dependent increase in hindpaw withdrawal latency. Morphine was most potent, followed by neostigmine, clonidine, carbachol, and edrophonium, in that order. Spinal pretreatment with atropine lessened the antinociceptive effects of carbachol, neostigmine, and edrophonium, but not those of morphine or clonidine. Intrathecal pretreatment with naloxone and yohimbine attenuated the effects of intrathecally administered morphine and clonidine, respectively. Mecamylamine, a nicotinic receptor antagonist, did not influence thermal nociception. Isobolographic analysis showed that mixtures of neostigmine with clonidine, edrophonium with clonidine, and edrophonium with morphine interacted synergistically. The effects of neostigmine and morphine were simply additive.

Conclusion.—The antinociceptive effects of intrathecally administered cholinomimetic and acetylcholinesterase-inhibiting drugs are mediated by spinal cholinergic muscarinic receptors. It appears that the various spinal receptor systems involved in nociceptive processing interact functionally.

▶ Spinal administration of cholinergic agonists produces analgesia in animals that is synergistic with intrathecal clonidine. Spinal administration of neostigmine in humans produces analgesia, but it is associated with a high incidence of nausea.—S.E. Abram, M.D.

Slowly Developing Placebo Responses Confound Tests of Intravenous Phentolamine to Determine Mechanisms Underlying Idiopathic Chronic Low Back Pain
Fine PG, Roberts WJ, Gillette RG, Child TR (Univ of Utah, Salt Lake City; RS Dow Neurological Sciences Inst, Portland, Ore)
Pain 56:235–242, 1994   101-95-23–4

Background.—Similarities between chronic back pain and distal, sympathetically determined dependent pain may reflect common pathophys-

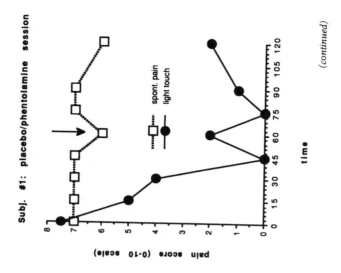

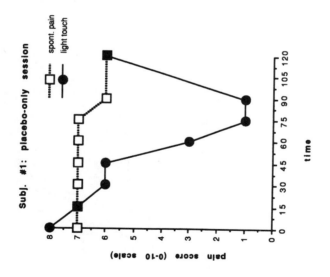

(continued)

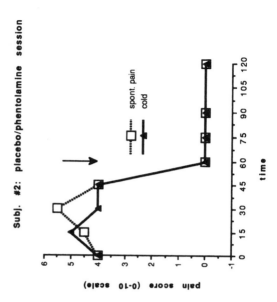

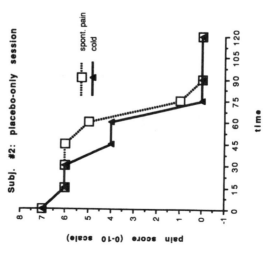

Fig 23-2 (cont).

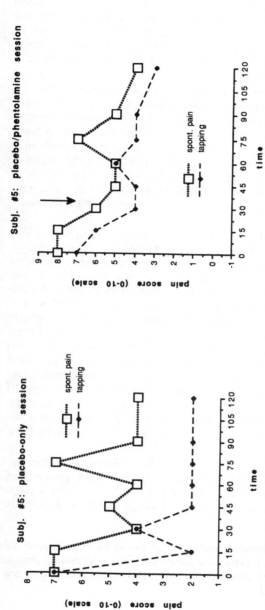

Fig 23–2.—Pain scores for different paralumbar evoked tests and spontaneous pain over time comparing placebo **(left)** with phentolamine **(right)** in 3 representative patients. The onset of IV phentolamine administration is depicted by the *arrows* above the record. (Courtesy of Fine PG, Roberts WJ, Gillette RG, et al: *Pain* 56:235–242, 1994.)

iologic mechanisms, including precipitation by deep-tissue injury, persistent pain in the apparent absence of continuing nociception, mechanical and cold allodynia, and unresponsiveness to opiates. Because previous reports have suggested that the α-adrenergic blocking actions of IV phentolamine serve as a diagnostic tool to test for sympathetically maintained pain, the ability of IV phentolamine to reduce the pain in idiopathic chronic low-back pain was assessed.

Study Design.—In a novel, placebo-controlled, crossover test, 6 healthy individuals, aged 27–44 years, with idiopathic chronic low-back pain were studied in 2 separate study sessions. In the placebo/phentolamine session, the participants were told that they would receive 6 separate infusions in random order. The study drug, 30 mg of phentolamine mesylate, was given either in the third or fifth infusions. In the placebo-only session, the patients received normal saline alone. The effects of infusions on spontaneous pain and evoked pains with touch, cold, tapping, and deep pressure were evaluated after each infusion at 15-minute intervals.

Outcome.—All participants showed strong placebo responses that prevented assessment of specific drug effects. Figure 23–2 shows the responses of 3 participants. During the placebo/phentolamine session, spontaneous pain increased during the first 2 assessments (15–30 minutes) and then decreased over the next 30 minutes. Ratings on all 4 stimulus-evoked pains decreased to 0 within the first 60 minutes. However, the phentolamine infusion began just after the 60-minute assessment; therefore, the decrease in pain ratings could not be attributed to the active drug. Overall, the placebo responses had onset latencies of 15–60 minutes, developed slowly over the next 15–45 minutes, and persisted for hours or several days. Except for the significant increase in heart rate with the active drug, there were no significant differences in ratings of spontaneous pain and stimulus-evoked pain between active drug and placebo. In fact, significant reductions in pain over time were reported before and in the absence of infusion of the active drug for most of the pain variables.

Conclusion.—The importance of understanding that placebo controls are essential in the evaluation of drugs and other palliative procedures on patients with chronic pain was reinforced. In addition, control paradigms must allow for placebo effects that develop slowly and are very persistent.

▶ The observation that substantial responses to placebos may require 30 minutes or more to develop is extremely important. This information should influence the manner in which placebo-controlled diagnostic procedures are conducted.—S.E. Abram, M.D.

Specific Enhancement by Fentanyl of the Effects of Intrathecal Bupivacaine on Nociceptive Afferent but Not on Sympathetic Efferent Pathways in Dogs

Wang C, Chakrabarti MK, Whitwam JG (Royal Postgraduate Med School, London)
Anesthesiology 79:766–773, 1993   101-95-23–5

Objective.—The combined effects of fentanyl and bupivacaine on spontaneous sympathetic activity, sensory afferent paths, and reflex-evoked efferent paths of somatosympathetic responses were examined in greyhound dogs to learn whether intrathecally administered bupivacaine causes more sensory than sympathetic blockade.

Methods.—Spontaneous activity was recorded in the renal sympathetic nerves. Reflex somatosympathetic responses were elicited by stimulating the tibial and radial nerves supramaximally. Bupivacaine was given intrathecally in doses of .5, 1, 2, 3.5, and 7 mg. Groups of dogs were pretreated with 5.4 mg of intrathecal fentanyl. This dose equalled the 25% effective dose for depressing C-fiber–mediated reflexes in the tibial nerve.

Results.—Bupivacaine inhibited both C-fiber– and Aδ-fiber–mediated somatosympathetic responses to tibial nerve stimulation in a dose-dependent manner. The effect of bupivacaine on the radial and tibial nerve reflexes resembled its action on spontaneous renal sympathetic activity. Pretreatment with intrathecal fentanyl depressed the tibial C-fiber reflex by 23.8% without significantly altering the tibial Aδ-response or the radial C-fiber or Aδ-responses. Administration of fentanyl markedly increased the effects of further doses of bupivacaine on the tibial Aδ- and C reflexes, but it did not further alter the radial nerve responses or the level of spontaneous sympathetic activity.

Conclusion.—Intrathecally administered bupivacaine depressed nociceptive reflexes in a dose-dependent manner. The spinal analgesia produced by bupivacaine may be enhanced by administering fentanyl as well. These agents act synergistically on the afferent pathway without further depressing efferent sympathetic activity.

▶ This study suggests that epidural local anesthetics but not opioids are likely to be effective in reducing sympathetic outflow in patients with reflex sympathetic dystrophy.—S.E. Abram, M.D.

Relationship Between Time of Treatment of Acute Herpes Zoster With Sympathetic Blockade and Prevention of Post-Herpetic Neuralgia: Clinical Support for a New Theory of the Mechanism by Which Sympathetic Blockade Provides Therapeutic Benefit
Winnie AP, Hartwell PW (Cook County Hosp, Chicago; Elmhurst Hosp Ctr, NY)
Reg Anesth 18:277–282, 1993   101-95-23–6

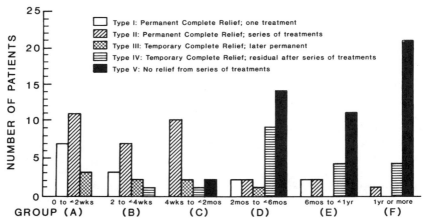

Fig 23–3.—Graphic representation of the relationship between time of treatment and type of response. (Courtesy of Winnie AP, Hartwell PW: *Reg Anesth* 18:277–282, 1993.)

Background.—The most common complication of herpes zoster is persistent pain, which is known as postherpetic neuralgia. Although the therapeutic benefit of sympathetic blocks in herpes zoster is well known in practice, it has not been fully studied. The relationship between the time of treatment of acute herpes zoster and the prevention of postherpetic neuralgia was examined.

Methods.—A retrospective chart audit was conducted of records of individuals who were treated for pain related to herpes zoster and had completed all follow-up, regardless of outcome. The patients were divided into 6 groups, according to the duration of symptoms before initiation of treatment, which ranged from fewer than 2 weeks after the onset of symptoms (group A) to more than 1 year (group F). All patients received stellate ganglion or epidural blocks, depending on the location of the pain. Patients' responses to treatment were classified as type 1 to type 5, which ranged from complete and permanent relief after a single block (type 1) to relief only for the duration of the local anesthetic (type 5).

Results.—A total of 122 patient records were reviewed. Response to treatment ranged from 100% in group A achieving complete relief of their pain to only 1 person (4%) in group F (Fig 23–3). Overall, the treatments were well tolerated, and there were no permanent sequelae or any side effects noted.

Conclusion.—The earlier sympathetic blocks are initiated, the more successful they will be in terminating the acute phase of the disease and preventing postherpetic neuralgia. It should be noted that acyclovir, although it is effective in terminating the acute phase of herpes zoster in a high percentage of patients, does not prevent the development of postherpetic neuralgia.

▶ Although most patients who were treated early in the course of their herpes zoster infection had eventual resolution of symptoms, it is not clear whether the blocks altered the course of their painful symptoms. Controlled studies are needed to determine the efficacy of blocks in treating postherpetic neuralgia. Perhaps the greatest importance of this study is that it demonstrates the futility of performing blocks more than a month or 2 after the onset of symptoms.—S.E. Abram, M.D.

Irradiation and Responsiveness to Pain Stimuli in Rats
Rutten EHJM, Dirksen R, Crul BJP, Oosterveld BJ, van Egmond J (Univ of Nijmegen, The Netherlands)
Life Sci 54:1815–1823, 1994   101-95-23-7

Objective.—Although radiotherapy has been used to alleviate pain in patients for 9 decades, no one has studied the benefit to the patient or the mechanism of analgesia. The extent of radiotherapeutic pain modification in the rat model was examined.

Methods.—The 66 rats in group 1 were irradiated; the 24 rats in group 2 were not. A tid-probe was inserted into the spinal columns of male Wistar rats that were then irradiated once with 4-MV photons from a linear accelerator. Final doses were 10 Gy, 15 Gy, or 17.5 Gy. Responses to hot-plate and tale-flick tests were recorded before and after irradiation. Baseline responses were measured 3 times at day 0; rats were then tested 3 times a day for 4 days.

Results.—Responses to the hot-plate test were delayed in irradiated rats at all doses. The tale-flick test responses were unaffected by irradiation at all doses. No side effects of radiation were observed.

Conclusion.—Irradiation may cause damage to neuronal systems that produce substances that transmit or conduct pain stimuli; this may also occur in humans.

▶ This study introduces the novel concept that irradiation that includes the spinal cord may produce analgesia independent of its effect on the tumor.—S.E. Abram, M.D.

Systemic Opioids Do Not Suppress Spinal Sensitization After Subcutaneous Formalin in Rats
Abram SE, Olson EE (Med College of Wisconsin, Milwaukee)
Anesthesiology 80:1114–1119, 1994   101-95-23-8

Background.—Noxious stimulation during surgery can produce postoperative hyperalgesia. Preoperative administration of intrathecal opioids before inhalation anesthesia can significantly reduce the severity of postoperative pain and postoperative systemic opioid requirements. Whether moderate doses of systemic opioids that were given before formalin injection would inhibit postoperative hyperalgesia was determined.

Methods.—A series of tests was carried out in 5 groups of male Sprague-Dawley rats. Flinches per minute were recorded 1 and 5 minutes after formalin injection during phase 1 analgesia and at 5-minute intervals thereafter for 1 hour during phase 2. All animals were given isoflurane 1% during formalin injection and for 6 minutes thereafter. Alfentanil, saline, and morphine were given to different groups before formalin injection, and naloxone and naltrexone were given to some groups 6 minutes after formalin injection to reverse the opioid effects.

Results.—The 3 saline-treated control groups showed nearly identical phase 2 activity. Neither alfentanil nor systemic opioids substantially blocked phase 2 activity. Total phase 2 activity in the morphine-pretreated animals was almost identical to that of the saline-treated controls.

Conclusion.—A combination of preoperative systemic opioid administration followed by inhalation anesthesia does not suppress postoperative hyperalgesia.

▶ There are now conflicting animal and human clinical data regarding the ability of systemic opioids to block spinal sensitization or "windup." The bulk of the evidence appears to suggest a lack of effect.—S.E. Abram, M.D.

Apnoea and Oximetric Desaturation in Patients Receiving Epidural Morphine After Gastrectomy: A Comparison of Intermittent Bolus and Patient Controlled Administration
Nozaki-Taguchi N, Oka T, Kochi T, Taguchi N, Mizuguchi T (Tochigi Cancer Centre Hosp, Chiba, Japan; Natl Cancer Centre, Chiba, Japan; Chiba Univ, Japan)
Anaesth Intensive Care 21:292–297, 1993   101-95-23–9

Introduction.—Arterial hypoxemia and apneas, with intervals of respiratory arrest of 12 seconds or greater, are common in patients who receive opioids after major abdominal surgery. The effects of different epidural opioid administrations on respiration have never been studied. Smaller dose requirements have been observed in epidural patient-controlled analgesia (PCA) compared with IV PCA.

Methods.—The incidence of respiratory abnormalities and episodic desaturations after gastrectomy was compared in 20 patients who received epidural morphine either by PCA with continuous infusion or by intermittent bolus injection preoperatively and for 60 hours after surgery. The morphine dose was similar in both groups. The patients were monitored with continuous-pulse oximetry, respiratory inductive plethysmography, and repeated arterial blood gas analysis. The average number of apneas per hour and the concomitant desaturation episodes

(SpO$_2$ < 90%) were counted; an SpO$_2$ below 80% was considered to be severe hypoxemia.

Results.—Episodes of apnea were greater in the bolus injection groups before surgery. However, the groups were not composed of the same patients who had many apneas after surgery. In the postoperative period, blood gas changes were similar, but central apneas (SpO$_2$ < 90%) and episodes of desaturation were significantly increased in most of the patients who received intermittent bolus injections. Only 1 patient in the PCA group showed an increase in the number of apneas and desaturation episodes. Severe desaturations to levels of less than 80% were seen in 3 patients of the bolus injection group, whereas none was seen in the PCA group.

Conclusion.—Postoperative apneas and episodic desaturations are greatly influenced by the mode of opioid administration. Patient-controlled epidural morphine with continuous infusions is associated with less frequent apnea, a lower incidence of episodic desaturations, and less severe desaturations compared with epidural intermittent bolus administration. A low-dose epidural infusion of morphine is known to keep the concentration of morphine near the respiratory center at a low constant level compared with high-volume bolus epidural morphine. Among the limitations of this study are the lack of a double-blind protocol design and of pain or sedative scores.

▶ The lower incidence of apnea with infusion may be related to lower peak CSF morphine levels.—S.E. Abram, M.D.

A Comparison of Epidural Catheters With or Without Subcutaneous Injection Ports for Treatment of Cancer Pain

de Jong PC, Kansen PJ (Dr Daniel den Hoed Cancer Ctr, Rotterdam, The Netherlands)
Anesth Analg 78:94–100, 1994   101-95-23–10

Objective.—The use of epidural analgesia for treatment of cancer pain has associated problems. The complications associated with the use of epidural catheters for treatment of such pain were analyzed in a retrospective study.

Methods.—Patients received either percutaneous catheters or subcutaneous injection ports. Morphine was the most commonly used opioid. Sufentanil was used in about 10% of the patients. Bupivacaine was added for all patients who were on continuous infusion. Clonidine was used in 6 patients. Incidences of dislodgement, infection, leakage, and occlusion were recorded.

Results.—A total of 149 patients received 250 catheters, 198 of which were percutaneous, including 41 that were tunneled and 52 that were subcutaneous. Approximately 21% of the percutaneous catheters be-

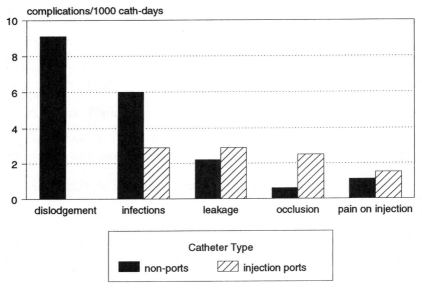

complications/1000 cath-days

Catheter Type
non-ports injection ports

Fig 23–4.—Number of complications per 1,000 catheter-days. (Courtesy of de Jong PC, Kansen PJ: *Anesth Analg* 78:94–100, 1994.)

came dislodged; no injection ports became dislodged. About 14% of the catheters became infected, with the nonport group having an incidence of infection twice that of the port group. There were significantly more leakage and occlusion incidents in the port group. There was no significant difference in the incidence of pain on injection between the 2 groups (Fig 23–4).

Conclusion.—The complication rate was lower for catheters equipped with injection ports.

▶ The 2 types of external epidural delivery systems have different complication profiles, but neither system appears to have a clear advantage. The lower cost and shorter procedure time of the simple tunneled catheter may give that system the edge.—S.E. Abram, M.D.

Comparative Local Anaesthetic Blocks in the Diagnosis of Cervical Zygapophysial Joint Pain
Barnsley L, Lord S, Bogduk N (Univ of Newcastle, Callaghan, Australia)
Pain 55:99–106, 1993   101-95-23–11

Background.—Diagnostic blocks are valuable in the investigation of chronic neck pain and are superior to morphologic, radiographic investigations. Comparative local anesthetic blocks have been recommended as

Patterns of Response in 45 Patients With Pain Relief After an Initial Diagnostic Nerve Block

Pattern of response	Description	No. of patients (%)	Cumulative %	Meet Criteria?
Concordant	Longer pain relief with bupivacaine Lignocaine lasted < 7 h and Bupivacaine lasted < 24 h	27 (60)	60	Yes
Concordant prolonged	Longer pain relief with bupivacaine Lignocaine lasted > 7 h and/or Bupivacaine lasted > 24 h	7 (16)	76	Yes
Discordant prolonged	Longer pain relief from lignocaine Lignocaine lasted > 7 h and/or Bupivacaine lasted > 24 h	6 (13)	89	No
Discordant	Longer pain relief from lignocaine Lignocaine lasted < 7 h and Bupivacaine lasted < 24 h	4 (9)	98	No
Discrepant	Pain relief on the first occasion, but no pain relief following a second injection	1 (2)	100	No

(Courtesy of Barnsley L, Lord S, Bogduk N: *Pain* 55:99–106, 1993.)

a substitute for normal saline control blocks used to identify patients' false positive responses. The usefulness of comparative local anesthetic blocks in the diagnosis of neck pain was explored.

Methods.—In a double-blind study, 47 patients with chronic neck pain were randomly assigned to receive controlled blocks of the cervical, zygapophyseal joints using 2% lidocaine or .5% bupivacaine. Patients' responses were recorded (table), and positive responses were followed by an additional block with the complementary anesthetic. Patients who felt longer pain relief from bupivacaine were considered to have true positive responses.

Results.—Of the 47 patients, 2 did not obtain any relief from the blocks. After the initial block, 45 patients reported pain relief; 1 of these did not obtain relief after confirmatory control blocks. Of the 44 patients who obtained pain relief after confirmatory control blocks, 34 had longer pain relief from bupivacaine; it was unlikely that this occurred by chance. A subgroup of 13 patients unexpectedly obtained pain relief for periods longer than the reported duration of action of either anesthetic.

Discussion.—Comparative local anesthetic blocks are convenient, valid tools for the identification of true positive responses to cervical zygapophyseal joint blocks and are a good alternative to normal saline controls.

▶ Although the use of 2 local anesthetic blocks of different duration is appealing for ethical reasons, the validity of the technique cannot be confirmed without comparison to a placebo (saline) injection. The risks of bupivacaine injections in the upper cervical region, with its proximity to the vertebral artery and subarachnoid space, are fairly significant.—S.E. Abram, M.D.

Comparison of the Analgesic Effects of Intrathecal Clonidine and Intrathecal Morphine After Spinal Anaesthesia in Patients Undergoing Total Hip Replacement
Fogarty DJ, Carabine UA, Milligan KR (Queen's Univ of Belfast, Northern Ireland; Royal Victoria Hosp, Belfast, Northern Ireland; Musgrave Park Hosp, Belfast, Northern Ireland)
Br J Anaesth 71:661–664, 1993   101-95-23–12

Background.—Opioids and α_2-agonists produce analgesia when administered spinally. Adjuvant drugs may be used to prolong the duration of blocks and provide postoperative analgesia. Clonidine is an α_2-agonist that prolongs spinal anesthesia, but there is little information about its analgesic properties as an adjuvant to intrathecal bupivacaine. The anesthetic and analgesic properties of intrathecal clonidine and intrathecal morphine were explored.

Methods.—Ninety patients undergoing total hip replacement were randomly assigned to receive intrathecal clonidine, morphine, or saline

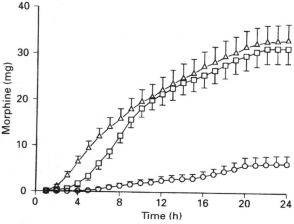

Fig 23–5.—Mean (standard error of the mean) postoperative cumulative morphine consumption after intrathecal saline (*triangle*), clonidine (*square*), or morphine (*circle*). (Courtesy of Fogarty DJ, Carabine UA, Milligan KR: *Br J Anaesth* 71:661–664, 1993.)

after administration of routine spinal anesthesia using .5% bupivacaine. Pain scores were recorded every 2 hours, and patient-controlled consumption of morphine was also recorded.

Results.—The time to the first request for analgesia was significantly longer in the group that received clonidine than in the group that received saline. Total morphine used the first night after surgery was significantly less in the group that received morphine (Fig 23–5). There were no differences between the group receiving clonidine and the group receiving saline. The duration of spinal analgesia was prolonged by clonidine, but morphine provided better postoperative analgesia.

Conclusion.—Intrathecal clonidine, 75–100 μg, offered little advantage in postoperative analgesia. There was no evidence of residual analgesia and no advantage in terms of postoperative side effects.

▶ It is unlikely that neuraxial clonidine will replace morphine for postoperative pain management, because of its shorter duration and frequent side effects. However, its best use may be combined with morphine. It is not clear whether the analgesic effects of the 2 classes of drug are synergistic, but there is some evidence that clonidine may slow the development of opioid tolerance.—S.E. Abram, M.D.

A Comparison of Caudal Epidural Bupivacaine With Adrenaline and Bupivacaine With Adrenaline and Pethidine for Operative and Post-operative Analgesia in Infants and Children

Kumar TPS, Jacob R (Christian Med College, Vellore, Tamil Nadu, South India)

Anaesth Intensive Care 21:424–428, 1993   101-95-23–13

Objective.—A randomized study was performed in 50 American Society of Anesthesiologists physical status I children 6 months to 12 years of age to compare 2 regimens of caudal epidural anesthesia: bupivacaine with epinephrine, and the same agents with meperidine added. The children were scheduled for elective surgery below the T10 level.

Methods.—Anesthesia was induced with nitrous oxide, oxygen, and halothane or with thiopental in larger children who preferred an injection. After endotracheal intubation, 25 children (group A) were randomized to receive .25% bupivacaine with 1:200,000 epinephrine epidurally. In addition to bupivacaine with epinephrine, the remaining 25 children (group B) received meperidine, .5 mg/kg. The amount of bupivacaine delivered was .5 mL/kg when only a saddle block was required and .75 mL/kg for other procedures that necessitated a sensory level of T10 or less.

Results.—There were no significant differences in cardiovascular or respiratory status between the 2 groups of children. Analgesia lasted significantly longer when meperidine was delivered (table). The time to first micturition also was prolonged in group B patients, and vomiting was considerably more frequent and severe than in group A children. Ten group B infants continued retching or vomiting for as long as 6 hours after surgery.

Conclusion.—Adding meperidine to caudally administered bupivacaine prolongs analgesia into the postoperative period, but it frequently results in prolonged vomiting and delayed micturition.

Assessment of Pain, Vomiting, and Micturition			
Clinical parameter	Group A	Group B	Significance
Duration of analgesia (in minutes)	381 + 95	501 + 71	$P<0.001$
First micturition from time of caudal (in minutes)	400 + 95	510 + 80	$P<0.001$
Vomiting	3/25	15/25	$P<0.001$

Note: For numerical continuous data, Student's *t*-test was used. For proportions, χ^2 test was used.

(Courtesy of Kumar TPS, Jacob R: *Anaesth Intensive Care* 21:424–428, 1993.)

▶ The high incidence of vomiting, which is often fairly prolonged (though not delayed, as with morphine), in the meperidine group is surprising because of the relatively high lipid solubility of the drug. The slight prolongation of analgesia does not appear to justify the use of the technique.—S.E. Abram, M.D.

The Effect of Epidural *Versus* General Anesthesia on Postoperative Pain and Analgesic Requirements in Patients Undergoing Radical Prostatectomy

Shir Y, Raja SN, Frank SM (Johns Hopkins Univ, Baltimore, Md)
Anesthesiology 80:49–56, 1994   101-95-23–14

Background.—The concept of preemptive analgesia was developed to minimize central sensitization after tissue injury. The technique reduces postinjury pain in animals, but studies in humans have yielded controversial results.

Objective.—The comparative effects of surgical epidural anesthesia using local anesthetics and general anesthesia on postoperative pain and demands for analgesia were examined in men who were scheduled to undergo radical retropubic prostatectomy.

Methods.—Thirty-five men received .5% bupivacaine, .25 mL/kg, epidurally. An infusion of .125% bupivacaine, .1 mL/kg/hr, was maintained during surgery, with the infusion rate adjusted to the individual patient's response. Thirty-four other patients received general anesthesia with 70% nitrous oxide and isoflurane in an end-tidal concentration of less than .5%. Bupivacaine was given epidurally after induction but before skin incision in a dose of .5% bupivacaine, .2 mL/kg, followed by .125% bupivacaine, .1 mL/kg/hr. Finally, 34 patients received general anesthesia only.

Results.—Patients who were given combined anesthesia received significantly less epidural bupivacaine than those who received only epidural anesthesia. The latter patients had a higher sensory level on arrival in the recovery room. Two patients in each group had moderate or severe pain at this time. Starting on the second postoperative day, the need for patient-controlled analgesia was significantly less in the epidural-only group than in the other groups. Pain scores were low in all 3 groups during patient-controlled analgesia. There were no clinically significant group differences in postoperative sedation or pain relief scores.

Conclusion.—In patients who were having a radical prostatectomy, epidural administration of bupivacaine during surgery lessened postoperative pain and reduced the need for postoperative analgesia.

▶ It appears that an intense local anesthetic block, as required for surgical anesthesia with epidural alone, is necessary for a preemptive analgesic effect. A partial block in conjunction with general anesthesia may offer no significant benefit with respect to postoperative pain.—S.E. Abram, M.D.

Long-Term Intrathecal Morphine and Bupivacaine in Patients With Refractory Cancer Pain: Results From a Morphine:Bupivacaine Dose Regimen of 0.5:4.75 mg/ml

Sjöberg M, Nitescu P, Appelgren L, Curelaru I (Sahlgrenska Hosp, Gothenburg, Sweden; Univ of Gothenburg, Sweden)
Anesthesiology 80:284–297, 1994   101-95-23–15

Background.—No clinical data are available on the concentrations and ratios in which intrathecal morphine and bupivacaine should be combined to optimize analgesia and minimize adverse effects. The efficacy and safety of a constant intrathecal infusion of morphine, .5 mg/mL, plus bupivacaine, 4.75 mg/mL (morphine:bupivacaine $\approx 1:10$), were assessed in the treatment of refractory cancer pain.

Methods.—In 53 patients with refractory cancer pain, this intrathecal morphine and bupivacaine combination was administered for as long as 6 months; the dosage was increased as needed. Patients could also use nonopioid analgesics and sedatives as needed. The efficacy of the treatment was measured using the following parameters: pain relief; total daily opioid doses; total daily nonopioid analgesic and sedative use, patient's sleep pattern, gait pattern, and body movements; and adverse effects.

Results.—During the intrathecal period, which was a median of 29 days, the median intrathecal daily dose was 6 mg for morphine and 50 mg for bupivacaine. Compared with previous intrathecal treatment, all patients had acceptable pain relief during treatment. The median total daily opioid use decreased from 120 mg to 10 mg. The use of nonopioid analgesics and sedatives decreased by about one half. The sleep pattern improved significantly, but the gait pattern did not. Urinary retention, paresthesias, and paresis/gait impairment were the most common side effects.

Conclusion.—Intrathecal administration of morphine, .5 mg/mL, plus bupivacaine, 4.75 mg/mL ($\approx 1:10$), can significantly relieve cancer pain, although side effects may occur as a result of the bupivacaine.

► Intrathecal morphine and bupivacaine are synergistic in animals. Several recent studies have shown this combination to be effective in large numbers of cancer patients who are relatively unresponsive to opioids alone.—S.E. Abram, M.D.

Single-Dose, Randomized, Double-Blind, Double-Dummy Cross-Over Comparison of Extradural and I.V. Clonidine in Chronic Pain
Carroll D, Jadad A, King V, Wiffen P, Glynn C, McQuay H (Univ of Oxford, England)
Br J Anaesth 71:665–669, 1993   101-95-23–16

Objective.—Because the clinical value of α_2-adrenergic agonists such as clonidine in relieving pain remains uncertain, the effects of clonidine, which was given extradurally and intravenously, were compared in 10 patients with chronic back pain who reportedly had previously gained relief from an extradural dose of clonidine, 150 µg, combined with a local anesthetic.

Methods.—A single dose of clonidine, 150 µg, was given either extradurally or intravenously using a randomized double-blind, double-dummy, crossover design. This approach had an 80% likelihood of detecting a difference in anlagesic effect with the 2 routes of administration. A nurse-observer estimated the pain intensity, the degree of relief, adverse side effects, and changes in mood and sedation for as long as 6 hours after injection.

Results.—Intravenous clonidine led to significantly greater relief of pain than extradural administration. Clonidine that was given by either route resulted in significant sedation and reductions in arterial blood pressure and heart rate. Eight patients had adverse effects from extradural clonidine and 7 from IV administration.

Conclusion.—There is no apparent advantage to administering clonidine extradurally rather than intravenously to patients with chronic pain.

▶ Clonidine appears to join the ranks of drugs such as fentanyl and alfentanil, which have little appreciable increase in analgesic effect when given epidurally rather than systemically. It is not clear whether the intrathecal route greatly increases the analgesic effect of these drugs. (See Abstract 101-95-23–32.)—S.E. Abram, M.D.

Effects of Combined Perioperative Epidural Bupivacaine and Morphine, Ibuprofen, and Incisional Bupivacaine on Postoperative Pain, Pulmonary, and Endocrine–Metabolic Function After Minilaparotomy Cholecystectomy
Dahl JB, Hjortsø N-C, Stage JG, Hansen BL, Møiniche S, Damgaard B, Kehlet H (Hvidovre Univ, Denmark)
Reg Anesth 19:199–205, 1994   101-95-23–17

Purpose.—There is experimental and clinical evidence that the additive or synergistic effects of a multimodal approach to pain management improve postoperative pain relief and that analgesia initiated before surgery may prevent postoperative pain. The effects of 2 anesthetic regimens for managing postoperative pain after minilaparotomy cholecystectomy were compared.

Methods.—Thirty-two healthy patients undergoing elective cholecystectomy were randomized to general anesthesia and continuous perioperative and postoperative thoracic epidural analgesia with bupivacaine and morphine for 38 hours after the operation or to general anesthesia with postoperative IM morphine every 6–8 hours. All patients took ibuprofen from the evening before the operation until 6 days after surgery. In addition, the surgical field was infiltrated with plain bupivacaine immediately before surgical incision.

Results.—Both anesthetic regimens almost abolished postoperative pain at rest. Patients in the epidural analgesia group had significantly less pain during cough 6 and 24 hours after the operation and during walking 24 hours after the operation than patients in the IM morphine group. This difference was no longer evident 48 hours after the operation, when epidural analgesia was discontinued. There was only a limited postoperative decrease in pulmonary function and no increase in plasma cortisol or glucose with either regimen. Most patients were discharged home within 2 days after surgery.

Conclusion.—Continuous epidural analgesia with bupivacaine and morphine provides better pain relief in the immediate postoperative period than IM morphine without adversely affecting pulmonary or endocrine-metabolic function.

▶ The inability to demonstrate substantial changes in pulmonary or endocrine-metabolic benefits of epidural analgesia in this study does not rule out the possibility of beneficial effects of the technique. A comparison was made to a technique of combined general anesthesia plus wound infiltration rather than to general anesthesia alone. Neither group demonstrated substantial pulmonary dysfunction.

It is unfortunate that we are increasingly being forced to demonstrate benefits in addition to improved analgesia. Third-party payers will probably require us to show cost benefits in the future, if they are to pay for added interventions. Patient comfort is no longer enough.—S.E. Abram, M.D.

Deafferentation Pain Exacerbated by Subarachnoid Lidocaine and Relieved by Subarachnoid Morphine: Case Report
Iacono RP, Boswell MV, Neumann M (Loma Linda Univ, California; Case Western Reserve Univ, Cleveland, Ohio)
Reg Anesth 19:212–215, 1994   101-95-23–18

Background.—Chronic neuropathic pain syndromes are often resistant to conventional drug therapy, including systemic opioids. Whether subarachnoid administration of opioids is effective for some forms of neuropathic pain was investigated.

Case Report.—Woman, 44, with a 16-year history of deafferentation pain of the legs, who had been resistant to multidisciplinary pain clinic management, including spinal cord stimulation, agreed to undergo differential spinal anesthesia with lidocaine and morphine. Evoked potential monitoring was used to evaluate the intensity of the spinal anesthetic block. Subarachnoid lidocaine injection exacerbated the leg pain, but subarachnoid morphine injection provided rapid pain relief. Long-term pain control has been maintained with an implanted spinal infusion device. At 18 months after pump implantation, the patient has continued to have satisfactory pain relief and has returned to work.

Conclusion.—The dramatic pain relief obtained with subarachnoid opioids in a patient with chronic deafferentation pain suggests involvement of a segmental, opioid-sensitive dorsal horn mechanism.

▶ This case gives an indication of the tremendous diversity of pathophysiologic and treatment responses that are encountered among chronic pain patients. Systematic trials of various treatment modalities can reveal surprising results.—S.E. Abram, M.D.

Comparative Spinal Neuropathology of Hydromorphone and Morphine After 9- and 30-Day Epidural Administration in Sheep
Coombs DW, Colburn RW, DeLeo JA, Hoopes PJ, Twitchell BB (Dartmouth-Hitchcock Med Ctr, Lebanon, NH)
Anesth Analg 78:674–681, 1994   101-95-23–19

Introduction.—Epidural opioid analgesia is widely used to control acute or chronic pain. However, the toxicity of high concentrations of morphine or hydromorphone and its effects on the epidural space and the adjacent neurologic structures have not been adequately studied. Therefore, the neurotoxicity of epidural morphine and hydromorphone was investigated in sheep.

Methods.—Ewes were randomly assigned to receive escalating epidural doses of morphine, hydromorphone, or normal saline solutions with implanted subcutaneous delivery systems for either 9 days or 30 days to evaluate neurotoxicity with both acute and chronic treatment. Neurologic behaviors, blood parameters, and CSF samples were analyzed at baseline and at the end of the study. After the animals were sacrificed, the spinal cord and epidural space were exposed and examined, and the tissues were analyzed histologically.

Results.—In the groups that were exposed to 9 days of epidural treatment, there were no significant differences between treatment groups in serum parameters, ambulatory behavior, or myelin basic protein levels in the CSF. There was no evidence of gross pathology. However, local inflammatory reaction was more pronounced in the tissues surrounding the catheters and in the epidural fat in the sheep that were given morphine or hydromorphone than in those that were given saline solutions.

In the sheep that were exposed to 30 days of epidural treatment, the groups receiving morphine and hydromorphone had hindlimb weakness that progressed with increasing doses. White cells were increased in the CSF of the sheep that were given morphine or hydromorphone. Severe fibrotic growth surrounded the epidural catheter in the 2 medicated groups. The inflammatory reactions were more localized in the 30-day controls than in the 9-day controls. In the other two 30-day groups, there were extensive fibrogranulomatous reactions in the catheter tracts, with lymphoid proliferation in various degrees that contained B and T lymphocytes, eosinophils, and eosinophilic granulomas. Some reactions extended through the dura, causing necrosis and fibrogranulomatous replacement of the spinal cord parenchyma; other reactions caused compression of the spinal cord.

Discussion.—Long-term escalating doses of epidural opioids were associated with severe neurologic pathology. The safety of chronic, high-dose epidural opioids should be reexamined.

▶ This study suggests that we may need to reexamine the safety of high-dose long-term intrathecal opioid administration. This issue may be especially important in patients with chronic nonmalignant pain who may be exposed to high spinal drug concentrations for a period of years.—S.E. Abram, M.D.

Lateral Popliteal Sciatic Nerve Block Compared With Subcutaneous Infiltration for Analgesia Following Foot Surgery
McLeod DH, Wong DHW, Claridge RJ, Merrick PM (Univ of British Columbia, Vancouver, Canada)
Can J Anaesth 41:673–676, 1994   101-95-23–20

Background.—Postoperative pain after foot surgery involving osteotomies is often severe and difficult to control with oral analgesics. A new lateral popliteal sciatic nerve block was recently described. The postoperative analgesia obtained with the lateral popliteal sciatic nerve block was compared with that obtained with subcutaneous wound infiltration using local anesthetic.

Patients.—Of the 40 women scheduled for foot surgery involving osteotomies, 21 were randomized to the new lateral popliteal sciatic nerve block and 19 to subcutaneous wound infiltration. Bupivacaine, .5%, was used for both treatments.

Results.—The median duration of analgesia was 1,082 minutes for patients who received the lateral nerve block and 373 minutes for those who were treated with wound infiltration with local anesthetic, a statistically significant difference. Only 1 patient (5%) in the nerve block group was dissatisfied with her postoperative analgesia compared with 8 patients (42%) in the wound infiltration group.

Conclusion.—The lateral approach to the sciatic nerve in the popliteal fossa of patients undergoing foot surgery provides effective, long-lasting postoperative analgesia and has a high level of patient satisfaction.

▶ Preoperative peripheral nerve blockade with bupivacaine is a low-risk technique and provides long-lasting postoperative analgesia. The technique requires almost no postoperative surveillance and is satisfactory for use with outpatients.—S.E. Abram, M.D.

Valproate for Treatment of Chronic Central Pain After Spinal Cord Injury: A Double-Blind Cross-Over Study
Drewes AM, Andreasen A, Poulsen LH (Viborg County Hosp, Denmark)
Paraplegia 32:565–569, 1994   101-95-23–21

Introduction.—Patients who have sustained spinal cord injury frequently experience chronic intractable pain, particularly central or phantom body pain. Recently, antiepileptic medications, particularly valproate, have been used to control central pain in these patients with some success. To determine the efficacy of valproate in treating chronic central pain in patients after they had spinal cord injuries, a double-blind, placebo-controlled, crossover study was undertaken.

Methods.—Twenty adult patients with nonprogressive spinal cord injuries who complained of central pain for longer than 1 month were assigned to receive either valproate or placebo for 3 weeks. After a 2-week washout period, the patients were given the other treatment for 3 weeks. The dose was adjusted weekly with monitoring of serum drug concentrations, liver function, pain intensity, and side effects. Treatment effect was assessed in each group.

Results.—Four patients experienced dizziness while taking valproate; no patients who took placebo experienced side effects. Pain improved in 6 patients who took valproate and in 4 patients who took placebo and worsened in 2 patients who took valproate and in 1 patient who took placebo. The median dose of valproate reached 1,800 mg, and the median serum drug concentration was 614 μmol/L.

Discussion.—Valproate did not produce significant analgesic effects in patient with central pain after spinal cord injury compared with placebo, despite the use of high doses and the achievement of high serum concentrations. The pharmacologic agents available may be more effective in treating mild or moderate pain. Further study of pain control in this patient population is needed, because there is a paucity of research in this area, although pain is common in patients with spinal cord injuries.

▶ As with almost all other treatments for the pain of spinal cord injury, this regimen provided little benefit for most patients.—S.E. Abram, M.D.

Preemptive Effect of Fentanyl and Ketamine on Postoperative Pain and Wound Hyperalgesia

Tverskoy M, Oz Y, Isakson A, Finger J, Bradley EL Jr, Kissin I (Rebecca Sieff Government Hosp, Safed, Israel; Univ of Alabama, Birmingham)
Anesth Analg 78:205–209, 1994   101-95-23–22

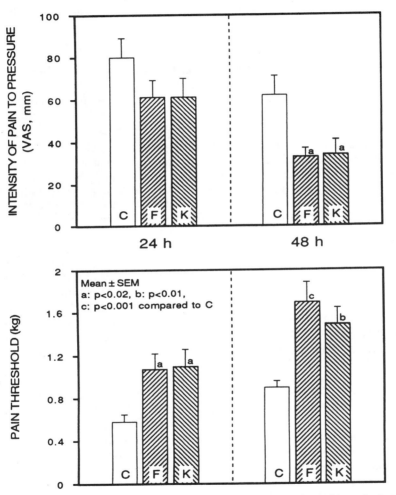

Fig 23–6.—Preemptive effect of fentanyl (F) and ketamine (K) on surgical wound hyperalgesia. **Top,** intensity of pain caused by 1.5 kg of pressure on the wound for 10 seconds, 24 hours (**left**) and 48 hours (**right**) postoperatively. **Bottom,** pain threshold to pressure on the wound 24 and 48 hours postoperatively. *Abbreviations:* C, control; VAS, visual analogue scale. (Courtesy of Tverskoy M, Oz Y, Isakson A, et al: *Anesth Analg* 78:205–209, 1994.)

Introduction.—Preemptive analgesia, administered before the painful stimulus, can potentially improve postoperative pain management. Patients who were scheduled for elective hysterectomy were used to test the hypothesis that fentanyl and ketamine would achieve this preemptive effect, reducing postoperative pain beyond the usual time of the drugs' analgesic action.

Methods.—The 27 women were randomized to fentanyl, ketamine, or control groups. Anesthesia in controls was induced with thiopental and maintained with isoflurane. In the other 2 groups, fentanyl or ketamine was added to both thiopental induction and isoflurane maintenance protocols. Postoperative pain medications were identical for the 3 regimens. A visual analogue self-rating method was used to measure the intensity of spontaneous incisional pain, movement-associated pain, and surgical wound hyperalgesia. An algometer was also used to assess wound pain.

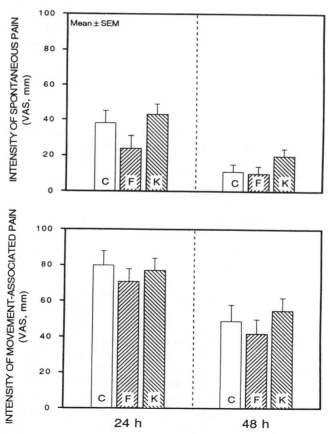

Fig 23–7.—Intensity of spontaneous and movement-associated pain 24 hours and 48 hours postoperatively. *Abbreviations:* C, control group; F, fentanyl group; K, ketamine group; VAS, visual analogue scale. (Courtesy of Tverskoy M, Oz Y, Isakson A, et al: *Anesth Analg* 78:205–209, 1994.)

Results.—The fentanyl and ketamine groups required significantly less meperidine than controls during the first 3 hours after surgery but not during hours 3–6. At 48 hours, the pain threshold was .9 kg in controls, 1.69 kg in the fentanyl group, and 1.49 in the ketamine group. Both groups showed a decrease in the intensity of pain to suprathreshold pressure on the wound compared with controls (Fig 23–6). Measures of spontaneous incisional or movement-associated pain were similar for the 3 groups (Fig 23–7).

Conclusion.—The effects of fentanyl and ketamine on wound hyperalgesia long outlast the direct analgesic action of these drugs when administered before induction of anesthesia and throughout the surgical procedure. This preemptive quality can be attributed to the prevention of central sensitization.

▶ Animal studies indicate that preemptive treatment with intrathecal opioids and N-methyl-D-aspartate (NMDA) antagonists is effective in reducing postinjury hyperalgesia. Studies involving systemic administration of these drugs are less impressive. High spinal levels of substances that block neurotransmitter release or the intracellular events initiated at the NMDA receptor may be required. It is still not clear how important the concept of preemptive analgesia is in the development of postoperative pain.—S.E. Abram, M.D.

Caudal Buprenorphine for Postoperative Analgesia in Children: A Comparison With Intramuscular Buprenorphine

Girotra S, Kumar S, Rajendran KM (Maulana Azad Med College, New Delhi, India; Associated LNJPN Hosp, New Delhi, India)
Acta Anaesthesiol Scand 37:361–364, 1993   101-95-23–23

Introduction.—Providing adequate postoperative analgesia for children is a priority, and opioids such as morphine have been used previously. Intramuscular buprenorphine was tested for its effectiveness as a postoperative analgesia in children after lower-extremity orthopedic surgery.

Methods.—Forty-four children, aged 1–10 years, were divided into groups: 23 received buprenorphine caudally and 21 received the drug intramuscularly. The dose for both groups was 4 $\mu g/kg^{-1}$ of body weight. During the first 24 hours after surgery, an observer used a 5-point pain scoring scale to evaluate the quality and duration of postoperative analgesia. Supplemental analgesia was administered for a pain score of more than 3, and the time elapsed until its administration was noted.

Results.—Caudal buprenorphine as an analgesia lasted significantly longer (median, 20.2 hours) than intramuscular buprenorphine (median, 5.2 hours). In the caudal group, 43% of patients did not require any supplemental analgesia during the first 24 hours, whereas all the patients in the intramuscular group required supplements within 10 hours. The incidence of nausea and vomiting was significantly higher in the intramuscular group (43%) than the caudal group (13%). All the children were easily arousable.

Conclusion.—Caudal buprenorphine had fewer side effects and provided from 10.8 hours to more than 24 hours of analgesia for children who had orthopedic surgery in a lower limb. Buprenorphine was preferred to other opioids because it is a mixed narcotic agonist-antagonist that has high lipid solubility and a high affinity for opioid receptors.

▶ Although the narcotic antagonist properties of buprenorphine may reduce the possibility of respiratory depression, its high receptor affinity may limit the reversibility of respiratory depression if it occurs.—S.E. Abram, M.D.

Epidural Clonidine Decreases Postoperative Requirements for Epidural Fentanyl
Delaunay L, Leppert C, Dechaubry V, Levron JC, Liu N, Bonnet F (Hôpital Henri Mondor, Créteil, France)
Reg Anesth 18:176–180, 1993   101-95-23–24

Background.—Although they provide efficient postoperative analgesia, epidural opioids are associated with side effects, including urinary retention, pruritus, and respiratory depression. Epidural clonidine has been shown in human studies to induce analgesia, and animal studies have shown that clonidine decreased the side effects of opioids and enhanced their analgesic effect. The effectiveness of a combination of epidural opioids and clonidine for postoperative analgesia was investigated.

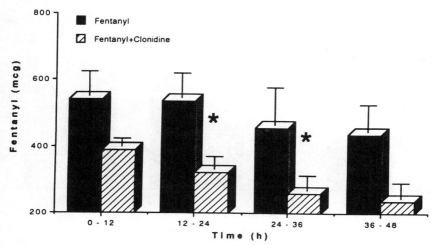

Fig 23–8.—Mean ± standard deviation values of the amounts of fentanyl administered over 12-hour periods in the 2 groups of patients. $P < .05$ intergroup significant difference. (Courtesy of Delaunay L, Leppert C, Dechaubry V, et al: *Reg Anesth* 18:176–180, 1993.)

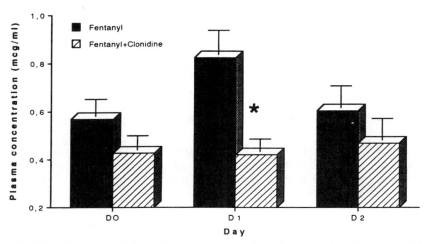

Fig 23–9.—Mean ± standard deviation values of plasma fentanyl concentrations when patients left the recovery room (day 0) and at 8 A.M. on day 1 and day 2. P < .05 intergroup significant difference. (Courtesy of Delaunay L, Leppert C, Dechaubry V, et al: *Reg Anesth* 18:176–180, 1993.)

Methods.—A randomized, double-blind trial was conducted in 25 patients during the first 72 hours after major abdominal surgery. In 1 group, on arrival in the recovery room, patients received a bolus of epidural fentanyl, 1 μg/kg⁻¹, diluted in a 10-mL isotonic saline solution followed by a continuous epidural infusion of fentanyl, 1 μg/kg⁻¹/hr⁻¹, in isotonic saline at a rate of 5 mL/hr. Patients in the second group received the same epidural fentanyl bolus dose followed by fentanyl, .5

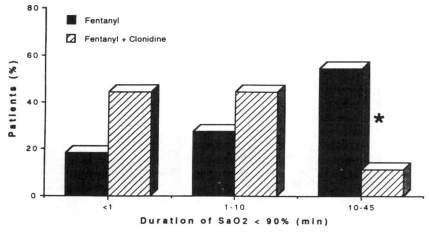

Fig 23–10.—Percentage of patients who experienced less than 1 minute or no duration. The arterial hemoglobin saturation (SaO₂) decreased < 90%, 1–10 minutes' duration. SAO₂ < 90%, 10–45 minutes' duration. SaO₂ < 90%, P < .05, intergroup significant difference. (Courtesy of Delaunay L, Leppert C, Dechaubry V, et al: *Reg Anesth* 18:176–180, 1993.)

$\mu g/kg^{-1}/hr^{-1}$, plus a continuous infusion of clonidine, .3 $\mu g/kg^{-1}/hr^{-1}$, diluted in isotonic saline at a rate of 5 mL/hr. Postoperative pain was assessed on a visual analogue scale at set intervals through the third postoperative day. Sedation, arterial blood pressure, heart rate, arterial partial pressure of carbon dioxide, arterial hemoglobin saturation (SaO_2), and plasma fentanyl concentrations were monitored during the same period.

Results.—Twelve patients were in the fentanyl group, and 13 were in the fentanyl and clonidine group. Significantly high amounts of fentanyl were administered in the fentanyl-only group at 12–24 and 24–36 hours (Fig 23–8). On day 1, plasma fentanyl concentrations were significantly lower in the fentanyl-plus-clonidine group (Fig 23–9). During the first postoperative night, the percentage of patients who documented a greater than 10-minute cumulative period of SaO_2 of less than 90% was significantly higher in the fentanyl group (Fig 23–10).

Conclusion.—Epidural fentanyl plus clonidine produces satisfactory analgesia after abdominal surgery with only a few side effects. The appropriate analgesic regimen that combines these 2 agents should be determined in further studies.

▶ Whereas the addition of epidural clonidine to the infusion of epidural fentanyl reduces the fentanyl requirement, it is not clear whether there is a synergy between the drugs. It is also unclear whether either drug is working through direct spinal or systemic effects.—S.E. Abram, M.D.

Hemodynamic and Analgesic Profile After Intrathecal Clonidine in Humans

Filos KS, Goudas LC, Patroni O, Polyzou V (Univ of Patras, Greece; Corinth Gen Hosp, Greece; Med Society of Analgesia, Patras, Greece; et al)
Anesthesiology 81:591–601, 1994   101-95-23–25

Introduction.—Respiratory depression limits the use of opioids for spinal analgesia. Studies of intrathecal clonidine administration have shown it to have fewer side effects and to require lower doses than epidural clonidine. Animal studies indicate that low doses of intrathecal clonidine have a depressor effect on systemic blood pressure (BP), but larger doses elicit a pressor effect with marked bradycardia. Human studies on intrathecal clonidine as the sole postsurgical analgesic indicated minimal BP reduction. The hemodynamic and analgesic dose-response to the use of intrathecal clonidine as the sole postsurgical analgesic was analyzed.

Methods.—Thirty healthy women undergoing elective cesarean section were randomly assigned in double-blind fashion to 1 of 3 equal groups. Anesthesia was achieved with thiopental, halothane, and nitrous oxide, with no other analgesics or tranquilizers given immediately after surgery. Intrathecal clonidine was administered 45 minutes after tracheal extubation. Group 1 was given 150 μg, group 2 received 300 μg, and 450 μg was given to group 3. Pain before and after coughing was assessed using a visual analogue scale at various intervals after administration. Hemodynamic and respiratory measurements were also variously recorded.

Results.—Significant pain reduction before and after coughing occurred almost immediately, followed by a significant dose-dependent response in all groups. Sedation occurred in all groups, with significantly more sedation in group 3 than groups 1 or 2. Immediate BP depressor effects occurred only in group 1. Heart rate was not reduced significantly in any group, and there were no delayed responses of bradycardia or hypotension.

Conclusion.—Administration of intrathecal clonidine in doses as great as 450 μg may be considered appropriate in a postoperative setting because of the hemodynamic stability and analgesic effect they confer.

▶ This study is unusual because there was very little hypotension or bradycardia associated with intrathecal clonidine administration.—S.E. Abram, M.D.

Pain and Its Treatment in Outpatients With Metastatic Cancer

Cleeland CS, Gonin R, Hatfield AK, Edmonson JH, Blum RH, Stewart JA, Pandya KJ (Univ of Wisconsin, Madison; Dana-Farber Cancer Inst, Boston; Carle Cancer Ctr, Urbana, Ill; et al)

N Engl J Med 330:592–596, 1994   101-95-23–26

Background.—Even when treated, pain in patients with cancer is often severe enough to impair functioning. Both patients and health care providers agree that pain is frequently poorly managed. The proportion of patients with cancer who have substantial pain, types of pain treatment, and the characteristics of patients who are at greater risk for undermedication with analgesic drugs was studied.

Methods.—Fifty-four centers contributed data on a total of 1,308 outpatients with recurrent or metastatic cancer. The patients rated their pain severity in the preceding week, the degree of pain-related functional impairment, and the degree of relief provided by analgesic agents. Physicians also provided data on the causes of pain, pain treatment, and their estimates of the impact of pain on patients' ability to function.

Findings.—Sixty-seven percent of the patients said they had experienced pain or had taken analgesics daily in the preceding week. Thirty-six percent had functional impairments caused by pain. Forty-two percent of patients with pain did not receive adequate analgesic treatment. Patients who were treated at centers that served mostly minority populations were 3 times more likely to have insufficient pain management than patients who were treated elsewhere. A discrepancy between the patient and the physician in judging the severity of pain predicted insufficient pain management. Other factors that were predictive of insufficient pain treatment were pain that was not attributed to cancer by physicians, better performance status, age 70 years or older, and female gender. Patients with less adequate analgesia had less relief and greater functional impairment.

Conclusion.—Many patients with cancer have considerable pain and receive inadequate analgesia, despite published guidelines for pain management. In this series, many patients had pain that was severe enough to impair functioning.

▶ This study suggests that cancer pain as well as chronic nonmalignant pain should be managed by individuals who are specifically trained in pain management techniques. All too often, the cancer subspecialists mistakenly assume that they are providing optimal care. Patients who are being cared for by primary care physicians may be even more likely to experience inadequate pain control. The statistics regarding minorities, women, and older patients are particularly distressing.—S.E. Abram, M.D.

Neurolytic Superior Hypogastric Plexus Block for Chronic Pelvic Pain Associated With Cancer

de Leon-Casasola OA, Kent E, Lema MJ (State Univ of New York at Buffalo)
Pain 54:145–151, 1993   101-95-23–27

Introduction.—Patients with tumor extension into the pelvis may have incapacitating pain that does not respond to administration of oral or parenteral opioids. Such patients require a more invasive approach to control the pain and improve their quality of life. The efficacy of neurolytic superior hypogastric plexus blocks in these patients was examined.

Patients.—During a 1-year period, 26 patients with cancer-associated pelvic pain were enrolled in the study. Twenty women had gynecologic cancer had 6 men had prostatic or colorectal carcinomas. All patients had disease progression that necessitated other modes of therapy. Each patient underwent a bilateral percutaneous neurolytic superior hypogastric plexus block with 10% phenol. Pain was assessed using a 10-point visual analogue pain score.

Results.—Eighteen patients (69%) obtained satisfactory pain relief, 15 after 1 block and 3 after a second block. The remaining 8 patients (31%) obtained only moderate pain control after 2 blocks, and they were then treated with epidural bupivacaine-morphine therapy, which ultimately diminished their pain. There were no intraoperative or long-term complications. All patients experienced significant reductions in oral opioid therapy after undergoing neurolytic blocks, but the reduction in usage was significantly greater when the neurolytic block had been successful.

Conclusion.—Neurolytic superior hypogastric plexus block is an effective technique for the relief of pelvic cancer pain in a high proportion of patients.

▶ As with a celiac block, this technique appears to offer significant improvement in symptoms without an appreciable risk of neurologic dysfunction. It is likely to be most helpful in patients with pelvic visceral pain who no longer experience satisfactory analgesia or who have intolerable side effects from systemic opioids. As with a celiac plexus block, it is not clear whether early intervention, before opioids become ineffective, provides better long-term pain management.—S.E. Abram, M.D.

Is Disease Progression the Major Factor in Morphine 'Tolerance' in Cancer Pain Treatment?

Collin E, Poulain P, Gauvain-Piquard A, Petit G, Pichard-Leandri E (Institut Gustave Roussy, Villejuif, France)
Pain 55:319–326, 1993   101-95-23-28

Background.—Physicians often limit the use of opioids for cancer-related pain because they fear that tolerance will develop and that the drugs will not then be effective when patients "really need" them. However, it is not clear to what extent tolerance occurs in humans who are given opioids as analgesics. The contribution of pharmacologic tolerance to escalating doses of morphine in patients with cancer was investigated.

Methods.—Twenty-nine patients who required oral morphine for cancer pain were studied by 2 independent teams. One team evaluated physical impairment, pain intensity, and pain treatment, and the other team evaluated depressive disorders and emotional and behavioral depressive patterns. All patients were seen at the initiation of morphine therapy and were followed up to the first morphine dose modification.

Findings.—Progressive disease was recorded in 24 of the 25 patients for whom morphine doses were increased. In the 4 patients with no dose increases, the disease was stable or in remission. Changes in depressed mood were not associated with pain intensity.

Conclusion.—The main factor resulting in increases in oral morphine doses in patients with cancer pain seems to be an increase in pain as a result of disease progression, not pharmacologic tolerance. These findings are consistent with previous results suggesting that opioid tolerance develops at a slower rate and to a lesser degree in animals in chronic pain than in pain-free animals.

▶ Cancer pain and opioid requirements generally escalate dramatically during the final few days of life, as tumor infiltration and nociception increase. This study adds further evidence that the opioid requirement correlates well with increased tumor invasion.—S.E. Abram, M.D.

Enhancement of Opiate Analgesia by Nimodipine in Cancer Patients Chronically Treated With Morphine: A Preliminary Report

Santillán R, Maestre JM, Hurlé MA, Flórez J (Univ Hosp M de Valdecilla, Santander, Spain; Univ of Cantabria, Santander, Spain)
Pain 58:129–132, 1994   101-95-23-29

Introduction.—Previous studies in rats indicate that nimodipine, a calcium channel blocker with a relatively high affinity for the CNS, potentiates the analgesic effect of μ-opioid agonists in naive and tolerant conditions. The ability of nimodipine to enhance morphine analgesia and/or modify the development of tolerance in cancer pain management was evaluated.

Treatment.—Twenty-three patients, aged 35 to 79 years, with stable tumor pain syndrome were treated. All patients needed successive increments of morphine for 21–780 days. Oral nimodipine was introduced with an initial dose of 60 mg, increasing to as much as 120 mg/day in 4 doses. Assessment of daily morphine consumption was the primary effect measurement of the study.

Outcome.—Nimodipine successfully reduced the daily dose of morphine in 16 (69.5%) patients, including 13 who received oral morphine and 3 who received intrathecal morphine (Fig 23–11). The daily dose of morphine was significantly reduced from 282 mg to 158 mg (Fig 23–12), and the intrathecal dose of morphine was reduced by 1–5 mg. The minimum dose of morphine was attained in 17.5 days of treatment and maintained for 73.4 days in 9 of 13 patients. Use of nimodipine did not result in a modification of the daily dose of morphine in 2 patients and

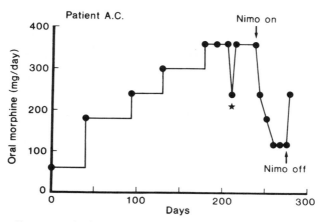

Fig 23–11.—Variations in the daily dose of oral morphine required to relieve pain in a patient with cancer before and after nimodipine (120 mg/day) is added. The *star* indicates that an unsuccessful attempt was made to reduce the morphine dose. (Courtesy of Santillán R, Maestre JM, Hurlé MA, et al: *Pain* 58:129–132, 1994.)

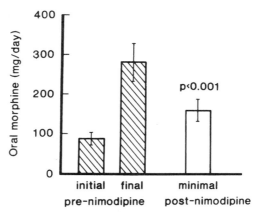

Fig 23–12.—Changes in the requirements of the daily dose of oral morphine (means and standard deviation) in 13 patients with cancer pain, before and after nimodipine (120 mg/day) is added. (Courtesy of Santillán R, Maestre JM, Hurlé MA, et al: *Pain* 58:129–132, 1994.)

was withdrawn in 5 patients during the first week of treatment because of intolerance or aggravation of the disease.

Conclusion.—Nimodipine enhanced the analgesic activity of long-term treatment with morphine in patients with cancer who required regular increments of the opiate to relieve pain. It controls the progressive increment in the daily dose of morphine and substantially reduces the daily dose of morphine for several weeks. Sustained channel blockade may disrupt some of the calcium-related mechanisms involved in the development of tolerance to morphine.

▶ At least 4 subtypes of calcium channels have been identified. The drugs currently used in clinical practice represent only 1. Because of the importance of calcium flux in the transmission of pain and the development of hyperalgesia, the calcium channel antagonists may represent a fertile area of analgesic research.—S.E. Abram, M.D.

Subarachnoid Adrenal Medullary Transplants for Terminal Cancer Pain: A Report of Preliminary Studies
Winnie AP, Pappas GD, Das Gupta TK, Wang H, Ortega JD, Sagen J (Univ of Illinois at Chicago)
Anesthesiology 79:644–653, 1993   101-95-23-30

Background.—Drug treatment often fails to control intractable cancer pain. Some patients rapidly become tolerant of parenteral opioids, and use of the epidural and subarachnoid routes for opioid treatment involves some potential mechanical problems as well as a risk of infection. Laboratory studies in rodents indicate that transplanting adrenal medullary tissue into the spinal subarachnoid space can significantly lessen pain without tolerance developing. The chromaffin cells secrete catecholamines and opioid peptides, which independently, and possibly synergistically, reduce pain.

Objective and Methods.—Five patients with intractable pain from unresectable cancer received adrenal medullary tissue from otherwise-healthy adults who had died of traumatic causes. Two cc of tissue was placed in the lumbar subarachnoid space, and the patient was discharged the next day.

Results.—Four patients had progressively decreasing pain scores and required smaller amounts of opioid. Three of them remained free of pain—2 for longer than 10 months—whereas 1 patient had recurrent pain after surgery for metastatic spinal cord compression 10 weeks after the transplant procedure. The spinal CSF contained increased levels of met-enkephalin and catecholamines after transplantation of adrenal medullary tissue.

Conclusion.—Transplanting adrenal medullary tissue to the subarachnoid space may provide an effective means of controlling intractable cancer pain.

▶ Although the results of this preliminary study of an intriguing technique are of interest, a much more meticulous and better-controlled study should have been undertaken. The potential for unanticipated complications is high, and the risks are not warranted unless efficacy can be better documented.—S.E. Abram, M.D.

Disposition and Respiratory Effects of Intrathecal Morphine in Children

Nichols DG, Yaster M, Lynn AM, Helfaer MA, Deshpande JK, Manson PN, Carson BS, Bezman M, Maxwell LG, Tobias JD, Grochow LB (Johns Hopkins Univ, Baltimore, Md; Children's Hosp and Med Ctr, Seattle; Vanderbilt Univ, Nashville, Tenn)
Anesthesiology 79:733–738, 1993   101-95-23–31

Introduction.—Safely administering opioid analgesics after surgery to infants has been a goal, particularly because the hormonal stress response associated with pain in children is similar to that of adults. Infants may be particularly vulnerable to respiratory depression after opioid administration; however, the extent and duration in infants and children have been poorly defined.

Methods.—In 10 children, aged 4 months to 15 years, who had repair of craniofacial defects, the disposition and respiratory effects of intrathecal morphine were studied. Before the end of surgery, morphine, .02 mg/kg, was administered intrathecally. After surgery, the minute ventilation in response to the increasing partial pressure of end-tidal carbon dioxide during carbon dioxide rebreathing was determined. The slope and intercept of the carbon dioxide response curve were calculated at 6, 12, and 18 hours after morphine was administered. Using radioimmunoassay, CSF and blood were analyzed for morphine concentration.

Results.—The carbon dioxide response curve slope decreased from a preoperative value of 35.1 to 16.3 mL/kg^{-1}/min^{-1}/mm Hg^{-1} at 6 hours after morphine and remained depressed to 23.4 at 12 hours and 23.5 at 18 hours. The mean minute ventilation decreased from 874 to 276 mL/kg^{-1}/min^{-1} at 6 hours, but then it recovered at 18 hours to 567. The mean CSF morphine concentration was 2,860 ng/mL at 6 hours and decreased to 640 ng/mL at 12 hours and 220 ng/mL at 18 hours.

Conclusion.—The ventilatory response to carbon dioxide was depressed with intrathecal morphine, .02 mg/kg, for as many as 18 hours; at the same time, greater CSF morphine concentrations were observed, which may result from the rostral spread of morphine in the CSF rather than from systemic absorption. Patients who are treated with intrathecal morphine require regular monitoring for respiratory depression during the first 18 hours after a single dose. The infants, aged 4 to 12 months, did not have greater ventilatory depression than the older children aged 2 to 15 years.

▶ Intrathecal morphine appears to carry the same risks of delayed, prolonged respiratory depressant effects in children.—S.E. Abram, M.D.

Prolonged Intrathecal Fentanyl Analgesia Via 32-Gauge Catheters After Thoracotomy
Guinard J-P, Chiolero R, Mavrocordatos P, Carpenter RL (Centre Hospitalier Universitaire Vaudois, Lausanne, Switzerland; Virginia Mason Med Ctr, Seattle)
Anesth Analg 77:936–941, 1993   101-95-23–32

Background.—Thoracic placement of epidural fentanyl has not resulted in better analgesia, reduced doses of fentanyl, or reduced side effects compared with lumbar catheter placement or IV administration. Intrathecal injection of opioids can produce excellent and prolonged analgesia, although single injections have an unpredictable and limited duration. Continuous intrathecal opioid infusion was evaluated for its analgesic effects after thoracotomy.

Methods.—Twelve patients were studied for 48 hours after thoracotomy. After awakening from anesthesia, patients rated their pain, and pulmonary function tests were measured. Ineffective analgesia was defined as a pain score greater than 30/100. Pruritus, nausea, sedation, and other measurements were recorded.

Results.—Fentanyl was infused intrathecally in a mean dose of .81 μg/kg^{-1}/hr^{-1}. Plasma fentanyl concentrations ranged from .49 to .72 ng/mL. Four patients required a supplementary bolus of intrathecal fentanyl. Within 1 hour at rest, but after 24 hours during coughing, pain scores declined to less than 30/100. Within 1 hour of fentanyl infusion, pulmonary function tests returned to about 50% of their preoperative values. The mean respiratory rates averaged 19; no apnea was noted. Pruritus occurred in 4 patients and nausea occurred in 1 patient. One catheter broke outside the patient.

Discussion.—Intrathecal infusion can provide safe, rapid, and intense analgesia. Current 32-gauge intrathecal catheters are not convenient for use during prolonged periods postoperatively.

▶ It is surprising that such large doses of intrathecal fentanyl are needed compared with the doses required for epidural or IV fentanyl analgesia (roughly three fourths). This technique seems to have relatively little advantage.—S.E. Abram, M.D.

Postoperative Analgesia in Children Using Continuous S.C. Morphine

McNicol R (Royal Hosp for Sick Children, Glasgow, Scotland)
Br J Anaesth 71:752–756, 1993   101-95-23–33

Objective.—Morphine, given by continuous subcutaneous infusion, has proved effective in relieving postoperative pain in adults. This approach was evaluated in 60 children with a mean age of 6½ years who underwent major abdominal, urologic, or orthopedic surgery under balanced general anesthesia.

Methods.—Analgesia was established intraoperatively after induction of anesthesia, using extradural or peripheral bupivacaine to produce a regional nerve block. Postoperatively, morphine, 1 mg/kg^{-1}, in 20 mL of sodium chloride was infused subcutaneously at rate of 3–5 mL/hr for a mean period of about 39 hours. Pain, sedation, and nausea/vomiting were monitored along with oxygen saturation.

Results.—Only 6% of the pain scores indicated more than mild pain (table). Eleven patients had severe pain at some time postoperatively. None of the children were unrousable at any time. All but 3% of the oxygen saturation values exceeded 94%. Thirteen of the 60 patients had varying degrees of nausea or vomiting. There were no cannula-related complications.

Discussion.—Nursing staff have been enthusiastic about the use of subcutaneous morphine infusion to control postoperative pain in children. Pulse oximetry should be used routinely if it is available.

▶ The benefits seen with the technique described may have occurred because all the patients received regional anesthesia intraoperatively.—S.E. Abram, M.D.

Analysis of Recordings From Postoperative Pain Charts

Number of patients: 60
Total number of recordings: 2361
Duration of infusion (Hrs) 17–80 (38.8)—Range (mean)

Pain scores
   0–1 $n = 2220$ (94%)
   2     $n = 120$ (5%)
   3     $n = 21$ (1%)
  Mean pain score of all recordings = 0.47

Sedation scores
   0–1 $n = 2353$ (99.7%)
   2     $n = 8$ (0.3%)
   3     $n = 0$ (0%)
  Mean sedation score of all recordings = 0.45

Sp_{O_2} (%)
  Minimum for each patient: mean 93% (range 86–98%)
  $Sp_{O_2} < 94\%$ $n = 75$ (3%)
  $Sp_{O_2} < 93\%$ $n = 30$ (1%)
  $Sp_{O_2} < 90\%$ $n = 1$ (0.04%)

Nausea scores ($n = 1248$)
   0 $n = 1213$ (97.2%)
   1 $n = 18$ (1.4%)
   2 $n = 16$ (1.3%)
   3 $n = 1$ (0.1%)

Abbreviation: Sp_{O_2}, pulse oximetry.
(Courtesy of McNicol R: *Br J Anaesth* 71:752–756, 1993.)

Effects of Retrobulbar Bupivacaine on Post-Operative Pain and Nausea in Retinal Detachment Surgery

Gottfreósdóttir MS, Gíslason I, Stefánsson E, Sigurjónsdóttir S, Nielsen NChr (Univ of Iceland, Reykjavik)
Acta Ophthalmol 71:544–547, 1993   101-95-23-34

Background.—Postoperative pain and nausea are common after retinal detachment surgery. The effects of retrobulbar bupivacaine block were evaluated for their impact on postoperative pain and nausea and on intraoperative and postoperative use of oral and parenteral pain medication.

Methods.—Thirty-two patients who were scheduled for scleral buckling surgery were randomly selected to receive general anesthesia with or without retrobulbar bupivacaine. After surgery, patients were questioned about their degree of pain and nausea at 2, 4, 8, 10, 24, and 48 hours.

Results.—Two hours after surgery, pain scores were significantly lower in the group that received the retrobulbar block. Patients who received the retrobulbar block complained less of nausea and vomiting and required significantly less parenteral pain relief. Men complained about postoperative pain more than women did. There were no complications associated with the retrobulbar injections.

Conclusion.—General anesthesia plus retrobulbar block provides optimal anesthesia and is recommended for relieving postoperative pain and reducing use of parenteral pain medications.

▶ With few exceptions, peripheral nerve blocks that are initiated before the incision appear to reduce the severity of postoperative pain. When they are used for ophthalmic surgery, modification of the severity of nausea, which may be more distressing than the pain, is an added benefit.—S.E. Abram, M.D.

Radiological Examination of the Intrathecal Position of Microcatheters in Continuous Spinal Anaesthesia
Standl T, Beck H (Univ Hosp Eppendorf, Hamburg, Germany)
Br J Anaesth 71:803–806, 1993   101-95-23–35

Background.—The intrathecal position of spinal catheters can affect the clinical outcome of continuous spinal anesthesia, but few studies have examined the position of large-gauge spinal catheters. The intrathecal position of spinal catheters was investigated using conventional radiography.

Methods.—Volunteers who were undergoing elective orthopedic surgery were randomly assigned to 1 of 2 groups: Group A patients had lumbar puncture and intrathecal insertion of the catheter performed

Intrathecal Position of 68 Microspinal Catheters Dependent on Interspace of Lumbar Puncture, Patient's Position During Catheter Insertion, and Intrathecal Insertion Depth

	Intrathecal position		
	Cranial	Puncture site	Caudal
Interspace			
L2–3	3 (33%)	3 (33%)	3 (33%)
L3–4	24 (53%)	15 (33%)	6 (13%)
L4–5	7 (50%)	5 (36%)	2 (14%)
Patient's position			
Sitting (group A)	22 (69%)	8 (25%)	2 (6%)
Right lateral (group B)	12 (33%)	15 (42%)	9 (25%)
Insertion depth (cm)			
2.0–3.0	6 (28%)	13 (62%)	2 (10%)
3.1–4.0	20 (59%)	9 (26%)	5 (15%)
> 4	8 (61%)	1 (8%)	4 (31%)

(Courtesy of Standl T, Beck H: *Br J Anaesth* 71:803–806, 1993.)

while in the sitting position, and group B patients had the same procedure performed while in the right lateral position. A 28-gauge spinal catheter was inserted 2–5 cm into the subarachnoid space and secured at the puncture site, and the catheter was left in place postoperatively. One day postoperatively, the position of the catheter was compared with the preoperative level. The position was tested statistically in respect to the point of entrance into the subarachnoid space, the position of the patient during insertion, and the catheter insertion depth.

Results.—Sixty-eight volunteers participated in the study, 32 in group A and 36 in group B, and all were adequately anesthetized. In all patients, there was no change in position noted between the level of the catheter that was marked at the level of the skin immediately after insertion and the level 1 day postoperatively. There was no statistical dependence of the intrathecal position of the catheters based on the lumbar interspace of insertion. The position of the catheters was significantly different between the groups, based on the position the patient assumed during insertion. For example, in group A (seated patients), 69% of the catheters were directed cephalad compared with 33% in group B. The intrathecal depth of insertion of the catheters also revealed significant differences between insertion depths: 31% of those inserted 4 cm or more were positioned more caudally, whereas 15% of those inserted 3.1–4 cm and 10% of those inserted 2–3 cm were positioned caudally (table).

Conclusion.—Despite the intent to position all spinal catheters cranially, only 50% were successfully directed in that manner, 34% remained at the level of the puncture site, and 16% were passed caudally. A greater number of cranially directed catheters were found in patients who were seated during insertion. A systematic investigation of the clinical consequences of the different intrathecal positions has not yet been reported.

▶ The cephalad direction of microspinal catheters appears to be important in reducing the likelihood of sequestration of high concentrations of local anesthetic.—S.E. Abram, M.D.

Interscalene Block for Pain Relief After Shoulder Surgery: A Prospective Randomized Study
Kinnard P, Truchon R, St-Pierre A, Montreuil J (Laval Univ, Québec)
Clin Orthop 304:22–24, 1994   101-95-23–36

Objective.—In a retrospective study of outpatient orthopedic surgeries involving the shoulder, the hospitalization rate was 11.8%. The safety and effectiveness of postoperative interscalene block in decreasing the hospitalization rate for patients undergoing outpatient shoulder surgery was determined.

Methods.—Thirty patients, with an average age 51.5 years, underwent decompressive acromioplasties. Fifteen patients had a postoperative interscalene block with 20 mL of .25% bupivacaine, and 15 had no block.

Results.—The group that received the block had significantly less pain than the other group. Mood and sleep duration were significantly improved in the group that received the block. There were 2 hospitalizations among the group that received no block and 1 hospitalization in the group that received the block; the difference was not significant. There were no complications in either group.

Conclusion.—For patients having shoulder surgery, an interscalene block is recommended to improve the postoperative recovery period.

▶ To say that there were no significant differences between groups with respect to incidence of hospitalization is meaningless in this study, which lacks adequate numbers to provide statistical power to demonstrate an effect.—S.E. Abram, M.D.

The Effect of Balanced Analgesia on Early Convalescence After Major Orthopaedic Surgery
Møiniche S, Hjortsø N-C, Hansen BL, Dahl JB, Rosenberg J, Gebuhr P, Kehlet H (Hvidovre Univ, Copenhagen)
Acta Anaesthesiol Scand 38:328–335, 1994   101-95-23–37

Objective.—An attempt was made to lessen postoperative pain and shorten the convalescence period after major orthopedic surgery using a balanced epidural analgesic regimen of low-dose bupivacaine and morphine in addition to systemic piroxicam, a nonsteroidal anti-inflammatory agent.

Study Plan.—Twenty patients who were to have total knee arthroplasty and 22 who were scheduled to have total hip arthroplasty were assigned to receive either continuous epidural anesthesia plus oral piroxicam for 48 hours postoperatively or general anesthesia followed by IM opioid and acetaminophen. General anesthesia included fentanyl, midazolam, and nitrous oxide in oxygen.

Results.—The patients who were given epidural analgesia had significantly less pain when mobilized within 48 hours of surgery, but no significant difference was noted after the withdrawal of epidural analgesia. However, reduction in pain did not appear to influence postoperative ambulation or patient activity, and it did not lessen fatigue or shorten the hospital stay. The most important factors limiting movement and activity were late postoperative pain, fatigue, and a conservative approach to postoperative management.

Conclusion.—Although epidural analgesia combined with systemic piroxicam enhances pain relief after major orthopedic operations, it does not allow patients to ambulate better or to be substantially more active, and it does not shorten the hospital stay.

▶ Here is yet another study that attests to reductions in pain but no measurable improvement in function associated with epidural analgesia. Is improved pain management reason enough to use the technique?—S.E. Abram, M.D.

Meperidine for Patient-Controlled Analgesia After Cesarean Section: Intravenous *Versus* Epidural Administration

Paech MJ, Moore JS, Evans SF (King Edward Mem Hosp for Women, Subiaco, Western Australia, Australia)
Anesthesiology 80:1268–1276, 1994   101-95-23–38

Introduction.—Both patient-controlled IV analgesia (PCIA) and patient-controlled epidural analgesia (PCEA) are effective methods of managing pain after cesarean section. Meperidine has been used successfully in this setting for both routes of administration. The existence of differences in quality of analgesia, side effects, patient satisfaction, dose requirement, or plasma drug concentration when meperidine is administered as PCEA or as PCIA after cesarean section was studied.

Methods.—Fifty women scheduled for elective cesarean section were enrolled in the study. At the first request for postoperative analgesia, they were randomly assigned to receive PCEA for an initial 12-hour period, followed by PCIA for a second 12-hour period (group 1) or to receive the opposite sequence (group 2). Group 1 received a loading dose of 25 mg of meperidine in 10 mL of saline epidurally and 10 mL of IV saline; group 2 received similarly formulated and administered IV meperidine and saline. All patients completed a series of visual analogue pain scales for pain at rest and with coughing over the 24-hour study. Venous blood samples were taken from 20 patients for plasma meperidine and normeperidine assays.

Results.—Results were available for 24 patients in group 1 and 21 patients in group 2. The time to onset of analgesia was similar for the 2 groups, but those receiving PCEA subsequently had significantly lower pain scores both at rest and with coughing. During the first 12 hours, the PCEA and PCIA groups reported similar nausea and pruritus scores; however, sedation scores were significantly higher in patients receiving PCIA. Meperidine use was reduced approximately 50% with the epidural route, and plasma meperidine and normeperidine concentrations were also significantly lower during PCEA.

Conclusion.—Almost 90% of the women who had elective cesarean section preferred PCEA over PCIA for postoperative pain relief. High-quality analgesia in the early postdelivery period allows mothers to care for their infant and ambulate freely. The epidural route also had significant advantages over the IV route in terms of side effects and dose requirements. However, neonatal effects in breast-feeding mothers have yet to be evaluated.

▶ In comparison to epidural fentanyl, epidural meperidine provides better analgesia and has lower drug requirements than systemic meperidine. The improved epidural effect may be related to better drug access to spinal cord opiate receptors or to the local anesthetic effect of the drug.—S.E. Abram, M.D.

Pre-Emptive Analgesia From Intravenous Administration of Opioids: No Effect With Alfentanil
Wilson RJT, Leith S, Jackson IJB, Hunter D (York District Hosp, England)
Anaesthesia 49:591–593, 1994   101-95-23–39

Objective.—Whether IV opioid alfentanil, when given preemptively before surgical incision, reduces the postoperative need for opioid analgesia compared with administering the same dose after surgery begins was studied.

Methods.—Forty American Society of Anesthesiologists physical status I or II patients, aged 25 to 65 years, scheduled for total abdominal hysterectomy through a transverse lower abdominal incision participated in the study. All patients received temazepam as premedication and propofol for induction. The patients were assigned to receive either alfentanil, 40 µg/kg, or physiologic saline at the time of induction. Anesthesia was maintained with 1% to 2% enflurane in oxygen and 65% to 70% nitrous oxide. Controls received the same dose of alfentanil 1 minute after surgical incision, and patients in both groups received morphine, .1 mg/kg, at this time. Patient-controlled analgesia with morphine was used postoperatively.

Results.—The groups did not significantly differ in the amount of morphine used during surgery, in the recovery room, or for as long as 24 hours postoperatively. At 24 hours, controls had significantly lower visual analogue pain scores while at rest, but scores on movement were identical in the 2 groups.

Conclusion.—Preemptive analgesia in which conventional doses of parenteral opioid are used was not clinically useful.

▶ This study presents results that agree with animal studies that fail to show a preemptive analgesic effect from systemic opioids (1).—S.E. Abram, M.D.

Reference

1. Abram SE, Olson EE: *Anesthesiology* 80:1114, 1994.

Interactions Between Fluoxetine and Opiate Analgesia for Postoperative Dental Pain

Gordon NC, Heller PH, Gear RW, Levine JD (Univ of Calif, San Francisco; Kaiser Found Hosp, Hayward, Calif)
Pain 58:85–88, 1994   101-95-23–40

Objective.—The role of serotonergic mechanisms in opiate analgesia was investigated in a double-blind, placebo-controlled study that compared the analgesic efficacy of combinations of fluoxetine, a serotonergic tricyclic antidepressant, with either the μ-opiate morphine or the κ-opiate pentazocine.

Methods.—Seventy patients whose impacted third molar teeth were to be extracted were randomly assigned to receive either fluoxetine in an oral dose of 10 mg or a placebo each day for 1 week before surgery. Pain was recorded on a visual analogue scale, and when pain of at least one fourth (2.5 cm) was recorded—but no sooner than 80 minutes after the onset of local anesthesia—the patients received a single-blind, open IV injection of either 6 mg of morphine sulfate or 45 mg of pentazocine.

Results.—In placebo recipients, pain was reduced by about 2 cm on the visual analogue scale. Morphine analgesia lasted about 2–3 hours, and pentazocine analgesia lasted about $1\frac{1}{2}$ hours. Pretreatment with fluoxetine did not affect pentazocine analgesia, but it significantly lessened the analgesic effect of morphine. After 90 minutes, patients who were given fluoxetine and morphine had more pain than they did at baseline.

Conclusion.—The attenuating effect of fluoxetine on μ-opiate analgesia probably reflects an alteration in the serotonergic circuits that modulate pain.

▶ Unlike tricyclic antidepressants, the new serotoninergic antidepressants (fluoxetine, sertraline, and paroxetine) do not appear to produce analgesia for neuropathic pain and, as shown in this study, may actually interfere with the analgesic effect of opioid analgesics.—S.E. Abram, M.D.

Analgesic Effect of Intra-Articular Morphine After Arthroscopic Meniscectomy

Dierking GW, Østergaard HT, Dissing CK, Kristensen JE (Silkeborg County Hosp, Denmark; Hvidovre Univ, Copenhagen)
Anaesthesia 49:627–629, 1994   101-95-23–41

Objective.—Data from clinical studies of local administration of opioids are still inconclusive. The analgesic effect of 2 mg of intra-articular morphine in patients having elective arthroscopic meniscectomy was evaluated.

Treatment.—In all patients, anesthesia was induced with propofol and alfentanil and was maintained with alfentanil, enflurane, and nitrous oxide oxygen. At the end of surgery, 18 patients received 2 mg of morphine hydrochloride in 40 mL of normal saline solution intra-articularly and 1 mL of normal saline intramuscularly, and 15 received 40 mL of normal saline intra-articularly and 2 mg of morphine hydrochloride intramuscularly; the latter group served as a control for any potential systemic effects of morphine. If requested, patients received supplemental IV morphine, .1 mg/kg, after surgery.

Outcome.—On a visual analogue scale of 0–100 mm, pain scores at rest and during active flexion of the knee 1–6 hours after surgery were low (less than 20 mm), but they did not differ significantly between patients receiving intra-articular morphine and those receiving IM morphine. Although pain during walking 6 hours after surgery was more pronounced, it was only slightly reduced from 31 mm in the IM morphine group to 25 mm in the intra-articular morphine group. Six patients in the intra-articular group and 2 patients in the IM group requested supplemental morphine within the first hour after surgery.

Conclusion.—Local analgesic effects of intra-articular morphine after arthroscopic meniscectomy were not observed when patients were at rest or when they were ambulatory.

Intraarticular Morphine for Postoperative Analgesia Following Knee Arthroscopy

Björnsson A, Gupta A, Vegfors M, Lennmarken C, Sjöberg F (Univ Hosp, Linköping, Sweden)

Reg Anesth 19:104–108, 1994   101-95-23–42

Introduction.—Studies of the intra-articular injection of local anesthetics have had conflicting results. Intra-articular injection of morphine can provide analgesia for as long as 6 hours postoperatively, but the effect can be reversed by a local injection of naloxone, which suggests that naloxone acts specifically with opioid receptors. A 2-stage, prospective, randomized, double-blind, controlled study assessed the postoperative analgesic effects of intra-articular injections of morphine or bupivacaine after minor arthroscopic knee procedures.

Methods.—After induction of standardized general anesthesia, 149 patients were divided into 2 study groups. The first group was randomly assigned to receive postoperative intra-articular injections of 1 mg of morphine, saline, 20 mL of .25% bupivacaine, or both morphine and bupivacaine. The second group was randomly assigned to receive intra-articular morphine, 5 mg; intra-articular saline; or IM morphine, 5 mg, and intra-articular saline. The patients rated their pain intensity using a visual analogue scale at 30, 60, 90, and 120 minutes and at 8, 24, and 48 hours after surgery and reported the number of analgesic tablets taken within a 48-hour period.

Results.—There were no significant differences between the groups in pain intensity as measured by the visual analogue scale or in the number of analgesic tablets taken in either arm of the study.

Conclusion.—Neither 1 mg nor 5 mg of morphine nor 50 mg of bupivacaine had a significant analgesic effect when it was injected directly into the articular space after minor diagnostic arthroscopic surgery.

▶ There is evidence accumulating that intra-articular opioids are not particularly effective in controlling postarthrotomy pain.—S.E. Abram, M.D.

Immediate and Prolonged Effects of Pre- Versus Postoperative Epidural Analgesia With Bupivacaine and Morphine on Pain at Rest and During Mobilisation After Total Knee Arthroplasty
Dahl JB, Daugaard JJ, Rasmussen B, Egebo K, Carlsson P, Kehlet H (Hvidovre Univ, Denmark; Univ Hosps in Århus, Denmark)
Acta Anaesthesiol Scand 38:557–561, 1994   101-95-23–43

Introduction.—Some recent studies have suggested that preoperative induction of analgesia may improve postoperative pain control, but results of comparative trials have varied. The immediate and prolonged analgesic effects of preoperative initiation vs. immediately postoperative initiation of intensive epidural administration of bupivacaine and morphine were compared.

Methods.—Thirty-two patients undergoing total knee arthroplasty were randomly assigned to receive identical epidural blockades that were initiated either 30 minutes preoperatively and after the induction of general anesthesia or during surgical closure. The patients assessed their pain using both a visual analogue scale and a verbal scale at rest and during elevation of the limb. Pain scores and requests for additional pain medication during a 7-day observation period were compared for the 2 groups.

Results.—There were no significant differences between the 2 groups in either visual analogue or verbal scale pain scores. The need for additional morphine or ketobemidone/morphine was comparable in the 2 groups throughout the 7 days. Only the use of postoperative fentanyl differed, with more patients in the postoperative epidural block group receiving it.

Discussion.—Immediate and prolonged pain control did not significantly differ between patients who received preoperative initiation and those who received postoperative initiation of the epidural blockade.

► The issue of preemptive analgesia and its clinical relevance in postoperative pain control is far from being settled.—S.E. Abram, M.D.

Postoperative Epidural Analgesia and Oral Anticoagulant Therapy
Horlocker TT, Wedel DJ, Schlichting JL (Mayo Clinic, Rochester, Minn)
Anesth Analg 79:89–93, 1994   101-95-23-44

Background.—Anticoagulants are used in patients undergoing major orthopedic procedures to prevent deep venous thrombosis (DVT) and pulmonary embolism. The relative safety of epidural analgesia in patients who are anticoagulated with low-dose heparin has been well documented, but there is little information about the safety of postoperative epidural analgesia in patients receiving low-dose warfarin.

Methods.—During a 5-year period, 192 epidural catheters were placed in 188 patients undergoing total knee replacement. Epidural catheters were placed through an 18-gauge needle. All patients received prophylactic oral warfarin to prolong the prothrombin time (PT) approximately 1.3–1.5 times the baseline PT.

Results.—The mean daily postoperative warfarin doses ranged from 2.6 to 4.6 mg. In addition to warfarin, 36 patients were treated with nonsteroidal anti-inflammatory drugs. Epidural catheters were left in place from 13 to 96 hours; the mean period of epidural analgesia was 37.5 hours. Blood was noted during catheter placement in 13 patients, but none of them showed signs of spinal hematoma. The mean PT did not increase until the third postoperative day, and it did not reach 15 seconds until the seventh postoperative day. The mean PT at the time of catheter removal was 13.4 seconds.

Conclusion.—Prophylactic low-dose warfarin given to patients with an indwelling epidural catheter for postoperative analgesia appears to be safe. Although the anticoagulant effect usually is not exhibited until after the epidural catheter has been removed, the PT must be measured daily to prevent major neurologic events.

► This study is helpful in establishing the risk-benefit ratio of epidural anesthesia in patients who are receiving oral anticoagulants for deep venous thrombosis prophylaxis.—S.E. Abram, M.D.

Intrathecal Infusional Analgesia for Nonmalignant Pain: Analgesic Efficacy of Intrathecal Opioid With or Without Bupivacaine
Krames ES, Lanning RM (San Francisco Ctr for Comprehensive Pain Management)
J Pain Symptom Manage 8:539–548, 1993   101-95-23-45

Introduction.—Despite mixed reports, intrathecal opioid therapy for nonmalignant pain is believed to be enhanced when it is combined with local anesthetics. Sixteen consecutive ambulatory outpatients who were receiving intrathecal infusions of opioids alone or in combination with bupivacaine for severe intractable nonmalignant pain were studied retrospectively.

Methods.—All patients had previously been given conventional pain therapy, and some had received invasive therapies; neither gave adequate analgesic effect. Psychological evaluations were done before implantation of an opioid infusion pump. Three patients had nociceptive pain, 5 had neuropathic pain, and 8 had pain of mixed nociceptive-neuropathic origin. A 3-day inpatient trial using opioids alone was conducted on 15 patients; the 16th patient started with morphine and bupivacaine combined. Thirteen of 16 patients experienced either poor control or side effects. Bupivacaine was added to their pumps in doses ranging from 3 to 4.5 mg to enhance analgesic effect or to reduce the opioid dosage so as to decrease side effects.

Results.—The mean treatment time was 27.8 months. Two of 3 patients with nociceptive pain, 2 of 2 with neuropathic pain, and 6 of 8 with mixed pain experienced an enhanced analgesic benefit or a decrease in opioid side effects with the opioid-analgesia combination. Subjective patient reports indicated that 13 patients (81%) had excellent results and 3 (19%) had fair results. No patients reported poor results during opioid treatment with or without bupivacaine.

Conclusion.—An opioid-analgesia combination can be efficacious in treating nonmalignant pain, particularly in patients with neuropathic pain. Controlled studies should be done to confirm that tolerance does not develop and that dosage levels appear to stabilize with this treatment.

▶ As with many uncontrolled reports of the efficacy of treatment modalities, the criteria for treatment success are vague. That most patients required local anesthetic suggests a low response rate to opioids alone.—S.E. Abram, M.D.

Respiratory Depression Associated With Patient-Controlled Analgesia: A Review of Eight Cases
Etches RC (Univ of Alberta, Edmonton, Canada)
Can J Anaesth 41:125–132, 1994   101-95-23–46

Introduction.—Patient-controlled analgesia (PCA) is often viewed as an effective alternative to conventional IM opioid analgesia and as being free of respiratory depression. However, there is little actual evidence that severe respiratory depression is less frequent than when epidural opioids are used.

Series.—Eight patients receiving PCA had severe respiratory depression, and 3 other patients were observed. All the patients had received morphine as well as at least 1 dose of naloxone. Three patients were subsequently excluded because their respiratory problems had begun shortly after surgery, before any opioid had been delivered by PCA. The incidence of severe respiratory depression associated with PCA in this population was .5%. Most patients cared for by the acute pain management service were adults who had major orthopedic or general surgery.

Risk Factors.—Two of the patients were elderly women; 3 had received other infusions concurrently. One patient's respiratory function was compromised, and another received sedative/hypnotic therapy at the same time as PCA. Use of a background infusion with PCA increased the risk that severe respiratory depression would develop. It is often difficult to use PCA safely in the elderly; patients with sleep apnea may also be problematic.

Conclusion.—Patient-controlled analgesia is a safe procedure when it is used appropriately, but it poses a risk of severe respiratory depression.

▶ The incidence of respiratory depression with PCA in this study was higher than the incidence with epidural opioids.—S.E. Abram, M.D.

Evaluation of Intravenous Ketorolac Administered by Bolus or Infusion for Treatment of Postoperative Pain: A Double-Blind, Placebo-Controlled, Multicenter Study
Ready LB, Brown CR, Stahlgren LH, Egan KJ, Ross B, Wild L, Moodie JE, Jones SF, Tommeraasen M, Trierwieler M (Univ of Washington, Seattle; Waikato Analgesic Research, Hamilton, New Zealand; St Joseph Hosp, Denver)
Anesthesiology 80:1277–1286, 1994   101-95-23–47

Background.—Previous studies have shown a reduction in morphine requirements in patients who are treated with IM ketorolac for postoperative analgesia after major surgery. Intravenous ketorolac is not yet marketed in the United States, but its safety has previously been documented. The analgesic efficacy and safety of IV ketorolac for postoperative analgesia were evaluated in a double-blind, randomized, multicenter trial.

Patients.—The study population consisted of 207 adult patients undergoing major surgery, of whom 65 were randomized to receive a ketorolac infusion, 68 to an IV ketorolac bolus, and 68 to placebo during the first 24 postoperative hours. All patients had access to supplemental IV morphine through a patient-controlled analgesia (PCA) pump. Pain intensity was assessed at study entry and at 2, 4, 6, and 24 hours, using categoric pain intensity scores and visual analogue scale (VAS) scores. The amount of morphine used during the 24-hour study was also measured.

Results.—Sixty-five patients (32%) did not complete the study. Categoric pain intensity scores and VAS pain scores in both ketorolac groups were significantly lower at various points in time during the study than those in the placebo group. The average amount of PCA morphine used in the ketorolac infusion group was significantly lower than that used in the placebo group, but the difference in morphine use between the bolus group and the placebo group did not reach statistical significance. There were no significant differences in sedation scores among the 3 groups at any point in time, but vomiting was significantly less frequent in both ketorolac groups. Study observers reported less nursing difficulty in the ketorolac infusion group. Overall, patient and observer ratings were statistically greater for both ketorolac groups.

Conclusion.—Patients who receive PCA morphine after major surgery will use less morphine if they are also given an IV ketorolac infusion. Intravenous ketorolac infusion and IV ketorolac bolus doses both improve the response to PCA morphine when compared with placebo.

▶ It appears that ketorolac infusion is associated with superior analgesia compared with bolus injection, despite the long duration of action of the drug.—S.E. Abram, M.D.

Postoperative Epidural Bupivacaine-Morphine Therapy: Experience With 4,227 Surgical Cancer Patients

de Leon-Casasola OA, Parker B, Lema MJ, Harrison P, Massey J (State Univ of New York, Buffalo; Univ of Pittsburgh, Pa)
Anesthesiology 81:368–375, 1994   101-95-23–48

Background.—The synergistic analgesic effects of epidural bupivacaine and morphine combination therapy for postoperative pain control have been demonstrated in earlier studies. However, the method is not widely accepted in surgical wards because of potential complications such as hypotension and catheter migration. The safety and effectiveness of postoperative epidural morphine-bupivacaine analgesia were assessed.

Patients.—During a 4-year period, patients undergoing surgery for cancer received general and epidural anesthesia followed by continuous epidural analgesia with .05% or .1% bupivacaine and .01% morphine. The goal was to maintain a dynamic visual analogue pain score (VAPS) of less than 5. The catheter was removed and patient-controlled analgesia was started in the event a sensory block did not develop. If a sensory block developed, supplemental IV morphine was administered as needed until the VAPS was less than 5.

Results.—Of 4,510 patients who entered the study, 283 (6.3%) were withdrawn for intraoperative catheter malposition. Of the remaining 4,227 patients, 2,248 (53.18%) had lumbar epidural catheters and 1,979 (46.82%) had thoracic catheters. The mean patient age was 68 years, and

61% of the patients were women. The mean duration of epidural analgesia was 6.3 days and the range was 2–19 days. Three patients (.07%) experienced respiratory depression and 126 (3%) had hypotension. Nausea or vomiting occurred in 929 patients (22%), but most had single episodes during the first 24 hours after surgery. Twenty-four patients (.57%) had infection at the catheter insertion site. There were no perioperative deaths associated with epidural analgesia and no cases of apparent catheter migration.

Conclusions.—Continuous epidural analgesia with bupivacaine and morphine is effective for postoperative pain management. Epidural analgesia can be safely administered on the surgical ward without special monitoring equipment.

▶ The combination of epidural morphine and bupivacaine appears to be rational and effective. As opposed to fentanyl, epidural morphine provides selective spinal effects, and the combination has been shown to be synergistic in animals.—S.E. Abram, M.D.

Preoperative Naproxen Sodium Reduces Postoperative Pain Following Arthroscopic Knee Surgery
Code WE, Yip RW, Rooney ME, Browne PM, Hertz T (Royal Univ, Saskatoon, Sask, Canada)
Can J Anaesth 41:98–101, 1994   101-95-23-49

Introduction.—Although arthroscopy offers a number of advantages over open orthopedic surgical procedures, there are few studies of post-arthroscopic pain. Some studies have suggested that nonsteroidal anti-inflammatory drugs may decrease the inflammation associated with arthroscopic procedures, probably through inhibition of prostaglandin synthesis. The efficacy of preoperative naproxen sodium in reducing postoperative pain and the length of day surgery stay in patients undergoing arthroscopic knee surgery was investigated in a randomized, double-blind trial.

Methods.—Of 66 American Society of Anesthesiologists physical status I and II patients undergoing outpatient arthroscopic knee surgery, 26 were assigned to receive 2 capsules of 275-mg naproxen sodium, whereas the other 40 received placebo. Outcome measures included preoperative and postoperative visual analogue pain scores, postoperative analgesic requirements before discharge and 24 hours afterward, and length of day-surgery stay.

Results.—Postoperative pain was decreased with naproxen, both in the hospital and after discharge. The groups did not differ in their need for inpatient postoperative analgesics or time to discharge. However, 71% of the placebo group required analgesics after discharge compared with 30% of the naproxen group.

Conclusion.—A single preoperative dose of naproxen sodium, 550 mg, can reduce postoperative pain in patients undergoing arthroscopic knee surgery. Significant pain reductions were noted both before discharge and for as long as 24 hours afterward.

▶ Although nonsteroidal anti-inflammatory drugs are effective in reducing postoperative pain, there is no evidence that preemptive administration (before incision) is more effective.—S.E. Abram, M.D.

Does Postoperative Epidural Analgesia Increase the Risk of Peroneal Nerve Palsy After Total Knee Arthroplasty?

Horlocker TT, Cabanela ME, Wedel DJ (Mayo Clinic, Rochester, Minn)
Anesth Analg 79:495–500, 1994   101-95-23–50

Introduction.—Peroneal nerve palsy, a rare complication after total knee arthroscopy (TKA), is generally attributed to surgical causes, particularly perioperative traction. Whether epidural analgesia could increase the risk of peroneal palsy in these patients, both by delaying diagnosis and allowing constrictive postoperative dressings and poor positioning in the continuous passive motion (CPM) machine, was studied retrospectively. The surgical and anesthetic risk factors that could contribute to the development of peroneal nerve palsy in patients undergoing TKA were identified.

Methods.—The records of all patients who underwent TKA during a 1-year period were examined. The data analyzed included demographic information, date and type of surgery, preexisting neuropathy, previous laminectomy, history of diabetes, preoperative flexion and valgus deformities, previous knee surgery, total tourniquet time, excessive postoperative bleeding, use of a CPM machine, and anesthetic technique, type, and duration.

Results.—There were 361 TKAs performed on 292 patients and 8 cases of peroneal nerve palsies in 7 patients. The diagnosis of peroneal nerve palsy was made on the day of surgery in 1 case, on the second postoperative day in 3, on the fourth postoperative day in 3, and on the sixth postoperative day in 1. The complication was associated with excessive postoperative bleeding, longer total tourniquet time, 10-degree or greater preoperative valgus deformity, and preexisting neuropathy. Although the anesthetic technique was not identified as a significant risk factor, the incidence of peroneal nerve palsy was higher in patients who had postoperative epidural analgesia. All those who had motor deficits or incomplete recovery had received postoperative epidural analgesia.

Discussion.—Although epidural analgesia was not a statistically significant risk factor for peroneal nerve palsy after TKA, the more profound deficits experienced by patients who received epidural analgesia suggests that it may be a relative risk factor. Therefore, patients with other risk factors for peroneal nerve palsy should receive epidural opioids rather than local anesthetics or minimum concentrations of epidural local anesthetic infusions. These patients should also be carefully positioned to prevent peroneal nerve compression or traction and should undergo frequent neurologic examinations.

▶ This study suggests that postoperative local anesthetic blockade does not predispose patients to compressive nerve injury. Nevertheless, meticulous attention should be paid to anatomical areas that are susceptible to nerve injury during the period of anesthetic blockade.—S.E. Abram, M.D.

Epidural Administration of Liposome-Associated Bupivacaine for the Management of Postsurgical Pain: A First Study
Boogaerts JG, Lafont ND, Declercq AG, Luo HC, Gravet ET, Bianchi JA, Legros FJ (Reine Fabiola Hosp, Montignies-sur-Sambre, Belgium; Free Univ of Brussels, Belgium; Institut Médical de Traumatologie et Revalidation, Loverval, Belgium)
J Clin Anesth 6:315–320, 1994   101-95-23–51

Objective.—Liposomes have been used as carriers for biologically active drugs. A liposomal encapsulation system for delivering bupivacaine was examined to determine whether there are analgesic advantages to this delivery system.

Methods.—After surgery, 2 groups of 13 patients received either bupivacaine plus epinephrine or liposomal encapsulated bupivacaine by epidural catheter. The onset and quality of analgesia, the quality of motor block, and the sympathetic block were measured every 5 minutes for the first 15 minutes after injection.

Results.—The average time to analgesia was approximately 4 minutes for both groups. In liposomal bupivacaine patients (group 2), 9 patients had no pain, and 5 patients had endurable pain. For those in group 1, who received plain .5 bupivacaine with 1:200,000 epinephrine, 6 patients were pain-free and 6 patients had endurable pain. The duration of analgesia was almost twice as long for group 2 as for group 1. Patients who underwent abdominal aortic surgery had analgesia durations of approxi-

---

Duration of Analgesia (Hours) in Aortic Abdominal Surgery Patients

BP 0.5% + Epi (n = 6)	2.42 ± 0.35
LIPO-BP 0.5% (n = 5)	10.6 ± 1.4

Note: Data are means ± standard error of the mean.
Abbreviations: *BP*, bupivacaine; *Epi*, epinephrine; *LIPO*, liposome.
(Courtesy of Boogaerts JG, Lafont ND, Declercq AG, et al: *J Clin Anesth* 6:315–320, 1994.)

mately 2.5 hours for group 2 and more than 10.5 hours for group 1 (table); there were no adverse events in either group.

Conclusion.—Liposomal-associated bupivacaine appears to significantly prolong postoperative epidural analgesia.

▶ There was a wide range in the duration of sensory blockade in the group that received liposomal bupivacaine (1.5–12 hours). The modest increase in analgesic duration associated with liposomal encapsulation does not seem to recommend this technique for routine postoperative use.—S.E. Abram, M.D.

Epidural Bupivacaine/Sufentanil Therapy for Postoperative Pain Control in Patients Tolerant to Opioid and Unresponsive to Epidural Bupivacaine/Morphine
de Leon-Casasola OA, Lema MJ (State Univ of New York, Buffalo)
Anesthesiology 80:303–309, 1994   101-95-23-52

Introduction.—Patients with cancer who require chronic pain control with large doses of opioids could pose a difficult problem in ensuring postoperative pain control. Even large doses of epidural bupivacaine and morphine may be inadequate. That sufentanil may have a greater analgesic effect than morphine in patients with opioid tolerance was studied.

Methods.—Twenty patients in whom chronic pain was controlled with large doses of oral morphine sulfate underwent abdominal surgery. With postoperative epidural morphine infusion, all patients rated their pain intensity to be at least 5 of 10 on a visual analogue pain scale (VAPS) for 6 hours or when the morphine infusion had been increased to at least 2 mg/hr^{-1}. At this point, 50 μg of sufentanil in 10 mL of normal saline was given as an epidural bolus. Thereafter, the epidural infusion contained sufentanil and bupivacaine at a rate required to maintain a VAPS score of less than 5 of 10. Signs of withdrawal or overdose were assessed, and pain control was monitored. Morphine and sufentanil doses were compared.

Results.—Before the patients were changed to the sufentanil protocol, they were given a mean epidural morphine dose of 1.8 mg/hr^{-1}, which produced pain intensity scores of 7–10 of 10 at a mean time of 5 hours after surgery. They also self-administered 39 mg of morphine using IV patient-controlled analgesia (PCA). After the switch, the patients received a mean of 17 μg of sufentanil per hr^{-1} in the first 4 hours, as they used only 8 mg of morphine with PCA, which produced pain intensity scores of 0–3 of 10. There were no signs of opioid withdrawal.

Discussion.—Adequate pain control can be achieved in patients in whom opioid tolerance has developed with epidural bupivacaine-sufentanil. Further study that compares the relative effectiveness of sufentanil and morphine should evaluate the effects of sufentanil in both opioid-naive and opioid-tolerant patients.

▶ This study examined the concept of intrinsic drug efficacy. Sufentanil required occupancy of fewer opiate receptors than morphine to produce a given level of analgesia. Under conditions of tolerance, many receptors become unresponsive, and a drug with a higher intrinsic efficacy, such as sufentanil, will be more likely to provide adequate analgesia.—S.E. Abram, M.D.

Treatment of Sympathetically Maintained Pain With Terazosin
Stevens DS, Robins VF, Price HM (Univ of Massachusetts, Worcester)
Reg Anesth 18:318–321, 1993   101-95-23-53

Background.—Sympathetically maintained pain can be diagnosed and treated with sympathetic nerve blocks. These blocks require invasive procedures, involve a certain amount of risk, and may not have long-lasting effects. Oral α-adrenergic antagonists are valuable in diagnosis and treatment of sympathetically maintained pain. A patient showed a rapid, complete, and long-lasting response to the oral α_1-antagonist terazosin.

Case Report.—Woman, 24, experienced acute onset of pain in the right levator scapulae muscle. The right arm turned bluish and cool. The initial diagnosis was right levator scapulae strain and right arm vasospasm from sympathetic overactivity. A right stellate ganglion block using 10 mL of 1% lidocaine at the C6 level provided total relief from symptoms, but shoulder pain returned after 1.5 hours. The color and temperature of the arm worsened during the next 5 days. A second stellate ganglion block using 10 mL of .25% bupivacaine at the C6 level provided total relief for only 5 hours. Only mild improvement was noted with oral opioids, nonsteroidal anti-inflammatory agents, muscle relaxants, transcutaneous electrical nerve stimulation, and physical therapy. Nifedipine was started, but it was discontinued because it did not decrease pain or vasospasm. A third and fourth right stellate ganglion block again produced temporary relief. Terazosin, 1 mg, was started on day 44. Within 2 days, all allodynia and vasospasm disappeared and shoulder girdle pain decreased. Within 5 days, the patient experienced only mild tenderness in the right levator scapulae muscle. Terazosin was increased to 2 mg for 60 days, during which all symptoms disappeared. The patient was symptom-free at 6 months after terazosin had been discontinued.

Discussion.—Terazosin has a 12-hour elimination half-time and a duration of action that may extend for longer than 18 hours. A single daily dose has excellent therapeutic effects on hypertension. Dosing at bedtime is recommended because orthostatic hypotension may occur, especially after the first dose. Terazosin has only minor side effects.

▶ Adrenergic-blocking agents, including α_1-antagonists, have been used for many years in treating sympathetically maintained pain (1), but there have been few reports of clinical success. For most patients, the doses required to produce adequate sympathetic blockade produce intolerable orthostatic hypotension. Intravenous phentolamine may be useful in predicting which patients will respond, but no such correlative studies have been undertaken.—S.E. Abram, M.D.

Reference

1. Abram SE, Lightfoot RW: *Reg Anesth* 6:79, 1981.

Signs and Symptoms of Reflex Sympathetic Dystrophy: Prospective Study of 829 Patients
Veldman PHJM, Reynen HM, Arntz IE, Goris RJA (Univ Hosp Nijmegen, The Netherlands)
Lancet 342:1012–1016, 1993   101-95-23–54

Background.—The pathogenesis of reflex sympathetic dystrophy (RSD) is not understood. Diagnosing and treating patients with this disorder are difficult. The signs and symptoms of RSD were studied prospectively.

Patients and Findings.—Eight hundred twenty-nine patients were included in the analysis. Early RSD was characterized by regional inflammation that increased after muscular exercise. Ninety-three percent of the patients reported pain, 69% had hypoesthesia, and 75% had hyperpathy. With time, tissue atrophy, involuntary movements, muscle spasms, or pseudoparalysis occurred in some cases. Forty-nine percent of the patients had tremor and 54% had a lack of muscular coordination. Sympathetic signs such as hyperhidrosis were uncommon and had no diagnostic value. In these patients, the disease did not manifest itself in 3 phases.

Conclusion.—The concept of an exaggerated regional inflammatory response to injury or operation in patients with RSD was not supported. The early symptoms of this disorder indicate an inflammatory reaction rather than disturbance of the sympathetic nervous system.

▶ This survey emphasized the complex pathophysiology and wide variation in symptoms among RSD patients. Motor dysfunction (tremors, weakness, atrophy), which is ignored in many discussions, is emphasized. The authors suggest that many of the changes seen are inflammatory in nature, but they fail to provide direct evidence for this assumption.—S.E. Abram, M.D.

Reflex Sympathetic Dystrophy of the Hand: An Excessive Inflammatory Response?
Oyen WJG, Arntz IE, Claessens RAMJ, Van der Meer JWM, Corstens FHM, Goris RJA (Univ Hosp Nijmegen, The Netherlands)
Pain 55:151–157, 1993   101-95-23–55

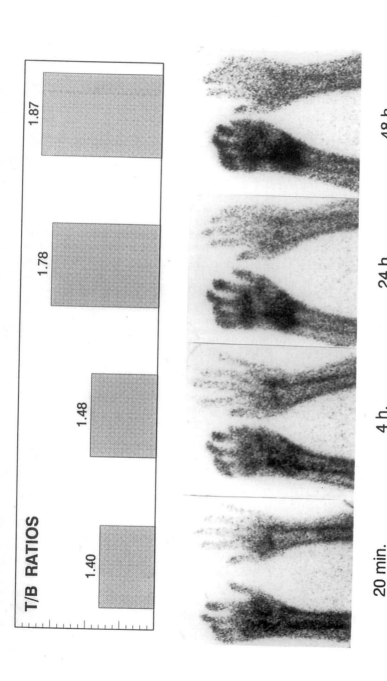

Fig 23-13.—Indium-111-IgG scintigraphy of a female patient, 34 years of age, who sustained fractures of metacarpals II–IV of the right hand 2 months before scintigraphy. A painful, swollen right hand developed with loss of function. Maximal exercise of the right hand: 5 times inflation of the manometer to 150 mm Hg. From **left** to **right:** images and target-to-background (T/B) ratios after 20 minutes and 4, 24, and 48 hours. Note the relative increase of activity over time in the affected right hand. (Courtesy of Oyen WJG, Arntz IE, Claessens RAMJ, et al: *Pain* 55:151–157, 1993.)

Background.—Reflex sympathetic dystrophy can occur after injury to extremities, in myocardial infarction, and in neurologic and rheumatologic diseases. It can be induced by fracture, surgery, or minimal trauma to an extremity. The pathophysiologic mechanism of reflex sympathetic dystrophy is unclear. A possible inflammatory component in patients with early reflex sympathetic dystrophy of the upper limb was investigated.

Methods.—In 23 patients with reflex sympathetic dystrophy of the hand, scintigraphy with indium-111–labeled human nonspecific polyclonal IgG was performed. After injection, images were made at 5 and 20 minutes and at 4, 24, and 48 hours (Fig 23–13). Blood flow and accumulation were assessed for 48 hours.

Results.—Flow increased in the affected hand in 19 patients and decreased in 3. One patient had bilateral reflex sympathetic dystrophy. Symptoms were aggravated by exercise in all patients. Before and after exercise, there was no significant change in the affected-nonaffected hand ratio. These ratios were significantly higher 48 hours after injection in patients who had early reflex sympathetic dystrophy. The affected-nonaffected hand ratios after 24 and 48 hours did not correlate with the flow-affected–nonaffected hand ratios. In 2 of 3 patients with decreased flow, late images showed excess accumulation. Significantly more patients with early reflex sympathetic dystrophy had positive scintigraphy.

Discussion.—The steadily increasing activity of indium-111–labeled human nonspecific polyclonal IgG suggests there is a flow-independent, inflammatory component in early reflex sympathetic dystrophy. The findings do not suggest that altered sympathetic activity and subsequent vasomotor tone changes are the only somatic factors involved in the development of reflex sympathetic dystrophy.

▶ The results of this study indicate that there is more to the pathophysiology of reflex sympathetic dystrophy than simply autonomic nervous system dysfunction. Indium-111–IgG scintigraphy may prove to be a useful diagnostic tool.—S.E. Abram, M.D.

Effects of Colchicine Applied to the Peripheral Nerve on the Thermal Hyperalgesia Evoked With Chronic Nerve Constriction

Yamamoto T, Yaksh TL (Univ of California, San Diego, La Jolla)
Pain 55:227–233, 1993   101-95-23–56

Background.—Topical application of colchicine to sensory nerves can prevent transsynaptic changes in spinal cord morphology and biochemistry that otherwise occur after nerve section. The role of colchicine-sensitive axonal transport in the thermal hyperalgesia noted after sciatic nerve constriction injury in rats was defined.

Methods.—Loose ligatures were placed around sciatic nerves in rats. Solutions of 5 or 50mM colchicine were applied proximal or distal to the nerve constriction injury. The effects of colchicine on thermal hyperalgesia and on levels of substance P, calcitonin gene–related peptide, and vasoactive intestinal polypeptide in the spinal cord and sciatic nerve were examined.

Results.—The solution of colchicine 50mM functioned as an axonal transport blocker. Colchicine that was applied proximal to the constriction injury eliminated hyperalgesia in a concentration-dependent manner. Colchicine that was applied distal to the injury had no effect on hyperalgesia. In rats without injuries, colchicine had no effect on motor function or paw-withdrawal response. Application of colchicine resulted in accumulation of substance P, calcitonin gene–related peptide, and vasoactive intestinal polypeptide in the nerve. In the dorsal horn, colchicine resulted in a modest reduction of substance P and calcitonin gene–related peptide levels, whereas vasoactive intestinal polypeptide levels were elevated.

Discussion.—Changes in spinal function evoked by nerve constriction may result from local generation of active factors that are transported centrally by a colchicine-sensitive mechanism.

▶ This study adds yet another piece to the puzzle of injury-induced hyperalgesia and suggests possibilities for future clinical research.—S.E. Abram, M.D.

Increased Venous Alpha-Adrenoceptor Responsiveness in Patients With Reflex Sympathetic Dystrophy
Arnold JMO, Teasell RW, MacLeod AP, Brown JE, Carruthers SG (Victoria Hosp, London, Ont, Canada)
Ann Intern Med 118:619–621, 1993   101-95-23-57

Background.—Reflex sympathetic dystrophy is considered to be a manifestation of sympathetic nervous system dysfunction and is characterized by vasomotor instability, hyperesthesia, and pain. Alpha-adrenoceptors have been implicated as mediators of sympathetically mediated pain. The responsiveness of the vascular α-adrenoreceptor in the dorsal superficial hand vein of patients with reflex sympathetic dystrophy to local infusions of norepinephrine was studied.

Methods.—Eleven patients with unilateral upper-limb reflex sympathetic dystrophy were injected first with saline then with .1 mL of norepinephrine per minute diluted from .5 to 256 ng/min in saline. Hand vein distention was measured after each injection. The median ED_{50} was defined as the estimated effective dose of norepinephrine that caused 50% constriction in the hand vein.

Results.—The norepinephrine ED_{50} was markedly reduced in the affected limbs of patients. There was no difference in the ED_{50} of affected limbs of patients with hemiplegia and those with trauma. The ED_{50} was lower in the unaffected limbs of patients with reflex sympathetic dystrophy than in age-similar controls. In unaffected limbs, the ED_{50} was lower in patients with hemiplegia than in those with trauma.

Discussion.—In limbs affected by reflex sympathetic dystrophy, increased responsiveness of venous α-adrenoceptors to locally infused norepinephrine occurs. The demonstration of this responsiveness may help in understanding the pathogenesis of this disorder.

▶ This study helps dispel the simplistic theory that reflex sympathetic dystrophy (RSD) is associated with a reflex increase in sympathetic outflow to the affected limb. Microneurographic recordings of sympathetic efferents in RSD patients generally fail to show a substantial alteration in activity.—S.E. Abram, M.D.

Segmental Reflex Sympathetic Dystrophy: Clinical and Scintigraphic Criteria
Kline SC, Holder LE (Union Mem Hosp, Baltimore, Md)
J Hand Surg (Am) 18A:853–859, 1993   101-95-23–58

Introduction.—Radionuclide scintigraphy is one of the most sensitive and specific tests for regional reflex sympathetic dystrophy (RSD). The potential of 3-phase radionuclide bone scanning (TPBS) to provide objective evidence of segmental RSD was evaluated.

Methods.—During a 6-month period, 133 patients underwent TPBS for a variety of upper-extremity problems. Eight patients met the clinical criteria for regional RSD, but they had involvement that was limited to only a portion of the hand. These criteria included diffuse pain, loss of function, and autonomic dysfunction. Twenty-three patients had regional RSD, 8 had diffuse pain but not RSD, 89 had focal pain, and 5 had other disorders.

Findings.—All 8 patients who met the strict criteria for segmental RSD showed a recognizable scan pattern, consisting of diffuse increased uptake in the involved ray, including periarticular uptake at the interphalangeal and metacarpophalangeal joints. The TPBS had a sensitivity of 100% and a specificity of 98% for segmental RSD, with positive and negative predictive values of 73% and 100%, respectively. There were 3 false positive scans, including 2 with a diffuse pattern of regional RSD with more intense segmental uptake in isolated rays.

Summary.—Recognition and documentation of a more localized form of RSD enable earlier recognition and treatment. The TPBS is both highly sensitive and specific for the diagnosis of segmental RSD.

▶ Documentation of these unusual RSD presentations helps catalogue the various subtypes of this group of disorders.—S.E. Abram, M.D.

Painful Symptoms Reported by Ambulatory HIV-Infected Men in a Longitudinal Study
Singer EJ, Zorilla C, Fahy-Chandon B, Chi S, Syndulko K, Tourtellotte WW (West Los Angeles VA Med Ctr)
Pain 54:15–19, 1993   101-95-23–59

Background.—Quality of life is an increasingly important issue for patients who are infected with HIV, because the life span of these patients can be prolonged by antiretroviral therapy and prophylaxis for opportunistic infections. The incidence of pain was studied in ambulatory patients infected with HIV.

Methods.—A total of 191 adult male volunteers were recruited from local sources and were positive for HIV. Data were collected during a 5-year period. The men reported symptoms of pain at baseline and every 6 months. Painful conditions were categorized as HIV-related, treatment-related, or unrelated to HIV.

Results.—At baseline, the most common painful conditions were HIV-related headaches, herpes simplex, peripheral neuropathy, back pain, herpes zoster, 3'-azido-3'-deoxythymidine–induced headaches, throat pain, and arthralgia. Headaches related to HIV, painful neuropathy, and herpes zoster were significantly more frequent in the advanced stages of the disease. The frequency of multiple pains was associated with increased disability and depression. Low CD_4 cell counts were associated with the use of multiple analgesics.

Conclusion.—Pain is a common symptom of ambulatory, indepedent individuals who are infected with HIV, even in the early stages of the disease.

▶ The prevalence of certain pain syndromes varies according to the type of population considered. Patients with a history of IV drug abuse may be more difficult to treat because of tolerance to opioids. Use of invasive procedures such as long-term neuraxial analgesics is often problematic because of the risk of infection.—S.E. Abram, M.D.

The Results of Operations on the Lumbar Spine in Patients Who Have Diabetes Mellitus
Simpson JM, Silveri CP, Balderston RA, Simeone FA, An HS (Tuckahoe Orthopaedic Associates, Richmond, Va; Long Island Jewish Med Ctr, Mineola, NY; Pennsylvania Hosp, Philadelphia; et al)
J Bone Joint Surg (Am) 75A:1823–1829, 1993   101-95-23–60

Clinical Findings for the Patients Who Were Available for Long-Term Follow-Up

	Diabetic Patients		Non-Diabetic Patients	
	Herniated Disc	Stenosis	Herniated Disc	Stenosis
Total no. of patients	20	24	33	22
Motor weakness				
Present	10	9	15	10
Absent	10	15	18	12
Sensory changes	12	12	18	11
Compression neuropathy	9	7	18	11
Diabetic neuropathy	3	5	NA	NA
Result at latest follow-up visit				
Excellent	3 (7%)	3 (7%)	27 (49%)	14 (25%)
Good	4 (9%)	7 (16%)	5 (9%)	6 (11%)
Fair	7 (16%)	12 (27%)	0	1 (2%)
Poor	6 (14%)	2 (4%)	1 (2%)	1 (2%)

Abbreviation: NA, not applicable.
(Courtesy of Simpson JM, Silveri CP, Balderston RA, et al: *J Bone Joint Surg (Am)* 75A:1823–1829, 1993.)

Objective.—The influence of diabetes on the outcome of posterior decompressive surgery for lumbar disk disease or spinal stenosis was examined in 62 patients who were compared retrospectively with the same number of patients who were not diabetic and of similar age and gender who underwent comparable operations. Twenty-one of the patients with diabetes were insulin-dependent. Forty-four patients with diabetes and

55 patients without diabetes were followed up for mean periods of 5 and 7 years, respectively.

Outcome.—Patients with diabetes spent an average of 8 days in the hospital after surgery compared with 5 days for the controls; the difference was chiefly the result of operative and medical complications. Six patients with diabetes had wound infections, and 1 of them died of myocardial infarction. The operative results were excellent or good in 39% of the patients with diabetes who were followed up, fair in 43%, and poor in 18%. By contrast, all but 5% of controls had excellent or good results (table). All 5 patients with diabetes who had severe weakness preoperatively were among the 8 with a poor outcome.

Conclusion.—Patients with lumbar disk disease or spinal stenosis who had diabetes did not do nearly as well as patients without diabetes after posterior decompressive surgery. Those who were weak or had findings of sensory neuropathy preoperatively were especially likely to do poorly.

▶ Diabetic patients appear to be much more susceptible to compressive neuropathies and are much more susceptible to infection. Most of the few reported cases of epidural abcesses reported after epidural steroid injections have occurred in diabetics. Management of diabetic patients with disk disease is problematic, and outcome studies of various treatment modalities should be carried out for this patient population.—S.E. Abram, M.D.

Outcomes in Treatment of Pain in Geriatric and Younger Age Groups
Cutler RB, Fishbain DA, Steele Rosomoff R, Rosomoff HL (Univ of Miami, Miami Beach, Fla; South Shore Hosp, Miami Beach, Fla)
Arch Phys Med Rehabil 75:457–464, 1994   101-95-23–61

Objective.—Because of continuing uncertainty regarding whether patients with chronic pain who are older than age 65 years benefit as much as younger patients from management at a pain center, a large number of patients were asked to rate themselves when they were admitted to a pain center and again when they were discharged.

Study Plan.—The 153 "geriatric" patients, who were older than 65 years of age, were compared with 126 "middle-aged" patients, 45–64 years of age, and with 191 "younger" patients, aged 21–44 years. No fewer than 43 rating scales were used to evaluate the pain itself, functional status, behavioral variables, and management goals. Change scores were compared using analysis of covariance and pairwise post hoc tests.

Findings.—The geriatric patients improved on all but 1 of the 43 self-rating scales, and the degree of improvement on 37 scales was significant—usually at a level of .001. The elderly patients differed significantly from the other age groups on most baseline variables, and their scores when admitted were better than those for the younger patients. Geriatric patients exhibited a significantly better change on 2 scales and a significantly worse change on 4.

Implications.—Geriatric patients with chronic pain clearly benefit from multidisciplinary treatment at a chronic pain center. At the same time, they appear to be a distinct group in many respects; therefore, they should be considered separately in outcome studies.

▶ Older patients are becoming disenfranchised by some segments of the medical community (see Abstract 101-95-23-26). Some of the unwillingness to treat them relates to low and delayed Medicare reimbursement and some to perceptions that they respond poorly to treatment. This study and several previous articles indicate that this group of patients responds at least as well as younger patients to pain management and rehabilitative interventions.—S.E. Abram, M.D.

Spinal Cord Stimulation in Belgium: A Nation-Wide Survey on the Incidence, Indications and Therapeutic Efficacy by the Health Insurer
Kupers RC, Van den Oever R, Van Houdenhove B, Vanmechelen W, Hepp B, Nuttin B, Gybels JM (Univ of Leuven, Belgium; Natl Alliance of Christian Benefit Societies, Brussels, Belgium)
Pain 56:211–216, 1994   101-95-23-62

Background.—For the past decade, spinal cord stimulation (SCS) has become an increasingly used means of treating some types of chronic

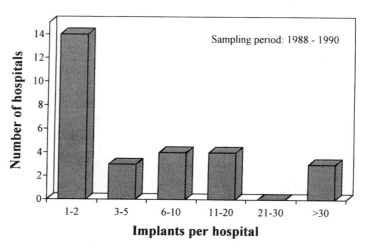

Fig 23–14.—Number of spinal cord stimulation (SCS) implants per hospital during a 3-year sampling period (1988–1990). In 28 hospitals, SCS was performed. In 14 of them, a maximum of 2 patients was implanted over the examined 3-year period. Only in 7 hospitals were more than 10 patients implanted during the investigated period. (Courtesy of Kupers RC, Van den Oever R, Van Houdenhove B, et al: *Pain* 56:211–216, 1994.)

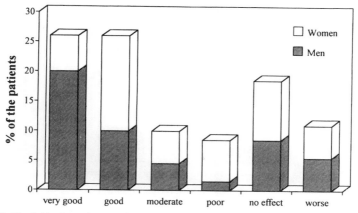

Fig 23–15.—Subjective evaluation of spinal cord stimulation (SCS) by the patient. In 70 patients (35 men and 35 women), the effect of SCS was evaluated by a third party (the sickness fund). In 52% of the patients, the effect was judged as good to very good. Men scored significantly better than women. (Courtesy of Kupers RC, Van den Oever R, Van Houdenhove B, et al: *Pain* 56:211–216, 1994.)

pain. Initially practiced only at university teaching hospitals, SCS is now practiced in a number of pain treatment centers within general hospitals. Initially, the method was used to treat pain of central neurogenic origin that was resistant to behavioral, pharmacologic, and surgical measures. A positive response to 1 week of trial stimulation was required, and psychiatric contraindications were ruled out by an independent psychiatrist.

Objective.—A nationwide survey was carried out in Belgium for 1983–1992 to document the frequency of SCS, the indications for which it was used, and its effectiveness.

Demographic Aspects.—Nearly 700 SCS devices were implanted in the decade reviewed in a population of fewer than 10 million persons. The

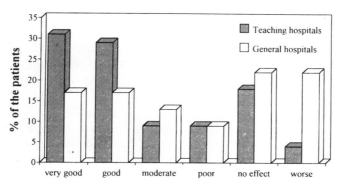

Fig 23–16.—Evaluation of the efficacy of spinal cord stimulation in 45 university teaching hospitals and in 23 general hospitals. Patients receiving implants in the teaching hospitals scored significantly better than patients receiving implants in the general hospitals. (Courtesy of Kupers RC, Van den Oever R, Van Houdenhove B, et al: *Pain* 56:211–216, 1994.)

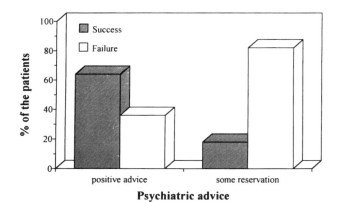

Fig 23–17.—Outcome of spinal cord stimulation (SCS) with respect to psychiatric advice. The effect of SCS was evaluated 6 months after implantation. Before the decision of implantation, patients were assessed by an independent psychiatrist. Of the 100 patients screened, 36 were withheld from implantation. Of the 48 patients who received positive advice (no psychiatric contraindication), 64% were considered as successes, whereas for the 16 patients for whom the psychiatrist made some reservations, only 18% were considered as successes. (Courtesy of Kupers RC, Van den Oever R, Van Houdenhove B, et al: *Pain* 211-216, 1994.)

number of implants increased rapidly after 1986 and stabilized somewhat in 1992. More than 80% of recipients were 31–60 years of age. Only one fourth of hospitals did more than 10 implantations in a 3-year period (Fig 23–14). The most common indication was failure to improve after back surgery, which accounted for 61% of implantations.

Efficacy.—Just more than half the 70 patients evaluated were considered to have had very good to good results (Fig 23–15), whereas in 27% of cases, the outcome was poor or SCS had no effect. Eleven percent of patients reported that stimulation made their pain worse. Better results were achieved in teaching hospitals than in general hospitals (Fig 23–16). Fewer than 5% of patients resumed their occupational activities. When the consulting psychiatrist had some reservations about whether SCS was indicated, the chances of a successful outcome were substantially reduced (Fig 23–17).

Conclusion.—Spinal cord stimulation was effective in about half the patients, but they were not likely to return to work. Adequate psychiatric screening can improve the overall outcome of SCS.

▶ With the rising cost of health care and our increasing inability to fund basic health care for a large segment of the population, it is critical that we not waste resources on the inappropriate use of expensive treatment modalities.

Spinal cord stimulation has been used indiscriminately in a number of treatment centers. Studies such as this help to concentrate use of SCS on patients for whom it is most likely to be of help. Previous studies have shown that certain conditions, such as unilateral chronic radiculopathy, are more likely to respond than others, such as postherpetic neuralgia. This study indicates that attention to psychopathology is important and that certain medical centers may be better able than others to use the modality effectively.—S.E. Abram, M.D.

Long Term Follow Up of Dorsal Root Entry Zone Lesions in Brachial Plexus Avulsion

Thomas DGT, Kitchen ND (Natl Hosp for Neurology and Neurosurgery, London)

J Neurol Neurosurg Psychiatry 57:737–738, 1994   101-95-23–63

Objective.—Dorsal root entry zone (DREZ) lesioning is indicated for pain relief in a number of injuries. The long-term results of 44 patients who underwent the DREZ procedure to relieve pain caused by brachial plexus avulsion injury were reported.

Methods.—The 44 patients, aged 19 to 66 years, had unilateral deafferentation pain. Drug therapy, stellate ganglion blockade, surgery, and transcutaneous stimulation had not been effective in relieving pain.

Results.—After an average of 63 months of follow-up, 30 patients said they had good pain relief, 5 had fair pain relief, and 9 had poor pain relief. Ten patients had postoperative motor deficits.

Conclusion.—In 64% of patients who had the DREZ procedure, pain relief was good or fair. Only 1 patient had decreasing pain relief a year after the procedure.

▶ It is reassuring that this very invasive procedure appears to provide continued benefit over a period of years for a condition that typically fails to respond to less drastic interventions. The results of this procedure are in contrast to those of cordotomy, a procedure that typically loses efficacy over a period of months.—S.E. Abram, M.D.

Reduction of Morphine Dependence and Potentiation of Analgesia by Chronic Co-Administration of Nifedipine

Antkiewicz-Michaluk L, Michaluk J, Romańska I, Vetulani J (Polish Academy of Sciences, Kraków, Poland)

Psychopharmacology 111:457–464, 1993   101-95-23–64

Introduction.—Calcium channel blockers are a class of drugs that when administered with morphine and other opioids offer promise in counteracting some of the problems associated with long-term administration of opioids. The effects of the channel-blocking agent nifedipine was studied in opiate-tolerant rats.

Methods.—Tolerance of or dependence on morphine was induced in male Wistar rats by a daily dose of 20 mg/kg for 8 consecutive days. Nifedipine, 5 mg/kg, was given 15 minutes before morphine in the experiments. For assessing responsiveness to a painful stimulus, morphine was administered acutely in doses of 2.5–10 mg/kg in the tail-flick test and in doses of 5–15 mg/kg in the hot-plate test, usually 30 minutes before the tests.

Results.—Long-term administration of high-dose morphine led to the development of the abstinence syndrome and a significant inhibition of body weight gain. Pretreatment with nifedipine did not affect inhibition of weight gain, but the abstinence syndrome was prevented in the animals that received pretreatment. Co-administration of nifedipine potentiated the morphine-induced analgesia measured in the hot-plate test but not in the tail-flick test. Nifedipine pretreatment partially restored the analgesic action of morphine in rats that were tolerant of morphine. In a long-term experiment, co-administration of nifedipine did not prevent the loss of morphine efficiency or the debilitating effect of long-term morphine treatment. A test performed 24 hours after the injection of nifedipine showed that the calcium channel–blocking agent prevented the naloxone-induced withdrawal syndrome. The combined treatment of morphine and nifedipine significantly increased the density of the cortical [^{3}H]prazosin-binding site. When the drugs were given individually in long-term treatment, the density of [^{3}H]naloxone- or [^{3}H]prazosin-binding sites in the cortex and in the rest of the brain did not significantly decrease.

Conclusion.—Two undesired effects of long-term treatment with opiates are the loss of effectiveness through development of tolerance and physical dependence. Co-administration of nifedipine may be a way to separate opiate tolerance and physical dependence. It may be possible to reduce the initial dose of morphine and to enhance the effectiveness of the opioid in tolerant patients. Prevention of the formation of physical dependence could lessen the danger of habit formation.

▶ A number of interesting interactions between spinal opioids and nonopioid analgesics are under investigation. They involve synergistic analgesic effects, blockade of nociception-induced hyperalgesia, and prevention of tolerance and physical dependence.—S.E. Abram, M.D.

Effects of the Serotonin-Receptor Agonist Sumatriptan on Postdural Puncture Headache: Report of Six Cases
Carp H, Singh PJ, Vadhera R, Jayaram A (Oregon Health Sciences Univ, Portland; Baylor College of Medicine, Houston)
Anesth Analg 79:180–182, 1994   101-95-23–65

Background.—Postdural puncture headache (PDPH) is commonly treated with caffeine and an epidural blood patch. However, caffeine provides only short-term relief, and the epidural blood patch is an invasive procedure. Subcutaneous sumatriptan injection has been approved for the treatment of migraine headache but not for PDPH. The effectiveness of sumatriptan injection for PDPH was assessed in a pilot study.

Patients.—Five women and 1 man who had received accidental dural punctures and had PDPH develop were treated with a 6-mg subcutaneous injection of sumatriptan. The headache resolved within 30 minutes of treatment in all 6 patients. Two patients had a recurrence of the headache and were given a second injection of sumatriptan, which again relieved the headache within 30 minutes. One of these 2 patients was also treated with an epidural blood patch. None of the patients showed a change in vital signs after the injection or complained of chest discomfort or pain at the injection site.

Conclusion.—Cutaneous sumatriptan injection appears to be effective for PDPH. Further studies are needed to establish its safety and efficacy for this new indication.

▶ This treatment is appealing, particularly for immunocompromised patients for whom the risk of epidural abscess after a blood patch may be high. Cutaneous sumatriptan injection will probably have its greatest application after small-bore dural puncture, and it is less likely to be of lasting benefit after accident dural puncture with large-bore epidural needles.—S.E. Abram, M.D.

Do Agents Used for Epidural Analgesia Have Antimicrobial Properties?

Feldman JM, Chapin-Robertson K, Turner J (Temple Univ, Philadelphia; Univ of South Alabama, Mobile; Yale Univ, New Haven, Conn)
Reg Anesth 19:43–47, 1994   101-95-23–66

Objective.—There is a low incidence of infection resulting from catheter placement in the epidural space, possibly because the local anesthetics used have anti-infective properties. The capability of lidocaine and bupivacaine in combination with fentanyl and sufentanil to inhibit bacterial growth was evaluated.

Methods.—Cultured specimens from epidural catheters yielded 53 bacterial isolates (table). Isolates were grown for 24 hours on Mueller-Hinton agar alone or in the presence of 2%, 1.5%, and 1% lidocaine; .5%, .25%, and .125% bupivacaine; .125% bupivacaine plus fentanyl, 2 μg/mL; .125% bupivacaine plus sufentanil, 3 μg/mL; and fentanyl, 5 μg/mL; fentanyl, 2 μg/mL; and sufentanil, .3 μg/mL.

Results.—Significantly fewer isolates grew in the presence of all concentrations of lidocaine and bupivacaine, although there was a significant increase in bacterial growth with a decrease in the lidocaine or bupivacaine concentration. Neither opioid inhibited bacterial growth, and neither opioid plus bupivacaine significantly inhibited bacterial growth when compared with bupivacaine alone.

Number of Isolates by Species That Grew in the Presence of the Study Agents

	Catheter Isolates								Noncatheter Isolates (sterile sites)
	Staph. Coagulase (−)	Staph. aureus	Strep. spp.	Micrococcus	Coryn	Bacillus spp.	Fastidious GNR	Growth Total	Staph. aureus
Agar alone	38	1	2	2	1	8	1	53	11
Lido 2%	0	0	0	0	0	0	0	0	0
Lido 1.5%	4	0	0	0	0	2	0	6	2
Lido 1.0%	15	1	0	1	1	4	0	22	6
Bup 0.5%	2	0	0	0	0	0	0	2	0
Bup 0.25%	2	1	0	0	0	0	0	3	6
Bup 0.125%	32	1	0	0	1	3	0	37	6
Bup 0.125% plus Fent 2	35	0	0	0	0	3	0	38	6
Bup 0.125% plus Sufent 0.3	32	0	0	0	0	3	0	35	6
Fent 5	38	1	2	2	1	8	0	53	11
Fent 2	38	1	2	2	1	8	1	53	11
Sufent 0.3	38	1	2	2	1	8	1	53	11

Abbreviations: Bup, bupivacaine; Coryn, Corynebacterium; Fent, fentanyl; GNR, gram-negative rod; Lido, lidocaine; Staph, Staphylococcus; Strep, Streptococcus; Sufent, sufentanil.
(Courtesy of Feldman JM, Chapin-Robertson K, Turner J: Reg Anesth 19:43–47, 1994.)

Conclusion.—Anesthetics appear to decrease the already low risk of infection from epidural catheters. More studies should be done to determine whether anesthetics can decrease the infection risk for at-risk patients.

▶ This study reconfirms the bacteriostatic properties of local anesthetics and provides an additional reason for combining local anesthetic with epidural opioids.—S.E. Abram, M.D.

Altered Sexual Function and Decreased Testosterone in Patients Receiving Intraspinal Opioids
Paice JA, Penn RD, Ryan WG (Rush-Presbyterian-St Luke's Med Ctr, Chicago)
J Pain Symptom Manage 9:126–131, 1994   101-95-23–67

Background.—Sexual dysfunction and reduced serum testosterone levels have been described in heroin addicts and methadone users, but the effects of intraspinal opioids on sexual function have not been well studied.

Patients.—Six men, aged 34–50 years, who were receiving intraspinal opioids, were questioned regarding their present libido and sexual function. Indications for intraspinal opioid therapy included failed back surgery syndrome and reflex sympathetic dystrophy. The average duration of spinal opioid therapy was 47.7 months. Men with reduced libido, sexual dysfunction, or low serum testosterone levels were offered testosterone therapy or a reduction in the opioid dose.

Results.—All 6 patients reported some reduction in libido. Four patients had consistent difficulty obtaining or maintaining an erection. Four patients sought treatment for the sexual dysfunction, and 3 of them agreed to IM testosterone cypionate therapy. Testosterone supplementation increased the serum testosterone levels and improved sexual function to near normal in all 3 men.

Conclusion.—Patients should be informed of the possibility of sexual dysfunction before spinal opioid therapy is initiated.

▶ Although sexual dysfunction may be a risk in chronic spinal opioid administration in men, apparently it can be corrected with testosterone replacement.—S.E. Abram, M.D.

Success Rates in Producing Sympathetic Blockade by Paratracheal Injection
Hogan QH, Taylor ML, Goldstein M, Stevens R, Kettler R (Med College of Wisconsin, Milwaukee; St Joseph's Hosp, Milwaukee, Wis)
Clin J Pain 10:139–145, 1994   101-95-23–68

TABLE 1.—Success of Horner's Syndrome and
Unilateral Warming

	$\Delta Ti \geq 1.5°C$	
	Yes	No
+ Horner's	57	27
− Horner's	3	13

(Courtesy of Hogan QH, Taylor ML, Goldstein M, et al: *Clin J Pain* 10:139-145, 1994.)

Objective.—There are no standards for judging the effectiveness of a sympathetic block. One hundred anterior paratracheal injections were examined and eye changes and hand temperatures were evaluated to determine the physiologic effectiveness of the block.

Methods.—Fingertip temperature was taken. A lidocaine block was administered into the anterior tubercle of the sixth cervical vertebra.

Results.—Forty patients had 100 blocks for a variety of indications. Horner's syndrome occurred in 84 blocks. Using hand-warming as the standard, in 60 blocks the injection side hand warmed by at least 1.5°C. In 31 blocks, the opposite hand also warmed by at least 1.5°C. Therefore, only 27 of the blocks, all of which had Horner's syndrome develop, were considered successful (Table 1). Using an ipsilateral temperature of at least 34°C as the standard, 28 of 70 blocks were considered successful, including 1 without Horner's syndrome (Table 2).

Conclusion.—The presence of Horner's syndrome plus a temperature increase that was higher on the injection side verified a successful block.

▶ A C6 anterior tubercle injection produces a unilateral increase in skin temperature in less than half of patients, despite ipsilateral Horner's syndrome in most cases. The same authors, using MRI scanning, previously showed that 15 mL of solution generally does not spread downward and posteriorly to surround the stellate ganglion (1). It is important to document skin tempera-

TABLE 2.—Success of Horner's Syndrome and Warming of
the Ipsilateral Hand by 1.5°C More Than the
Contralateral Hand

	$\Delta Ti-\Delta Te \geq 1.5°C$	
	Yes	No
+ Horner's	27	57
− Horner's	0	16

(Courtesy of Hogan QH, Taylor ML, Goldstein M, et al: *Clin J Pain* 10:139-145, 1994.)

ture or other signs of sympathetic denervation in the affected extremity when assessing the results of stellate ganglion block.—S.E. Abram, M.D.

Reference

1. Hogan Q, et al: *Am J Roentgen* 158:655, 1992.

Long-Term Continuous Intrathecal Administration of Morphine and Bupivacaine at the Upper Cervical Level: Access by a Lateral C1–C2 Approach

Crul BJ, van Dongen RT, Snijdelaar DG, Rutten EH (Univ of Nijmegen, The Netherlands)
Anesth Analg 79:594–597, 1994   101-95-23–69

Introduction.—Because the pain caused by progressive tumor growth in the head and neck is rarely one-sided or affecting only 1 nerve, it usually cannot be managed with nerve blocks or neuroablative procedures. These patients are usually treated with oral morphine combined with co-analgesics, such as antidepressants or anticonvulsants, and corticosteroids. Recently, a combination of morphine and bupivacaine, which was administered intrathecally, was used to control persistent, severe pain in 2 patients with head and neck tumors.

Case 1.—Woman, 50, who had an inoperable, advanced, progressive squamous cell carcinoma of the base of the tongue, experienced severe aching pain in her right neck and severe stabbing pain in her right ear, which could not be relieved with oral analgesics. An intrathecal catheter was placed in the C1-2 interspace, using a left lateral approach, for morphine infusion. However, the pain control was insufficient, and bupivacaine was added to the morphine on the fifth day, which produced acceptable pain control. There were no reported or observed side effects.

Case 2.—Woman, 48, with a recurrence of a squamous cell carcinoma of the floor of the mouth, had severe piercing pain in her left ear and pain with swallowing. Her pain was not controlled with high doses of oral analgesics, and she was having drug-related side effects. An intrathecal catheter was inserted at C1-2, and the catheter tip was positioned at the foramen magnum. Some pain relief was achieved with morphine 4.8 mg/day. The addition of 2 mg of bupivacaine per mL to the morphine solution produced adequate pain control. The initial infusion of bupivacaine produced dizziness and vertigo, which disappeared with subsequent lower doses.

Discussion.—The technique of intrathecal catheter insertion at the C1-2 level was similar to that used in percutaneous cervical cordotomy. Because the safety of this use of bupivacaine is not known, the patient should be carefully monitored for 2–3 days after a stable dose has been reached. These results justify further study of continuous intrathecal infusion at the upper cervical level.

▶ This technique obviously has a high potential for complications and should be reserved for desperate situations.—S.E. Abram, M.D.

Survey of Opioid Use in Chronic Nonmalignant Pain Patients
Jamison RN, Anderson KO, Peeters-Asdourian C, Ferrante FM (Brigham and Women's Hosp, Boston; Univ of Massachusetts, Worcester)
Reg Anesth 19:225–230, 1994   101-95-23–70

Introduction.—Although opioids are well accepted as appropriate therapy for acute and cancer pain, there are concerns about efficacy, side effects, tolerance, and addiction when they are used to treat chronic nonmalignant pain. Nevertheless, opioids are increasingly used for that purpose. Patients who took oral opioids to manage chronic nonmalignant pain were surveyed to assess the frequency of medication use, the incidence of side effects, and the patients' perceptions of benefit.

Methods.—Patients from 2 university hospital pain centers who had taken opioids to control their pain were asked to complete a 10-item questionnaire documenting their medication type, dosage, length of time taken, perceived benefit, perceived tolerance, increases in dosage, and adverse side effects. The questionnaire was also sent to randomly chosen patients in other pain centers.

Results.—Questionnaires were completed and returned by 109 of the patients who were known to have used opioids, of whom 102 reported current use of opioids, and by 108 randomly chosen patients, of whom 10 reported using opioids for pain control. The most common diagnosis in these patients was low-back pain (45.1%), followed by extremity (39.4%), abdominal (8.5%), myofascial (4.2%), and neuropathic (2.8%) pain. Patients who took oral opioids reported greater pain intensity and were more likely to be taking other pain medications as well than were patients who were not using opioids. Of those who were taking oral opioids, 83% reported that the opioids relieved their pain, 25% perceived no decline in the medication's ability to relieve pain, 35% did not need to increase the dose, 36% did not fear addiction or dependence, and 56% reported no adverse side effects.

Discussion.—Most of the opioid users perceived their pain as being more intense than the nonusers and were more likely to seek additional pain medication. Most of the patients who were taking opioids experienced some drug tolerance, although most reported that the medication was beneficial and were not concerned about addiction or side effects. Controlled trials are required to identify the patient and pain factors that predict the greatest benefit from opioid therapy.

▶ Unfortunately, this study, and most others that examine this topic, fails to identify factors that predict satisfactory long-term results with oral opioids in noncancer patients.—S.E. Abram, M.D.

Cardiovascular Toxicity Associated With Intraarticular Bupivacaine
Sullivan SG, Abbott PJ Jr (Summit Surgery Ctr, Frisco, Colo; Vail-Summit Orthopaedics and Sports Medicine, Colo)
Anesth Analg 79:591–593, 1994   101-95-23–71

Introduction.—Several studies have reported the safe use of intra-articular bupivacaine for analgesia at doses greater than 60 mL of .25% bupivacaine solution with 1:400,000 or 1:200,000 epinephrine. Although cardiovascular toxicity has not been previously reported in association with intra-articular injection of bupivacaine, 2 such cases occurred in patients undergoing outpatient knee arthroscopy.

Case 1.—Man, 38, with no drug allergies, underwent knee arthroscopy. After sedation with 2.5 mg of midazolam and 100 μg of fentanyl, 60 mL of .25% bupivacaine was injected slowly with 1:400,000 epinephrine and 2 mg of morphine. Before the injection was complete, the patient developed slurred speech, increased heart rate, paleness, shaking hands, and increased arterial blood pressure. He had tachycardia with a wide QRS and inverted T waves. Blood drawn revealed serum drug levels of 3.9 μg/mL. He was given oxygen and recovered normal sinus rhythm within 10 minutes. The surgery was completed. The patient experienced 2 episodes of bradycardia 2 hours after the injection, which resolved with IV administration of glycopyrrolate the first time and atropine the second time.

Case 2.—Man, 19, was first sedated with 4 mg of midazolam and 100 μg of fentanyl. Arthroscopy was performed with epidural administration of lidocaine with epinephrine. Intra-articular injection of 30 mL of .25% bupivacaine was used for postoperative analgesia. Within 1 minute, the patient was unconscious, had an oxygen saturation of 78%, and experienced several episodes of ventricular tachycardia. He regained consciousness with stimulation and recovered normal sinus rhythm within 3 minutes. He had no postoperative complications.

Discussion.—These are the first reports of cardiovascular toxicity with intra-articular injection of standard doses of bupivacaine. Serious consequences may have been averted because of the youth and the health of the patients, previous sedation with midazolam, prompt oxygenation or stimulation, and co-administration of epinephrine. The immediacy of the toxic reactions suggests that the intra-articular pathology may have allowed direct access to the systemic circulation. Therefore, intra-articular bupivacaine should be used cautiously when blood-tinged joint effusion or intra-articular cartilaginous trauma is found or suspected.

▶ The high vascular uptake of local anesthetic from inflamed joints has been recognized for many years as a potential hazard. Apparently, this lesson must be relearned periodically.—S.E. Abram, M.D.

Local Anesthetic Lidocaine Inhibits the Effect of Granulocyte Colony-Stimulating Factor on Human Neutrophil Functions

Ohsaka A, Saionji K, Sato N, Igari J (Hitachi Gen Hosp, Ibaraki, Japan; Juntendo Univ, Tokyo)
Exp Hematol 22:460–466, 1994   101-95-23–72

Background.—Lidocaine reportedly inhibits a number of neutrophil functions in vitro, including phagocytosis and the release of superoxide and lysosomal enzyme. Lidocaine also inhibits the adherence of neutrophils to nylon fiber both in vitro and in vivo. Because increased neutrophil adherence and release of oxygen radicals are thought to play key roles in inflammatory disease, suppression of these functions might limit neutrophil-mediated tissue destruction.

Objective and Methods.—Neutrophils from healthy adults were studied to learn whether lidocaine inhibits the actions of granulocyte colony-stimulating factor (G-CSF) on superoxide release by neutrophils and the expression of cellular adhesion molecules. Superoxide was assayed spectrophotometrically, and cell-surface antigens were detected by indirect immunofluorescence.

Findings.—When neutrophils were stimulated by the chemotactic peptide N-formyl-methionyl-leucyl-phenylalanine, the release of superoxide was enhanced by recombinant human G-CSF. In addition, the cytokine downregulated the expression of leukocyte adhesion molecule-1 on the surface of activated neutrophils and upregulated the expression of CDE11b/CD18 leukocyte integrin. Exposure of neutrophils to lidocaine inhibited all these responses in a dose-dependent manner.

Conclusion.—Lidocaine inhibits the function of human neutrophils by countering the expression of cellular adhesion molecules. It might conceivably be an effective anti-inflammatory agent through the inhibition of the effects of inflammatory cytokines.

▶ Infiltration with local anesthetic may reduce postoperative wound pain by limiting the local inflammatory response. However, there is concern that the effect of local anesthetic on neutrophil function may retard wound healing or predispose to wound infection.—S.E. Abram, M.D.

Local Anesthetic Myotoxicity: A Case and Review

Hogan Q, Dotson R, Erickson S, Kettler R, Hogan K (Med College of Wisconsin, Milwaukee; Univ of Wisconsin, Madison)
Anesthesiology 80:942–947, 1994   101-95-23–73

Introduction.—Local anesthetic can be injected into muscle tissue to treat myofascial pain, into the wound margins as surgery proceeds, and to produce neural blockade during surgical anesthesia. Myotoxic complications have seldom been reported.

Case Report.—Woman, 40, who had previously received local anesthesia without complications, underwent capsular release of the shoulder under neural blockade with .5% bupivacaine containing epinephrine, which was administered by a catheter placed in the interscalene groove at the level of the cricoid cartilage. Injection of 45 mL produced sensorimotor blockade of the shoulder, arm, and hand. The patient received isoflurane, fentanyl, and nitrous oxide for general anesthesia during the 4-hour operation. Shoulder pain was described 16 hours postoperatively. Another bupivacaine injection, totaling 1,140 mg, was ultimately ineffective. Anesthesia persisted in the neck, and, after 3 days, the sternocleidomastoid muscle became tender and minimally swollen. Electromyography on postoperative day 19 showed reduced recruitment in the muscle. Persistent pain prompted an MRI study on day 45 that demonstrated increased signal intensity in the affected muscle tissue. A biopsy specimen revealed degenerating and regenerating muscle fibers as well as myophagia, splitting of muscle fibers, and inflammatory infiltration with many eosinophils. The patient received prednisone, 60 mg/kg, for 1 month, and her symptoms gradually resolved.

Discussion.—A localized myopathy caused by bupivacaine injection of the muscle tissue is the most likely explanation for the myotoxic effect. The histologic findings were typical of local anesthetic myopathy. Damage can result from the repeat administration of doses that, singly, are safe.

▶ The implications of the myotoxic effect of local anesthetics for the treatment of myofascial pain are obvious. It is not clear whether local anesthetic myotoxicity is related to the therapeutic effect of trigger-point injections. The most myotoxic drug is bupivacaine, and the least toxic is procaine.—S.E. Abram, M.D.

Epidural Analgesia in the Management of Severe Vaso-Occlusive Sickle Cell Crisis

Yaster M, Tobin JR, Billett C, Casella JF, Dover G (Johns Hopkins Hosp, Baltimore, Md)
Pediatrics 93:310–315, 1994   101-95-23–74

Objective.—Whether continuous epidural analgesia could effectively treat the pain of vaso-occlusive crisis in children with sickle cell disease who were unresponsive to conventional analgesic therapy was determined.

Treatment.—Nine children were treated with a 5 mg continuous epidural infusion of lidocaine (1.5 mg/kg/hr) during 11 painful vaso-occlusive crises. If pain returned, fentanyl, .5–1.5 µg/kg/hr, was added or bupivacaine, .2–.4 mg/kg/hr, was substituted for lidocaine. All patients had severe pain that was unresponsive to high-dose systemic opioids, nonsteroidal anti-inflammatory drugs, and adjunctive measures. Pain on a numerical scale from 0 to 10 (0 = no pain, 10 = worst pain) and oxygen saturation were monitored.

Outcome.—Analgesia was immediate, with pain scores decreasing from 9 to 1 within 15 minutes in 8 of 9 patients. Analgesia was continuously effective in 9 of 11 crises, and it dramatically improved arterial oxygen saturation from 91% to 99% in 7 of 9 patients. Plasma lidocaine levels ranged from 1.1 to 4.6 mg/L and dose-related toxicity did not occur. Five patients had tachyphylaxis to lidocaine develop and required either the addition of fentanyl or the substitution of bupivacaine for lidocaine to maintain analgesia for 2–5 days. Catheters remained in place for 1.5–5 days. One patient became acutely hypotensive secondary to high sympathetic blockade (T4) but responded to IV fluids and epinephrine. Four catheter-related complications occurred: 1 inadvertent dural puncture during insertion of the catheter, 1 fell out, 1 failed placement, and 1 was removed for fever. Epidural analgesia was not associated with sedation, respiratory depression, or limitation of movement. All epidural catheters were cultured on removal, and none showed any bacteriologic growth.

Conclusion.—The first documented successful use of epidural analgesia in the management of severe vaso-occlusive crises in children with sickle cell disease was reported. Continuous epidural analgesia with local anesthetics, alone or in combination with fentanyl, effectively and safely treated the pain of sickle cell vaso-occlusive crises without causing sedation, respiratory depression, or significant limitation of ambulation. Furthermore, early treatment of the painful crisis with this technique improves oxygenation, a critical factor in the evolution of further sickling. Until more information is available, epidural analgesia should be administered using very conservative infusion rates and be limited to patients for whom conventional therapy has failed.

▶ Although epidural analgesia is effective at controlling the pain of sickle cell crisis, there is no evidence of any advantage to epidural analgesia over systemic opiates.—S.E. Abram, M.D.

Dose-Related Antagonism of the Emetic Effect of Morphine by Methylnaltrexone in Dogs

Foss JF, Bass AS, Goldberg LI (Univ of Chicago)
J Clin Pharmacol 33:747–751, 1993   101-95-23–75

Introduction.—Emesis occurs in 20% to 30% of patients who are given opioids for analgesia. In animal studies, the quarternary narcotic antagonist N-methylnaltrexone bromide (MNTX) does not reverse or prevent morphine analgesia, but its potential to antagonize morphine-induced emesis still must be established. The effects of MNTX on emetic response were investigated in adult male mongrel dogs.

Study Design.—Eighty-five animals were assigned to one of 11 groups that were challenged with morphine alone or with morphine and various doses of MNTX that were given either intramuscularly or intravenously.

Results.—The administration of MNTX prevented morphine-induced emesis in the dog in a dose-related manner. Intramuscular doses of .25 mg/kg or greater or IV doses of .2 mg/kg completely blocked the emetic response for about 60 minutes. By contrast, MNTX did not prevent emesis induced by apomorphine, an agent that triggers vomiting through stimulation of dopaminergic receptors.

Conclusion.—The quarternary narcotic antagonist MNTX prevents morphine-induced emesis. The findings suggest that the opioid receptors that produce emesis may function outside the blood-brain barrier and that the peripherally acting MNTX prevents opioid-induced emesis by blocking these receptors, without affecting analgesia. The ability of MNTX to prevent emesis may be clinically useful, but these effects must be proven in humans before MNTX can add safety and comfort to the treatment of patients in pain.

▶ A narcotic antagonist that affects peripheral but not CNS opiate receptors may have clinical potential, particularly for constipation and urinary retention. It is actually surprising that MNTX reduced the incidence of emesis after systemic morphine because nausea and vomiting are thought to be related to effects on the brain-stem chemoreceptor trigger zone.—S.E. Abram, M.D.

Prolonged Analgesia With Liposomal Bupivacaine in a Mouse Model

Grant GJ, Vermeulen K, Langerman L, Zakowski M, Turndorf H (New York Univ)
Reg Anesth 19:264–269, 1994   101-95-23–76

Purpose.—None of the current local anesthetics produce long-lasting analgesia when administered in a single dose. Catheterization techniques are commonly used to prolong the effective duration of local anesthetics in lengthy surgical procedures, but systemic toxicity has been reported.

Sensory block duration and systemic toxicity of an ultralong-acting local anesthetic produced by encapsulating bupivacaine into liposomes were assessed.

Methods.—A liposomal formulation containing 1.1% bupivacaine was synthesized, and the median lethal dose (LD_{50}) of plain and liposomal bupivacaine was measured in mice by intraperitoneal injection. The duration of sensory block obtained with equivalent concentrations of 1.1% liposomal bupivacaine, 1.1% plain bupivacaine with or without 1:200,000 epinephrine, and normal saline solution was determined using the tail-flick test.

Results.—The LD_{50} was 61 mg/kg for plain bupivacaine and 291 mg/kg for liposomal bupivacaine, confirming that liposomal encapsulation significantly decreases systemic toxicity. The addition of epinephrine to plain bupivacaine increased the duration of sensory block from 46 minutes to 81 minutes, but injection of liposomal bupivacaine increased the duration of analgesia to 130 minutes, a statistically significant difference.

Conclusion.—Liposomal bupivacaine is an ultralong-lasting local anesthetic with significantly enhanced efficacy and safety when compared with the duration of sensory block obtained using equivalent doses of plain bupivacaine with or without epinephrine.

▶ Liposomal encapsulation of local anesthetic may provide a useful analgesic technique for prolonged epidural local anesthetic infusion. In addition to chronic toxicity studies, it will be necessary to determine whether the motor, sympathetic, and sensory-blocking characteristics are altered by encapsulation.—S.E. Abram, M.D.

24 Psychological Aspects in Anesthesiology and Pain

A Measure of Consciousness and Memory During Isoflurane Administration: The Coherent Frequency

Munglani R, Andrade J, Sapsford DJ, Baddeley A, Jones JG (Cambridge Univ, England; MRC Applied Psychology Unit, Cambridge, England)

Br J Anaesth 71:633–641, 1993   101-95-24-1

Objective.—Some objective measure of the depth of anesthesia is needed to allow detection of conscious awareness during light anesthesia with neuromuscular block. Changes in cognitive function produced by increasing isoflurane concentrations were assessed for comparison to a new measurement of depth of anesthesia using the coherent frequency (CF) of the auditory evoked response (AER).

Methods.—Seven anesthetists breathed isoflurane at increasing doses of 0%, .2%, .4%, and .8% end-tidal concentrations. Doses were then decreased from .8% to 0%. At each concentration, auditory clicks were presented at frequencies of 5 to 47 Hz for assessment of CF, which was derived from the AER after Fourier transform. Psychological performance was evaluated using a within-list recognition (WLR) test and a category recognition (CR) test.

Results.—As the isoflurane dose increased, CF and WLR and CR scores all decreased. Changes in CF were correlated with scores on both psychological tests. For some participants, a painful stimulus given during .4% isoflurane inhalation caused an increase in CF, WLR, and CR. However, this finding was not significant for the group overall, although the short-word interval scores of the WLR indicated an increase in attention. There was no response at the .8% isoflurane dose before or after a painful stimulus. As the isoflurane dose decreased from .8% to 0%, CF increased and WLR and CR scores improved. On recovery, there was no evidence of implicit learning of words presented during .8% isoflurane. On post-trial memory testing, the CF obtained during anesthesia was related to subsequent memory. Associations were noted between conscious awareness with explicit memory and a median CF of 33 Hz; conscious awareness without explicit memory and a CF of 25 Hz; and absence of both responsiveness and implicit memory and a mean CF of

15 Hz. The CFs associated with these different categories of memory were significantly different.

Conclusion.—The CF of the AER appears to reflect the likelihood of awareness during isoflurane inhalation. Psychological tests support the presence of consistent changes with anesthetic administration and stimulation. The results suggest a possible relationship between responsiveness during the trial, post-trial memory, and a particular range of CF.

▶ I included this paper and several others on the subject of "level of consciousness" monitoring in this edition of the YEAR BOOK because we are rapidly approaching a time when we can—with confidence and without too much in the way of massively expensive electronics—monitor level of consciousness and even awareness during anesthesia. When we can do this (and these authors have made a significant step in that direction), the next step should be obvious to everyone. We should be able to develop computer linkages to our "awareness or consciousness monitors" that, in turn, will administer rapidly acting, volatile anesthetics in a more or less closed-loop fashion, i.e., I am talking about the development of a true anesthesia controller. The computer would "fiddle" with the inspired concentration of the volatile agent(s) and not only keep the patient asleep, but also do so in the most cost-effective manner, minute-by-minute. I do not think this is far-fetched. If we had an "anesthesia controller," who would run it? Where would *that* development take us in the controversy over the level of training required to provide anesthesia?—J.H. Tinker, M.D.

Midlatency Auditory Evoked Potentials and Explicit and Implicit Memory in Patients Undergoing Cardiac Surgery

Schwender D, Kaiser A, Klasing S, Peter K, Pöppel E (Ludwig-Maximilians-Univ, Munich)
Anesthesiology 80:493–501, 1994   101-95-24–2

Introduction.—Many reports have described intraoperative awarenesss in patients undergoing cardiac surgery. One recently used indicator of awareness in these patients has been midlatency auditory evoked potentials (MLAEPs). Explicit and implicit memory for information presented during anesthesia, as well as MLAEP as an experimental indicator, were assessed in 45 patients undergoing elective cardiac surgery.

Methods.—All patients received general anesthesia maintained with high-dose fentanyl, 1.2 mg/hr^{-1}. In addition, 10 patients received flunitrazepam, 1.2 mg/hr^{-1} (group 1); 10 received isoflurane, .6 to 1.2 vol% (group 2); and 10 received propofol, 4 to 8 mg/kg^{-1}/hr^{-1} (group 3). The remaining 15 patients served as controls (group 4), and were randomized to 1 of the anesthetic regimens. For the first 3 groups, an audiotape including an implicit memory task—to associate the name "Robinson Crusoe" with the word "Friday"—was played after sternotomy but before cardiopulmonary bypass. While the patients were awake and while they were under anesthesia—both before and after the audiotape was played—auditory evoked potentials were recorded for measurement of the latencies of the brain-stem peak V and the early cortical potentials Na and Pa.

Results.—When assessed 3 to 5 days after surgery, none of the patients had any clear explicit memory of events during surgery. However, the groups differed significantly in their incidence of implicit recall. Five patients in group 1 had implicit memory of Robinson Crusoe, compared with 1 each in groups 2 and 3 and none in group 4. On potentials recorded in the awake state, MLAEPs showed high peak-to-peak amplitudes and a periodic waveform. For patients with implicit memory, the pattern persisted during general anesthesia. This group had no increase in latency or decrease in amplitude in Na and Pa before or after the audiotape was played. Patients without implicit memory had severe attenuation or abolition of the MLAEP waveform, together with marked increases in latencies and decreases in amplitudes or complete suppression of Na and Pa. For 9 patients, including all 7 who had implicit memory, the latency of Pa increased by less than 12 ms. For 21 of the 23 patients without implicit memory, the latency of Pa increased by more than 12 ms during anesthesia and the audiotape presentation.

Conclusion.—Preservation of the early cortical potentials of MLAEPs during general anesthesia may be associated with processing of auditory information and postoperative recall of an implicit memory task. A Pa latency increase of more or less than 12 ms is 100% sensitive and 77% specific in identifying patients who do and do not have implicit memory after surgery.

▶ Cardiac surgical patients are, of course, among the highest-risk patients for awareness during anesthesia because of the times during which myocardial depressant anesthetics cannot be easily used. I strongly believe that we are near a legitimate understanding of how to monitor for—and therefore, hopefully, block—awareness and/or memory of awareness during anesthesia. I have included several papers on this subject in this edition of the YEAR BOOK because I think these are among the most important developments in recent years in our field.—J.H. Tinker, M.D.

The Subjective, Behavioral and Cognitive Effects of Subanesthetic Concentrations of Isoflurane and Nitrous Oxide in Healthy Volunteers
Zacny JP, Sparacino G, Hoffmann PM, Martin R, Lichtor JL (Univ of Chicago)
Psychopharmacology 114:409–416, 1994   101-95-24-3

Introduction.—Although it is known that nitrous oxide has analgesic, amnestic, and anxiolytic effects and that isoflurane has amnestic effects, isoflurane's analgesic and anxiolytic abilities have not been widely studied. Therefore, the degree to which nitrous oxide and isoflurane impair psychomotor and cognitive functioning was assessed and compared.

Methods.—Nine patients participated; none had a history of significant psychiatric disorder or substance use disorder or were taking any prescription medication. The patients were exposed to alternating anesthetics, each in 2 subanesthetic concentrations and 2 placebos, with the order determined randomly. Isoflurane concentrations were .3% and .6% and nitrous oxide concentrations were 20% and 40%, which produced equivalent anesthesia. Each of the 6 sessions was separated by at least 3 days. Tests measuring the subjective effects, psychomotor performance, memory, and physiologic effects were administered before inhalation, then at 2, 15, and 29 minutes during inhalation, and 5, 30, and 60 minutes after inhalation was discontinued.

Results.—The participants reported stronger drug effects with the higher concentrations of both drugs; the 2 anesthetics had a similar duration of effects. Some disliked the odor of isoflurane. Participants felt similarly stimulated, dizzy, spaced out, drunk, and hungry with both drugs, but isoflurane induced significantly greater confused, sedated, and carefree feelings and significantly less feelings of being in control of thoughts and body. Both drugs caused diminished cognitive functioning. Isoflurane inhalation had a significantly greater effect on psychomotor impairment than nitrous oxide, although normal psychomotor performance was recovered within 5 minutes after each drug was discontinued. Both immediate and delayed free recall were impaired similarly with both drugs.

Discussion.—Although participants disliked its odor, isoflurane had other attributes that recommend it for conscious sedation procedures. It produced sedation and had amnestic effects but did not produce increased anxiety or airway irritation. Psychomotor function returned to normal levels quickly after inhalation ended. Because it has an odor, exposure to medical personnel can be controlled, thereby limiting any possible toxic effects of repeated exposure. Further study of volatile anesthetics should explore the suitability of isoflurane and the rest of that class of agents for use in conscious sedation procedures.

▶ I chose this paper because we should be aware of the effects of our drugs in subanesthetic concentrations in outpatients who have passed from our care to the home environment. Most of us say to our outpatients something rather flippant such as, "Don't make any major decisions or sign any mortgages, etc., during the next 24–48 hours." Actually, we have little idea as to how long these various subanesthetic effects of our agents really last. Nor do we understand which agents really are better than others in this regard. Even if we knew which agents were better than others in this regard, do these subanesthetic effects constitute reasons for choosing one agent over another? I hope to see considerable additional research in this area. This paper is a helpful start.—J.H. Tinker, M.D.

Reducing Smoking: The Effect of Suggestion During General Anaesthesia on Postoperative Smoking Habits

Hughes JA, Sanders LD, Dunne JA, Tarpey J, Vickers MD (Morriston Hosp, Swansea, Wales; Univ of Wales, Cardiff; St James's Univ, Leeds, England; et al)

Anaesthesia 49:126–128, 1994

101-95-24–4

Rationale.—There is evidence that intraoperative events are processed by patients even when the depth of anesthesia is adequate. Attempts have been made to suggest to patients that recovery will improve or pain will be less severe, but their efficacy is uncertain. Because about one third of patients given general anesthesia are smokers, perioperative suggestions might be an effective and inexpensive means of reducing smoking.

Objective.—A recorded message was played to patients during general anesthesia in an attempt to reduce their dependence on tobacco.

Methods.—Patients who smoked and who wished to stop were offered the chance to participate. The 122 women accepted into the study were 18–66 years of age and in American Society of Anesthesiologists class I or II; all were to have elective operations. An active message was designed to encourage listeners to stop smoking, whereas the control message used the same voice counting numbers. A double-blind design was used. The tape was played through earphones, starting when the induction agent was injected. Patients were visited at home about 1 month after surgery.

Results.—Eighty-five of the 100 assessable women underwent gynecologic surgery. All 8 patients who abstained totally from tobacco use had heard the active message. Of 28 patients who had continued smoking but at a lower level, 18 had heard the active message. Only 1 of 7 patients who reported smoking more than previously had been in the active group. No patient recalled hearing a message.

Conclusion.—Anesthetists, through suggestions to unconscious patients, may be able to help them to stop smoking.

▶ I included this study because I want to state, again, "Beware of enthusiastic positive early reports." There is no question that patients can "learn" during general anesthesia yet not have recall. The "learning" studies have been, for the most part, simple word-association tests. I think it is a gigantic leap of faith to suppose that patients might "learn" to stop smoking or change some other destructive behavior during general anesthesia. If I am wrong (after valid confirmative reports), I will subject myself to general anesthesia with a "stop eating" tape! Please understand that my "beware of enthusiastic positive early reports" is not meant in any way to impugn the integrity of these or any other investigators. We want things to happen, and this desire tends to introduce biases of which we are, perhaps, not aware, despite high integrity and the best of intentions. These authors are first-class folks, and I surely hope their report is followed by others that are confirmatory, but I hope they will pardon me if I don't hold my breath.—J.H. Tinker, M.D.

The Effect of Intravenous Ranitidine and Metoclopramide on Behavior, Cognitive Function, and Affect

Schroeder JA, Wolfe WM, Thomas MH, Tsueda K, Heine MF, Loyd GE, Vogel RL, Hood GA (Univ of Louisville, Kentucky)
Anesth Analg 78:359–364, 1994   101-95-24–5

Background.—Ranitidine can produce neuropsychiatric side effects because of its action on histamine (H_2) receptors in the CNS. Metoclopramide, a dopamine D_2-receptor antagonist, may produce disorders of both movement and affect through effects on dopaminergic neurons in the striatum and mesocortex.

Study Plan.—The effects of these drugs, alone and in combination, were studied in 123 women scheduled to have bilateral tubal occlusion. None had a history of psychiatric illness or were receiving medication chronically. Patients were randomly assigned to receive placebo, 50 mg of ranitidine, 10 mg of metoclopramide, or both drugs. The drugs were diluted in normal saline and given IV over 2 minutes. Cognitive function was assessed from patients' responses to questions about their views of anesthesia and the operation.

Findings.—Cognitive function remained intact in all groups. Patient attitudes toward anesthesia and surgery were generally more positive after the injection. Five patients appeared drowsy after receiving ranitidine, and 1 was restless. These patients described feelings of agitation and restlessness. Akathisia developed in 6 patients after they received metoclopramide. Restlessness was more prevalent in the metoclopramide recipients than in the ranitidine recipients, and one fourth of patients appeared drowsy after receiving metoclopramide. These patients reported feeling uncomfortable and "jumpy." Various combinations of these changes were noted after both ranitidine and metoclopramide were injected. The akathisia associated with metoclopramide was more prominent in patients who also received ranitidine. Patients who had both restlessness and movement disorder responded to IV midazolam injection.

Suggestions.—Akathisia is unacceptably frequent when both metoclopramide and ranitidine are administered. When a preanesthetic medication is not administered, it may be best to give metoclopramide only when it is clearly indicated.

▶ Cimetidine, an H_2-receptor antagonist, produces dose-related neuropsychiatric disturbances of confusion, slurred speech, delirium, and coma, which commonly occur when the plasma concentration increases to above 1.5 ng/ mL. These side effects occur more commonly in elderly patients and in those with impaired renal function because excretion by the kidney accounts for

80% of total elimination. Neuropsychiatric side effects have been said to be less with ranitidine administration, but this study suggests caution in the concomitant use of metoclopramide and ranitidine.—M. Wood, M.D.

Propofol and Thiopental Anesthesia: A Comparison of the Incidence of Dreams and Perioperative Mood Alterations
Oxorn D, Orser B, Ferris LE, Harrington E (Sunnybrook Health Science Centre, Toronto; Univ of Toronto)
Anesth Analg 79:553–557, 1994   101-95-24–6

Purpose.—When healthy volunteers were given subanesthetic doses of propofol in an earlier study, half of the participants reported experiencing pleasant subjective effects. There are also reports of perioperative dreams after propofol anesthesia. Perioperative mood profiles and dream patterns after anesthesia with either propofol or thiopental, combined with nitrous oxide, were compared.

Methods.—A prospective, randomized, double-blind study was undertaken in 56 women undergoing outpatient diagnostic dilatation and curettage. Twenty-nine patients were randomly selected to receive propofol anesthesia and 27 to receive thiopental anesthesia. Patients were assessed by a trained nurse who collected information in the outpatient department before surgery, at least 1 hour after surgery, and the next day by telephone. Mood was assessed with the Multiple Affect Adjective Check List–Revised, a self-administered questionnaire that measures anxiety, depression, hostility, positive affect, and sensation seeking. Perioperative sleep and recall of dreams were assessed by a questionnaire for surgical patients.

Results.—After surgery, all patients were significantly less anxious than before surgery, regardless of which anesthetic was used. The incidence of dreams, both pleasant and unpleasant, was small and equal in both groups. However, patients in the propofol group had significantly higher sensation-seeking scores compared with patients in the thiopental group. There was no difference in any of the other mood variables between the 2 groups.

Conclusion.—Patients who receive propofol anesthesia induction are more likely to demonstrate adventurous tendencies in the postoperative period than patients who receive thiopental induction.

▶ Patients seem to like propofol anesthesia. I have had patients who have requested propofol for a second anesthetic, and this study does seem to suggest that subanesthetic doses of propofol may well affect patient mood. Please see my comments for Abstract 101-95-26–2 regarding the mood and abuse potential of subanesthetic doses of propofol.—M. Wood, M.D.

Awareness During Total I.V. Anaesthesia

Sandin R, Nordström O (Länssjukhuset, Kalmar, Sweden)
Br J Anaesth 71:782–787, 1993   101-95-24-7

Objective.—The incidence of awareness during anesthesia, which appears to be most common with anesthetic techniques using neuromuscular block, was addressed. There have been surprisingly few reports of awareness during total IV anesthesia (TIVA). Five patients with awareness during TIVA were reported.

Patients.—The cases were identified from an experience of about 2,500 patients undergoing TIVA with mechanically controlled ventilation and neuromuscular block. In 2 cases, the problem resulted from inability to deliver the target anesthetic dose. In the other 3, the patients had a greater-than-anticipated need for anesthetics. All 5 cases were deemed preventable and attributed to lack of experience.

Conclusion.—All incidents related to patient awareness during TIVA should be published in detail, including a judgment as to whether the information in the anesthesia record is reliable. Preoperative, perioperative, and postoperative data on the most recent 1,727 TIVA patients have been gathered into a data base, including questioning about unpleasant experiences during anesthesia on a second occasion, after leaving the postoperative care unit.

▶ The problem of awareness during IV anesthesia and the question of whether subconscious learning occurs during anesthesia have recently become focuses of attention for anesthesiologists. Although I recognize that awareness during anesthesia is a real problem, I am not sure what to believe regarding memory and learning during anesthesia. It is certainly a topical subject, and I await further animal and human studies. Interested readers are referred to the review by Ghoneim and Block (1).—M. Wood, M.D.

Reference

1.   Ghoneim MM, Block RI: *Anesthesiology* 76:279, 1992.

Awareness Under Anaesthesia: The Patients' Point of View

Cobcroft MD, Forsdick C (Ipswich, Queensland, Australia)
Anaesth Intensive Care 21:837–843, 1993   101-95-24-8

Objective.—Although awareness during surgery is rare, the symptoms of patients after such occurrences are problematic and are poorly managed by medical personnel. The awareness experience during surgery of 227 patients in Australia and New Zealand was documented.

Methods.—The contents of letters were analyzed by key words. A total of 187 letters were analyzed. The most common procedure was cesarean section. Sensations, psychological experiences, reactions, postoperative reactions, and responses of others were noted.

Results.—The overall awareness incidence ranges from .2% to .9%. Others have estimated the incidence of recall at .9% and the incidence of "dreams" at 6.1%. Only 1 patient initiated a lawsuit. Most patients had pain, and most had their pain experience trivialized. Most patients were told that their experiences were imaged or dreamed. Most described their awareness symptoms only in terms of apprehension. Eleven patients described more than 1 instance of awareness.

Conclusion.—As a result of these experiences, patients are angry, resentful, fearful, and traumatized.

▶ Although the subject has recently been reviewed in the American literature by Ghoneim and Block (1), this article makes several informative points: First, over half the episodes of awareness were during cesarean section and were much less common in virtually any other form of surgery/anesthesia; second, the incidence of awareness does not appear to be declining as we reach the modern age; and third, such awareness can cause severe psychological trauma postoperatively, such as women not wanting to have another child because of the problem or being too frightened to experience another anesthetic. The response of others to these feelings was disbelief, ignoring the situation, or listening without comment. This article heightens our awareness that we need to be better trained to deal with awareness in patients and to be able to comfort them and reassure them regarding its rarity and its lack of recurrence in any one individual. It is apparent from the letters reviewed in this article that the persons who were aware wanted to establish a bond of empathy with someone who believed them and could talk openly about the events.

Although we are reassured that very few patients have recurrent episodes of awareness, there were 11 cases of patients claiming to have experienced more than 1 episode of awareness, meaning that there may be a hard core of patients who are really "resistant to anesthetics." The authors of this article and I believe that the excellent summary of Ghoneim and Block should be compulsory reading for all anesthesiologists, and its practical recommendations should be discussed protocol in every operating room in every hospital and a personal code of conduct for every anesthesiologist.—M.F. Roizen, M.D.

Reference

1.   Ghoneim MM, Block RI: *Anesthesiology* 76:279, 1992.

Effects of Background Stress and Anxiety on Postoperative Recovery
Liu R, Barry JES, Weinman J (United Medical and Dental School, London)
Anaesthesia 49:382–386, 1994   101-95-24–9

Background.—Although stress is known to have many physical consequences, there has been very little research on the effects of stress on recovery. The effects of background stress and anxiety on postoperative recovery in dental patients were investigated.

Methods.—Thirty healthy outpatients undergoing anesthesia for dental extractions were in American Society of Anesthesiologists status I and ranged in age from 16 to 50 years. Questionnaires were administered before surgery to assess trait and state anxiety and stress levels. State anxiety was assessed again after surgery. Recovery was evaluated with a preoperative and postoperative battery of cognitive tasks.

Findings.—The level of background stress in the 6 months preceding surgery was associated with physical parameters of recovery, such as time needed for patients to open their eyes, perceived pain, and increased postoperative morbidity. High levels of state anxiety after surgery were associated with pain after surgery. Preoperative trait and state anxiety were unrelated to any parameter of recovery or postoperative morbidity.

Conclusion.—Patients with high levels of stress were at an increased risk of delayed recovery and increased morbidity. Such patients may, therefore, need to have surgery delayed or to be treated as inpatients for whom rapid recovery is not imperative and where they may benefit from reassurance and premedication. Although further research is needed to confirm these findings, a brief assessment of the psychological health of patients appears to be warranted.

▶ When reading this article, I wish there were more data than just correlations and coefficients; rather, did these correlations imply a clinical difference? In other words, it is fine to say that the anxiety correlates with the time to opening eyes, but we don't know whether these changes are seconds, minutes, or hours; whether they really make a difference; or whether the correlation between anxiety and postoperative pain means that anxiety could be treated and postoperative pain relieved. Like all good studies, this one poses more questions than it answers.

One further comment: The authors state that at 4 hours postoperatively, the patients had significant defects in their ability to retain new visual and verbal information and in their level of attentiveness, and this after a propofol/suxamethonium/isoflurane anesthetic. These results regarding the return of attentiveness and ability to retain visual and verbal information are different from those that Zacny, Lichtor, Apfelbaum, and colleagues have obtained in patients in our psychomotor laboratory at the University of Chicago, with the main difference in drugs and drug therapies being the use of muscle relaxant and the use of ibuprofen. Although I wonder whether these are small differences, and I really cannot tell from the data provided in this paper, I also wonder whether the difference is in the ibuprofen and/or suxamethonium, or the testing strategy, or some other factor.—M.F. Roizen, M.D.

Psychologic Testing as an Aid to Selection of Residents in Anesthesiology

McDonald JS, Lingam RP, Gupta B, Jacoby J, Gough HG, Bradley P (Ohio State Univ, Columbus; Univ of California, Berkeley)
Anesth Analg 78:542–547, 1994

101-95-24-10

Background.—The objective criteria used in the process of selecting residents focus on factors other than personality. For anesthesiology residents, achievement is associated more with personality than with academic factors. Interviewers on selection committees have their own opinions and intuitions regarding psychological qualities that will differentiate between good and unacceptable candidates. However, it would help to have an objective guide based on measures of relevant personality factors. Personality traits and interests were identified among residents and were related to job performance.

Methods.—At the beginning of a 3-year program, 95 residents in anesthesiology completed a set of psychological tests and questionnaires. Personality and occupational interests were assessed. The residents' clinical performance ratings obtained from faculty supervisors at 2 years were compared with the psychological tests.

Results.—Residents with high clinical performance scored better than residents with low performance in dominance, independence, empathy, responsibility, socialization, achievement motivation, and well-being. The highest performance ratings were given to Alpha personalities with high levels of ego integration.

Conclusion.—Anesthesiology relies on personal commitment, ability to work with a team, willingness to put the patient's welfare first, attention to detail, and superior vigilance. Selection should pay special attention to factors of empathy, reliability, independence, and ability to work in both structured and unstructured situations.

▶ This article by McDonald et al. seems to parallel that by Clarke et al. (1) in that the high-performance residents were those who were dominant, independent, and responsible; could empathize with patients; and had high achievement motivation, high socialization, well-being, and self-discipline. My guess is that people with these traits will succeed in any field.

Will we be able to use these traits in segregating out anesthesiologists for our programs? I don't know whether the field is ready for it, and because we are all involved in residency recruitment and not selection now, I don't know whether the medical students would view this as a favorable trend. However, the California Psychological Inventory and other tests may well be helpful in identifying applicants for residency who will perform well later on in the specialty. Maybe such tests should be given in the third year of medical school, but my guess is that every specialty would want the better-performing students, and their success in anesthesia would also mean success in any other field.—M.F. Roizen, M.D.

Reference

1. Clarke IM, et al: *Can J Anaesth* 41:393, 1994.

Personality Factors and the Practice of Anaesthesia: A Psychometric Evaluation
Clarke IMC, Morin JE, Warnell I (Univ of Calgary, Alta, Canada)
Can J Anaesth 41:393–397, 1994   101-95-24-11

Background.—The use of questionnaires to assess personality is an important part of selecting personnel. The personality profiles of Canadian anesthetists were examined and the roles of personality variables in job satisfaction determined.

Methods.—Seven hundred eighty senior Canadian anesthetists were sent the Cattell 16PF Form "C" and a short demographic questionnaire. Usable responses were received from 330 physicians (42.3%).

Findings.—Most anesthetists reported that they were very happy with their work and were not thinking of a career change. The least satisfied physicians were, on average, 7 years younger than the satisfied physicians. The former tended to be United Kingdom–qualified physicians practicing in Ontario. On the Catell 16PF, age and years of practice were positively correlated with several personality components. Increasing age was associated with higher means on emotional stability, conscientiousness, and self-sentiment integration. The mean scores on insightfulness, fast learning, and adaptability declined significantly with an increase in years of service. Female physicians were more tender-minded, sensitive, and overprotective than their male counterparts, as well as more insecure, self-reproaching, and apprehensive. Married anesthetists had a higher mean score on carefulness, showed less practicality and more imaginative traits, and had lower mean scores on the openness-shrewdness dimension. Work satisfaction was positively associated with emotional stability and negatively associated with years of service. Work satisfaction was also negatively associated with traits of suspicion, jealously, and pretension.

Conclusion.—The personality profiles of these respondents showed them to be intelligent, somewhat dominant yet sensitive, independent yet somewhat unsure and rather tense, and tolerant but shy and serious. Emotional stability and self-esteem increased with age. Some differences were found between women and men.

▶ This article bodes well for anesthesiologists in health care reform. Those in Canada have gone through health care reform, but the job satisfaction rate for most anesthesiologists was very high—63.9 ± 20 on a visual analogue scale. Those least satisfied tended to be younger and practicing in Ontario where much more health care reform and health care rationing appear to have taken place than in the rest of Canada. Perhaps the most notable characteristics of anesthesiologists were independence, tenseness, and brightness. Both emotional stability and self-esteem in this specialty increased with age, but this did not lead to complacency, as conscientiousness was also more often seen in older anesthesiologists.—M.F. Roizen, M.D.

Call Mosby Document Express at **1 (800) 55-MOSBY** to obtain copies of the original source documents of articles featured or referenced in the YEAR BOOK series.

25 Anesthesia Training and Continuing Education

Recruitment in Anaesthesia: Results of Two National Surveys
Yang H, Wilson-Yang K, Raymer K (McMaster Univ, Hamilton, Ont, Canada)
Can J Anaesth 41:621–627, 1994   101-95-25–1

Background.—In 1987, a 2-pathway system for licensure was introduced in Quebec. In this system, physicians are licensed only after certification in family medicine or in a Royal College specialty. To better understand the dynamics of anesthesia recruitment, 2 national surveys were conducted.

Methods.—In the first survey, undergraduate anesthesia curricula were documented in Canadian medical schools. The number of students from each school entering anesthesia at the first-year postgraduate level in 1993 was also recorded. This number was then correlated with the undergraduate anesthesia exposure in that school. In the second survey, residents' reasons for choosing anesthesia were elicited. Reasons for specializing in anesthesia were classified into 5 groups, and residents were told to indicate as many reasons as they wished. Residents were also asked to give 2 or 3 principal reasons for specializing in anesthesia.

Findings.—Although all medical schools offered anesthesia electives, the annual total anesthesia lecture time, length of anesthesia rotations, and level at which they occurred varied greatly. The number of students entering anesthesia in 1993 was unassociated with the aspects of anesthesia exposure that were surveyed. For residents specializing in anesthesia, "hands-on," "time-off," "physiology/pharmacology," and "immediate gratification" were among the most selected reasons and the principal reasons for their choice. Five reasons were among both the least-selected reasons and principal reasons for choosing anesthesia: "research," "role model," "earning potential," "technology," and "pain management."

Conclusion.—Anesthesia recruitment does not appear to be related to the duration of undergraduate exposure. Rather, it seems to be influenced by technical, applied basic sciences, and life-style considerations.

▶ It appears that the United States will be going to a type of system somewhat like the Canadian's; that is, a 2-pathway system in which family practitioners get licensed more quickly and see greater financial rewards sooner than do nonfamily practitioners. That system has led to a reduction in specialty residency slots (previously done in Canada) and decreased the desirability of all the specialties. This survey was undertaken to determine whether there was a correlation between the number of students entering anesthesia and aspects of anesthesia exposure during medical school. The authors found no such correlation; that is, anesthesia recruitment is not related to the duration of anesthesia exposure in undergraduate medical school, but is influenced by the technical, applied basic science, and life-style factors of anesthesia.

I believe the message is that to recruit into anesthesia, we need to position ourselves and make ourselves a specialty that teaches the basic science of pain and cardiovascular physiology, that exposes the "hands on" and immediate effects of our work, and that has control over our work schedules. That is why many of us between the ages of 45 and 55 went into anesthesia. We did not see the financial rewards or they were not where they were for the later generation, but we saw the fun of dealing daily with real-life physiology and pharmacology and the immediate satisfaction in helping someone. I think that we can make the specialty as good as we want it to be, and when the financial gratification of going into anesthesia will not be the motivator it was in the 80s, anesthesia should be a fun specialty to practice.—M.F. Roizen, M.D.

Resident Supervision in the Operating Room: Does This Impact on Outcome?

Fallon WF Jr, Wears RL, Tepas JJ III (Univ of Florida, Jacksonville)
J Trauma 35:556–561, 1993   101-95-25-2

Background.—In resident training programs, greater autonomy is granted to residents of greater ability and seniority. However, this decision typically is left completely to the judgment of supervising faculty, without the assistance of objective, quantifiable standards. The impact of resident supervision in the operating room was evaluated by exploring associations between complications and death and the involvement of an attending physician during surgery.

Methods.—The degree of faculty involvement in all resuscitations and surgeries was objectively graded during a 12-month period at 1 medical center. The outcome of each procedure was evaluated, relative to mortality and complication rates, and associations between outcome and faculty involvement were determined.

Results.—When all services were evaluated together, physicians were scrubbed or present during surgery or resuscitation in 91.8% of the cases. Mortality occurred in 6.7% and complications occurred in 7% of the cases. When an attending physician was present or scrubbed, mortality and complication rates were significantly lower. When results were stratified by individual service, the effect of attending physician involvement was not significant. However, when services were categorized as "elective" (otolaryngology, plastic surgery, and urology) and "nonelective" (general trauma, vascular, cardiac, and pediatric surgeries), the association among faculty involvement and decreased mortality and complication rates was highly significant. The greatest impact of attending physician involvement was noted in the surgical subspecialty services.

Conclusion.—Close supervision of general surgery residents during subspecialty rotations is vital. Mortality evaluations in trauma patients should include probability of survival data to determine whether greater involvement of the attending physician may improve outcome. Finally, the impact of supervision by senior residents vs. faculty must be further explored, and standard for appropriate supervision levels should be established.

▶ This important article directly states that the more time an attending physician spends in the operating room, the lower will be the complication rate. Although one assumes this is true, this is the first documentation of it in absolute morbidity and mortality studies. Can we in anesthesia learn from this study in surgery? Would it mean that any senior physician (not necessarily an attending, but any other senior physician) could also perform the same checking function, such as 2 residents or 2 attendings being better than one? I would think the answer is yes, but I am not sure. I would urge those who wish to read this paper to read the comments by the other senior surgeons and by the authors at the end of this paper as well.—M.F. Roizen, M.D.

Basic Simulations for Anaesthetists: A Pilot Study of the ACCESS System
Byrne AJ, Hilton PJ, Lunn JN (Morriston Hosp, Swansea, Wales; Univ Hosp of Wales, Cardiff)
Anaesthesia 49:376–381, 1994   101-95-25-3

Introduction.—As in the training of pilots, simulators might be useful in the training of anesthetists. Previous simulators have been criticized as being either expensive or unrealistic. The development and initial testing of the Anaesthetic Computer Controlled Emergency Situation Simulator (ACCESS) system—an economical and realistic new device for the training of anesthetic trainees—were reported.

Methods.—The simulations used a resuscitation manikin connected to a standard anesthetic machine, an IV cannula, and a modified breathing system. Trainees were introduced to each simulated scenario as though they were taking over a case from a colleague and asked to manage the anesthetics as though the patient were real. A single tutor was present in the role of an interested but unhelpful anesthetic assistant; the trainee had to perform any required actions. A computer screen displayed images of 4 commonly used instruments—an automatic blood pressure recorder, pulse oximeter, ECG monitor, and oxygen analyzer/capnograph—all of which behaved as though connected to a real patient. Each simulated scenario was constructed as a series of discrete, numbered states with defined therapeutic interventions. The tutor controlled each simulation, observing the actions of the trainee and entering the appropriate response into the computer by means of a keypad. Each simulation was followed through until the patient stabilized or died.

Results.—The preliminary evaluation used 4 scenarios: contamination of the oxygen supply with nitrous oxide, ventricular tachycardia with cardiovascular collapse, bradycardia in a child, and hypotension resulting from an overdose of anesthetic at induction. A total of 64 simulations were tested on 5 trainees with fewer than 12 months of anesthetic experience and on 11 experienced anesthetists. The trainees caused 2 "deaths" and solved the problems in a median of 2.5 minutes; the experienced anesthetists caused 1 "death" and solved the problems in 1.8 minutes. All the deaths occurred in the oxygen contamination scenario. The pupils rated the ACCESS system as easy to use, realistic, and educationally valuable.

Conclusion.—The ACCESS system is a potentially useful tool for anesthetic training. It is affordable and fully portable; it requires only 1 tutor, with no need for previous experience or skills in its operation. New scenarios are easily constructed. An attempt is being made to collect enough data to determine how well the simulator can distinguish among different grades of anesthetists.

▶ The interesting part of the ACCESS simulator system developed by Byrne, Hilton, and Lunn is that it was developed to be within the budget of any British department of anesthesia, to be fully portable, to use standard anesthesia equipment wherever possible, and to be operated by a single tutor without any special training in either education or computer application. In addition, the aim was to produce a realistic environment for trainees. In this first report of a test of the system, it appears that it did produce a realistic display and that it seems to have met the criteria proposed. Will we all be judged by simulators before too long? I don't know, but perhaps the goal of the simulator should be not only to train us and to retrain us, but also to have us master the simulations before we practice anesthesia.—M.F. Roizen, M.D.

An Objective Methodology for Task Analysis and Workload Assessment in Anesthesia Providers

Weinger MB, Herndon OW, Zornow MH, Paulus MP, Gaba DM, Dallen LT

(Univ of California, San Diego; Stanford Univ, Calif)
Anesthesiology 80:77–92, 1994

101-95-25–4

Objective.—In anesthesiology, equipment failure or human error can have serious results. Understanding the anesthesia provider's job can lead to better evaluation and more effective training. Performance evaluation techniques for anesthesia providers were developed.

Methods.—The type of activity, number of activities, time per activity, and work load of 5 novice and 8 experienced anesthesia providers were noted by observers.

Results.—Experienced anesthesia providers spent significantly more preintubation time conversing with the patient, inserting the IV catheter, adjusting and observing monitors, and securing and manipulating airways. Post intubation, experienced anesthesia providers spent significantly more time observing monitors, recording, and watching the surgical field. Before intubation, the novice group took significantly more time intubating patients, securing airways, observing monitors, and talking with the attending anesthesiologist. During the postintubation period, novices spent most of their time observing monitors, recording, and talking with the anesthesiologist. They focused on fewer activities and took more time to perform them. Both groups thought that their work load was heavier during the preintubation period.

Conclusion.—This objective task analysis of the job of anesthesia provider may provide an understanding of performance parameters that could prove helpful in assessing progress in training.

▶ Because the method of analysis involved a click-and-point system using an Apple Macintosh computer, I wonder how much the results were biased by anticipation of the observer. Nevertheless, an important set of data and an important methodology have been developed to assess workload. Perhaps this could also be compared with other specialties in determining intensivity of workload for relative value–based systems.—M.F. Roizen, M.D.

Assessment of an Interactive Learning System With "Sensorized" Manikin Head for Airway Management Instruction

From RP, Pearson KS, Albanese MA, Moyers JR, Sigurdsson SS, Dull DL
(Univ of Iowa, Iowa City; Univ of Arkansas, Little Rock; Michigan State Univ, East Lansing)
Anesth Analg 79:136–142, 1994

101-95-25–5

Objective.—Airway management is difficult to teach because of the lack of favorable teaching environments for most emergency situations. Trainees need some basic motor skills to receive the greatest benefit from actual patient care, but these skills are difficult to acquire without previous experience. An interactive, self-study learning system for airway-management instruction, using a "sensorized" manikin head developed by the American Heart Association, is now commercially available. The teaching efficacy and patient safety of this learning system were assessed by comparison to traditional, preclinical classroom airway-management instruction.

Methods.—Before 97 third-year medical students performing anesthesia rotations were allowed to participate in airway management on anesthetized patients, they were randomized to receive either instruction on the Actronics learning system or a lecture with guided practice on a standard tracheal intubation manikin. As the students progressed to actual airway management on anesthetized patients, their performances were rated on 22 variables. The assessments were completed in blinded fashion by anesthesia faculty, residents, and nurse-anesthetists.

Results.—The 2 groups were comparable in experience with airway management at the beginning of the study. The patients on whom the learning-system group performed airway management were older, had a larger average body mass index, and had higher Mallampati classifications. In no case did the students' performances result in patient morbidity or mortality. The 2 groups showed no differences in the quality of airway management efforts or in the self-appraisal of their performance. Psychomotor skills developed with equal speed, and there were no differences between the groups in satisfaction with the methods of instruction.

Conclusion.—The Actronics interactive learning system appears to work just as well as didactic instruction for introducing airway management to third-year medical students during anesthesia rotations. However, its current cost makes it difficult to justify the use of the simulator. The cost is about $14,000, including hardware and software; the device is warranted, and technical support is readily available.

▶ Well, does this article mean that the faculty can be replaced by interactive learning tools? I don't know, but the future promise of excellent teaching with less faculty involvement because of interactive media, or better learning because of reinforcement by interactive media, seems to be highlighted by some successful tests. All of those in anesthesia interested in studying the educational process and the science of education are urged to read this article, as it is a model first step in designing tests of the interactive learning modules.—M.F. Roizen, M.D.

Video Analysis of Two Emergency Tracheal Intubations Identifies Flawed Decision-Making
Mackenzie CF, Craig GR, Parr MJ, Horst R, Level One Trauma Anesthesia Simulation Group (Univ of Maryland, Baltimore; Man-Made Systems Corp,

Ellicott City, Md)
Anesthesiology 81:763–771, 1994

101-95-25–6

Introduction.—It may be difficult to reconstruct exactly what happened during a critical incident involving anesthesia because recall of the event is incomplete, self-serving accounts are offered, or the incident is perceived differently by various participants. Videotaping offers the possibility of documenting such incidents to promote quality assurance. It can also be used as an educational tool.

Methods.—Two episodes involving emergency airway management were videotaped with the consent of those who provided anesthesia care. Images and sound were recorded by miniature cameras and microphones suspended from the ceiling of the admitting areas of a trauma center, and the tapes were analyzed using a commercial video analysis software package.

Observations.—In one instance, monitoring of oxygen saturation and the end-tidal carbon dioxide was inadequate to establish the cause of chest inflation that accompanied ventilation. A laryngoscopist could have made this diagnosis. The supervising anesthesiologist failed to communicate his findings on listening to the chest, and, as a result, the esophageal airway was removed before protection against aspiration was established through placement of a cuffed tracheal tube. In the other case, more extensive monitoring could have led to the continuance of mask ventilation until IV access was achieved, and succinylcholine could have been given by this route rather than by the less predictable IM route.

Suggestions.—Incidents such as these could be lessened by more comprehensive skills training and by better training in the areas of communication and coordination. In addition, it might be helpful to rehearse previous difficult cases and to use stress reduction techniques in clinical practice.

▶ I thought that this was a most original and interesting article and it represents a new avenue of anesthesia research. All of us want to improve our handling of emergency situations, and constructive analysis of why we did or did not do something can be very helpful. Never forget that it is always easy to be wise in retrospect when viewing the videotape.—M. Wood, M.D.

26 Ethical Issues in Anesthesiology/Critical Care

Psychoactive Substance Use Among American Anesthesiologists: A 30-Year Retrospective Study
Lutsky I, Hopwood M, Abram SE, Jacobson GR, Haddox JD, Kampine JP
(Med College of Wisconsin, Milwaukee)
Can J Anaesth 40:915–921, 1993   101-95-26-1

Background.—Psychoactive substance use is a problem among medical students, residents, and practicing physicians. Anesthesia is a high-risk medical specialty for the development of chemical dependence. The cumulative incidence of substance use among anesthesiologists during training and practice, the effect of stress on drug use, and the deterrent efficacy of institutional prevention programs were investigated.

Methods.—Two hundred sixty anesthesiologists who had trained between 1958 and 1988 at the Medical College of Wisconsin were surveyed by mail regarding the use of psychoactive substances. More than 70% of the questionnaires were returned.

Findings.—Ninety-two percent of the respondents reported using alcohol; 31% used marijuana; and 9% used cocaine. Twenty-nine (16%) were identified as being substance-dependent: 19 were alcoholic, 6 were drug-impaired, and 4 were dependent on both drugs and alcohol. The prevalence of impairment was greater among anesthesiologists who finished their training after 1975. Fifty-eight (32%) of anesthesiologists had used illicit drugs to "get high." Eleven respondents said they used drugs daily for 2 weeks or more, and 8 admitted being dependent. The parents of impaired anesthesiologists were more likely to have substance abuse problems than the parents of unimpaired anesthesiologists. The divorce rate for impaired anesthesiologists was 24.1%, compared with 5.2% for unimpaired anesthesiologists. Increased substance use did not reflect increased stress during training. Few anesthesiologists recalled having any drug counseling. Seventy percent of the respondents thought that hospital drug control policies were fair or poor. Respondents born after 1951 were more critical of drug control programs than were older respondents. Both residents and faculty reported incidents of substance abuse.

Conclusion.—Substance abuse appears to be rather common among anesthesiologists. About half the survey respondents who admitted to impairment reported substance abuse problems that began before residency. Alcohol was the substance most commonly abused. None of the anesthesiologists admitting impairment was ever required to give up a medical license. Most respondents thought that programs created to identify and treat substance abuse problems during specialty training were inadequate.

▶ The impressive thing is that 15.8% of anesthesiologists admitted to being substance-dependent. Although the authors state that this percentage is greater than for the general population, my understanding is that similar studies showed somewhere between 15% and 20% of the general population to have the same addictions. The parental history of substance abuse is worrisome, and perhaps we should do something in an aggressive, interventional way with people who enter anesthesia or people in anesthesia who have parents or grandparents who have been subject to drug abuse.

It is also important to understand that it was not clear from this survey how aggressively the University of Wisconsin educated their residents and staff about the problems of drug abuse and how to avoid them. Because most of these residents trained during the period when education regarding drug abuse was not prevalent, it is not clear how much drug counseling was done. This absence of education and counseling is substantiated by the fact that fewer than 15% of the anesthesiologists in the survey received any counseling whatsoever. I hope this has changed at the University of Wisconsin, but we don't know whether counseling is an effective deterrent. Like most good articles, this one stimulates more questions than it answers.—M.F. Roizen, M.D.

Propofol at a Subanesthetic Dose May Have Abuse Potential in Healthy Volunteers
Zacny JP, Lichtor JL, Thompson W, Apfelbaum JL (Univ of Chicago)
Anesth Analg 77:544–552, 1993   101-95-26–2

Objective.—Both patient reports and laboratory studies suggest that propofol may have the potential to be abused. Accordingly, the rewarding effects of propofol were examined in normal persons using a discrete-trials choice procedure.

Methods.—Twelve healthy participants drank alcohol regularly and 4 of these reported using marijuana. Most of the participants had had some experience with stimulants, marijuana, and hallucinogens but had not used them heavily. The participants were exposed in a blinded manner to 2 acute bolus injections of propofol in a dose of .6 mg/kg and 2 injections of Intralipid. In 3 more sessions, they chose which color-coded injection they wished to receive.

Results.—Four of the 12 participants chose propofol on all 3 occasions, and 2 others chose it twice. Five participants chose Intralipid on all 3 choice occasions, and 1 chose it twice. Those who chose to receive propofol described pleasant effects and no unpleasant residual effects. The participants who did not prefer propofol described sudden dizziness and/or disorientation after injection of propofol and/or dysphoric residual effects.

Implication.—Propofol acts as a reward in some individuals, suggesting the need for further studies to determine whether it is a drug of abuse.

▶ Many patients have reported euphoria and elation on awakening from propofol anesthesia as propofol concentrations decline to subanesthetic levels. Only 12 subjects were studied, and to use the authors' words, "most had a history of some use of illegal drugs." The importance of this article lies in the idea that subanesthetic doses of propofol may have abuse potential. If this is indeed the case, then storage and accountability procedures for this drug may have to be changed. Subhypnotic doses of propofol have been suggested to have antiemetic properties that may be useful for patients undergoing chemotherapy, and I wonder about the abuse potential for propofol in this situation.—M. Wood, M.D.

Use of Refractometry to Identify Opioid-Containing Solutions
Eagle CJ, Maltby JR, Kryski S, Hardy D (Univ of Calgary, Alta, Canada)
Can J Anaesth 41:248–252, 1994   101-95-26-3

Background.—Various methods are used to control abuse of opioids and other substances by anesthesia personnel. The value of refractometry in identifying the contents of different opioid-containing solutions was investigated.

Methods.—A handheld refractometer was used to determine the refractions of various opioids at ampule levels and solutions commonly used in the operating room. In addition, refractions were measured for serial dilutions of each opioid in each solution. Refractions were studied in the undiluted content of alfentanil, fentanyl, morphine, and sufentanil ampules and in solutions of Ringer's lactate, .9% saline, 3.3% dextrose in .3% saline, and distilled water. The opioids were serially diluted in 1:2, 1:4, and 1:8 dilutions for each solution. Blinded identification of various diluted opioid solutions was then attempted.

Findings.—Refractometric values for undiluted fentanyl and sufentanil were identical to the values for distilled water. Refractometric values for undiluted alfentanil and morphine were nearly identical to one another and 1:2 and 1:4 dilutions of either drug in Ringer's lactate or .9% saline.

Conclusion.—The nature of refraction of light makes the refractometer unreliable for identifying the tampered contents of syringes and ampules. The use of the refractometer will probably not result in better narcotic control or earlier detection of drug-dependent anesthesia personnel.

▶ This article shows that addicts can defeat almost anything, and the defeating of refractometry for routinely identifying opioids seems to be fairly simple; the user just switches distilled water for fentanyl or sufentanil. It is likely that such routine screening would only benefit the very early addict, who, soon after addiction started, would probably read the literature and find out what would defeat the system.—M.F. Roizen, M.D.

Physicians' Behavior and Their Interactions With Drug Companies: A Controlled Study of Physicians Who Requested Additions to a Hospital Drug Formulary
Chren M-M, Landefeld CS (Case Western Reserve Univ, Cleveland, Ohio)
JAMA 271:684–689, 1994   101-95-26-4

Introduction.—Physicians can have a large impact on the sales of a drug by their prescribing practices, their influence on the prescribing behavior of colleagues and physicians in training, and their choice of research. The null hypothesis that interactions with drug companies are not associated with physician behavior was tested.

Participants and Methods.—In a teaching hospital, 40 full-time attending physicians who requested addition of a drug to the hospital formulary from January 1989 through October 1990 were studied. The 80 randomly selected control physicians had not made such requests. Drugs were classified according to whether they had a major therapeutic advantage, a modest advantage, or no advantage over therapies existing in the formulary. All physicians completed a survey regarding their interactions with drug companies in the past year.

Results.—The survey response rate was 88%. Physicians who requested formulary additions interacted with drug companies more than the other physicians. They were also more likely to request drugs manufactured by a specific company if they had met with pharmaceutical representatives or accepted money from these companies. Controlling for 4 physician characterictics did not alter these associations between drug company interactions and formulary additions. Of 55 requested drugs, 29 were independently classified as having little or no advantage over therapies existing in the formulary.

Conclusion.—There was a strong association between physicians' requests for a hospital formulary addition and their interactions with drug companies. Physicians who had an interaction with a specific company were 9 to 21 times more likely than other physicians to request a drug supplied by that company.

▶ Although this article seems to indicate that physicians are susceptible to motivation from drug companies, it is hard to get excited about this because of some obvious problems with the data as they relate to anesthesia and critical care. For instance, the authors state:

This study does not prove that interactions with drug companies influenced the behavior of the interacting physician; alternative explanations are possible. The temporal direction may have been reversed—ie, physicians, by virtue of their expertise or interest, may have first requested that drugs be added to the formulary and then interacted with the companies whose drugs they had requested. Or, unknown confounding factors may have contributed to our findings. Neither of these alternative explanations is likely, however, given the fact that most of the requested drugs represented little or no therapeutic advantage over drugs already in the formulary. . . .

When scanning the list, I was struck by 2 that relate to anesthesia—esmolol and propofol—that are listed as drugs having little or no advantage. I would venture to say that virtually everyone in anesthesia would think that propofol and esmolol represent major therapeutic advances over anything that went before in the anesthesia intensive care armentarium. Thus, because the only assumptions I know about in this study have little credibility, I have to question all the data.—M.F. Roizen, M.D.

The Clinical Management of Dying Patients Receiving Mechanical Ventilation: A Survey of Physician Practice

Faber-Langendoen K (Univ of Minnesota, Minneapolis)
Chest 106:880–888, 1994   101-95-26–5

Objective.—Although mechanical ventilation is widely used today, little guidance is available in the literature regarding ventilatory assistance for patients who refuse life-sustaining treatment. Accordingly, a survey dealing with this issue was sent to 513 randomly selected critical care physicians and was returned by 308 of them. Of these, 273 were involved in ventilator management. They included internists, surgeons, pediatricians, and anesthesiologists.

Findings.—Fifteen percent of physicians reported almost never withdrawing ventilation from a patient who was to forego life-sustaining treatment and who was expected to die. Another 15% nearly always withdrew ventilator therapy. Thirty-seven percent withdrew ventilation less than half the time. Factors involved in the decision are listed in the table. One fourth of respondents recognized a moral difference between deciding not to intubate and withdrawing ongoing ventilation. Subspecialists and those who were experienced in managing ventilated patients were more likely to see no such moral difference. One third of physicians preferred terminal weaning, 13% used extubation for withdrawal, and the rest used both these methods. Most of those who preferred terminal weaning believed it to maximize patient comfort. The medications

Factors Influencing Decisions to Withdraw Ventilatory Support

	N/T*	%
Factors reported to *increase* the probability of ventilator withdrawal		
Underlying, terminal diagnosis	240/267	90
Living will requesting no prolonged ventilator support†	195/224	87
Obtunded mental status	196/266	74
An involved family	134/259	52
Advanced age†	114/222	51
Factors reported to *decrease* the probability of ventilator withdrawal		
Alert mental status	205/265	77
Coexistence of a treatable condition	186/266	70

* Number citing this factor/total number answering this question.
† Responses of nonpediatricians only.
(Courtesy of Faber-Langendoen K: Chest 106:880–888, 1994.)

most often used when withdrawing ventilatory support were morphine and benzodiazepines.

Discussion.—For many reasons, physicians may be more reluctant to discontinue mechanical ventilatory assistance than to not initiate it. Some physicians prefer to extubate as the most direct method, whereas others prefer to terminally wean patients because they believe it to be more acceptable to the family.

▶ This study raises some very important concerns regarding the ethical practices among apparently experienced intensivists. That 15% of those responding would almost never withdraw ventilator support and that 26% still believe that withholding support and withdrawing support are not ethical equivalents lead me to believe that there is a knowledge deficit in our intensive care community. Another concern is that some physicians, albeit just a few, apparently use or maintain paralytic agents during terminal weaning or terminal extubations from mechanical ventilation (another reason to strictly regulate the use of neuromuscular blocking agents in the ICU). And finally, I am shocked by the revelation that a large percentage of intensivists delegate the responsibility for termination of mechanical ventilation to nurses or respiratory therapists. I can only conclude that these "doctors" are only capable of talking about what should be done but are incapable of being at the patient's bedside when the task is at hand.—D.M. Rothenberg, M.D.

Attitudes Toward Assisted Suicide and Euthanasia Among Physicians in Washington State

Cohen JS, Fihn SD, Boyko EJ, Jonsen AR, Wood RW (Univ of Minnesota,

Minneapolis; Univ of Washington, Seattle)
N Engl J Med 331:89–94, 1994

101-95-26–6

Introduction.—Although there has been considerable public debate among physicians and the general population regarding physician-assisted suicide and euthanasia, little is known about the opinions of most physicians. Randomly selected physicians practicing in Washington State were surveyed concerning their opinions on the ethics and legalization of assisted suicide and euthanasia.

Methods.—A random selection of 1,416 physicians from several medical specialties and subspecialties were mailed questionnaires.

Results.—There were 938 respondents (69%). Of these, 48% could find no ethical justification for euthanasia, and 42% could. Although 54% thought that legalized euthanasia would be appropriate in certain situations, only 33% would be willing to euthanize a patient. Physician-assisted suicide could not be ethically justified in any circumstance for 39% of the respondents, whereas 50% could find ethical justification. Whereas 53% would legalize assisted suicide in some circumstances, only 40% would be willing to assist a patient themselves. There were significant differences among specialties in the support of these practices, with psychiatrists voicing the most support and hematologists/oncologists voicing the least.

Both physicians who opposed these practices and those who supported them considered their views consistent with the role of the physician. Religious beliefs were more frequently cited as the reasons for opposing than for supporting euthanasia and assisted suicide. Most of those who supported the practices cited respect for the patients' right to self-determination and reduction of the patient's fears as reasons for their views. Safeguards suggested included an impartial witness to the patient's request, confirmation of the patient's mental competence, agreement of 2 physicians with the decision, and an established relationship between the patient and the assisting physician.

Discussion.—The views of physicians are polarized on the issues of assisted suicide and euthanasia. However, there is considerable belief that medical treatment may be inadequate for patients who are terminally ill. Support from the medical community for legislation permitting euthanasia or assisted suicide will require the incorporation of substantial safeguards.

▶ Previous articles have suggested that if physician-assisted suicide (i.e., the patient pulls the trigger) or physician-assisted death (i.e., the doctor pulls the trigger) were to be legalized (as it recently was in Oregon), the anesthesiologists should be at the forefront in safeguarding this practice from abuse. Unfortunately, such proposals, along with surveys similar to this one, fail to ask anesthesiologists their opinions of such matters. Curious about the feelings of our specialty, I surveyed more than 1,200 American Society of Anesthesiologists members and found that over 56% believed in the concept of physician-assisted death, and of those, over 90% stated that they would be willing to participate in some manner if requested (1). Whether these respondents truly understood the ramifications of their statements is uncertain. What is certain is that, as members of a profession that specializes in the ability to ease pain, we have a responsibility to ensure that neither individuals nor society in general uncritically embrace physician-assisted death or physician-assisted suicide as appropriate methods of dealing with suffering.—D.M. Rothenberg, M.D.

Reference

1. Rothenberg DM, McCarthy RJ: *Anesthesiology* 77:1082A, 1992.

Call Mosby Document Express at 1 (800) 55-MOSBY to obtain copies of the original source documents of articles featured or referenced in the YEAR BOOK series.

Subject Index*

A

Abdomen
  compression, interposed, with
    cardiopulmonary resuscitation,
    outcome during asystole and
    electromechanical dissociation,
    94: 188
  interventions, screening laboratory tests
    before, 93: 66
  lower, surgery
    pain after, continuous epidural
      methadone for, 93: 386
    pre-emptive lumbar epidural block
      reducing pain after, 94: 461
  surgery
    bupivacaine 0.1% not improving
      epidural fentanyl after, 93: 388
    effects on liver blood flow, 93: 50
    major, epidural vs. IV sufentanil for,
      epidural fentanyl analgesia in,
      95: 214
    major, recovery after, propofol,
      nitrous oxide and isoflurane in,
      95: 26
    oxygen desaturation risk during sleep,
      93: 265
    pain relief for infant undergoing,
      morphine vs. bupivacaine, 94: 465
Abortion
  prostaglandin-induced, metoclopramide
    enhancing analgesia for, 94: 106
Abuse
  cocaine, nonmedical, detracting from
    availability in hospital, 93: 7
  nicotine and alcohol, in postoperative
    bacterial infection, 95: 175
  potential of subanesthetic dose of
    propofol, 95: 498
  sexual and physical, and chronic pelvic
    pain, 94: 443
ACCESS system
  basic simulations anesthetists, 95: 491
ACE
  inhibitors
    calcium antagonists and low systemic
      vascular resistance after
      cardiopulmonary bypass, 95: 207
    premedication attenuating
      sympathetic responses during
      surgery, 95: 104
Acetaminophen
  perioperative effects in children
    undergoing myringotomy, 93: 231
Acetazolamide

in acute mountain sickness, and gas
  exchange, 93: 304
Acetylcholine
  receptors, tolerance and upregulation
    after d-tubocurarine, 93: 39
Acid
  aspiration
    at emergency cesarean section,
      omeprazole reducing risk of,
      95: 289
    of gastric contents at emergency
      cesarean section, IV ranitidine
      reducing risk of, 94: 304
  gastroesophageal reflux, and ranitidine,
    94: 107
Acid-base
  management with carbon dioxide in
    phosphate concentration in
    hypothermic cardiopulmonary
    bypass, 94: 224
  status of newborn after spinal and
    extradural anesthesia for cesarean
    section, 93: 198
  variables, maternal and fetal, with
    propofol and thiopental (in
    pregnant ewe), 94: 286
Acidity
  gastric, preoperative anxiety influencing,
    93: 69
Acidosis
  intramyocardial hypercarbic, correction
    with sodium bicarbonate, 95: 190
  lactic
    bicarbonate effects on hemodynamics
      and tissue oxygenation in, 93: 329
    hypoxic, Carbicarb, sodium
      bicarbonate and sodium chloride in
      (in dog), 94: 341
  metabolic
    contractile dysfunction during, and
      energy metabolism impairment,
      93: 300
    mild, sodium bicarbonate for, vs. IV
      Carbicarb for surgery, 95: 366
Acquired immunodeficiency syndrome (see
  AIDS)
Acupuncture
  discriminative sensation and, 93: 238
  like transcutaneous electrical nerve
    stimulation, 94: 401
  somatosensory evoked potentials by,
    and tactile skin stimulation, 93: 238
Adductor
  muscle of larynx and adductor pollicis
    rocuronium at, 93: 46
  pollicis muscle

---

* All entries refer to the year and page number(s) for data appearing in this and previous
editions of the YEAR BOOK.

oncology patient, epidural anesthesia for postoperative analgesia, 93: 108
outpatients, propofol reducing emesis in airway obstruction in, 94: 323
oximetry, pulse, 93: 228
modified sensor for, 95: 137
preoxygenation, how long, 93: 224
propofol vs. thiopentone for, IV, cardiovascular effects, 94: 322
pulmonary edema complicating upper airway obstruction, 93: 224
reflex sympathetic dystrophy, clinical characteristics and follow-up, 93: 434
respiratory failure, extracorporeal life support for, survival predictors, 94: 223
respiratory tract infection, upper, and general anesthesia, 93: 226
sevoflurane concentration for, end-tidal, and minimum alveolar concentration, 95: 313
sevoflurane pharmacology in, 95: 311
spinal fusion, normovolemic hemodilution and intraoperative autotransfusion in, 93: 183
surgery, ambulatory, preoperative screening with telephone questionnaire method, 93: 221
tonsillectomy
bupivacaine for, 94: 459
ondansetron decreasing emesis after, 95: 89
tracheobronchomalacia and airway collapse, 93: 229
trauma
drugs in emergency airway management in, 93: 219
endotracheal intubation in, 93: 221
upper extremity fracture, IV regional anesthesia for, 93: 106
vancomycin, perioperative, hypoxia after, 94: 114
venipuncture, EMLA patch vs. EMLA 5% cream for, single unit dose package, 95: 103
vs. adult anesthesia closed malpractice claims, 94: 149
young, outpatient tonsillectomy for, 93: 223
Chloride
sodium, in lactic acidosis, hypoxic (in dog), 94: 341
Chloroprocaine
bupivacaine and, 93: 199
for dorsal penile nerve block in newborn circumcision vs. lidocaine, 93: 211

inhibiting clonidine, 93: 199
not symptomatic marker of IV injection in labor, 95: 242
Chlorpromazine
decreasing muscle pain, 93: 48
Cholecystectomy
laparoscopic
diaphragmatic function before and after, 95: 61
lung function tests before and after, 95: 8
and nitrous oxide, 93: 232
during pregnancy, 94: 249
minilaparotomy, perioperative bupivacaine, morphine and ibuprofen in, 95: 413
Cholinesterase
activity
and cocaine toxicity, 93: 60
and mivacurium induced neuromuscular blockade recovery, 94: 123
atypical plasma, in mivacurium induced neuromuscular blockade, 94: 121
inhibition, spinal, antinociceptive effects of, 95: 395
Chromaffin
cell transplant for chronic pain (in rat), 93: 440
Chymopapain
activity after chemonucleolysis in intervertebral disc (in dog), 93: 412
Cimetidine
in midazolam recovery, IV, 94: 105
Circadian
variation in vascular tone and α-sympathetic vasoconstrictor activity, 93: 71
Circuit
tubing, anesthetic uptake and washout characteristics of, and decontamination techniques, 94: 174
Circulation
arrest, hypothermic, barbiturates impairing cerebral metabolism during (in animals), 94: 227
cerebral, in ischemic cerebrovascular disease, and sevoflurane, 95: 86
failure, acute, splanchnic oxygenation assessment by gastric tonometry in, 94: 361
hypothermic arrest vs. low flow cardiopulmonary bypass in infant heart surgery, 95: 197
microcirculation during dorsal column stimulation and sympathectomy (in rat), 93: 415

maternal
after intrathecal sufentanil, 94: 271
during spinal anesthesia, prophylactic
angiotensin II vs. ephedrine
infusion to prevent, 95: 286
in spinal block vs. spinal epidural
block for cesarean section, 95: 275
prevention during spinal anesthesia with
ephedrine vs. crystalloid, 94: 34
during ritodrine infusion, ephedrine as
vasopressor of choice for, 95: 297
spinal clonidine-induced, neostigmine
counteracting (in sheep), 94: 447
in torso injuries, penetrating, immediate
vs. delayed fluid resuscitation in,
95: 330
Hypotensive
anesthesia to avoid homologous
transfusion in spinal fusion,
93: 182
Hypothermia
accidental, cardiopulmonary bypass for
resuscitation in, 93: 328
anesthesia-induced, prevention, 95: 97
during aortic aneurysm repair,
abdominal, 95: 220
for circulatory arrest vs. low flow
cardiopulmonary bypass for infant
heart surgery, 95: 197
deep regional, of spinal cord protecting
against ischemia during thoracic
aorta cross-clamping, 95: 217
in hand causing pulse oximetry
inaccuracy, 93: 247
malignant, 94: 175
in preterm infant, 93: 213
Hypothermic
cardiopulmonary bypass, acid-base
management and carbon dioxide in
phosphate concentration in,
94: 224
circulatory arrest, barbiturates impairing
cerebral metabolism during (in
animals), 94: 227
spinal cord transection, anesthetic
potency not altered after (in rat),
95: 67
Hypotonia
perilymphatic, hearing loss after spinal
anesthesia as, 93: 104
Hypoxemia
fetal, intrapartum, monitoring fetal heart
rate in, 94: 316
hypercapnic, buffering in (in pig),
94: 340
pulse oximetry to detect, 94: 134
reduction by pulse oximetry monitoring,
93: 248

respiratory tract infection in children
and, upper, 93: 227
Hypoxia
after vancomycin, perioperative, 94: 114
Hypoxic
lactic acidosis, Carbicarb, sodium
bicarbonate and sodium chloride in
(in dog), 94: 341
lung vasoconstriction in perfused lung,
sevoflurane in (in rabbit), 95: 62
pulmonary vasoconstriction, inhaled
nitric oxide reversing, without
systemic vasodilation, 94: 74
ventilatory response, propofol
depressing, during conscious
sedation and isohypercapnia,
95: 229
Hysterectomy
abdominal, morphine after, 93: 368
analgesia after, epidural morphine and
fentanyl for, 94: 318
general anesthesia for, therapeutic
suggestions, 93: 91
meperidine after, intranasal, 94: 445

I

Ibuprofen
perioperative, with bupivacaine and
morphine in cholecystectomy,
minilaparotomy, 95: 413
Identification, 94: 180
Immune
response
effects of anesthesia and surgery on,
93: 26
literature on, summary of, 93: 27
system, and halothane, 93: 80
Immunological
assay after halothane exposure, 93: 80
Immunotherapy
in herpes zoster prevention in aged,
94: 400
Implant
spinal cord stimulation, evoked
potential monitoring during,
lidocaine and tetracaine, 93: 414
Incontinence
stress, after delivery, with epidural
anesthesia during labor, 94: 266
Indocyanine green
clearance after prolonged halothane vs.
isoflurane, 93: 33
Indomethacin
in thoracotomy, preoperative vs.
postoperative, 94: 416
Induction

partial pressure differences,
inspiratory-arterial, components of,
95: 60
prolonged, in children during
mechanical ventilation, 94: 374
propofol and sevoflurane, 93: 13
rapid increase in concentration, giving
less transient cardiovascular
stimulation than desflurane rapid
increase concentration, 95: 71
recall of music and, 94: 474
recovery after major abdominal surgery
and, 95: 26
remifentanil effects and (in dog), 94: 89
rocuronium with, continuous IV,
94: 126
for sedation in ICU, 93: 298
in status epilepticus, convulsive, 93: 28
subanesthetic concentrations
effects on memory and
responsiveness, 94: 475
subjective, behavioral and cognitive
effects of, 95: 477
sympathetic hyperactivity during, vs.
desflurane, 94: 59
vs. barbiturate, in thoracic aorta
cross-clamping, with paraplegia
after (in dog), 94: 239
vs. desflurane, for coronary artery
surgery, 93: 32
vs. nitrous oxide, for intra-operative
monitoring of somatosensory
evoked potentials, 95: 146
Isohypercapnia
propofol depressing hypoxic ventilatory
response during, 95: 229
Isotonic
hemodilution in hematocrit
determination, 94: 143
Isovolemic
hemodilution, effects on left ventricular
myocardial function in
compromised coronary blood flow
(in dog model), 94: 57
IVOX
for extrapulmonary gas exchange,
94: 369

J

Jaw
relaxation after halothane
succinylcholine in children, 95: 131
Joint
facet, injection, for low back pain,
93: 409
zygapophyseal

cervical, pain, local anesthetic blocks
in, 95: 406
pain, cervical, prevalence of, 93: 410
Jugular vein
aneurysm, causing vagal nerve palsy,
complicating catheterization,
95: 41
cannulation, internal, valve injury
complicating, 95: 42
catheterization, Seldinger method for,
93: 244
internal, cannulation of, very high
approach, 94: 138

K

K+ channel agonists
lipid-soluble, for pain, 93: 453
Kallikrein-kinin system
heparin during coronary bypass and,
93: 154
Karnofsky scale
function and chronic pain, 93: 408
Ketamine
with fentanyl for postoperative pain and
wound hyperalgesia, 95: 418
Ketoconazole
for ARDS prophylaxis, 95: 360
Ketorolac, 93: 20, 94: 77
inducing bronchospasm, 94: 78
IV, by bolus or infusion, for
postoperative pain, 95: 443
in migraine, vs. meperidine and
hydroxyzine, 93: 417
nasal polyposis and bronchial asthma,
94: 77
perioperative effects in children
undergoing myringotomy, 93: 231
for sickle cell vaso-occlusive crisis pain,
93: 20
tromethamine, for postoperative
analgesia after ambulatory surgery,
94: 452
vs. meperidine for migraine, 93: 20
Kidney
effect on, of enflurane, nicardipine and
atrial natriuretic peptide for
intraoperative hypertension, 94: 96
failure, chronic, mivacurium and,
prolonged duration, 94: 122
function, 94: 390
after cardiac surgery, and
"renal-dose" dopamine, 94: 200
after major vascular surgery,
postoperative low dose dopamine
in, 95: 355

Author Index